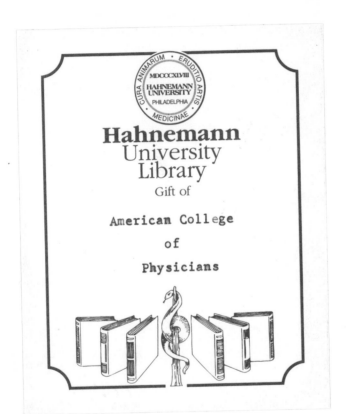

Hypertension and Renal Disease in the Elderly

EDITED BY

Manuel Martinez-Maldonado MD

Professor and Vice Chairman of Medicine
Emory University School of Medicine
Chief, Medical Service
Atlanta VA Medical Center
Atlanta, Georgia

BOSTON

Blackwell Scientific Publications

OXFORD LONDON EDINBURGH
MELBOURNE PARIS BERLIN VIENNA

© 1992 by Blackwell Scientific Publications, Inc.
Editorial offices:
238 Main Street, Cambridge
    Massachusetts 02142, USA
Osney Mead, Oxford OX2 0EL, England
25 John Street, London WC1N 2BL
    England
23 Ainslie Place, Edinburgh EH3 6AJ
    Scotland
54 University Street, Carlton
    Victoria 3053, Australia

Other Editorial offices:
Librairie Arnette SA
2, rue Casimir-Delavigne
75006 Paris
France

Blackwell Wissenschafts-Verlag
Meinekestrasse 4
D-1000 Berlin 15
Germany

Blackwell MZV
Feldgasse 13
A-1238 Wien
Austria

First published 1992

Set by Setrite Typesetters Ltd, Hong Kong
Printed in the United States of America
by Hamiltons, Albany, New York

93 94 95   5 4 3 2 1

DISTRIBUTORS

USA
    Blackwell Scientific Publications, Inc.
    238 Main Street, Cambridge
    Cambridge, Massachusetts 02142
    (Orders: Tel: 800 759-6102
                 617 876-7000)

Canada
    Times Mirror Professional Publishing, Ltd
    5240 Finch Avenue East
    Scarborough, Ontario M1S 5A2
    (Orders: Tel: 416 298-1588
                 800 268-4178)

Australia
    Blackwell Scientific Publications
    (Australia) Pty Ltd
    54 University Street
    Carlton, Victoria 3053
    (Orders: Tel: 03 347-0300)

    Outside North America and Australia
    Marston Book Services Ltd
    PO Box 87
    Oxford OX2 0DT
    (Orders: Tel: 0865 791155
                 Fax: 0865 791927
                 Telex: 837515)

Library of Congress
Cataloguing-in-Publication Data

Hypertension and renal disease in the elderly
    edited by Manuel Martinez-Maldonado.
          p.   cm.
    Includes bibliographical references and index.
    ISBN 0−86542−093−9
    1. Kidney diseases in old age.
    2. Hypertension in old age.
    I. Martinez-Maldonado, Manuel.
    [DNLM: 1. Hypertension—in old age.
    2. Kidney Diseases—in old age.
    WJ 300 H998]
    RC903.H96   1992
    618.97′661 −dc20
    DNLM/DLC

Contents

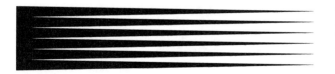

Contributors

George L. Bakris, MD
Assistant Professor of Medicine and Pharmacology, Department of Medicine, Division of Nephrology, University of Texas Health Sciences Center, Renal Division, San Antonio, TX, USA

D. Craig Brater, MD
Professor of Medicine and Pharmacology, Director of Clinical Pharmacology, Wisbard Memorial Hospital, Indianapolis, IN, USA

Jan A. Bruijn, MD, PhD
Assistant Professor in Pathology, Laboratory of Pathology, University of Leiden, Leiden, The Netherlands

John C. Burnett Jr, MD
Associate Professor of Medicine and Physiology, Division of Cardiovascular Diseases, Mayo Clinic, Rochester, MN, USA

José L. Cangiano, MD
Chief, Hypertension Section, VA Medical Center; Professor of Medicine, University of Puerto Rico School of Medicine, San Juan, Puerto Rico, South America

Patricia G. Cavero, MD
Assistant Professor of Medicine, Cardiology Division, Moffit Hospital, University of California, San Francisco, CA, USA

Ramzi S. Cotran, MD
F.B. Mallory Professor of Pathology, Harvard Medical School; Chairman, Department of Pathology, Brigham and Women's Hospital, Boston, MA, USA

Barbara S. Daniels, MD
Assistant Professor of Medicine, Division of Renal Diseases, Department of Medicine, University of Minnesota, Minneapolis, MN, USA

Gerald F. DiBona, MD
Professor and Vice Chairman, Department of Internal Medicine, University of Iowa, College of Medicine; Chief, Medical Service, Iowa VA Hospital, Iowa City, IA, USA

Harriet P. Dustan, MD
Emeritus Professor of Medicine, VA Distinguished Physician, Veterans Administration, Birmingham, AL, USA

Garabed Eknoyan, MD
Professor of Medicine, Renal Section, Department of Medicine, Baylor College of Medicine, Houston, TX, USA

Alberto U. Ferrari, MD
Established Investigator, National Research Council of Italy, Milano, Italy

Annette E. Fitz, MD
Professor of Internal Medicine, Department of Internal Medicine, University of Iowa College of Medicine, Iowa City, IA, USA

Agnes Fogo, MD
Assistant Professor of Pathology and Paediatrics, Department of Pathology, Vanderbilt University School of Medicine, Nashville, TN, USA

Edward D. Frohlich, MD
Vice President and Professor of Medicine, Department of Medicine, Sections of Nephrology and Hypertensive Diseases, Alton Ochsner Medical Foundation and Ochsner Clinic, New Orleans, LA, USA

Richard J. Glassock, MD
Professor and Chairman, Department of Medicine, University of Kentucky College of Medicine, Lexington, KY, USA

Thomas H. Hostetter, MD
Professor of Medicine; Director, Division of Renal Diseases, University of Minnesota School of Medicine, Minneapolis, MN, USA

Priscilla Kincaid-Smith, MD
Professor, Department of Medicine, University of Melbourne; Director of Nephrology, Department of Nephrology, Royal Melbourne Hospital, Melbourne, Victoria, Australia

Ulla C. Kopp, PhD
Assistant Professor, Department of Internal Medicine, University of Iowa College of Medicine and VA Medical Center, Iowa City, IA, USA

Neil A. Kurtzman, MD
Chairman, Department of Internal Medicine, Division of Nephrology, Texas Tech University, Health Sciences Center, School of Medicine, Lubbock, TX, USA

Moshe Levi, MD
Assistant Professor of Internal Medicine, University of Texas Southwestern Medical Center, Dallas, TX, USA

Robert D. Lindeman, MD
Chief, Division of Geriatric Medicine; Professor of Medicine, Department of Medicine, University of New Mexico School of Medicine, Albuquerque, NM, USA

Manuel Martinez-Maldonado, MD
Professor and Vice Chairman of Medicine, Emory University School of Medicine; Chief, Medical Service, Atlanta VA Medical Center, Atlanta, GA, USA

W. Scott McDougal, MD
Chief of Urology, Massachusetts General Hospital; Professor of Surgery, Harvard Medical School, Boston, MA, USA

Kenneth L. Minaker, MD, FRCP(C)
Associate Professor of Medicine, Division on Aging, Harvard Medical School; Director, Geriatric Research Education and Clinical Center, Brockton/West Roxbury DVAMC; Associate Physician, Department of Medicine, Division of Gerontology, Beth Israel Hospital; Associate Director, Clinical Research Center, Beth Israel Hospital, Boston, MA, USA

Stephen H. Norris, MD
Associate Professor of Medicine, Division of Nephrology, Department of Internal Medicine, Texas Tech University, Health Sciences Center, School of Medicine, Lubbock, TX, USA

C. Venkata S. Ram, MD
Professor of Internal Medicine, Director of Hypertension Clinics, St Paul Medical Center and Parkland Memorial Hospital, University of Texas Southwestern Medical Center, Dallas, TX, USA

John W. Rowe, MD
President of Mount Sinai School of Medicine, Mount Sinai Hospital, New York, NY, USA

Antonio Santoro, MD
Associate Professor, Department of Nephrology and Dialysis, Malpighi S. Orsola-Malpighi Hospital, Bologna, Italy

William J. Stone, MD
Professor of Medicine, Department of Medicine, Vanderbilt University School of Medicine; Chief, Nephrology Section, VA Medical Center, Nashville, TN, USA

John W. Warren, MD
Professor of Medicine and Head, Division of Infectious Diseases, University of Maryland School of Medicine, Baltimore, MD, USA

William E. Yarger, MD
Professor and Vice Chairman, Duke University Medical Center; Chief, Medical Service, Durham Department of VA Medical Center, Durham, NC, USA

Alessandro Zuccala, MD
Associate Professor, Department of Nephrology and Dialysis, Malpighi S. Orsola-Malpighi Hospital, Bologna, Italy

Pietro Zucchelli, MD
Chief, Department of Nephrology and Dialysis; Professor of Medicine, Malpighi S. Orsola-Malpighi Hospital, Bologna, Italy

Foreword

It is particularly satisfying to me to see the publication of this volume on hypertension and renal disease in older people and to have the opportunity to help introduce it. My own career began in the field of renal physiology and diseases; it may not be out of place to note that as a medical student I helped carry out the first renal dialysis done at the Massachusetts General Hospital. As I moved on into more concerns with chronic diseases in general and with aspects of aging, I have continued to see the importance of the range of topics covered in this book.

Hypertension is one of the most common conditions affecting older people and contributes in major ways to the chronic disabilities and mortality from stroke and myocardial infarctions, two of the three leading causes of death in older people. This book addresses thoroughly the various underlying pathologies which contribute to hypertension and relate these changes to physiologic and pathologic aspects related to aging itself. Similarly, chapters in the book address both aging-related renal changes and the diseases of the kidney which may afflict older people. Each chapter combines basic knowledge with guidance for clinical applications. Discussions of pharmacologic interventions are particularly helpful and useful.

In almost every aspect of aging, including those covered in this book, it is always important to recognize the considerable individual variability in older people; a sizable number of older people simply do not show the changes with age which may appear to be present when only averages are looked at. Furthermore, given the fact that the variability between individuals is usually a life-long characteristic, it is important to obtain longitudinal data on individuals. For example, as pointed out in several of these chapters, when longitudinal measurements of glomerular filtration rates are studied, a third or more of individuals show no changes in their glomerular filtration rates even in later years, when compared with their earlier test results. One of the most challenging general questions in aging research, in the areas of the vascular and renal systems as well as in other systems, is the question of why is there such variability, and why do some people maintain good function in later years when others do not?

In addition to providing up-to-date, critically reviewed information about what is known of the characteristics of renal function and diseases with aging, and the characteristics of hypertension, as well as providing practical clinical guidance for evaluation and treatment, the authors of the chapters in this book have pointed out the many frontiers calling for further research. This volume should be of much interest and usefulness to scholars concerned with all aspects of these topics as well as its usefulness to clinicians, both general and specialized, who are working with more and more older people faced with these common conditions.

T. Franklin Williams

Preface

The major developments in detection, classification, and treatment of hypertension in the population at large undoubtedly have been responsible for the reduction in cardiovascular morbidity and mortality achieved in the previous decade. Meanwhile, lengthened survival has swollen the ranks of the elderly in most industrial societies. It is expected that in the middle of the next century, baby-boomers in this country will enter their dotage and increase the numbers of our elderly to 18%; and that Japan, 11% of whose population is already 65 or older, will increase its aged citizens to 17% by the year 2000 and to 21% by 2010 [1]. Among the illnesses that affect the aged, hypertension is easily detectable and controllable. We can predict with equal certainty that renal function declines with age and that attempts to curtail the ruin of filtering units are mandatory if life is to be prolonged gracefully.

In this volume, we have assembled world experts in the fields of hypertension and renal disease who have a special interest in the pathophysiology and management of these conditions in the elderly. Throughout their medical/scientific careers, it has been their mission to develop knowledge that may alleviate the renal deterioration and/or elevations of blood pressure that stalk the unwary. Their contributions to this book are based on their vast experience as contributors to the literature that has provided most of the base of our knowledge of the problems of high blood pressure and renal function in the elderly. In some cases, not enough information existed; therefore, some overlap has occurred in the content of chapters. As editor, I must apologize for any inconvenience this may cause our reader. As a practical man, I hope for forgiveness in view of the possibility that repetition often leads to knowledge. A larger *mea culpa* must be admitted in relation to insufficient knowledge of a particular condition in relation to the elderly, a situation totally out of the control of the authors. Nevertheless, they have all been diligent in providing outstanding chapters that I hope serve as guides in the uncharted seas of renal disease and hypertension in the aged.

While this book was in production, a landmark study in the management of hypertension in the elderly has appeared: the so-called Systolic Hypertension in the Elderly Program (SHEP) involving a multicenter, randomized, double-blind, placebo-controlled study of 4736 people 60 years or older [2]. This group represented 1.06% of the population screened; the subjects were characterized by systolic hypertension (160−219 mmHg) and diastolic pressures >90 mmHg. Women represented 57% of the group, and 14% of the subjects were black. Stepped care treatment was conducted with chorthalidone (12.5−25 mg/dl = Step 1) and atenolol (25−50 mg/dl = Step 2). During an average followup of 4.5 years, there was a dramatic reduction of fatal and nonfatal strokes with no significant reduction in quality of life. Reductions in major cardiac and cardiovascular events were also achieved by SHEP with a low order excess of adverse effects. While larger scale, long-term studies are required, the results of SHEP provide critical and rational information for the treatment of isolated systolic hypertension where mostly anecdotal reports existed. Efficacious therapy of both systolic and diastolic hypertension by hydrocholothiazide (or step care diuretic and hydralazine, methyldopa, metropolol, or reserpine) in men past the age of 60 has also been presented, although large-scale, long-term studies of hypertension in the elderly are equally lacking [3]. Vast areas of inquiry remain beyond these studies.

We enter this last decade of the century equipped with powerful investigative techniques, an improved and expanded pharmacologic armamentarium, and information such as that provided by SHEP. It is our hope that the chapters that make up this volume will spark readers into action. Perhaps the contents of this tome will ignite a dormant idea, or create the urge to look further into the vast mysteries of what goes awry in hypertension and renal disease. If the outcome improves understanding and treatment of the diseases of the elderly, we will feel that our mission has been fulfilled.

I would like to thank the authors for their contributions, particularly Dr T. Franklin Williams, former director of the National Institute of Aging, for his splendid foreword to the volume. My editor, Dr Victoria Reeders, has been patient and extremely helpful with the development of the project since we first discussed it one lovely summer afternoon in an austere room in Oxford, England. To her I owe my gratitude *siempre eterna*. Lastly to Mike Snider at Blackwell Scientific Publications, whose help and cooperation carried the project over some of its hurdles.

References

1 Dentzer S. The graying of Japan. US World and News Report, 1991;111(14):65−74.
2 SHEP Cooperative Research Group. Prevention of stroke by antihypertensive drug treatment in older persons with isolated systolic hypertension: Final results of the Systolic Hypertension in the Elderly Program (SHEP). J Am Med Assoc 1991; 265:3255−3264.
3 Department of Veterans Affairs Cooperative Study Group on Antihypertensive Agents. Treatment of hypertension in the elderly. I. Blood pressure and clinical changes. Results of a Department of Veterans Affairs Cooperative Study. Hypertension 1990;15:348−369.

Notice

The indications and dosages of all drugs in this book have been recommended in the medical literature and conform to the practices of the general medical community. The medications described do not necessarily have specific approval by the Food and Drug Administration for use in the diseases and dosages for which they are recommended. The package insert for each drug should be consulted for use and dosage as approved by the FDA. Because standards for usage change, it is advisable to keep abreast of revised recommendations, particularly those concerning new drugs.

1

The aging kidney: pathologic alterations

Jan A. Bruijn
Ramzi S. Cotran

Introduction

The development of renal functional and structural abnormalities with aging has been described in humans [1–5] and in several animal species [6–8]. Functional changes have been related to morphologic alterations in glomeruli, tubules, and blood vessels. The pathogenesis of these structural abnormalities in humans, except as it relates to vascular disease, is unknown but several mechanisms have been suggested by studies of renal aging in experimental animals.

The purpose of this chapter is to describe the anatomic changes in the aging human kidney. The underlying pathogenetic pathways will be referred to only briefly, since most of these will be discussed elsewhere in this book.

Gross appearance

A decline in glomerular filtration and renal blood flow rates usually starts at around the age of 30 [1,9,10] and is accompanied by the gradual development of morphologic changes, which involve blood vessels, glomeruli, tubules, and the interstitium. The combined weight of both kidneys, which has a peak of 250–270 g in young adults, decreases to 180–200 g by the age of 90 [11]. Grossly, there is usually symmetric contraction of the kidneys [12,13]. The renal capsule is often adherent to the renal surface, especially over areas of old scarred infarcts. The kidneys of most humans over 60 years of age show a fine granular appearance of the subcapsular surface at gross inspection, a picture resembling benign nephrosclerosis. In more severe cases the weight is further reduced and larger surface craters may be observed, which have been related to local infarction or ischemic atrophy induced by atheroemboli. The decrease in renal mass is predominantly cortical, as can be observed on cross-sectioning [14]. Depending upon the severity of the glomerular damage the interstitium may show a fibrotic appearance with loss of the normal "stripened" architecture. The scarred areas are usually wedge-shaped and may extend into the medulla. Older kidneys may show some small cortical adenomas or cysts. In the most severe cases a completely atrophic or "end-stage" kidney may be found.

Glomerular alterations

Histologically the characteristic lesion in the aging kidney is glomerular sclerosis. The incidence of sclerotic glomeruli related to age has been the subject of a number of studies [15–17]. Kaplan *et al.* [2] quantitated the incidence of sclerotic glomeruli in kidneys from 122 patients without clinical evidence of primary renal disease or hypertension. Their study was based on examination of large sections of kidney generally containing over 200 glomeruli. They found that less than 10% of the glomeruli would be expected to be sclerotic in 95% of people up to age 40–45 years. In patients over 45–50 years of age they found an increasingly broad scatter of the incidence of sclerotic glomeruli, with the upper 95% population limit exceeding 10%, making the distinction between age-related and disease-related sclerosis less clear for this age group (Fig. 1.1). In another study Kappel & Olsen [3] measured the relative amount of cortical interstitial tissue and sclerosed glomeruli in 123 normal human kidneys, and related their results to age and sex.

They found no differences related to sex. Both the percentage of interstitial tissue and the amount of obsolescent glomeruli increased with age. A small number of sclerotic glomeruli (0–1%) was found until the age of 40, and thereafter it increased to about 30% in persons over 80 years of age.

In most studies described the sclerotic glomeruli are usually found scattered between essentially normal glomeruli, and are present diffusely throughout the renal cortex, except for the scarred areas related to earlier infarction. The remaining glomeruli may show hypertrophy. The structural changes in the sclerotic glomeruli consist of wrinkling and thickening of the glomerular basement membrane with shrinkage and eventual collapse of the glomerular tuft, accompanied by expansion of the extracellular matrix, later followed by global sclerosis [15,18–20]. Electron microscopic studies show a loss of epithelial cell foot processes around the shrinking glomerular capillaries, and sometimes reduplication of Bowman's capsule [21,22]. During the process of collapse of the glomerular tuft, formation of a fibrotic scar internal

Fig. 1.1 Percentage sclerotic glomeruli in kidneys from 122 autopsied patients plotted against age. (a) Observed percentage sclerosis (arithmetic scale). (b) Observed and predicted percentage sclerosis (arcsine scale) with upper and lower limits containing 95% of the population. The regression line is given by the equation $y = 0.0084x$, where x = age in years and y is an angle (in radians) determined by the transformation $y = 2 \arcsin \sqrt{PSG/100}$. Thus, for example, when $x = 55$, $y = 0.0085(55) = 0.462$. Therefore, $PSG/100 = 0.052$ or the predicted mean $PSG = 5.2\%$. (Each digit represents the number of cases at any given point; solid triangles, medical examiner cases (MEC); solid circles, hospital cases (HC); circled solid triangles, MEC and HC at the same point.) (From Kaplan *et al.* [2].)

(a)

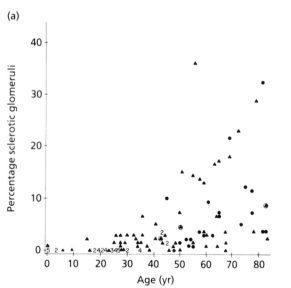

(b)

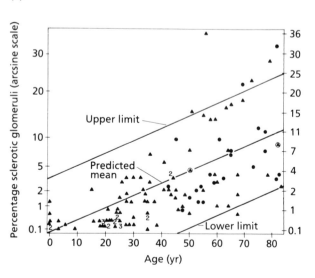

to Bowman's capsule may be observed due to the deposition of collagen [22–24]. Complete obsolescence of the glomerulus may lead to a direct communication between the preglomerular and postglomerular capillaries [19].

The pathogenesis of the glomerulosclerosis seen in aging humans is unknown, but it has been assumed to be related to the ischemia caused by the vascular sclerosis. In the past decade, however, it has been proposed that hemodynamic and dietary factors, akin to those which play a role in experimental models of glomerulosclerosis in rats, may also be relevant to the glomerulosclerosis of human aging.

In rats of certain strains progressive glomerulosclerosis and proteinuria develop spontaneously with age, eventually leading to end-stage renal insufficiency [5,8,25]. Elema & Arends described a lesion which spontaneously develops in kidneys of rats of the Wistar strain, first in local areas of some glomeruli, gradually spreading with time and involving larger parts and more glomeruli [8]. Proliferative changes were not present but in the early lesions accumulation of hyaline, eosinophilic material in the subendothelial areas of the capillary loops with positive staining for IgM and complement was observed. This was later followed by increase in mesangial matrix and development of adhesions, reminiscent of focal and segmental glomerulosclerosis. Similar lesions were described by Couser & Stilmant in aging Sprague–Dawley rats [25]. Fifty percent of 12-month-old animals and 90% of 24-month-old animals of this strain were found to be proteinuric (more than 20 mg/day). Mesangial deposits of IgM in occasional lobules of some glomeruli and slight mesangial hyperplasia were found in 3-month, 6-month, and nonproteinuric 12-month-old rats. In 25–30% of proteinuric 12-month-old rats focal and segmental areas of glomerular sclerosis were present with adhesions to Bowman's capsule, foamy cells, intraluminal eosinophilic deposits, and capillary wrinkling and collapse. These lesions were more advanced in 24-month-old Sprague–Dawley rats. Further studies on laboratory rats have shown that focal and segmental sclerosis-like lesions develop spontaneously with aging in most rat strains, although a considerable strain-dependent variability in the severity of the lesions and of the accompanying clinical symptoms exists [25–31]. In further studies on these models the spontaneous development of sclerotic lesions in aging rats has been related to hemodynamic, dietary, and genetic factors [8,31,32].

Although focal and segmental sclerosis is not the typical morphologic lesion occurring in aging human glomeruli, as described above the observations in aging rats have led to extensive studies on the role of hemodynamic, dietary, and genetic factors in renal deterioration in aging humans as well. The possible role of these factors in the sclerosis of aging glomeruli in humans is discussed in detail in Chapters 14 and 15. Other risk factors, when superimposed on aging, may accelerate the process of renal deterioration. These factors include glomerulonephritis, diabetes mellitus, systemic hypertension, nephrolithiasis, vesicoureteral reflux, and reduction of renal mass due to, for example, infarction or surgery. Deterioration of renal function may also be aggravated by interstitial nephritis due to drug reactions or immunologic mechanisms. Of note, the spectrum of glomerulonephropathies seen in the elderly is essentially similar to that which occurs in children and young adults [11].

Much has been learned recently of the nature and composition of sclerotic glomeruli. Glomerulosclerosis is characterized by the accumulation of extracellular matrix synthesized by glomerular cells upon injury [33–38]. An interesting point to note is that although indistinguishable by routine histologic methods, the composition of the sclerotic lesions differs between the models studied with regards to the extracellular matrix molecules present [39,40]. Studies on the steady-state levels of mRNA encoding for extracellular matrix molecules suggest that the increased production of extracellular matrix leading to glomerulosclerosis is regulated at the transcriptional level [39,41,42]. Transcription of sequences encoding for extracellular matrix molecules is regulated by DNA binding proteins, as was recently shown for collagen Type IV by Killen et al. [43], and is further influenced by cytokines. It is now believed that cytokines determine not only the quantity of extracellular matrix expansion, but also the exact biochemical composition of the sclerotic lesions. Whether these factors play a role in the genesis of sclerotic aging glomeruli in humans deserves further study.

Vascular alterations

Renal vascular alterations in the aging kidney run the gamut from typical atherosclerotic lesions in the large arteries to hyaline arteriolar sclerosis characteristic of small arterioles. Depending upon the degree of generalized disease, large- and medium-sized renal arteries may show the characteristic changes of atherosclerosis. The main renal artery and segmental arteries may show true atheromas consisting of fibrofatty intimal plaques. While occasionally such plaques may also be present in the more peripheral arterial branches and the arcuate arteries, changes in these vessels are characterized by irregular thickening of the vessel walls due to fibrosis of the intima and sometimes of the media, which may lead to stenosis. In the walls of the interlobular arteries fibroelastic intimal thickening is the most characteristic alteration. In these lesions concentric layers of elastin form due to reduplication of the lamina elastica interna. Smooth-muscle cells show hyperplasia in the intima and hypertrophy in the media [22].

In the smaller arterioles, including the afferent arterioles, the most common change is hyaline arteriolar sclerosis. The characteristic lesion consists of homogeneous hyaline depositions in the intima and media of small arteries and arterioles. These changes lead to thickening of the vessel wall and stenosis of the lumen. The lesions of hyaline arteriosclerosis, which affect mostly the proximal part of the afferent arteriole [44], have been related to endothelial damage. Presumably, damage to the endothelial cells results in leakage of plasma contents followed by subendothelial deposition of these molecules in the form of eosinophilic hyaline material. Electron microscopic studies of the hyaline material show that it may contain either different types of plasma protein-like granules [21,22,45,46], or confluent endothelium and smooth-muscle basement membranes [47]. Extracellular matrix production by smooth-muscle cells would further contribute to the thickening of the vessel wall. It is believed that the resultant arteriolar stenosis underlies the glomerular ischemia described earlier in this chapter and, indeed, the occurrence of atrophic nephrons has been shown to increase in patients with small-artery and arteriolar disease [48].

Although hyaline arteriolosclerosis is present to some degree in normotensive patients and increases with age it is more severe in patients with hypertension and diabetes. Autopsy studies show that in the absence of hypertension only approximately 15% of human individuals older than 50 years show appreciable morphologic changes of arteriolar nephrosclerosis, whereas such changes are present in 97% of kidneys after exposure to high blood pressures for some years [13,49,50]. The relationship of hyaline arteriosclerosis to hypertension has been the subject of much discussion and controversy [4,21,44,50–54], and it remains as yet to be determined whether the renal microvascular changes contribute to the genesis of hypertension, or are the cause of the decline in renal function observed repeatedly with aging [4].

Atheroembolic disease

In addition to atherosclerosis and arteriolar sclerosis, a vascular abnormality which may be found in the aging kidney is atheroembolic renal disease. This disorder is restricted mostly to patients over 50 years of age suffering from severe atherosclerosis, and shows a preferential occurrence in whites [55]. The presence of atheromatous plaques in larger vessels predisposes to thrombosis and embolism [56]. In a study on post-mortem kidneys, Gore et al. [57] found cholesterol emboli in 4.7% of men and 2.7% of women older than 50 years of age, while the incidence was 14.7% in patients with severe atherosclerosis [58,59]. The most common site for atheromatous plaques is the lower descending aorta, predominantly around the ostia of the major branches, including the renal arteries. Disconnection of an embolic mass from the main plaques may occur spontaneously, or may be triggered by trauma, angiographic procedures [60,61], or surgical manipulation [62]. Subsequently, atheroemboli or cholesterol emboli are transported to the intrarenal interlobular, arcuate, or even smaller vessels, leading to arterial obstruction, ischemia, and sometimes infarction. The size of the infarct will depend on its age and the size of the vessel involved.

In atheroembolic disease an acute and a chronic form are distinguished. In acute or subacute atheroembolic disease clinical manifestations are characterized by the development of renal insufficiency, associated with hypertension, minimal abnormalities observed on urinalysis, eosinophilia, hypocomplementemia, and typical skin lesions within days to weeks following the ischemic insult [63–67]. Over time, the number of infarcts may increase and contribute significantly to nephron loss and decreasing renal function. Depending upon the extent of the cumulative injury, chronic renal atheroembolic disease may develop, characterized clinically by chronic renal failure and hypertension. Hyperfiltration in the remaining nephrons perpetuates renal deterioration by mechanisms described elsewhere in this book (see Chapter 2).

On gross examination of cases of acute atheromatous emboli, multiple recent cortical infarcts are observed, as has been described in post-mortem studies [63]. The multiplicity of the lesion with subsequent ischemic degeneration and scarring of nephrons leads to "pitting" of the renal surface and eventually generalized atrophy of the kidney in the chronic disease [11]. Microscopical studies of atheromatous emboli at different stages after the onset have been described by a number of authors in humans and in experimental models [11,63–65,67–72]. From these reports the following sequence of events can be deduced. Crystals of cholesterol or esters of cholesterol with or without associated cellular material embolize to small arteries and cause damage to the vascular endothelium, resulting in an inflammatory response including edema in the vessel wall [63]. In fresh emboli (30 min to 2 days) cholesterol clefts are found occluding the lumina of arcuate and intralobular arteries and afferent arterioles. Cholesterol crystals may also be found in the glomeruli, and in three different case reports a relationship between acute atheroembolic renal disease and necrotizing glomerulonephritis has been suggested [73–75]. The crystals tend to show rounded corners and often have an elliptical shape in paraffin-embedded material, while they assume rhomboidal shapes with sharper corners after epoxy embedding [63]. In the early phase endothelial injury can be detected at the ultrastructural level by the presence of cytoplasmic hydropic vesicles and cytoplasmic blebs [63]. There is edema of intimal stroma, and some fibrin and slight platelet aggregation can be seen, but thrombosis is not a characteristic feature of the embolic lesions [63,64,69]. An influx of leukocytes around the cholesterol crystals is observed within 1–3 days [64,67]. Subsequently, macrophages and foreign-body giant cells appear, followed by proliferative changes in the endothelium, intimal intercellular fluid accumulation separating cells and extracellular elements, and intimal fibrosis [63,64,67]. This leads to the typical appearance of emboli in which the crystals are embedded in a thickened, proliferated intima and in which foreign-body giant cells or histiocytic aggregates may still be present. In a period of weeks to months after the embolization, partial dissolution of occlusive thrombi may occur with recanalization of the vessel lumina by endothelium growing over the embolus [63,67]. Older lesions observed show crystals embedded deep in the outer intima without surrounding cellular reaction [63]. Thus in chronic atheroembolic disease, thickened vessel walls possibly containing resolved emboli, constitute the typical morphologic lesion. In addition, both global glomerulosclerosis and focal and segmental sclerosis of glomeruli have been found in chronic renal atheroembolic disease. These alterations have been ascribed to ischemia secondary to the vascular stenosis, and to compensatory hyperfusion, respectively [58,62,67,76,77]. The chronic lesion is further characterized by the occurrence of interstitial fibrosis and tubular atrophy accompanying nephron loss.

Tubulointerstitial alterations

Foci of tubular atrophy, interstitial fibrosis, and chronic inflammation are found in most aging kidneys, commonly associated with areas of glomerular sclerosis. In a study of 123 kidneys from humans without clinical signs of kidney disease Kappel & Olsen found a significant increase of interstitial fibrosis with age [3]. Others reported similar findings [78–80]. A number of morphometric studies on biopsies from patients with glomerular dysfunction have shown that a deteriorating glomerular filtration rate (GFR) correlates better with progressive changes in the interstitial architecture than with morphologic alterations in the glomerulus [81–85]. This may be explained by the fact that the interstitial fibrosis in itself damages the postglomerular capillary network, leading to a further decrease in GFR [21]. Several other theories have also been put forward to explain why interstitial damage should affect glomerular function, and these were extensively discussed elsewhere [85] (see Chapter 16).

Cysts and adenomas

One or more acquired cysts may be found in the kidneys of about 50% of all people 40 years and older [21,86]. Although often localized in the cortex, they may be found in the medulla as well, and it is believed that their distribution may in fact be random [87]. Their size may vary, and although half are less than 1 cm in diameter [21] very large cysts measuring almost 30 cm in diameter have been described [88,89]. They are usually asymptomatic, although in rare cases their presence may lead to rupture, hemorrhage, or ureteral obstruction. Some cysts have been found to coincide with the presence of a benign or malignant tumor either structurally related to the cyst itself, or elsewhere in the same kidney [90–92]. Some have cysts related to hypertension, possibly due to compression of a blood vessel leading to ischemia of renal parenchyma and concurrent activation of the renin–angiotensin cascade [93–95].

Grossly, the cysts are most often unilocular and round or oval. The cyst wall is one or several millimeters thick, grayish white with a smooth outer and inner surface. The wall may be traversed by several blood vessels and fibrous bands. The cysts usually contain a clear, yellowish fluid resembling transudate [88,96,97]. In some cases the contents may be hemorrhagic due to bleeding. On microscopic examination the cyst wall is most often lined by simple flattened epithelium, sometimes with focal papillary formations. The subepithelial stroma consists mostly of collagen in which some leukocytes may be dispersed and sometimes hemosiderin-laden macrophages may be found. The adjacent renal parenchyma may appear compressed. Simple cysts are believed to arise from a dilated tubule or glomerulus. Some believe that they arise from tubular diverticula which are found in increasing incidence with age [87,92,98,99]. The pathogenesis of cyst formation in aging is unknown, but theories that attempt to explain cystogenesis in congenital or acquired cystic disease on the basis of tubular basement membrane alterations [100–106] may also be relevant to renal cyst formation in the elderly.

Renal adenomas, also called renal adenocarcinomas of low metastatic potential [107], are small tumors, histologically indistinguishable from carcinomas, which are found in up to 7% of kidneys at autopsy [108,109]. The epidemiology of renal adenomas is similar to that of renal carcinomas, and the incidence of these tumors is highest in the 50–70 age group [11,110,111]. On gross examination, renal adenomas are usually reasonably well demarcated with a mostly pale to yellow cut-surface area. They can be found throughout the whole renal cortex and may sometimes contain small cysts. Histologically, they are composed of sheets of large cells with a clear, vacuolated cytoplasm containing glycogen and lipid. The nuclei are relatively small and little nuclear polymorphism, polychromasia, and anisokaryosis are seen, while mitotic figures are rare. Areas of necrosis may be found, although they are usually absent in small tumors.

References

1 Davies DF, Shock NW. Age changes in glomerular filtration rate, effective renal plasma flow, and tubular excretory capacity in adult males. J Clin Invest 1950;29:496–507.

2 Kaplan C, Pasternack B, Shah H, et al. Age-related incidence of sclerotic glomeruli in human kidneys. Am J Pathol 1975;80:227–234.

3 Kappel B, Olsen S. Cortical interstitial tissue and sclerosed glomeruli in the normal human kidney, related to age and sex. A quantitative study. Virchows Arch (Pathol Anat) 1980;387:271–277.

4 Lindeman RD, Tobin JD, Shock NW. Association between blood pressure and the rate of decline in renal function with age. Kidney Int 1984;26:861–868.

5 Anderson S, Brenner BM. Effects of aging on the renal glomerulus. Am J Med 1986;80:435–442.

6 Saxton JA Jr, Kimball GC. Relation of nephrosis and other diseases of albino rats to age and to modifications of diet. Arch Pathol 1941;32:951–965.

7 Guttman PH, Anderson AC. Progressive intercapillary glomerulosclerosis in aging and irradiated beagles. Radiat Res 1968;35:45–60.

8 Elema JD, Arends A. Focal and segmental glomerular hyalinosis and sclerosis in the rat. Lab Invest 1975; 33:554–561.

9 Shock NW. Kidney function tests in aged males. Geriatrics 1946;1:232–239.

10 Olbrich O, Ferguson MH, Robson JS, et al. Renal function in aged subjects. Edinb Med J 1950;57:117–127.

11 Frocht A, Fillit H. Renal disease in the geriatric patient. J Am Geriatr Soc 1984;32:28–43.

12 Zollinger HU. Niere und Ableitende Harnwege. In Doerr W, Uehlinger E, eds. Spezielle Pathologische Anatomie, vol. 3. Berlin: Springer-Verlag, 1966:577.

13 Kincaid-Smith P. Parenchymatous disease of the kidney and hypertension. In Genest J, Koiw E, Kuchel O, eds. Hypertension: Physiopathology and Treatment. New York: McGraw-Hill, 1977:794.

14 Tauchi H, Tsuboi K, Okutomi J. Age changes in the human kidney of the different races. Gerontologia 1971;17:87–97.

15 McGregor L. Histological changes in the renal glomerulus in essential (primary) hypertension. A study of fifty-one cases. Am J Pathol 1930;6:347–366.

16 Howell TH, Piggot AP. The kidney in old age. J Gerontol 1948;3:124–128.

17 Emery JL, Macdonald MS. Involuting and scarred glomeruli in the kidneys of infants. Am J Pathol 1960;36:713–723.

18 McManus JFA, Lupton CH Jr. Ischemic obsolescence of renal glomeruli. The natural history of the lesions and their relation to hypertension. Lab Invest 1960;9:413–434.

19 Ljungqvist A, Lagergren C. Normal intrarenal arterial pattern in adult and ageing human kidney. A micro-angiographical and histological study. J Anat 1962;96:285–300.

20 Takazakura E, Sawabu N, Handa A, *et al.* Intrarenal vascular changes with age and disease. Kidney Int 1972;2:224−230.

21 Heptinstall RH. Hypertension. II. Essential hypertension. In Heptinstall RH, ed. *Pathology of the Kidney*. Boston: Little, Brown & Co., 1983:181−246.

22 Jones DB. Arterial and glomerular lesions associated with severe hypertension. Light and electron microscopic studies. Lab Invest 1974;31:303−313.

23 Nagle RB, Kohnen PW, Bulger RE, *et al.* Ultrastructure of human renal obsolescent glomeruli. Lab Invest 1969;21:519−526.

24 Thoenes W, Rumpelt HJ. The obsolescent renal glomerulus-collapse, sclerosis, hyalinosis, fibrosis. A light- and electron microscopical study on human biopsies. Virchows Arch (Pathol Anat) 1977;377:1−15.

25 Couser WG, Stilman MM. Mesangial lesions and focal glomerular sclerosis in the aging rat. Lab Invest 1975;33:491−501.

26 Medlar EM, Blatherwick NR. The pathogenesis of dietary nephritis in the rat. Am J Pathol 1937;13:881−895.

27 Blatherwick NR, Medlar EM. Chronic nephritis in rats fed high protein diets. Arch Intern Med 1937;59:572−596.

28 Linkswiler H, Reynolds MS, Bauman CA. Factors affecting proteinuria in the rat. Am J Physiol 1952;168:504−508.

29 Kennedy GC. Effects of old age and overnutrition on the kidney. Br Med Bull 1957;13:67−70.

30 Bolton WK, Benton FR, Maclay JG, *et al.* Spontaneous glomerular sclerosis in aging Sprague−Dawley rats. I. Lesions associated with mesangial IgM deposits. Am J Pathol 1976;85:277−302.

31 Weening JJ, Beukers JJB, Grond J, *et al.* Genetic factors in focal segmental glomerulosclerosis. Kidney Int 1986;29:789−798.

32 Grond J, Beukers JJB, Schilthuis MS, *et al.* Analysis of renal structural and functional features in two rat strains with a different susceptibility to glomerular sclerosis. Lab Invest 1986;54:77−83.

33 Striker LMM, Killen PD, Chi E, *et al.* The composition of glomerulosclerosis. I. Studies in focal sclerosis, crescentic glomerulonephritis and membranoproliferative glomerulonephritis. Lab Invest 1984;51:181−192.

34 Adler S, Striker LJ, Striker GE, *et al.* Studies of progressive glomerular sclerosis in the rat. Am J Pathol 1986;123:553−562.

35 Border WA. Distinguishing minimal change from mesangial disorders. Kidney Int 1988;34:419−434.

36 Bruijn JA, Hogendoorn PCW, Hoedemaeker PhJ, *et al.* The extracellular matrix in pathology−a review. J Lab Clin Med 1988;111:140−149.

37 Diamond JR, Karnovsky MJ. Focal and segmental glomerulosclerosis: analogies to atherosclerosis. Kidney Int 1988;33:917−924.

38 Fries JWU, Sandstorm DJ, Meyer TW, *et al.* Glomerular hypertrophy and epithelial cell injury modulate progressive glomerulosclerosis in the rats. Lab Invest 1989;60:205−218.

39 Bruijn JA, Munaut C, Baelde JJ, *et al.* Extracellular matrix (ECM) expansion and mRNA levels in the development of experimental glomerular sclerosis (abstr.). Kidney Int 1990;37:409.

40 Hogendoorn PCW, Bruijn JA, Gelok EWA, *et al.* Development of progressive glomerulosclerosis in experimental chronic serum sickness. Nephrol Dial Transplant 1990;5:100−109.

41 Border WA, Okuda S, Languino LR, *et al.* Suppression of experimental glomerulonephritis by antiserum against transforming growth factor betal. Nature 1990;346:371−374.

42 Border WA, Okuda S, Languino LR, *et al.* Transforming growth factor-beta regulates production of proteoglycans by mesangial cells. Kidney Int 1990;37:689−695.

43 Killen PD, Long R, DeMeester CA, *et al.* Transcriptional regulation of collagen IV genes (abstr.). Kidney Int 1990;37:220.

44 Smith JP. Hyaline arteriolosclerosis in the kidney. J Pathol Bacteriol 1955;69:147−168.

45 Biava CG, Dyrda I, Genest J, *et al.* Renal hyaline arteriosclerosis. An electron microscope study. Am J Pathol 1964;44:349−363.

46 Fisher ER, Perez-Stable E, Pardo V. Ultrastructural studies in hypertension. I. Comparison of renal vascular and juxtaglomerular cell alterations in essential and renal hypertension in man. Lab Invest 1966;15:1409−1433.

47 McGee WG, Ashworth CT. Fine structure of chronic hypertensive arteriopathy in the human kidney. Am J Pathol 1963;43:273−299.

48 Heptinstall RH. Renal biopsies in hypertension. Br Heart J 1954;16:133−141.

49 Williams RH, Harrison TR. A study of the renal arteries in relation to age and to hypertension. Am Heart J 1937;14:645−658.

50 Moritz AR, Oldt MR. Arteriolar sclerosis in hypertensive and non-hypertensive individuals. Am J Pathol 1937;13:679−728.

51 Bell ET. *Renal Diseases*, 2nd edn. Philadelphia: Lea & Febiger, 1950.

52 Tracy RE, Toca VT. Nephrosclerosis and blood pressure. I. Rising and falling patterns in lengthy records. Lab Invest 1974;30:20−29.

53 Tracy RE, Toca VT. Nephrosclerosis and blood pressure. II. Reversibility of proliferative arteriosclerosis. Lab Invest 1974;30:30−34.

54 Miller PL, Rennke HG, Meyer TW. Hypertension and progressive glomerular injury caused by focal glomerular ischemia. Am J Physiol 1990;259:F239−F245.

55 Saklayen MG. Atheroembolic renal disease: preferential occurrence in whites only. Am J Nephrol 1989;9:87−88.

56 Flory CM. Arterial occlusions produced by emboli from

eroded atheromatous plaques. Am J Pathol 1945; 21:549−565.

57 Gore I, McCombs HL, Lindquist RL. Observations on the fate of cholesterol emboli. J Atheroscler Res 1964; 4:527−535.

58 Gore I, Collins DP. Spontaneous atheromatous embolization. Am J Clin Pathol 1960;33:416−426.

59 Schornagel HE. Emboli of cholesterol crystals. J Pathol Bacteriol 1961;81:119−122.

60 Wagner RB, Martin AS. Peripheral atheroembolism: Confirmation of clinical concept, with a case report and review of the literature. Surgery 1973;73:353−359.

61 Ramirez G, O'Neill WM, Lambert R, et al. Cholesterol embolization. A complication of angiography. Arch Intern Med 1978;138:1430−1432.

62 Thurlbeck WM, Castleman B. Atheromatous emboli to the kidneys after aortic surgery. N Engl J Med 1957; 257:442−447.

63 Jones DB, Iannaccone PM. Atheromatous emboli in renal biopsies. An ultrastructural study. Am J Pathol 1975; 78:261−276.

64 Cosio FG, Zager RA, Sharma HM. Atheroembolic renal disease causes hypocomplementemia. Lancet 1985; 2:118−121.

65 McGowan JA, Greenberg A. Cholesterol atheroembolic renal disease. Report of 3 cases with emphasis on diagnosis by skin biopsy and extended survival. Am J Nephrol 1986; 6:135−139.

66 Kasinath BS, Corwin HL, Bidani AK, et al. Eosinophilia in the diagnosis of atheroembolic renal disease. Am J Nephrol 1987;7:173−177.

67 Williams HH, Wall BM, Cooke CR. Case report: Reversible nephrotic range proteinuria and renal failure in atheroembolic renal disease. Am J Med Sci 1990;299:58−61.

68 Kassirer JP. Atheroembolic renal disease. N Engl J Med 1969;280:812−817.

69 Warren BA, Vales O. The ultrastructure of the stages of atheroembolic occlusion of renal arteries. Br J Exp Pathol 1973;54:469−478.

70 Jeynes BJ. Combined streptokinase and taurochenodeoxycholate action on experimentally induced atherothromboemboli. Arch Pathol Lab Med 1986;110:1143−1148.

71 Dumazer PH, Modesto A, Bonafe JL, et al. Les embolies renales de cholesterol: a propos de 6 observations. Nephrologie 1988;9:67−72.

72 Aujla ND, Greenberg A, Banner BF, et al. Atheroembolic involvement of renal allografts. Am J Kidney Dis 1989;13: 329−332.

73 Goldman M, Thoua Y, Dhaene M, et al. Necrotizing glomerulonephritis associated with cholesterol microemboli. Br Med J 1985;290:205−206.

74 Hannedouche T, Godin T, Courtois M, et al. Necrotizing glomerulonephritis and renal cholesterol embolization. Nephron 1986;42:271−272.

75 Remy P, Jacquot C, Nochy D, et al. Cholesterol atheroembolic renal disease with necrotizing glomerulonephritis. Am J Nephrol 1987;7:164−165.

76 Tilley WS, Harston WE, Siami G, et al. Renal failure due to cholesterol emboli following PTCA. Am Heart J 1985;110: 1301−1302.

77 Smith MC, Ghose MK, Henry AR. The clinical spectrum of renal cholesterol embolization. Am J Med 1981; 71:174−180.

78 Dunnill MS, Halley W. Some observations on the quantitative anatomy of the kidney. J Pathol 1973;110:113−121.

79 Bohle A, Grund KE, Mackensen S, et al. Correlations between renal interstitium and level of serum creatinine. Virchows Arch (Pathol Anat) 1977;373:15−22.

80 Hestbech J, Hansen HE, Amdisen A, et al. Chronic renal lesions following long-term treatment with lithium. Kidney Int 1977;12:205−213.

81 Risdon RA, Sloper JAC de, De Wardener HE. Relationship between renal function and histologic changes found in renal biopsy specimens from patients with persistent glomerulonephritis. Lancet 1968;2:363−366.

82 Schainuck LI, Stricker GE, Luther RE, et al. Structural-functional correlations in renal disease. II. The correlations. Hum Pathol 1970;1:631−641.

83 Bohle A, Mackensen-Haen S, Gise HV. Significance of tubulointerstitial changes in the renal cortex for excretory function and concentration ability of the kidney: a morphometric contribution. Am J Nephrol 1987;7:421−433.

84 Grund KE, Mackensen S, Gruner J, et al. Renal insufficiency in nephrosclerosis (benign nephrosclerosis resp. transition from benign to secondary malignant nephrosclerosis). Correlations between morphological and functional parameters. Klin Wochenschr 1978;56:1147−1154.

85 Neilson EG. Pathogenesis and therapy of interstitial nephritis. Kidney Int 1989;35:1257−1270.

86 Tada S, Yamagishi J, Kobayashi H, et al. The incidence of simple renal cysts by computed tomography. Clin Radiol 1983;34:437−439.

87 Welling LW, Grantham JJ. Cystic diseases of the kidney. In Tisher CC, Brenner BM, eds. Renal Pathology, 1st edn. Philadelphia: Lippincott, 1989:1233−1277.

88 Fish GW. Large solitary serous cysts of the kidney. Report of 32 cases including two cases cured by aspiration and instillation of 50 percent dextrose solution. J Am Med Assoc 1939;112:514−518.

89 Braasch WF, Hendrick JA. Renal cysts, simple and otherwise. J Urol 1944;51:1−10.

90 Levine SR, Emmett JL, Wooner LB. Cyst and tumor occurring in the same kidney. J Urol 1964;91:8−9.

91 Lang EK. Coexistence of cyst and tumor in the same kidney. Radiology 1971;101:7−16.

92 Dunnill MS, Millard PR, Oliver D. Acquired cystic disease of the kidneys: A hazard of long-term intermittent maintenance haemodialysis. J Clin Pathol 1977;30:868−877.

93 Rockson SG, Stone RA, Gunnells JC. Solitary renal cyst with segmental ischemia and hypertension. J Urol 1974; 112:550−552.

94 Churchill D, Kimoff R, Pinsky M, *et al*. Solitary intrarenal cyst: Correctable cause of hypertension. Urology 1975; 6:485−488.

95 Kala R, Fyhrquist F, Halttunen P, *et al*. Solitary renal cyst: hypertension and renin. J Urol 1976;116:710−711.

96 Bricker NS, Patton JF. Cystic disease of the kidneys. A study of dynamics and chemical composition of cyst fluid. Am J Med 1955;18:207−219.

97 Clarke BG, Hurwitz ES, Dudinsky E. Solitary serous cysts of the kidney: Biochemical, cytologic and histologic studies. J Urol 1956;75:772−775.

98 Fetterman GH. Microdissection in the study of normal and abnormal renal structure and function. Pathol Annu 1970; 5:173−205.

99 Baert L, Steg A. Is the diverticulum of the distal and collecting tubules a preliminary stage of the simple cyst in the adult? J Urol 1977;118:707−710.

100 Milutinovic J, Agodoa LY. Potential causes and pathogenesis in autosomal dominant polycystic kidney disease. Nephron 1983;33:139−144.

101 Thaler MM, Ogata ES, Goodman JR, *et al*. Congenital fibrosis and polycystic disease of liver and kidneys. Am J Dis Child 1973;126:374−380.

102 Carone FA, Rowland RG, Perlman SG, *et al*. The pathogenesis of drug-induced renal cystic disease. Kidney Int 1974;5:411−421.

103 Carone FA, Hollenberg PF, Nakamura S, *et al*. Tubular basement membrane change occurs pari passu with the development of cyst formation. Kidney Int 1989;35: 1034−1040.

104 Kanwar YS, Carone FA. Reversible changes of tubular cell and basement membrane in drug-induced renal cystic disease. Kidney Int 1984;26:35−43.

105 Ojeda JL, Ros MAA, Icardo JM, *et al*. Basement membrane alterations during development and regression of tubular cysts. Kidney Int 1990;37:1270−1280.

106 MacKay K, Striker LJ, Pinkert CA, *et al*. Glomerulosclerosis and renal cysts in mice transgenic for the early region of SV40. Kidney Int 1987;32:827−837.

107 Peterson RO. *Urologic Pathology*. Philadelphia: Lippincott, 1986.

108 Newcomb WD. The search for truth, with special reference to the frequency of gastric ulcer-cancer and the origin of Grawitz tumours in the kidney. Proc R Soc Med 1936; 30:113−136.

109 Fite GL. Classifications of tumors in the kidney. Arch Pathol 1945;39:37−41.

110 Brodsky GL, Garnick MB. Renal tumors in the adult patient. In Tisher CC, Brenner BM, eds. *Renal Pathology*, 1st edn. Philadelphia: Lippincott, 1989:1467−1504.

111 Garnick MB, Richie JP. Renal neoplasia. In Brenner BM, Rector FC, eds. *The Kidney*, 4th edn. Philadelphia: WB Saunders, 1991.

2

Renal hemodynamics and glomerular filtration and their relationship to aging

Robert D. Lindeman

Introduction

The accuracy and simplicity with which renal clearances can be performed, requiring only timed urine samples and blood samples drawn at the midpoints of these periods, has made the kidney an ideal organ system for studying the physiologic changes that occur with aging. Cross-sectional studies in humans suggest that there is a progressive decline with age after the age of 40 years. The Baltimore Longitudinal Study on Aging [1] confirmed these observations in a cross-sectional analysis of their study population, and then showed a comparable decline in these subjects followed longitudinally. However, when these subjects were subsequently studied by calculating regression equations for each individual, one-third of the subjects showed no decline over periods up to 23 years [2]. The decrease in mean creatinine clearance was due primarily to the other two-thirds which had decreases in renal function, some of which were very remarkable. There has been a growing awareness, confirmed in various functional tests of other organ systems that a decline in function with age is not inevitable, i.e. there is not a progressive involutional (physiologic) process whereby kidney function deteriorates with age. A recent editorial [3] has used the terms "successful" vs. "usual" aging to distinguish between what is seen in some subjects who age well and the usual picture seen using mean values in any aging population. The latter would be due to the superimposition of pathology, often asymptomatic or at least undetected.

Changes in glomerular filtration rate with age

A number of cross-sectional studies have been published showing an age-related decline in renal function after the age of 30–40 years [4–13]. Lewis & Alving [4] were the first to recognize this decrease which they documented by quantifying urea clearances. Davies & Shock [5] were the first to report inulin clearances, generally accepted as the most accurate and precise measure of glomerular filtration rate (GFR), in aging individuals free of cardiovascular, renal, and acute illnesses by history and physical examination. Seventy male subjects between the ages of 40 and 80 years showed a decline in clearance rates which approximated 1 cm³/min per year of age. Wesson [11] incorporated these findings with data collected from

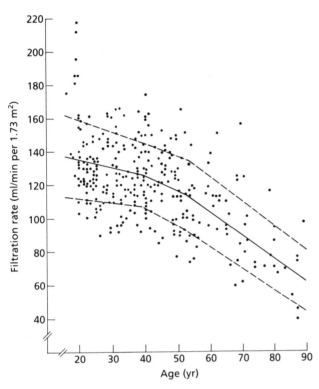

Fig. 2.1 Glomerular filtration rates (inulin clearances) per 1.73 m² in normal men vs. age from 38 studies. The solid and broken lines represent the means plus one standard deviation. (From Wesson [11].)

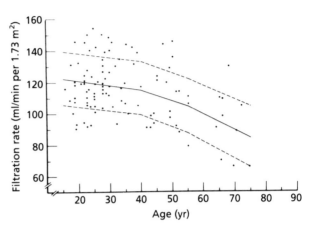

Fig. 2.2 Glomerular filtration rates (inulin clearances) per 1.73 m² in normal women vs. age from 38 studies. The solid and broken lines represent the means plus one standard deviation. (From Wesson [11].)

37 additional studies where individual inulin clearances and age were recorded, and found an accelerating decrease in GFR with increasing age in both males and females (Figs 2.1 and 2.2). The rate of decline was more rapid in males.

Prior to the Rowe *et al.* [1] 10-year analysis of the Baltimore Longitudinal Study on Aging, all studies had been cross-sectional, comparing measurements made on subjects of various ages. Cross-sectional studies might not reflect true age changes as the elderly subjects might represent selected survivors not representative of the original cohort. Furthermore, the physiologic characteristics of cohorts could change appreciably over time.

These limitations of a cross-sectional study are avoided by following serial measurements in the same subjects over an extended period of time (longitudinal study). Even longitudinal studies have limitations, as subtle changes in laboratory techniques may develop over time

and increased familiarity (decreased stress) with physiologic tests can produce changes that may be difficult to separate from age-related changes.

In 1976, Rowe *et al.* [1] reported on serial creatinine clearances obtained on 884 community-dwelling volunteers studied at 12–18 month intervals. There was an accelerating decline in creatinine clearances similar to that observed in their cross-sectional analysis (Figs 2.3 and 2.4), indicating that selective mortality and cohort differences had had no significant impact on the cross-sectional results.

Although mean true creatinine clearance rates fell from 140 cm³/min per 1.73 m² at age 25–34 years to 97 cm³/ min per 1.73 m² at age 75–84 years, serum creatinine concentrations rose insignificantly from 0.81 to 0.84 mg/ 100 ml. This means that creatinine production falls at nearly the same rate as the renal clearance of creatinine reflecting the decrease in body muscle mass that occurs with age. The practical implication of this observation is that the serum creatinine concentration in the older patient must be interpreted with this in mind when used to determine or modify dosages of drugs cleared totally or partially by the kidney, for example digoxin and the aminoglycoside antibiotics.

The most recent observations on creatinine clearances published from this longitudinal study provide additional important information [2,14,15]. A separate regression equation plotting the serial creatinine clearances against

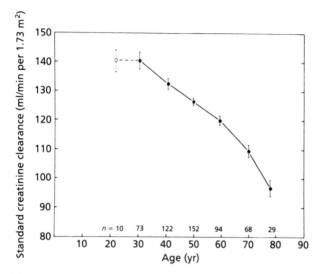

Fig. 2.3 Cross-sectional differences in standard creatinine clearance with age. The number of subjects in each age group is indicated above the abscissa. Values plotted indicate mean ± SEM. (From Rowe *et al.* [1].)

Fig. 2.4 Comparison of cross-sectional age differences and longitudinal age changes in creatinine clearance. The dots represent the mean values for each age decade obtained from cross-sectional data. Longitudinal results are represented by line segments which indicate the mean slope of changes in creatinine clearance for each decade. Lines are drawn with the midpoints at the mean clearance for each age decade, and with their lengths along the abscissa, representing the mean time span over which the longitudinal data were collected for each age group. (From Rowe *et al.* [1].)

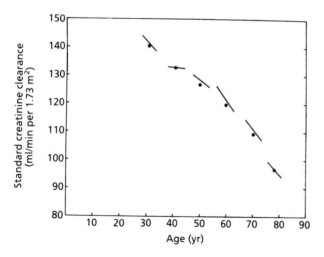

age for each of the 446 volunteers followed between 1958 and 1981 with five or more clearances at 12–18 month intervals was calculated. Subjects with any history or laboratory evidence to suggest renal or urinary tract disease (Group I) and subjects started on diuretics or antihypertensive agents (Group II) were separated out from the 254 "normal" subjects (Group III). The mean decrease in creatinine clearance in the last group was 0.75 ml/min per year of age, only slightly less than the 0.87 ml/min per year seen in the entire group and close to what has been previously reported in cross-sectional analyses.

Figure 2.5 illustrates one subject selected because he had the most studies [14]. A negative regression coefficient indicates the subject had a decrease in creatinine clearance over time; a positive regression coefficient indicates he had an increase in creatinine clearance. One-third of all subjects that were followed had a positive slope. The standard error of the mean is a measure of the dispersion of points around the regression line. Eighty percent of the individuals had smaller standard errors of the means than the subject illustrated meaning that this subject was more erratic in his values compared to most subjects.

Examples of some of the additional plots are shown in Figure 2.6. The six subjects at the top of the figure had substantial decreases in creatinine clearance ($>2\,cm^3$/ min per year). The six subjects in the middle had lesser decreases but still showed steady declines over time. Of

Fig. 2.5 Sample plot of creatinine clearance vs. age for one subject with 14 separate determinations over a 23-year period. (From Lindeman *et al.* [2].)

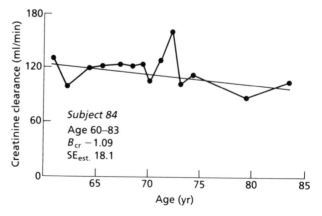

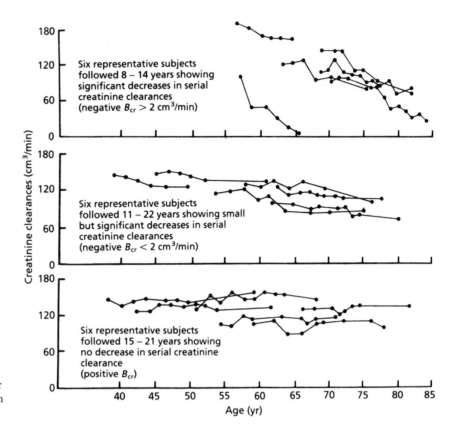

Fig. 2.6 Individual plots of serial creatinine clearances vs. age in years for representative subjects. (From Lindeman *et al.* [2].)

most interest were the six subjects at the bottom that exhibited positive slopes meaning there was an increase over the period of time studied (15−21 years).

Figure 2.7 shows the distribution of these regression coefficients for the 254 "normal" subjects plotted against age. Note again that patients with positive regression coefficients (B_{cr}) had no decrease in renal function over the time period studied and this includes a substantial number of individuals over the age of 60 years. These observations have important implications in understanding the pathophysiology of the decline in renal function observed with age and will be discussed later.

Renal blood and plasma flow

The quantity of blood (or plasma) perfusing the kidney, generally estimated by measuring *para*-aminohippurate (PAH) or diodrast clearances at low concentrations, decreases with age at a rate slightly greater than the decrease

Fig. 2.7 Regression coefficients plotting change in creatinine clearance vs. time in years (B_{cr}) vs. age in years for 254 normal subjects. Positive B_{cr}s (above the 0 line) represent increasing creatinine clearances over time; negative B_{cr}s (below the 0 line) represent decreasing creatinine clearances over time. (From Lindeman *et al.* [2].)

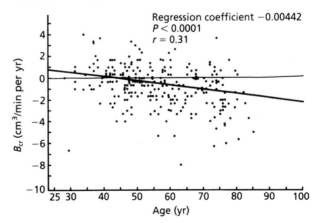

observed in the inulin clearances. In the studies reported by Davies & Shock [5], the effective renal plasma flow (ERPF) fell from a mean of 649 ml/min during the fourth decade to a mean of 289 ml/min during the ninth decade. Others have reported similar age-related decrements in ERPF [16–18]. When Wesson [11] combined reported data from 38 studies, he showed a decline in males from 610 ml/min at age 45 years to 350 ml/min at age 75 years, and in females from 565 ml/min at age 45 years to 300 ml/min at age 75 years. The extraction ratios at low arterial PAH concentrations were 92% in both young and old subjects in two studies [19,20].

The decrease in renal blood flow (RBF) with age without a proportionate decrease in blood pressure is indicative of either vascular impedence due to intraluminal pathology (atheromata) or an increase in renal vasculature resistance due to vasoconstriction. Since RBF can be increased transiently by administration of vasodilators (or pyrogen) in both young and elderly subjects, a vasoconstrictive (reversible) component must be implicated in the regulation of the renal circulation in both young and elderly as discussed in the next section.

The filtration fraction

The filtration fraction (FF), obtained by dividing the inulin clearance (GFR) by PAH clearance (ERPF), increases with age, although in most studies the increase is not impressive [21]. The series by McDonald et al. [16] studying young (mean age 36.6 years), middle-aged (mean age 58.8 years) and elderly (mean age 76.9 years) men, reported values of 0.189, 0.206, and 0.232, respectively (some of the subjects in the last group had hypertension and/or heart failure). These subjects were administered pyrogen intravenously. While GFR remained constant, all three groups showed an increase in ERPF which was proportionately greater with age resulting in FFs of 0.115, 0.123, and 0.122 for the young, middle-aged, and elderly groups, respectively. The disappearance of the age-related differential suggests that the relatively reduced RPF with age is a physiologic rather than an anatomic phenomenon. Calculations using Lamport's formula suggest that both the afferent and efferent arterioles are involved in the pressure regulation and that there is a physiologic increase in peripheral resistance (vasoconstriction) with age in the efferent arterioles of the kidneys.

Hollenberg et al. [22] studied RBF by the radioactive xenon washout technique, and although the method does not allow direct comparison their results are difficult to understand when compared with McDonald et al. [16]. The method provides data from which the flow/g of kidney tissue can be calculated. Filtration fractions can be calculated from their data indicating values of 0.185, 0.200, 0.217, and 0.237 for 20-, 40-, 60- and 80-year-old people, respectively [22]. In some of these subjects, the vasodilator acetylcholine was injected into the renal artery prior to the xenon resulting in vasodilatation and increased RBF but little change in GFR. In contrast to the studies by McDonald et al. the FFs (0.106, 0.115, 0.125, and 0.137, respectively) were not equalized. One possible explanation is that acetylcholine is not as effective a vasodilator as pyrogen. A 10-fold increase in the dose of acetylcholine further increased RBF and lowered the FF but did not change the previously described relationship.

The injection of the vasoconstrictor angiotension had comparable effects in young and elderly decreasing RBF similarly percentage-wise. The FFs were 0.251, 0.278, 0.312, and 0.358 in the 20-, 40-, 60- and 80-year-olds, respectively. Because the rapid or cortical component of flow decreased more rapidly than did the mean value for flow, it was assumed that cortical nephrons lose flow more rapidly than do the juxtamedullary nephrons. The authors point out that the juxtamedullary nephrons have a higher FF than do the cortical nephrons, and suggest that a selective loss of the latter would account for the increase in mean FF in the elderly. The other possible explanation would be that a relatively greater vasoconstriction of the efferent arteriole occurs in the elderly, perhaps because of the influence of angiotension.

The concept that changes in FF can be used to estimate relative alterations in preglomerular (afferent arteriole) and postglomerular (efferent arteriole) resistances is frequently cited to explain observed differences or changes in FF. It has been specifically suggested that the decrease in FF that occurs in response to angiotensin-converting enzyme (ACE) inhibition reflects preferential postglomerular vasodilatation [23,24]. Carmines et al. [25] recently cautioned that there are usually parallel changes in arteriolar afferent and efferent resistance resulting from pathophysiologic hemodynamic changes and from pharmacologic agents.

The influence of age on other renal functions

Maximum tubular transport capacity

The tubular maximum for diodrast or PAH secretory transport decreases with age at a rate nearly parallel to the decrease in inulin clearance [5,20,26]. The tubular maximum for glucose reabsorption also decreases with age at a rate closely paralleling the decrease in inulin clearance [27].

Although the reduction in the secretory and resorptive tubular maximums with age could be explained by a progressive loss of functional nephrons, animal experiments have shown fewer energy-producing mitochondria [28], lower enzyme concentrations [28−30], lower concentrations of total or sodium−potassium activated adenosine triphosphatase (ATPase) activity [31], decreased sodium extrusion and oxygen consumption [32], and decreased tubular transport capacity [28] in the tubular cells in old kidneys compared with young kidneys. Thus aging not only results in a reduction in the nephron population but produces detrimental changes in the basic biochemistry of the tubular cells. Available clearance techniques in humans are unable to detect these changes in tubular cell function, however, presumably because healthy nephrons are able to compensate for changes in diseased but still functional nephrons.

Concentrating and diluting ability

A decrease in urinary concentrating ability with age is well documented in humans [4,17,33−36]. Rowe *et al.* [36] showed that active community-dwelling men over a wide age range subjected to 12 hours of water deprivation increased urine osmolality to a mean of 1109 mosmol/liter in young subjects (mean age 33 years), 1051 mosmol/liter in middle-aged subjects (mean age 49 years), and 882 mosmol/liter in old subjects (mean age 68 years). Attempts to relate the decrease in concentrating ability to the more rapid decrease in GFR than solute load, presumably resulting in an increased solute load in surviving functional nephrons, have not been successful [17,36]. Rowe *et al.* [36] suggested the greater perfusion of juxtamedullary nephrons would increase medullary blood flow resulting in a "washout" of solute and a decrease in concentrating ability. The observations of Hollenberg *et al.* [22] would support such a contention.

Maximum diluting ability, as measured by minimum urine osmolality achieved with water loading, also decreases with age [17]. Another way to look at diluting ability in young vs. old subjects is to compare free water clearance (C_{H_2O}) corrected for nephron mass as shown in Table 2.1. Although free water clearance decreases with age, C_{H_2O} factored by inulin clearance changes little with age, suggesting there is no basic defect in the ability of the tubule to produce a dilute urine.

Maximum urine osmolality following high-dose pitressin infusion was significantly reduced in elderly subjects undergoing a water diuresis [34]. However, elderly people after water loading appear to respond normally to graded doses of antidiuretic hormone insufficient to maximally concentrate the urine [17]. In fact, it takes less pitressin to make the urine isotonic in older individuals

Table 2.1 Maximum diluting capacity in young, middle-aged, and elderly male subjects after ingestion of 20 cm³H₂O/kg body weight

	Young	Middle-aged	Elderly
No. of subjects	7	7	7
Mean age (year)	31	60	84
Mean GFR (cm³/min)	149 ± 9	92 ± 8	65 ± 4
Urine flow (cm³/min)	19.8 ± 1.7	11.1 ± 1.5	8.5 ± 1.2
Urine osmolality (mmol/liter)	52 ± 3	74 ± 6	92 ± 11
Total solute excretion/100 ml GFR	690	840	1120
C_{H_2O} (cm³/min)	16.2 ± 1.4	8.4 ± 1.3	5.9 ± 1.0
C_{H_2O}/100 ml GFR (cm³/min)	10.9	9.1	9.1

than in younger people. The observations in the first study appear most likely to be the result of a diminished medullary tonicity rather than a defect in the ability of the kidney to respond to pitressin.

Urine acidification

Despite the decrease in renal function with age, the blood pH, P_{CO_2}, and bicarbonate of aged people do not differ from the values observed in young subjects under basal conditions [37,38]. Following ingestion of an acid load (NH_4Cl), however, the decreases in blood pH and bicarbonate concentrations take longer to return to baseline [37–39]. The minimum urine pH achieved after an acid load is comparable in young and elderly subjects, but total acid excretion (ammonia plus titratable acid minus bicarbonate) in aging people decreases at a rate paralleling the decrease in GFR [38]. In other words, if total acid excretion is factored by GFR, similar excretion rates are obtained in young and elderly. There was an increase in the urinary buffers responsible for titratable acid (phosphate, creatinine, etc.) per unit GFR in the older subjects. Conversely, the younger subjects excreted a greater percentage of their acid load as ammonium. A deficiency of glutamine, the substrate responsible for ammonia production, could not be shown to be responsible for the lack of ammonia production in elderly subjects. Subsequently, Agarwal & Cabebe [40], selecting a group of elderly subjects with GFRs similar to those observed in younger subjects, showed a small pH gradient defect and reduced ammonium excretion in old compared to young subjects.

Glomerular permeability

Glomerular permeability does not appear to change with age in normal subjects. Van Zonneveld [41] found an increasing incidence of proteinuria in a population survey of people over 65 years of age. Nevertheless, by the age of 85 only a minority of patients had evidence of proteinuria. Glomerular permeability to free hemoglobin, determined by factoring free hemoglobin clearances by inulin clearances in healthy young and elderly subjects, did not change with age [42]. Furthermore, there was no difference in glomerular permeability to a spectrum of different molecular weight dextrans when young and elderly subjects were compared [43]. Finally, filtration characteristics of intact glomeruli showed no evidence of changing glomerular pore size with increasing age.

Changes with age in the renal response to alterations in the internal and external environment

The kidneys are responsible for maintenance of a constant internal environment of fluid volume and electrolyte concentrations. Imbalances result not from intrinsic renal changes with age but rather from extrarenal pathology affecting renal regulatory mechanisms. Cohn & Shock [44] showed no change with age in blood or plasma volumes in male subjects age 20–90 years. Serum sodium, potassium, chloride, calcium, and magnesium concentrations do not vary significantly with age nor does acid–base balance.

Epstein & Hollenberg [45] reported that older subjects failed to conserve sodium as rapidly and efficiently as did younger subjects (Fig. 2.8). Several investigators [46,47] have shown that elderly people have lower plasma renin activities and urinary aldosterone excretions both on restricted and unrestricted salt intakes and both standing and lying. Serum cortisol and renin substrate concentrations were not different in young and old subjects. Although the cause of the decreased renin and aldosterone in older subjects remains speculative, it probably accounts for the decreased ability to conserve sodium when challenged with a low-sodium diet. Furthermore, it also accounts for the greater tendency of the elderly subjects to develop potentially dangerous hyperkalemia when receiving potassium supplements [48].

The diurnal variations in urine sodium, potassium and chloride excretion, and GFR appear blunted in older subjects compared with young. One potential explanation might be that the normal daytime increases in each of these parameters is more blunted by the counter influence of posture in older subjects, i.e. there is a greater decrease in these parameters with standing in older subjects. Actually, when the response to tilt is compared in young and elderly subjects, there is little difference in the percentage decrease in sodium excretion and GFR in response to 1 hour of 45° tilt [49]. Finally, Armbrecht et al. [50] have demonstrated a marked decrease (10-fold) in the ability of the kidney to convert 25-OH vitamin D_3 to $1,25(OH)_2$ vitamin D_3 in young vs. adult rats. The decreased ability to hydroxylate 25-OH D_3 was also observed in isolated slices of rat kidney indicating a depletion in the kidney of the enzyme necessary for this conversion. The mechanism remains unclear.

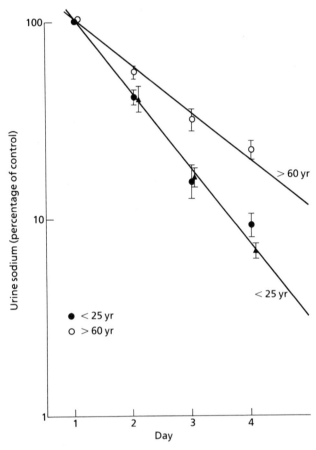

Fig. 2.8 Response of urinary sodium excretion to restriction of sodium intake in normal man. The mean half-time for eight subjects over 60 year of age was 30.9 ± 2.8 hours and was 17.6 ± 0.7 hours for subjects under the age of 25 years ($P < 0.01$). (From Epstein & Hollenberg [45].)

Pathophysiology of the decrease in renal function with age

Cross-sectional studies from "normal" aging populations have demonstrated a consistent decrease in renal function with age which tends to accelerate in the older age groups. Whether this is due to a progressive involutional change with loss of nephron units through attrition and a decline in cellular function through the life of the individual, or is due to "events" producing multiple, intermittent, often undetected acute and/or chronic injury, or both, remains unclear. Examples of the latter include undetected glomerulonephritis secondary to immunologic injury following an infection, pyelonephritis due to bacterial or viral infection, toxic tubular injury due to drugs or other nephrotoxins, vascular occlusions with resultant ischemic injury, and urinary tract obstruction. The evidence that the decrease is due to a progressive involutional change vs. it being due to superimposed pathology is reviewed. The fact that many individuals can go many years without showing a decrease in GFR [2] weighs against the former.

Evidence that renal changes with age are due to progressive and inevitable involution

Studies by Hayflick [51–53] have shown that cultured normal cells, such as diploid human fibroblasts, have a finite lifespan and that the population-doubling potential of these cells is inversely related to the age of the donor. Similar observations have been made of renal cells cultured *in vitro* [54].

As cultured normal cells approach the end of their *in vitro* lifetime, a number of biochemical decrements occur which herald the approaching loss of division capacity [51–53]. The animal studies reported earlier [28–32] showing that tubular cells have fewer energy-producing mitochondria, lower enzyme concentrations, lower concentrations of sodium–potassium activated ATPase activity, decreased sodium extrusion and oxygen consumption, and diminished tubular transport in old compared to young kidneys would be consistent with such a cellular aging phenomenon.

The observation of glomerular loss in the absence of overt lesions in the large and small vessels indicates that nephron loss occurs normally without an overt vascular cause. The sequence of glomerular obsolescence without shunting in the cortical glomeruli and with shunting in the juxtamedullary glomeruli appears to originate at the glomerular level, possibly associated with capillary lesions [55–57]. It is difficult to attribute these changes to specific disease entities in the absence of any characteristic observable pathologic abnormality.

Evidence that renal changes with age are due to superimposed pathology

Two representative studies are reported to document that pathologic changes, generally asymptomatic and undetected, must contribute, at least in part, to the observed decline in renal function with age. Friedman *et al.* [58]

utilized scintillation scanning techniques to localize defects in kidney function in elderly people with no past history of renal disease. They found abnormal scans in 25 out of 35 elderly patients with a mean age of 75 years and mean creatinine clearance of 53 cm³/min. Sixteen showed areas of diminished uptake which were felt to represent ischemic lesions.

Asymptomatic bacteriuria may be another contributor to decreased renal function in the aged. Dontas *et al.* [59] found that 27% of clinically healthy residents of the Athens House for the Aged had persistent bacteriuria and the mean inulin clearances (70 vs. 81 cm³/min) were lower in this group.

The studies reported earlier from the Baltimore Longitudinal Study of Aging [2,14,15] provide convincing evidence that the decrease in renal function observed with age is the result of intervening pathology as opposed to a relentless involutional process. One-third of the normal subjects, some of them elderly, showed no decrease in renal function over the period of the study (up to 23 years).

Compensatory renal hypertrophy

Unilateral nephrectomy causes compensatory hypertrophy in the normal remaining kidney. However, the rates of enlargement and increased function are much reduced in the old when compared to the young. Anatomic and physiologic increases parallel each other. Renal size and function increase rapidly the first 3−7 days postnephrectomy, more slowly the next 3 weeks, and then may show continued slight increases for many months in transplant donors [60]. The extensively studied roles of various renotropic (humoral) factors, ion fluxes, and other potential growth modulators have been reviewed elsewhere [61−63]. The role of epidermal growth factor (EGF) will be discussed later in this chapter.

The number of glomeruli does not increase after birth in humans so that the compensatory enlargement is not due to an increase in the number of nephrons. Rather, the glomeruli increase in volume and the tubules, chiefly the proximal convoluted segment, enlarge. In young animals, cellular hyperplasia predominates; in older animals, the chief response is that of cellular hypertrophy [64−70]. Even though the kidneys of older animals enlarge primarily by hypertrophy, the rate of hypertrophy is slower in old than in young animals. This is supported by studies

of cell counts [67], RNA/DNA ratios [64,68], counts of mitoses [65,66,70], and measures of double-stranded DNA replication [69].

Renal compensatory hypertrophy has been of clinical interest because of its importance in renal transplant donors. Ogden [71] found that in 28 donors the remaining kidney showed an inverse relationship between age at the time of nephrectomy and function 3 years later. Subsequently Boner *et al.* [60] showed that the single kidney GFR increased 48% in 20-year-old people compared to 30% in 60-year-old people. This phenomenon may be important in understanding the ability of the aging kidney to replace and repair cells in the nephron injured by a variety of pathologic processes.

Possible role of hyperperfusion and hyperfiltration in the loss of renal function with age

When the population of normal glomeruli is reduced by surgical ablation or renal disease in the rat model, the remaining glomeruli react with an "adaptive" hyperperfusion and hyperfiltration [72]. This glomerular hyperfiltration disrupts the integrity of the capillary membrane resulting in proteinuria, accumulation of mesangial deposits, and initiation or acceleration of the loss of renal function through a process of developing glomerular sclerosis. This same process is observed in aging animals of many species as well as in humans. The increases in glomerular capillary pressure and flow that follow uninephrectomy in the rat are accompanied by a moderate acceleration in the development of the glomerular sclerosis normally seen in the aging rat [73]. With the rat remnant kidney where much greater increases in pressure and flow are created, the structural changes develop even more rapidly.

In an attempt to elucidate the mechanisms responsible for the age-related glomerular sclerosis, a number of maneuvers have been performed aimed at modifying glomerular capillary pressures and flows. Most notable has been the dietary restriction of protein. Hostetter *et al.* [72] found that the single-nephron GFR in remnant kidney nephrons of rats fed a 24% protein diet was twice that of animals fed a 6% protein diet. Additional studies in rat and dog remnant kidney models have demonstrated that dietary protein restriction delays the development of proteinuria and the structural changes of glomerular sclerosis [74,75].

Significant increases in GFR and RPF occur acutely after ingestion of a high-protein (meat) meal; whereas dietary intake of isocaloric quantities of carbohydrate and fat have little effect on kidney function. The post-prandial increase in RBF after protein ingestion is un-related to changes in cardiac output indicating that there is a preferential increase in perfusion and GFR [76,77]. When animals are maintained continuously on protein-rich diets, there is a cumulative effect resulting in sus-tained increases in blood flow and FF resulting in renal hypertrophy [78].

Brenner et al. [79,80] have suggested that the protein-rich diet characteristic of modern western society itself induces chronic renal hyperperfusion and hyperfiltration, thereby contributing to the structural and functional deterioration of the aging kidney. According to this hypo-thesis, the high glomerular pressures and flows necessary to meet the demands of a protein-rich diet contribute to the development of glomerular sclerosis.

Similar changes are seen in both diabetic and hyper-tensive rat models. Both GFR and kidney size are in-creased in early Type I (insulin-dependent) diabetes mellitus producing changes in humans similar to those observed in animal models [81]. The state of glomerular hyperperfusion and hyperfiltration created by abnormal carbohydrate metabolism is corrected when the carbo-hydrate metabolism is normalized. Glomerular sclerosis with impairment of GFR develops in diabetics with hyperperfusion and hyperfiltration of long duration.

Hypertension in the animal model with underlying renal disease or diabetes hastens the development of glomerular sclerosis. When hypertension is experimen-tally induced in the diabetic animal using the two kidney Goldblatt model (clipped and unclipped renal arteries), asymmetry of the renal lesions is seen [82]. In the un-clipped kidney exposed to elevated systemic pressures, more severe glomerular sclerosis is observed compared to the clipped kidney with reduced systemic pressure. Similarly, normotensive diabetic rats have less severe lesions when compared with hypertensive diabetic animals [83]. Dietary protein restriction lowers glomeru-lar pressures and flows in diabetic rats [84]. It appears that the beneficial effects of protein restriction in diabetic animal models is related, at least in part, to this reduction in hyperfiltration.

Hypertension in humans results in an accelerated loss of renal function [14,15]. There may be a transient period of hyperfiltration in early hypertension, however, which tends to obscure for a time the impact of the elevated systemic pressures on kidney funciton [15].

Brenner et al. [79,80], based on these and additional observations, have proposed the progressive decline in renal function with age, as with primary renal disease, diabetes mellitus, hypertension, and renal ablation, is due to hyperperfusion and hyperfiltration resulting in glomerular sclerosis. The proposed mechanisms are illustrated in Figure 2.9.

Not all evidence supports the theory that hyperfiltration leads to glomerular sclerosis in man. Long-term follow-up studies of patients undergoing uninephrectomy for unilateral renal disease or kidney transplant donation are necessary to determine the consequences of a reduction of functioning nephrons on renal structure and function. It appears that renal function is reasonably well main-tained for periods up to 30 years [85–88]; however, there does appear to be a higher incidence of both proteinuria and hypertension in age- and sex-matched controls [85,86,88]. Fine [89] has proposed the concept that "glomerular tolerance" to injury as well as perfusion pressure determines whether or not glomerular sclerosis will develop.

Concept of renal reserve

Bosch et al. [90] quantified the increase in GFR and ERPF after an oral protein load and termed this increase the "renal functional reserve capacity." They theorized that this represented the abililty of the kidney under periods of stress to increase glomerular flow and filtration. Four normal young volunteers showed a mean increase in GFR (creatinine clearance) from 105 to 171 ml/min after an 80 g protein meal. They also showed using low-, normal-, and high-protein diets that the GFR varied directly with the protein intake from a mean of 101 ml/min on a low-protein diet to a mean of 127 ml/min on a high-protein diet. They speculated that if the kidney reaches the point where it is hyperperfusing and hyperfiltering at all times, i.e., it loses its "renal functional reserve capacity," that it would be susceptible to damage (glomerular sclerosis). They also felt that if one lowered GFR with a low-protein diet that this might allow the renal reserve to be re-established possibly explaining the beneficial effect of

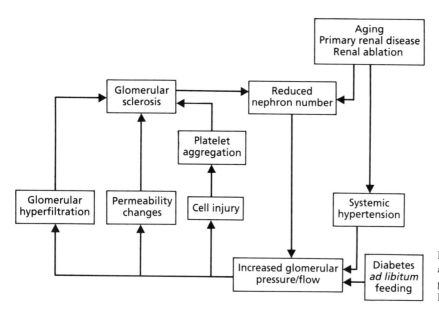

Fig. 2.9 Proposed role of hyperperfusion and hyperfiltration in the development of glomerular sclerosis. (From Anderson & Brenner [80].)

low-protein diets in patients with underlying progressive renal disease [91–95].

These same investigators [96] further demonstrated that patients with underlying renal disease lost some or all of this ability to increase their GFR after an oral protein load and suggested that loss of this ability meant they were already hyperfiltering. Rodriguez-Iturbe et al. [97] compared creatinine clearances before and after a high-protein meal in 25 kidney donors and 35 patients with poststreptococcal glomerulonephritis against 44 normal controls. The mean increase in the postacute nephritis and nephrectomy patients was 18% compared to 58% in the controls again suggesting the first two groups had a diminished renal reserve capacity.

Cassidy & Beck [98], however, found no difference in the percentage change in creatinine clearance after a standardized meat meal between kidney donors and normal controls. Rodriguez-Iturbe et al. [99] showed that moderate- to high-protein loads (1.1–1.4 g/kg body weight) increased inulin clearances much more than PAH clearances thereby significantly increasing FFs. This again would be consistent with the concept that afferent arteriolar vasodilatation occurs with acute protein loading which would make the kidney susceptible to damage from increased pressures. Two other groups, however, failed to show such an increase in FF after an acute protein load [100,101].

Infusions of amino acids and dopamine have been used to increase GFR and to quantify renal reserve [100,102,103] but offer no advantages other than more rapid onset of action. Of particular interest is the observation that somatostatin infusion abolishes the effect of amino acids on GFR suggesting the effect is mediated by some hormone(s) whose secretion is inhibited by somatostatin [103].

Effect of dietary protein restriction on renal hemodynamics and functional reserve capacity

The observation that acute protein loading in humans causes an increase in GFR, ERPF, FF, and presumably the glomerular capillary pressure suggests that protein restriction might have the appropriate effect of reducing renal hemodynamics and glomerular capillary pressure due to afferent arteriolar vasoconstriction, thereby modifying the progressive nature of renal function loss seen with renal disease and age. Whether protein restriction over a longer period of time actually has effects opposite to those of acute protein loading remains less clear.

At least four groups [103–106] have reported that normal subjects placed on short-term protein restriction decreased GFR and to a lesser extent ERPF and FF. In contrast, El Nahas et al. [107] showed that in patients with severe renal insufficiency, when switched from a high-protein to a low-protein diet, GFR remained unchanged and ERPF decreased, thereby increasing the FF. Wetzels *et al.* [108] and Rosenberg *et al.* [109] reported similar findings in patients with less severe renal insufficiency. Subsequently, this same group [110], using only modest dietary protein restriction (0.6 g/kg per day vs. 1.8 g/kg per day) in normal volunteers, showed that dietary protein restriction did not affect GFR while ERPF fell and therefore the FF increased. The reasons for these contradictory results remain unexplained.

A failure of GFR to decrease with dietary protein restriction does not necessarily mean that glomerular capillary pressure will not decrease and account for the protective effect of dietary protein restriction. In the rat remnant nephron model where hyperfiltration was established, several investigators [111,112] have demonstrated that protein restriction reduced glomerular capillary pressure but not GFR (or single-nephron GFR). The decrease in glomerular capillary pressure is offset by an increase in the ultrafiltration coefficient. Further evidence that this may be the case in humans is provided by the observation that protein restriction improved glomerular permselectivity without affecting GFR [109]. Therefore, a low-protein diet may exert its protective effects independent of an effect on glomerular hemodynamics, i.e. the findings are consistent with a reduction in glomerular capillary pressure but not flow.

The inverse relationship between dietary protein intake and response to an acute protein load ("renal functional reserve capacity") suggested in Bosch's studies [90,96] has not been confirmed in subsequent studies. The GFR increases as much or more in subjects on a high-protein diet after a high-protein (meat) meal than while on a low-protein diet [105,106,110]. These findings clearly fail to support the concept that there is a "ceiling" for GFR or "renal functional reserve capacity" which might be improved by placing subjects on a low-protein intake to lower GFR.

Measurements of renal hemodynamics in humans are insufficiently precise to define changes in glomerular capillary pressure, especially if changes in the ultrafiltration coefficient or RBF distribution should occur concurrently. Whether measurements of the effects of acute protein load or dietary protein restriction are of any physiologic significance in predicting the therapeutic effectiveness of protein restriction remains doubtful.

Role of EGF and other humoral mediators on compensatory hypertrophy and hyperfiltration

Epidermal growth factor is a 600 dalton peptide (53 amino acids) which is a potent multiplication (mitogenic) and maturation factor for cells and a modifier of many kinds of secretory cells. It was first isolated from mouse submandibular (salivary) glands but mouse and human EGF are very similar in structure and function. Epidermal growth factor receptors have been identified by immunostaining techniques in the thick ascending limb of Henle's loop and early distal convoluted tubule. Unilateral nephrectomy greatly increases EGF concentrations in these sites and in the urine [113]. Furthermore, pre-EGF mRNA also increases in these sites after unilateral nephrectomy suggesting EGF is synthesized there. It does not appear that this source of EGF contributes to the circulating EGF.

Although EGF has been reported to be synthesized in sites other than salivary glands, e.g. duodenum and kidney tubule, removal of the salivary glands in mice (sialoadenectomy) produces EGF-deficient mice [114]. Kidneys of EGF-deficient mice failed to undergo compensatory hypertrophy after unilateral nephrectomy causing renal insufficiency. The kidneys of animals receiving EGF replacement, as in animals without sialoadenectomy, developed compensatory hypertrophy without renal insufficiency.

An increase in dietary protein (from 6 to 24%) was associated with a doubling of urinary EGF [115]. Furthermore, protein feeding results in hypertrophy of the thick ascending limb of Henle's loop [116]. Finally, an age-related decrease in urinary EGF has been reported [117].

When one uses this information to construct a hypothesis, it appears the process of compensatory hypertrophy (which is probably the same as regeneration and repair of injured kidney tissue) must be mediated through stimulation of growth factors, e.g., EGF, and that the release of growth factor and/or response (receptor activity) is modified by age, making repair slower and perhaps less than optimal.

References

1 Rowe JW, Andres R, Tobin J, *et al.* The effect of age on creatinine clearance in men: a cross-sectional and longi-

tudinal study. J Gerontol 1976;31:155−163.

2 Lindeman RD, Tobin J, Shock NW. Longitudinal studies on the rate of decline in renal function with age. J Am Geriatr Soc 1985;33:278−285.

3 Rowe JW, Kahn RL. Human aging: usual and successful. Science 1987;237:143−149.

4 Lewis WH Jr, Alving AS. Changes with age in the renal function in adult men. Am J Physiol 1938;123:500−515.

5 Davies DF, Shock NW. Age changes in glomerular filtration rate, effective renal plasma flow, and tubular excretory capacity in adult males. J Clin Invest 1950;29:496−507.

6 Van Pilsum JF, Seljiskog L. Long-term endogenous creatinine clearance in man. Proc Soc Exp Biol Med 1958; 97:270−272.

7 Stewart CP. Renal function in aged. Gerontol Clin 1959; 1:160−167.

8 Pelz KS, Gottfried SP, Pog E. Kidney function studies in old men and women. Geriatrics 1965;20:145−149.

9 Beck H, Vignon JC. Clearance de la creatinine endogene, chez les personnes ages. Rev Fr Gerontol 1966;12:145−148.

10 Muether RO, Schnessler WP, Sommer AJ. Laboratory studies on the aging kidney. J Am Geriatr Soc 1967; 15:260−273.

11 Wesson LG Jr. Renal hemodynamics in physiological states. In Wesson LG Jr, ed. *Physiology of the Human Kidney*. New York: Grune & Stratton, 1969:98−100.

12 Hansen RM, Kampmann J, Laursen H. Renal excretion of drugs in the elderly. Lancet 1970;1:1170.

13 Lindeman RD, Goldman R. Anatomic and physiologic age changes in the kidney. Exp Gerontol 1986;21:379−406.

14 Lindeman RD, Tobin JD, Shock NW. Association between blood pressure and the rate of decline in renal function with age. Kidney Int 1984;26:861−868.

15 Lindeman RD. Hypertension and the kidney. Nephron 1987;47(Suppl. 1):62−67.

16 McDonald RK, Solomon DH, Shock NW. Aging as a factor in the renal hemodynamic changes induced by a standardized pyrogen. J Clin Invest 1951;5:457−462.

17 Lindeman RD, Lee TD Jr, Yiengst MJ, et al. Influence of age, renal disease, hypertension, diuretics, and calcium on the antidiuretic response to suboptimal infusions of vasopressin. J Lab Clin Med 1966;68:206−223.

18 Adler S, Lindeman RD, Yiengst MJ, et al. Effect of acute acid loading on urinary acid excretion by the aging human kidney. J Lab Clin Med 1968;72:278−289.

19 Bradley SE. *Transactions of the First Conference on Factors Regulating Blood Pressure*. New York: Josiah Macy Jr Foundation, 1947:118.

20 Miller JH, McDonald RK, Shock NW. The renal extraction of *p*-amino-hippurate in the aged individual. J Gerontol 1951;6:213−216.

21 Goldman R. Aging of the excretory system: kidney and bladder. In Finch CE, Hayflick L, eds. New York City: Van Nostrand Co., 1977:409−431.

22 Hollenberg NK, Adams DF, Solomon HS, et al. Senescence and the renal vasculature in normal man. Circ Res 1974;34: 309−316.

23 Bauer JH, Reams GP. Hemodynamic and renal function in essential hypertension during treatment with enalapril. Am J Med 1985;79(Suppl. 3c):10−13.

24 Zatz R, Dunn BR, Meyer TW, et al. Prevention of diabetic glomerulopathy by pharmacologic amelioration of glomerular capillary hypertension. J Clin Invest 1986;77: 1925−1930.

25 Carmines PK, Perry MD, Hazelbrig JB, et al. Effects of preglomerular and postglomerular vascular resistance alterations on filtration fraction. Kidney Int 1987;31(Suppl. 20):5229−5232.

26 Watkin DM, Shock NW. Age-wise standard value for C_{IN}, C_{PAH}, $^{om\ Tm}$$_{PAH}$ in adult males. J Clin Invest 1955;34:969.

27 Miller JH, McDonald RK, Shock NW. Age changes in the maximal rate of renal tubular reabsorption of glucose. J Gerontol 1952;7:196−200.

28 Barrows CH Jr, Falzone JA Jr, Shock NW. Age differences in the succin-oxidase activity of homogenates and mitochondria from the livers and kidneys of rats. J Gerontol 1960;15:130−133.

29 Wilson PD, Franks LM. Enzyme patterns in young and old mouse kidneys. Gerontologia 1971;17:16−32.

30 Burich RJ. Effects of age on renal function and enzyme activity in male C57BL/6 mice. J Gerontol 1975; 30:539−545.

31 Beauchene RE, Fanestil DD, Barrows CH Jr. The effect of age on active transport and sodium−potassium activated ATPase activity in renal tissue of rats. J Gerontol 1965; 20:306−310.

32 Proverbio F, Proverbio T, Marin R. Ion transport and oxygen consumption in kidney cortex slices from young and old rats. Gerontologia 1985;31:166−173.

33 Lindeman RD, VanBuren HC, Raisz LG. Osmolar renal concentrating ability in healthy young men and hospitalized patients without renal disease. N Engl J Med 1960; 262:1306−1309.

34 Miller JH, Shock NW. Age differences in the renal tubular response to antidiuretic hormone. J Gerontol 1953; 8:446−450.

35 Dontas AS, Marketos S, Papanayiotou NT. Mechanism of renal tubular defects in old age. Postgrad Med J 1972; 48:295−303.

36 Rowe JW, Shock NW, DeFronzo RA. The influence of age on the renal response to water deprivation in man. Nephron 1976;17:270−278.

37 Shock NW, Yiengst MJ. Age changes in the acid−base equilibrium of the blood of males. J Gerontol 1950;5:1−4.

38 Adler S, Lindeman RD, Yiengst MJ, et al. Effect of acute acid loading on urinary acid excretion by the aging human kidney. J Lab Clin Med 1968;72:278−289.

39 Hilton JG, Goodbody MF Jr, Krvesi OR. The effect of pro-

longed administration of NH_4Cl on the blood acid−base equilibrium of geriatric subjects. J Am Geriatr Soc 1955; 3:697−703.

40 Agarwal BN, Cabebe FG. Renal acidification in elderly subjects. Nephron 1980;26:291−293.

41 Van Zonneveld RJ. Some data on the genito-urinary system as found in old-age surveys in the Netherlands. Gerontol Clin 1959;1:167−173.

42 Lowenstein J, Faulstick DA, Yiengst MJ, et al. The glomerular clearance and renal transport of hemoglobin in adult males. J Clin Invest 1961;40:1172−1177.

43 Faulstick D, Yiengst MJ, Ourster DA, et al. Glomerular permeability in young and old subjects. J Gerontol 1962; 17:40−44.

44 Cohn JE, Shock NW. Blood volume studies in middle aged and elderly males. Am J Med Sci 1949;217:388−391.

45 Epstein M, Hollenberg NK. Age as a determinant of renal sodium conservation in normal man. J Lab Clin Med 1976; 87:411−417.

46 Crane MG, Harris JJ. Effect of aging on renin activity and aldosterone excretion. J Lab Clin Med 1976;87:947−959.

47 Weidman P, DeMyttenaere-Bursztein S, Maxwell MH, et al. Effect of aging on plasma renin and aldosterone in normal man. Kidney Int 1975;8:325−333.

48 Lawson DH. Adverse reactions to potassium chloride. Q J Med 1974;43:433−440.

49 Lee TD Jr, Lindergren RD, Yiengst MJ, et al. Influence of age on the cardiovascular and renal response to tilting. J Appl Physiol 1966;21:55−61.

50 Armbrecht HJ, Zenser RV, Davis BB. Effect of age on the conversion of 25-hydroxy vitamin D_3 to 1,25-dihydroxy vitamin D_3 by kidney of rats. J Clin Invest 1980; 66:1118−1123.

51 Hayflick L. The biology of human aging. Am J Med Sci 1973;265:432−445.

52 Hayflick L. Current theories of biologic aging. Fed Proc 1975;34:9−13.

53 Hayflick L. The cell biology of human aging. N Engl J Med 1976;295:1302−1308.

54 Soukupova M, Holeckova E, Cinnerova O. Behavior of explanted kidney cells from young, adult and old rats. Gerontologia 1965;11:141−152.

55 Ljungvist A, Lagergren C. Normal intrarenal arterial pattern in adult and aging human kidney. A microangiographical and histologic study. J Anat 1962;96:285−298.

56 Ljungvist A. Structure of the arteriole−glomerular units in different zones of the kidney. Nephron 1964;1:329−337.

57 Takazakura E, Wasabu N, Handa A, et al. Intrarenal vascular changes with age and disease. Kidney Int 1972;2:224−230.

58 Friedman SA, Raizner AE, Rosen H, et al. Functional defects in the aging kidney. Ann Intern Med 1972;76:41−45.

59 Dontas AS, Papanayiotou P, Marketos SG, et al. The effects of bacteriuria on renal functional patterns in old age. Clin Sci 1968;34:73−81.

60 Boner G, Shelp WD, Neton M, et al. Factors influencing the increase in glomerular filtration rate in the remaining kidney of transplant donors. Am J Med 1973; 55:169−174.

61 Austin H III, Goldin H, Preuss HG. Humoral regulation of growth. Nephron 1981;27:163−170.

62 Preuss HG. Symposium on compensatory renal growth. Kidney Int 1983;23:571−646.

63 Fine L. The biology of renal hypertrophy. Kidney Int 1986; 29:619−634.

64 Kennedy CG. Effects of old age and overnutrition on the kidney. Br Med Bull 1957;23:67−70.

65 Reiter RJ, McCreight CE, Sulkin NM. Age differences in cellular proliferation in rat kidneys. J Gerontol 1964; 19:485−489.

66 Phillips TL, Leong GF. Kidney cell proliferation after unilateral nephrectomy as related to age. Cancer Res 1967; 2:286−292.

67 Zumoff B, Pachter MR. Studies of rat kidney and liver growth using total nuclear counts. Am J Anat 1964; 114:479−493.

68 Johnson HA, Vera Roman JM. Compensatory renal enlargement: hypertrophy versus enlargement. Am J Pathol 1966; 49:1−13.

69 Levitsky EL. Age-dependent changes of DNA replication in rat spleen and kidney. J Gerontol 1980;26:321−326.

70 McCreight CE, Sulkin NM. Cellular proliferation in the kidneys of young and senile rats following unilateral nephrectomy. J Gerontol 1959;14:440−443.

71 Ogden DA. Donor and recipient function 2−4 years after renal homotransplantation. Ann Intern Med 1967; 67:998−1006.

72 Hostetter TM, Olson JL, Rennke HG, et al. Hyperfiltration in remnant nephrons: a potentially adverse response to renal ablation. Am J Physiol 1981;9:F85−F93.

73 Striker GE, Nagle RB, Kohnen PW, et al. Response to unilateral nephrectomy in old rats. Arch Pathol Lab Med 1969;87:439−442.

74 El-Nahas AM, Paraskevakou H, Zoob S, et al. Effect of dietary protein restriction on the development of renal failure after subtotal nephrectomy in rats. Clin Sci 1983;65: 399−406.

75 Polzin DJ, Osborne CA, Hayden DW, et al. Influence of reduced protein diets on morbidity, mortality, and renal function in dogs with induced chronic renal failure. Am J Vet Res 1984;45:506−517.

76 Avasti PS, Greene ER, Voyles WF. Noninvasive Doppler assessment of human postprandial renal blood flow and cardiac output. Am J Physiol 1987;252:F1167−F1174.

77 Fronek K, Stahlgren LH. Systemic and regional hemodynamic changes during food intake and digestion in non-anethetized dogs. Circ Res 1968;23:687−692.

78 Schoolwerth AC, Sandler RS, Hoffman PM, et al. Effects of nephron reduction and dietary protein content on renal ammoniagenesis in the rat. Kidney Int 1975;7:397−404.

79 Brenner BM, Meyer TW, Hostetter TH. Dietary protein intake and the progressive nature of kidney disease: the role of hemodynamically medicated glomerular injury in the pathogenesis of progressive glomerular sclerosis in aging, renal ablation, and intrinsic renal disease. N Engl J Med 1982;307:652–659.

80 Anderson S, Brenner BM. Effects of aging on the renal glomerulus. Am J Med 1986;80:435–442.

81 Mogensen CE, Anderson MJF. Increased kidney size and glomerular filtration rate in early juvenile diabetes. Diabetes 1973;22:706–712.

82 Mauer SM, Steffes MW, Azar S, et al. The effects of Goldblatt hypertension on development of the glomerular lesions of diabetes mellitus in the rat. Diabetes 1978;27: 738–744.

83 Bank H, Klose R, Aynedjian HS, et al. Evidence against increased glomerular pressure initiating diabetic nephropathy. Kidney Int 1987;31:898–905.

84 Zatz R, Meyer TW, Noddin JL, et al. Predominance of hemodynamic rather than metabolic factors in the pathogenesis of diabetic glomerulopathy. Proc Natl Acad Sci USA 1985;82:5963–5967.

85 Hakim RM, Goldszer RC, Brenner BM. Hypertension and proteinuria: long-term sequelae of uninephrectomy in humans. Kidney Int 1984;25:930–936.

86 Vincenti F, Amend WJC Jr, Kaysen G. Long-term renal function in kidney donors: Sustained compensatory hyperfiltration with no adverse effects. Transplantation 1983; 36:626–629.

87 Werland D, Sutherland DER, Chavers B, et al. Information on 628 living-related kidney donors at a single institution, with long-term follow-up in 472 cases. Transplant Proc 1984;16:5–7.

88 Miller IJ, Suthanthiran M, Riggio RR, et al. Impact of renal donation: long-term clinical and biochemical follow-up of living donors in a single center. Am J Med 1985; 79:201–208.

89 Fine LG. Preventing the progression of human renal disease: have rational therapeutic principles emerged? Kidney Int 1988;33:116–128.

90 Bosch JP, Saccaggi A, Lauer A, et al. Renal functional reserve in humans: effect of protein intake on glomerular filtration rate. Am J Med 1983;75:943–950.

91 Barsotti G, Morelli E, Giannoni A, et al. Restricted phosphorus and nitrogen intake to slow the progression of chronic renal failure: a controlled trial. Kidney Int 1983; 24(Suppl. 16):278–284.

92 Alvestrand A, Ahlberg M, Bergstrom J. Retardation of the progression of renal insufficiency in patients treated with low protein. Kidney Int 1983;24(Suppl. 16):268–272.

93 Oldrizzi L, Rigiu C, Valvo R, et al. Progression of renal failure in patients with renal disease of diverse etiology on protein restricted diet. Kidney Int 1985;27:553–557.

94 Rosman JB, TerWee PH, Meijer S, et al. Prospective randomized trial of early dietary protein restriction in chronic renal failure. Lancet 1984;2:1291–1295.

95 Williams AJ, Walls J. Metabolic consequences of differing protein diets in experimental renal disease. Eur J Clin Invest 1987;17:117–122.

96 Bosch JP, Lauer A, Glabman S. Short-term protein loading in assessment of patients with renal disease. Am J Med 1984;77:873–879.

97 Rodriguez-Iturbe B, Herrera J, Garcia R. Response to acute protein load in kidney donors and in apparently normal post acute glomerulonephritis patients: evidence for glomerular hyperfiltration. Lancet 1985;2:461–464.

98 Cassidy MJD, Beck RM. Renal functional reserve in live related kidney donors. Am J Kidney Dis 1988;11:468–472.

99 Rodriguez–Iturbe B, Herrera J, Garcia R. Relationship between glomerular filtration rate and renal blood flow at different levels of protein-induced hyperfiltration in man. Clin Sci 1988;74:11–15.

100 TerWee PH, Geerlings W, Rosman JB, et al. Testing renal reserve filtration capacity with an amino acid solution. Nephron 1985;41:193–199.

101 Hostetter TH. Renal hemodynamic response to a meat meal in humans. Am J Physiol 1986;250:F613–F618.

102 TerWee PM, Rosman JB, Van Der Giest S. Renal hemodynamics during separate and combined infusions of amino acids and dopamine. Kidney Int 1986;29:870–874.

103 Castellino P, Coda B, DeFronzo RA. Effect of amino acid infusion on renal hemodynamics in humans. Am J Physiol 1986;251:F132–F140.

104 Pullman TH, Alving AS, Dern RJ, et al. The influence of dietary protein intake on specific renal functions in normal man. J Lab Clin Med 1954;44:321–332.

105 Bergstrom J, Ahlberg M, Alvestrand A. Influence of protein intake on renal hemodynamics and plasma hormone concentrations in normal subjects. Acta Med Scand 1985; 217:189–196.

106 Viberti G, Bognetti E, Wiseman MJ, et al. Effect of a protein restricted diet on renal response to a meat meal in humans. Am J Physiol 1987;253:F388–F393.

107 El Nahas AM, Masters-Thomas A, Brady JA, et al. Selective effect of low protein diets in chronic renal disease. Br Med J 1984;289:1337–1341.

108 Wetzels JFM, Hoitsma AJ, Berden JHM, et al. Renal hemodynamic effects of a short-term high protein and low protein diet in patients with renal disease. Clin Nephrol 1988;30:42–47.

109 Rosenberg ME, Swanson JE, Thomas BL, et al. Glomerular and hormonal responses to dietary protein intake in human renal disease. Am J Physiol 1987;253:F1083–F1090.

110 Wetzels JFM, Wiltink PG, Van Diujnhoven EM, et al. Short-term protein restriction in healthy volunteers: effects on renal hemodynamics and renal response to a meat meal. Clin Nephrol 1989;31:311–315.

111 Nath KA, Kren SM, Hostetter TH. Dietary protein restric-

tion in established renal injury in the rat. Selective role of glomerular capillary pressure in progressive glomerular dysfunction. J Clin Invest 1986;78:1199−1205.

112 Meyer TW, Anderson S, Rennke HG, *et al*. Reversing glomerular hypertension stabilizes established glomerular injury. Kidney Int 1987;31:752−759.

113 Roll LB, Scott J, Bell GI, *et al*. Mouse preproepidermal growth factor synthesis by the kidney and other tissues. Nature 1985;313:228−231.

114 Uchida S, Tsutsumi O, Hise MK, *et al*. Role of epidermal growth factor in compensatory renal hypertrophy in mice

(abstr.). Kidney Int 1988;33:387.

115 Gung A, Badr KF, Orth DN, *et al*. Effect of dietary protein and uninephrectomy on urinary epidermal growth factor excretion (abstr.). Kidney Int. 1988;33:376.

116 Bouby N. Influence of dietary protein on adenylate cyclase activity of the medullary thick ascending limb (abstr.). Kidney Int 1987;31:430.

117 Uchihashi M, Hirota Y, Fujita T, *et al*. Age-related decrease in urinary excretion of human epidermal growth factor. Life Sci 1982;31:679−683.

3

Central and peripheral neural mechanisms regulating renal function and arterial pressure in the elderly

Annette E. Fitz
Ulla C. Kopp
Gerald F. DiBona

This chapter will review the central and peripheral neural mechanisms that regulate renal function and arterial pressure in the aged. To accomplish this, we will first review the normal physiology of the central and peripheral neural control of renal function and arterial pressure as requisite background for the subsequent consideration of the effects of the aging process on these control mechanisms.

Normal physiology of central and peripheral neural control of renal function

Neuroanatomy

The extensive and exclusive adrenergic innervation of the afferent and efferent glomerular arterioles, proximal and distal renal tubules, thick ascending limb of Henle's loop, and juxtaglomerular apparatus in the rat and monkey has been demonstrated by Barajas et al. [1,2]. By autoradiography, tritiated norepinephrine was observed in small dense-cored vesicles—the neurosecretory granules—of these adrenergic nerve terminals [3]. The greatest number of innervated profiles is in the proximal tubules, followed by the thick ascending limb of Henle's loop, the distal convoluted tubule, and the collecting duct [4]. It is interesting to note that the highest relative frequency of innervation (i.e., the ratio of the number of innervated profiles/the total number of profiles studied) is in the thick ascending limb of Henle's loop, followed by the distal convoluted tubules and the proximal tubule (Table 3.1). Recent studies further showed that the density of innervation along the thick ascending limb of Henle's

Table 3.1 Relative frequency of innervation of nephron segments. (Adapted from Barajas et al. [4])

Nephron segment	Profiles		
	Innervated	Total	Ratio (%)
Proximal tubule	608	25 602	2.4
Distal tubule (TALH/DCT)	493	7 579	6.5
TALH	51	712	7.2
DCT	38	844	4.5
Collecting duct	53	2 094	2.5

TALH, thick ascending limb of Henle's loop; DCT, distal convoluted tubule.

loop is heterogenous. The highest density of innervation is found in the thick ascending limb of Henle's loop of the juxtamedullary nephrons [5]. Adrenergic innervation of renal tubules has also been identified in the dog [6], human [7], and bullfrog kidney [8].

Catecholamine-containing terminals of postganglionic peripheral nerves are generally thought to utilize norepinephrine as a transmitter. Whether dopamine also serves as a neural transmitter has been an issue of controversy. The neuronal content of dopamine is small compared to that of norepinephrine (4−10%). However, levels of dopamine in the canine renal cortex have been found to be significantly higher than what could be predicted from the tissue norepinephrine level [9]. Histochemical examination suggested that the dopamine present in the tissue is primarily axonal. Furthermore, neural elements containing dopamine have been demonstrated in the glomerular vascular pole [10].

Electrical and reflex stimulation of the renal nerves results in a frequency-dependent renal venous overflow of norepinephrine and dopamine [11−15]. The renal venous outflow of dopamine is 15−20% of that of norepinephrine both at rest and during reflex or electrical renal nerve stimulation, arguing against a preferential activation of nonadrenergic or putative dopaminergic nerves during renal nerve stimulation.

Catecholamine receptors

In the renal vasculature of rats, dogs, and humans the predominating adrenoceptors are of the α1-subtype [16] (Table 3.2). The α2-adrenoceptors and β-adrenoceptors are sparsely distributed [17−19]. Dopamine-1 receptor mediated increases in cAMP production in dog and rat arteries and afferent arterioles have been suggested to be responsible for the renal vasodilatation produced by dopamine [20−22]. In the glomeruli, high concentrations of β1-adrenoceptor binding sites have been demonstrated in rats, dogs, and guinea pigs [23−26].

In the proximal tubules, α1- and α2-adrenoceptor binding sites [26,27] are concentrated in the basolateral membranes [28]. The α1- and α2-adrenoceptors are found on the convoluted but not on the straight portion of the proximal tubules [29,30]. In contrast, β2-adrenoceptors are found in the straight but not in the convoluted portion of the proximal tubules [25,31]. Dopamine and dopamine receptors have been localized to the proximal convoluted tubules in rats and rabbits [32−34].

Table 3.2 Localization of renal adrenoceptors

Structure	Adrenoceptors
Renal vasculature	α1-adrenoceptors and dopamine-1 receptors
Glomeruli	β1-adrenoceptors
Proximal tubules	α1- and α2-adrenoceptors
Convoluted tubules	α1- and α2-adrenoceptors, dopamine receptors
Straight tubules	β2-adrenoceptors
Cortical thick ascending limb of Henle's loop and distal convoluted tubules	β-adrenoceptors
Cortical and medullary collecting tubules	α2- and β2-adrenoceptors
Papillary collecting ducts	α2-adrenoceptors

In cortical thick ascending limb of Henle and distal convoluted tubules cAMP activity is increased by activation of β-adrenoceptors [35]. In cortical and medullary collecting ducts cAMP activity is increased by β2-adrenoceptor activation and decreased by α2-adrenoceptor activation [29,35−37]. In papillary collecting ducts α2-adrenoceptor mediated decreases in cAMP activity have been described [38].

Finally, radioligand studies have described the presence of β1-adrenoceptors in distal and cortical collecting tubules [18].

Since the nephron may be divided into approximately a dozen tubular segments with distinct morphologic, electrophysiologic, and transport characteristics, only microdissection studies will completely reveal the precise anatomic localization of adrenoceptors in relation to specific functions.

Renal circulation

Alterations in renal nerve activity

The relationship between the magnitude of increases in renal nerve activity and the magnitude of renal blood flow (RBF) responses has been studied in detail using electrical stimulation of the renal nerves in anesthetized animals. Whereas renal nerve stimulation at frequencies below 1 Hz has little or no effect on RBF, the slope of the stimulation frequency response curve is relatively steep at frequencies above 1 Hz with 50% and 70% reductions in RBF at average stimulation frequencies of 2 and 4 Hz, respectively [13,39−41]. Furthermore, the magnitude of the renal blood flow response to renal nerve stimulation is also related to the level of dietary sodium intake: compared to normal-sodium diet, low-sodium diet suppresses the renal vasoconstrictor response to renal nerve stimulation [41]. Surgical or pharmacologic renal denervation in conscious dogs or humans [42,43] does not affect RBF or renal vascular resistance suggesting that during basal conditions renal sympathetic nerve activity is low and plays no or only a minimal role in the control of basal RBF.

Whether renal nerve activity influences autoregulation of RBF has been the focus of many studies. However, as discussed by DiBona [44], current available evidence supports the concept that renal nerves do not play a role in the mechanisms involved in autoregulation of RBF.

Effector loci of renal nerves
The localization of the effector loci for renal nerves within the cortical microcirculation has been elucidated by micropuncture techniques. In euvolemic rats acute renal denervation does not affect single-nephron glomerular filtration rate (GFR) or its determinants [45]. In models of increased renal nerve activity, such as acute extracellular fluid volume depletion, congestive heart failure, and chronic sodium depletion, acute renal denervation increases single-nephron GFR in association with decreased afferent and efferent arteriolar resistance and increased glomerular ultrafiltration coefficient [46,47]. Conversely, electrical stimulation of the renal nerves at a frequency which causes marked decreases in RBF decreases single-nephron GFR and single-nephron plasma flow. The fall in single-nephron plasma flow is associated with significant increases in afferent and efferent renal vascular resistance, in particular with the former [48]. Recent studies by Kon [49] suggest that the marked fall in glomerular ultrafiltration coefficient caused by renal nerve stimulation is partly related to decreased surface area since morphologic studies show that glomeruli from the stimulated kidney are markedly smaller than glomeruli from the contralateral nonstimulated kidney, and partly related to narrowing of afferent and efferent arterioles in the stimulated kidney [49]. Results from *in vitro* perfusion studies suggest that the reductions in

afferent and efferent luminal diameter observed during electrical renal nerve stimulation are related to neurogenically released norepinephrine [50]. Norepinephrine causes severe focal constriction of afferent arterioles which cannot be attributed to pressure-induced autoregulatory responses in the renal vasculature [51].

Catecholamine receptors
The adrenoceptor subtype mediating renal vasoconstriction has been determined *in vivo* and *in vitro* using selective α1- and α2-adrenoceptor agonists and antagonists. The ratio between α1- and α2-adrenoceptor-mediated renal vasoconstriction seems to vary between species. In the rat, intrarenal administration of α1-adrenoceptor agonists causes large decreases in RBF; α2-adrenoceptor agonists are without effect [52]. In the dog, although selective α1-adrenoceptor antagonists completely block the renal vasoconstrictor response to intrarenal administered norepinephrine and renal nerve stimulation [53], agonists which activate α2-adrenoceptors can also cause a small but definite renal vasoconstriction [54,55]. In the rabbit, a combination of α1- and α2-adrenoceptor antagonists produces a greater attenuation of the renal vasoconstrictor responses to renal nerve stimulation or renal arterial administration of norepinephrine than that produced by α1-adrenoceptor antagonist alone, suggesting that both renal α1- and α2-adrenoceptors participate in the renal vasoconstrictor response [56].

The evidence supporting the existence of dopaminergic nerves has been reviewed [57,58]. It is well known that administration of dopamine results in an increase in RBF [59,60]. Although stimulation of the renal nerves results in an increase in renal venous output of dopamine [61], there is no physiologic evidence for the existence of renal vasodilator nerves [53]. Pharmacologic evidence for the existence of renal dopaminergic vasodilator fibers has been provided by the use of electrical stimulation of the midbrain [62] or intracerebroventricular administration of ouabain [63]. *In vitro* and micropuncture studies have shown that dopamine produces equal relaxation of rabbit afferent and efferent arterioles [64], increases single-nephron GFR and glomerular ultrafiltration pressure (the latter attenuated by a dopamine-2 antagonist [65]), suggesting a role for dopamine in the control of glomerular hemodynamics.

Renal tubular solute and water transport

Alterations in renal nerve activity

The presence of a denervation diuresis and natriuresis in conscious rats with chronic renal denervation clearly demonstrates a physiologic role for the renal nerves in the control of renal tubular solute and water transport [66,67]. The decreased proximal tubular reabsorption following acute or chronic renal denervation occurs independent of changes in renal interstitial pressure and peritubular oncotic and hydrostatic pressure [45,68]. Further studies have shown that the increased urine flow rate and urinary sodium excretion following renal denervation are associated with decreased sodium and water reabsorption in the loop of Henle and the distal tubule in addition to the proximal tubule [69]. Conversely, stimulation of the renal nerves can cause decreases in urine flow rate and sodium excretion in the absence of changes in RBF and GFR [70] which are due to increased sodium and water reabsorption in the proximal tubule [71–73] and the loop of Henle [40].

The role of the renal innervation in the renal excretory responses to intravascular volume expansion has been extensively studied [40,74]. One of the mechanisms involved in the natriuretic response to volume expansion derives from activation of atrial stretch receptors. Activation of left or right atrial stretch receptors by inflation of a balloon placed in the left atria in dogs [75] and the junction of the right atria and superior vena cava in rats [76] results in a natriuresis which is associated with a decrease in renal sympathetic nerve activity. Furthermore, the renal sympathetic nerve activity and natriuretic responses are abolished by bilateral cervical vagotomy [75]. Central hypervolemia induced by head-out water immersion stimulates cardiac and thoracic volume receptors and results in a diuresis and natriuresis in humans [77], primates [78], and dogs [79] which are associated with a fall in renal sympathetic nerve activity and are abolished by renal denervation [79]. The different mechanisms involved in the natriuretic response to isotonic saline volume expansion show a different sequence of events. Despite parallel increases in right atrial pressure, pulmonary wedge pressure, plasma atrial natriuretic peptide concentration, and urinary sodium excretion during isotonic saline volume expansion, only urinary sodium excretion shows a sustained increase when saline is continuously infused [80]. The sustained increase in urinary sodium excretion is associated with a sustained decrease in renal sympathetic nerve activity and is abolished by aortic denervation plus vagotomy [81]. The magnitude of the renal responses to volume expansion is related to the basal prevailing renal nerve activity which in turn, is a function of the steady-state sodium balance [82]. In rats on a low-sodium diet which have the highest renal sympathetic nerve activity and lowest right atrial pressure, saline volume expansion produces the greatest decrease in renal sympathetic nerve activity and greatest increase in urinary sodium excretion. The cause of the impaired cardiopulmonary baroreceptor reflex decrease in renal nerve activity during volume expansion in rats on a high NaCl diet is located in the afferent limb of the reflex arc [83].

Catecholamine receptors

Studies in sodium-replete humans show that changes in plasma norepinephrine concentration within the physiologic range reduce urinary sodium excretion in the absence of renal hemodynamic changes [84]. The accumulated evidence from studies in dogs [85], rabbits [86], and rats [87,88] indicates that the antidiuretic and antinatriuretic responses to increases in renal sympathetic nerve activity are mediated by postsynaptic α1-adrenoceptors located at neuroeffector junctions throughout the extent of the nephron. Smyth *et al.* [89] have suggested that α1-adrenoceptors which mediate the neurally induced water and sodium retention are located postjunctionally whereas α2-adrenoceptors which antagonize the renal actions of circulating hormones such as vasopressin are located extrajunctionally. *In vitro* and micropuncture studies have shown that the α2-adrenoceptor mediated blockade of the hydro-osmotic action of vasopressin is located in the cortical collecting tubule, and is mediated by a pertussis toxin-sensitive mechanism [90–92]. With respect to dopamine, available evidence argues against a role for dopamine-1 receptors in the antinatriuresis produced by low-frequency renal nerve stimulation which does not affect renal hemodynamics [93]. However, a recent study in rats showing a decrease in urinary sodium excretion in the acutely denervated but not in the contralateral innervated kidney, following administration of dopamine antagonists, suggest that renal dopamine may play a role in denervation natriuresis [94]. Whether dopamine antagonists influence the diuretic and natriuretic responses to intravenous volume loading is controversial as both positive and negative results have been reported in rats and dogs [95]. However, in humans dopamine antagonists have been shown to attenuate the natriuretic response to both lower body positive pressure [96] and head-out water immersion [97]. Since it has been suggested that the natriuresis observed during high-sodium diet is related to dopamine-mediated inhibition of proximal tubular $Na^+-K^+-ATPase$ activity [98], it may be argued that the blunted natriuretic responses to lower body positive pressure, head-out water immersion, and renal denervation following administration of dopamine antagonists may be related to a reduction of the dopamine-mediated inhibition of proximal tubular $Na^+-K^+-ATPase$ activity.

Renin secretion rate

Renin is found mainly in the cortex where it occurs as granules within the cytoplasm of modified smooth-muscle cells. The finding that juxtaglomerular granular cells containing renin extend proximally along the afferent arteriole, with only a minor portion of the juxtaglomerular granular cells in direct contact with the macula densa region of the distal tubule, suggest a diversity among the juxtaglomerular granular cell population with respect to stimuli for renin secretion. In fact, recent *in vitro* studies have shown that whereas juxtaglomerular granular cells responding to changes in sodium chloride concentration or transport are located within or close to the glomeruli, cells responding to β-adrenergic stimulation are located in the afferent arteriole at some distance from the glomerulus [99].

Three primary mechanisms are involved in the control of renin secretion rate: the renal vascular baroreceptor mechanism, the tubular macula densa receptor mechanism, and direct sympathetic neural control mechanism. These mechanisms have been the subject of several reviews [70,100−104].

Alterations in renal nerve activity
Electrical renal nerve stimulation results in a frequency-dependent increase in renal venous outflow of norepinephrine and renin secretion rate (Table 3.3) [12,39]. Similarly, graded reflex stimulation of the renal nerves produced by stepwise reductions of right atrial pressure [105] or carotid sinus pressure [106] results in proportional increases in renin secretion rate. Vagally innervated cardiopulmonary receptors exert a tonic inhibitory

Table 3.3 Influence of renal nerves on renin secretion

Renal nerve stimulation (Hz)	Effect on renin secretion rate
0.25	Modulation of nonneural mechanisms
0.50	Direct neural release from juxtaglomerular granular cells without alterations in stimuli to macula densa or baroreceptor
0.60−1.00	Alteration in stimulus to macula densa receptor
1.00	Alteration in stimulus to vascular baroreceptor

Effects become additive as frequency of renal nerve stimulation increases

influence on renin secretion rate as shown by increased renin secretion rate, following section, or cold block of the vagus nerves [107]. Nonhypotensive hemorrhage results in an increase in renin secretion rate which is greater from the innervated than the contralateral denervated kidney [108] and is abolished by either renal denervation [108], inflation of a balloon in the left atrium [109], or vagotomy [110]. In conscious dogs the renin secretion rate response to bilateral carotid occlusion with renal perfusion pressure held constant is associated with a relatively modest increase in renal nerve activity of 62% in contrast to the 500% increase observed in response to auditory stimulation. The 62% increase in renal nerve activity does not alter renal hemodynamic or excretory function [111−113]. The results from these and other studies would suggest a role for both low- and high-pressure baroreceptor reflexes in the physiologic control of renin secretion rate.

Recent studies have further shown that neurally mediated increases in renin secretion rate are influenced by the dietary sodium intake. Although it has long been known that low-sodium diet increases renin secretion rate [70], the mechanisms involved are still a matter of controversy. Whereas a recent study in conscious sodium-depleted dogs [114] failed to demonstrate an increase in renal venous outflow of norepinephrine—an index of renal nerve activity—other studies in anesthetized dogs and conscious restrained rats show increases in renal venous outflow of norepinephrine [11] and renal sympathetic nerve activity [82], respectively. Although it is conceivable that the differences in the results between these animal studies may be related to the additional stress related to the anesthesia [11] and the restrainer [82], a recent study in rats failed to show that the increased arterial plasma renin activity in low-sodium diet was related to a renal tubular mechanism [115]. Furthermore, it is known that dietary sodium restriction increases renal norepinephrine spillover in normal human subjects [116,117]. Following vagotomy, plasma renin activity is similarly elevated in low- and normal-sodium-diet rats to a level higher than in high-sodium-diet rats; it has been suggested that vagotomy (normal-sodium-diet rats) and dietary sodium restriction (low-sodium-diet rats) disinhibit a vagally mediated tonic suppression of renin secretion via pathways which are dependent on intact renal sympathetic nerves. An additional mechanism that may be involved in the enhanced renin secretion rate in animals or humans on a low-sodium diet is an increased number of renin-containing granules within the juxtaglomerular granular cells [118,119]. In support of this hypothesis are the studies by Osborn & Kinstetter [41] which showed that chronic ingestion of a low-sodium diet enhanced the renin secretion rate response to electrical renal nerve stimulation. Since the decrease in urinary sodium excretion produced by renal nerve stimulation was least in the low-sodium-diet dogs, it is unlikely that the enhanced renin secretion rate response was related to a macula densa mechanism but rather to a direct effect of chronic low-sodium diet on the renin content of juxtaglomerular granular cells.

Catecholamine receptors

It is well established that the renin secretion rate response to increases in renal nerve activity at intensities causing no or minimal changes in renal hemodynamics (low-level renal nerve stimulation) is mediated by activation of renal β1-adrenoceptors [39,85,120,121] — β2-adrenoceptors are not involved [85,122].

There has been substantial debate concerning the role of α-adrenoceptors in the control of neurally mediated renin secretion. Whereas there is little doubt that the increase in renin secretion rate produced by renal nerve stimulation at intensities causing marked decreases in urinary sodium excretion and RBF is partly related to activation of vascular and/or tubular α-adrenoceptors [123–125], the role of α-adrenoceptors in the increase in renin secretion rate produced by renal nerve stimulation at intensities causing minimal renal hemodynamic changes has been controversial. Early studies by Blair [126] showed that the increase in renin secretion rate produced by low-level renal nerve stimulation was inhibited by α-adrenoceptor antagonists when renal arterial pressure was controlled at 80–90 mmHg, i.e., 30–40 mmHg below spontaneous arterial pressure. However, these findings were not confirmed by other investigators who examined renin secretion responses to low-level renal nerve stimulation in the absence and presence of α-adrenoceptor antagonists at spontaneous renal arterial pressure [104,124]. More recent studies by Blair et al. [127] have confirmed that the differences in the results between her initial studies and those of others [104] were related to the level of renal arterial pressure and could be explained by an interaction between the neural and nonneural mechanisms regulating renin release which is dependent on the intensity of renal nerve stimulation and the level of renal arterial pressure (vide infra). Furthermore, a recent study in conscious rats demonstrates that the increase in plasma renin activity following administration of the α2-adrenoceptor antagonist yohimbine is a secondary consequence of a generalized increase in sympathetic nervous system activity [128].

The role of prostaglandins in neurally mediated renin secretion has been examined in detail. Although it is well established that renal nerve stimulation over a wide range of frequencies increases both renal prostaglandin and renin secretion rate, both of which are inhibited by the prostaglandin synthesis inhibitor indomethacin [104], the interaction between the two is still a matter of controversy. While the findings by Osborn et al. [129] suggest that prostaglandins and β1-adrenoceptor stimulation act in series to increase secretion rate during low-frequency renal nerve stimulation, the bulk of the current evidence fails to support the concept that β-adrenoceptor-stimulated renin secretion is mediated by the renal prostaglandin system [130]. Rather, most studies suggest that the prostaglandin-dependent increase in renin secretion rate is related to the α-adrenoceptor mediated renal vasoconstriction and/or sodium reabsorption [123].

Interaction between neural and nonneural mechanisms

In evaluating the role of each of the mechanisms involved

in the control of renin secretion rate early studies examined each mechanism in a fashion which allowed it to be evaluated independently of the influence of the other two mechanisms. More recent evidence indicates, however, that in many physiologic conditions there is an interaction between the neural and nonneural mechanisms in the control of renin secretion rate [102,131].

Some of the earliest studies suggesting an interaction between the renal nerves and the baroreceptor/macula densa mechanisms showed that intravenous furosemide or suprarenal aortic constriction elicits a greater renin secretion rate response in the innervated than in the denervated kidney [132,133]. Subsequent studies in dogs showed that the increase in renin secretion rate mediated by nonneural mechanisms can be influenced by the prevailing level of renal sympathetic nerve activity, as electrical renal nerve stimulation at a frequency of 0.25 Hz, which does not affect renin secretion rate at spontaneous renal perfusion pressure, enhances the renin secretion rate response to suprarenal aortic constriction or furosemide [134]. Further studies showed that the stimulus—response curve of nonneural mechanisms for renin secretion rate is shifted to the right (towards higher renal perfusion pressures) in the presence of renal nerve stimulation. The higher the renal nerve stimulation frequency the further the stimulus—response curve is shifted to the right [135]. Similarly, studies in conscious dogs [136] and rats [137] show that reflex renal nerve stimulation shift the stimulus—response curve relating plasma renin activity to renal arterial pressure to the right. Propranolol or renal denervation prevents the shift of the stimulus—response curve produced by reflex renal nerve stimulation [137]. In addition, studies in humans have shown that reflex renal nerve stimulation produced by cold pressor stress enhances the increase in renal venous plasma renin activity produced by renal arterial pressure reduction [138].

Normal physiology of central and peripheral control of arterial pressure

In general, neural mechanisms control the moment-to-moment modulation of cardiovascular responses to internal and external environmental stimuli. The coupling of cardiovascular activity to behavior may be one of the principal contributions of the central nervous system to the control of the circulation. An important development in integrated cardiovascular control is the finding that blood-borne substances can influence central neural and humoral regulation of the circulation by acting on specific central nervous system structures. The loci which mediate central neural actions of these substances are the circumventricular organs which lack a blood—brain barrier. The most widely studied substance in this respect is the peptide angiotensin II which, besides its peripheral action, also activates regions in the area postrema, subfornical organ, and organum vasculosum laminae terminalis (OVLT) [139,140].

Peripheral role of angiotensin II

Studies in isolated perfused rat kidney have suggested that intrarenal generation of angiotensin II facilitates renal venous outflow of norepinephrine during renal nerve stimulation [141]. Subsequent in vivo studies in rats by Handa & Johns [142] confirm this hypothesis by showing an attenuated antinatriuretic and antidiuretic response to low-frequency renal nerve stimulation following angiotensin-converting enzyme inhibition in rats. Further studies show that the degree of reduction of the antinatriuretic and antidiuretic responses to electrical or reflex renal nerve stimulation following angiotensin-converting enzyme inhibition is dependent on the prevailing level of renin—angiotensin system activity which was manipulated by changes in dietary sodium content [143,144]. However, several studies [145] have failed to report a physiologic role for the facilitatory effect of angiotensin II on neural release of norepinephrine. It was reported that urinary sodium excretion was similar in the denervated and contralateral innervated kidney in conscious dogs on low-sodium diet during control and angiotensin-converting enzyme inhibition plus angiotensin II infusion. Although these findings strongly argue against a role for the renal nerves in the sodium-retaining effects of angiotensin II during sodium restriction, the similar urinary sodium excretion from innervated and denervated kidneys during control may suggest that basal renal nerve activity was not increased to levels comparable to those during low-frequency renal nerve stimulation (0.5—1 Hz) [70].

Central role of angiotensin II

Since angiotensin II does not cross the blood—brain barrier the focus of many studies concerning the role of angiotensin II in blood pressure regulation has been the area postrema. Bilateral ablation or local cooling of the area postrema abolishes the pressor response to infusion of angiotensin II into the vertebral arteries [140]. The pressor response is mediated by increased central sympathetic vasoconstrictor outflow as demonstrated by the abolition of the response by either sympathetic blockade or spinal cord transection [146]. Evidence that area postrema participates in the regulation of blood pressure derives from studies in dogs, showing that electrical stimulation of area postrema increases blood pressure due to augmented sympathetic activity, and lesioning the area results in mild hypotension [147]. More recent studies [148] show similar hypotensive effects in rats following lesioning of area postrema.

The main stimulatory effects of blood-borne angiotensin II upon forebrain regions, such as the subfornical organ and/or the OVLT are to elicit thirst and cause the release of pituitary hormones.

Thus, changes in the blood concentration of angiotensin II may assume a powerful role in exerting both short-term (sympathoneuronal, via effects on area postrema) and long-term (hormonal, via effect on subfornical organ and OVLT) effects upon blood pressure regulatory mechanisms.

Hypertension

There is now considerable evidence to support the view that neurons of the ventrolateral medulla play a critical role in controlling blood pressure [139]. The C1-epinephrine-containing neurons of rostral ventrolateral medulla, projecting to the spinal cord, provide tonic excitatory vasomotor background. Lesioning the C1-area will lower blood pressure and stimulation of the area will increase blood pressure. A1-neurons do not project to the spinal cord but to other sites of the brain, e.g., the magnocellular portions of the paraventricular and supraoptic nuclei. A1-neurons also innervate C1-neurons. Excitation of the A1-neurons decreases blood pressure and lesioning of the A1-area increases blood pressure. The C1-neurons are inhibited by noradrenergic neurons of the A1-group. The action of the baroreceptors in inhibiting sympathetic outflow is mediated through projections into the C1-area. Reis *et al.* [139] have suggested that hypertension is the result of an increased sympathetic discharge due to an imbalance between the C1- and A1-neurons. Of interest in this context is the substantial evidence showing that the ventrolateral medulla surrounding the C1-neurons

is the site of action of α2-adrenoceptors agonists (e.g., clonidine) that act centrally to lower blood pressure.

Hypertension and renal nerves

Studies by Koepke [149] have shown the role of central α- and β-adrenoceptors in the enhanced renal response to environmental stress in spontaneous hypertensive rats (SHR). Administration of a β2-adrenoceptor antagonist into posterior hypothalamus or an α2-adrenoceptor agonist into the central amygdaloid nucleus prevents the increase in renal nerve activity and the decrease in urinary sodium excretion produced by acute environmental stress, which in turn is produced by an air jet stream directed to the rat's head. Similar air jet stress has no effect in normotensive Wistar Kyoto rats (WKY). Increased sympathetic activity and especially enhanced renal sympathetic nerve activity have been observed in SHR [150]. Renal denervation delays the onset of hypertension in SHR. The delay in the development of hypertension is associated with a greater percentage of ingested sodium excreted by renal denervated rats. Taken together these findings suggest that the efferent renal sympathetic nerves contribute to the development of hypertension in SHR.

In another model of hypertension, the one-kidney one-clip and two-kidney one-clip hypertensive rat, the afferent renal nerves from the clipped kidney contribute to the hypertension. The kidney is a sensory organ with sensory receptors which are sensitive to increases in intrarenal pressure and to changes in the chemical environment in the renal interstitium [151]. Studies by Katholi *et al.* [152] have suggested that the enhanced blood pressure in the Goldblatt hypertensive rat is related to increased renal levels of adenosine in the clipped kidney, activating renal sensory receptors. In support of this hypothesis are the studies showing that the fall in blood pressure following renal denervation is associated with a fall in plasma norepinephrine concentration and a decrease in hypothalamic norepinephrine content [153]. Furthermore, in contrast to SHR in which afferent renal denervation is without effect on the development of hypertension [154], afferent renal denervation in one-clip one-kidney hypertensive rats attenuates the development of hypertension [155].

Central and peripheral neuromechanisms regulating renal function and arterial pressure in the aged

Blood pressure tends to increase with age as has been noted in many socioeconomic groups from industrialized nations [156,157]. The age-related rate of rise of blood pressure in these large population samples does not differ greatly from population to population [156,157]. Less acculturated societies often show no appreciable blood pressure rise with age [156–161], until they come into contact with western culture, when they tend to display blood pressures similar to those noted in western societies. Differences in the slope of blood pressure changes with age appear to be strongly related to cultural influences [156]. The nature of the cultural influences or interaction of these influences in relationship to the age-related increase in blood pressure has not been identified, although major factors probably include dietary changes as well as factors related to the sympathetic nervous system, particularly with regard to stress and occupational hazards. The regression slope for blood pressure vs. dietary Na/K (by recall) increases with age, at least in the United States [162]. Whether "salt sensitivity" is a function of age, however, is not clear at this time [163,164]. To some degree the rate of increase in blood pressure is related to initial blood pressure level as shown by Svardsudd & Tibblin [165] as well as Rabkin et al. [166], who noted a similar positive correlation between initial blood pressure and rate of rise which was greater for systolic than for diastolic pressures, particularly in older age groups. Recently, however, a relatively small but age-, sex-, and race-matched 20-year study by Timio et al. in secluded nuns, compared to control lay women, suggested that living in a "stress-free" monastic environment prevented the age-related rise in systolic and diastolic blood pressures noted in controls [167]. Blood pressures, body habits, and diet were all similar between groups at the beginning of the study, and both weight and body mass index increased to a similar degree in both groups of subjects [167]. Dietary sodium also remained equal in the two groups. This data suggests that factors associated with the stress of an industrial society, beyond simple dietary and age factors may be significant in age-related blood pressure increase.

Effects of aging process on neural control of renal function

There is little anatomic or functional data available concerning the sympathetic nervous system as it relates to renal function in aging humans, or in animals. A number of changes in renal morphology occur with age such as loss of renal mass [168–170], development of nephron obsolescence [168,169,171], loss of glomeruli [168–173], changes in cortical tubular and glomerular basement membranes [171,174,175], mean proximal tubular length [176], development of distal tubular diverticuli in the region of the macula densa [176], development of aglomerular arterioles [174] and arteriographic changes in the renal vasculature [174,177] suggesting that parallel changes in renal innervation or renal nerve activity might be expected. However, studies of this nature have not been reported. Little work is available in animals, although Ljungqvist & Ungerstedt [178] report normal adrenergic innervation patterns in nonstenosed kidneys in rats in which two-kidney one-clip renal artery clip (Goldblatt) hypertension had been present for 2–11 months [178]. Galbusera et al. [179] found that while the total β-adrenoceptor number in the aging kidney were normal, the number of β2-adrenoceptors were reduced, as were the high affinity α1-adrenoceptors [179]. The number of α-adrenoceptors was slightly decreased and dopamine-1 receptors were significantly reduced in older rats [179]. These receptor studies were not accompanied by functional studies. We have noted little change in response to renal sensory receptor stimulation when young SHR (5–6 weeks) were compared to older SHR (14–15 weeks, treated with Captopril) [180], nor were changes noted in similarly treated WKY rats [180].

Functional evidence of renal nerve activity in aging adults is also difficult to obtain although indirectly, changes in functional activity may be inferred. Functional studies as a rule suffer from the unavailability of parallel microscopic data which might contribute to the understanding of the relationship of potential morphologic changes in the renal nerves which might occur with aging to the functional defects noted.

Glomerular filtration rate

In rats receiving an ad lib diet, GFR (C_{inulin}) decreased significantly with age (30 months) [181,182], but para-aminohippurate (PAH) clearance and filtration factor (FF) did not change significantly [181]. Sodium, potassium, calcium, and magnesium excretion reportedly tend to fall over time [182]. Lewis & Alving [183] and later Davies & Shock [184] using inulin clearances determined that GFR in humans declined between the ages of 40 and 80. The decline in GFR averaged approximately 0.75−1 ml/min per year of age. Wesson has suggested that there is an accelerated decrease in GFR with increasing age which is also more rapid in males [185]. These studies were cross-sectional, however, and in 1976 Rowe *et al.* reported an analysis of 10-year longitudinal determinations of renal function utilizing true creatinine clearances [186]. True creatinine clearances obtained at 12−18 month intervals on 884 community-dwelling volunteers in Baltimore were evaluated. An accelerating decline in creatinine clearance with increasing age similar to that observed in cross-sectional studies was noted [186]. Mean creatinine clearance fell from 140 ml/min per 1.73 m^2 at age 25−34 years to 97 ml/min per 1.73 m^2 at age 75−84 years. Serum creatinine concentrations rose slightly. The proportionate decrease in creatinine production, indicated by a modest increase in serum creatinine concentration in the face of declining creatinine clearance, probably reflects the decrease in lean body muscle mass that occurs with age. Most recently Lindeman *et al.* reanalyzed these data and showed that the decrease in creatinine clearance was not uniform in the group and that there were subjects at even older ages who had no decrease in their creatinine clearances studied serially over intervals of 5−7½ years [187,188]. In his study the average decline of creatinine clearance was approximately 0.75 ml/min per year; however, in subjects free of renal and urinary tract disease and untreated with diuretics or antihypertensives, the slopes of the creatinine clearance vs. time were normally distributed. One-third of all subjects had no decrease in creatinine clearance.

Renal blood flow, renal plasma flow, and filtration fraction
Renal blood flow estimated by PAH clearances decreases with age [184,187,188]. Miller *et al.* in 1961 showed that the extraction ratios of arterial PAH were approximately 92% and were not influenced by age [189]. However, as Davies & Shock have demonstrated, the PAH clearance in humans falls from a mean of 649 ml/min during the fourth decade to a mean of 289 ml/min in the ninth decade [184]. This decrease was proportionately slightly greater than the decrease in inulin clearance with age

resulting in an increase in FF from 0.19 to 0.25 over the age range studied. Similar increases have been confirmed by others [185,190]. Since glomeruli become obsolescent initially in the corticomedullary junction of the kidney, one might anticipate that GFR would decrease as rapidly or more rapidly than renal plasma flow. Indeed the age-related decrease in RBF in the presence of normal blood pressures suggests either vascular obliteration due to increasing blood vessel wall thickness, other intraluminal pathology, or progressive renal vasoconstriction [168,177].

Recalculation of the data of Davies & Shock suggests that renal vascular resistance also rises with age so that renal vascular resistance in the 80−89-year age group appeared to be substantially higher (more than double) that in the age group of 20−40 [184]. Although none of the subjects had primary hypertension a number of the individuals studied had other diseases which may have altered renal−neural or other hormonal functions. The study of McDonald *et al.* is of interest in this regard since they determined that the renal vasodilation in response to pyrogen administration appeared to be greater in older subjects (70−85 years) than in younger subjects suggesting the existence in older subjects of a greater functional resting renal vasoconstriction [190]. Administration of pyrogen to aminopyrine-treated patients did not alter GFR but produced marked increases in renal plasma flow with the disappearance of the age-related differences in FF [190].

Peripheral vascular resistance in the resting state generally increases with aging [191,192]. Cardiac output generally remains stable or decreases slightly with age. Landowne & Stanley [193] as well as Bender [194] have shown that the fraction of total cardiac output received by the kidney decreases with age. This coupled with the data on resting FF and renal vascular resistance, and the changes in these measurements that occur with pyrogen administration, suggest that the relatively decreased RBF and increase in renal resistance of aging are functional alterations rather than fixed anatomic changes.

Renal nerves and the reflex control of the systemic and renal vascular beds appear to be important factors in control of RBF and vascular resistance [70]. The evidence in aging individuals therefore may suggest either enhanced renal nerve activity with age similar to that noted for muscle sympathetic nerve activity [195] or a greater response of the renal vascular bed to change in renal nerve activity, or a combination of functional and anatomic factors.

Hollenberg et al. [177] using xenon washout techniques found that there was a selective decrease in renal cortical perfusion associated with aging and that acetylcholine administration resulted in increased RBF which was greater in younger subjects as compared to older subjects. In contrast the vasoconstrictor response to angiotensin II was similar in both age groups. This indirectly suggests that in contrast to the data cited above, the renal vasculature in the basal state in the older patient is relatively more vasodilated as compared to that in younger subjects. In this study the rapid or cortical component of RBF decreased more rapidly than mean RBF suggesting that cortical nephrons were more affected by age than the juxtamedullary nephrons [177]. Since juxtamedullary nephrons have a higher FF than do cortical nephrons, perhaps the selective loss of cortical nephrons explains the increase in FF observed with age. Alternatively, the increased FF observed with age could be caused by disproportionately greater vasoconstriction in the efferent arteriole as opposed to afferent arteriole in older subjects.

Hollenberg et al. also demonstrated that increases of sodium intake increased RBF in young individuals whereas in older subjects RBF was relatively unaltered by variations in sodium intake [177]. Since the renal effects of a sodium load are probably mediated by a number of factors including volume receptors, atrial natriuretic hormone, adrenergic receptors, central nervous system mechanisms, as well as local factors such as renin, angiotensin, and prostaglandins, the changes reported in this study may be a result of loss of integrative function rather than an alteration in renal nerve activity. Luft et al. [196] have reported an age-related decrease in the ability to excrete a sodium load, possibly because of age-related alterations in sympathetic activity such as the relation between norepinephrine and dopamine [164,196], or perhaps because of inability to increase RBF in an appropriate fashion following a sodium load [177].

Both GFR and RBF, as well as sodium excretion, are strikingly influenced by renal nerve activity in animals [82,85,197]. The diminished ability of the aging kidney to conserve sodium in response to sodium deprivation as shown by Epstein & Hollenberg suggests that the direct tubular effect of enhanced renal nerve activity which should theoretically occur with sodium deprivation may be diminished in the aging humans [198]. On the other hand Mizelle et al. recently demonstrated that compensatory adaptation to sodium deprivation can occur in the denervated canine kidney [199]. In addition the attenuation in renin and aldosterone response to sodium deprivation known to occur with age may also contribute to abnormal sodium conservation [200]. The elderly also exhibit defects in sodium excretion after a water or saline load reflected by a tendency to exaggerated natriuresis in these circumstances [168]. Maximum concentrating ability of the kidney, and maximum diluting ability also diminish with age [168]. This may, however, be a function of age-related changes in renal mass and filtration units since C_{H_2O} adjusted for GFR is similar in middle-aged and older subjects [168].

The head-out water immersion (HOI) studies of Tajima et al. [201] demonstrated that HOI produced an earlier and greater natriuresis and diuresis in older subjects, compared to younger individuals, as well as a blood pressure increase in older patients. Basal plasma atrial natriuretic factor was higher in the elderly, as has been reported by others [202], but no measurements of catecholamines were reported. While the natriuresis might have been related to the increased blood pressure, the lack of fall in blood pressure with diuresis might suggest an inability to appropriately suppress sympathetic activity and catecholamine levels in these subjects when volume is expanded [203–205]. Studies by Sowers & Mohanty, however, suggest that cardiopulmonary baroreflex control of vascular resistance is comparable in elderly and middle-aged men [192], even though circulating catecholamine levels are generally higher in older individuals [206–208].

The apparent conflicts between the older studies of McDonald, Solomon, Davies, Shock, and their colleagues, and the newer studies by Hollenberg and his coinvestigators may be partially explained by subject selection as well as by the techniques used in the studies presented. Shock et al. studied a wide range of elderly subjects and utilized conventional clearance techniques and a systemic vasodilator (pyrogen) in their studies. These studies may have been influenced by other factors such as pyrogen-induced changes in PAH extraction, or by other pyrogen-induced central or peripheral reflex changes, hormonal factors, etc. The studies of Hollenberg et al. included a narrower group of subjects in that these were all potential kidney donors. In addition, intrarenal artery injection of drugs was used which should reduce systemic effects, but their study techniques did not allow studies of clearance so that changes in GFR and/or FF could be evaluated. In addition, the marked heterogenous nature of the changes in renal function that occur with aging and the relatively small number of subjects used in these studies, suggests that further studies should be performed. In particular, studies of renal nerve activity, morphology, and function in aging animals would be of benefit. In addition, further studies of age-related functional changes in association with maneuvers designed to stimulate neural activity in humans would be of benefit. Certainly, known age-related changes in renal function in both animals and humans still leave open the question of the influence of the renal nerves in the renal effects of the aging process.

Renin—angiotensin system

The effects of aging on renin release supports the concept that diminished activity of renal sympathetic neural control may occur in individuals as they age, although at present, changes in renal nerve activity probably cannot be separated from anatomic changes occurring in the juxtaglomerular apparatus. A number of studies including the study of Weidmann et al. have demonstrated that plasma renin activity, serum renin concentration, and aldosterone concentrations tend to decrease with age [200,209—213]. Weidmann et al. showed that both upright posture and sodium depletion consistently cause significant increases in circulating renin and aldosterone in both young and old individuals. However, the mean renin levels achieved in response to these stimuli were almost always significantly less in older individuals than in younger individuals. Since plasma norepinephrine levels are generally higher than "normal" in older subjects [206—208], and epinephrine levels are usually not changed by age [208,214], the relative blunting of renin release in the older age group, in response to posture and changes in intravascular volume, suggest some decrease in end-organ responsiveness to normal renal nerve activity, diminution of adrenoceptor number or affinity as suggested by Galbusera et al. [179], or diminished formation or release of renin by the juxtaglomerular apparatus itself. Of interest is the study by Aoi & Weinberger [215] who showed that basal renin release decreased with increasing age in the SHR and Sprague—Dawley rat. The ability of kidney slices from SHR to demonstrate increased renin release in response to in-

cubation with norepinephrine was not however, impaired by age. In addition, in parallel experiments in WKY rats, basal renin release was unimpaired by age and norepinephrine-induced renin release was also not impaired by age [215]. These data suggest that in some species of aging rats, formation of renin may be decreased, while mechanisms for release of renin from the juxtaglomerular apparatus mediated by catecholamines remain relatively intact.

Some of the apparent decreases in plasma renin activity might be accounted for by a relative excess of less active high-molecular-weight renin as found in aging stroke-prone SHR [216]. Other components of the renin—substrate reaction appear to be unchanged by age [209]. The question of whether circulating angiotensin II levels may be altered by age has not been well studied, although angiotensin I and II levels are normal in aged normal subjects [217,218]. This is inconsistent, however, with what is generally known about renin in the aged. However, circulating and tissue levels of angiotensin II are likely to be important in both the control of blood pressure and possibly age-related changes in renal excretion of sodium [219,220]. If, as reported, sensitivity to angiotensin II may be increased with age [219], renal nerve activity might well influence GFR and sodium excretion in aging subjects both directly and indirectly through angiotensin II.

Catecholamines

It is difficult to determine either directly or indirectly the activity of renal nerves in aging adults; however, the data of Annat et al. suggesting that plasma levels of dopamine β-hydroxylase activity, an index of sympathetic nervous activity, were normal in both hypertensive and normotensive aging adults, are of interest [221]. Most studies have found that plasma norepinephrine level increases with aging in both normals and hypertensive [206—208]. Whether the increased plasma norepinephrine levels are related to increased production or increased release as suggested by Young et al. [222], decreased renal excretion, failure of receptors to bind norepinephrine, or failure to take up circulating norepinephrine is not clear, although all of these may be a factor. In addition, hypertension itself may alter age-related increases in circulating norepinephrine since Sowers & Mohanty have reported resting norepinephrine levels to be the same in younger (<55 years) and older (>55 years) hypertensives [192].

Esler *et al.* [223] have also reported higher than normal renal norepinephrine spillover but normal plasma norepinephrine levels in young hypertensives (<40 years) compared to normal subjects. In the over 60 age groups no difference was observed in plasma norepinephrine concentration when normals and hypertensives were compared, nor was renal norepinephrine spillover or clearance different [223,224]. Renal norepinephrine spillover was similar in old normals and hypertensives to younger normals as well [223]. These investigators attribute the increased plasma norepinephrine to a fall in norepinephrine clearance with increasing age in both normals and hypertensives, possibly related to a decrease in cardiac output. Esler *et al.*, using norepinephrine isotope dilution techniques, have determined in younger patients with essential hypertension that the greatest increase in norepinephrine spillover, and consequently selective activation of the sympathetic nervous system, appears to occur in the cardiac, and especially the renal beds [223,224]. Linares *et al.* [225] have suggested that both basal and stimulated plasma norepinephrine levels, stimulated by Na^+ deprivation, are higher in older subjects due at least in part to decreased removal of norepinephrine, as well as an age-related increase in norepinephrine release. Peroneal muscle sympathetic nerve activity was increased both in aging normals and hypertensives, circulating norepinephrine levels were much the same [195] in older subjects and only somewhat and insignificantly higher than in younger individuals.

Elliott *et al.* [226] studied the effect of age on systemic peripheral vascular α-adrenoceptor responsiveness in humans by administering the α-adrenoceptor antagonist prazosin and the α1-adrenoceptor agonist phenylephrine to young (22–32 years) and older individuals (66–78 years) [226]. While earlier studies by Amann *et al.* [227] appeared to suggest increased α-adrenoceptor responsiveness with aging, the finding by Elliott *et al.* that the blood pressure response to phenylephrine appeared attenuated in the aging individuals did not support enhanced α-adrenoceptor sensitivity in this group of individuals; however, it does not rule out reduced responsiveness to α-adrenoceptor agonist activity.

Feldman *et al.*, as well as other investigators, have found that the elderly have reduced β-adrenergic sensitivity to agonists, perhaps due to differences in receptor affinity [228–232]. These studies deal with β-adrenoceptors in nonrenal beds in humans. As noted above, the number of renal β-adrenoceptors is not altered in aging rat kidney, although the number of β-adrenoceptors in other tissues, including central nervous system tissue, are altered by age in SHR, WKY, and standard laboratory rats [233,234]. On the other hand, renin release in response to adrenalin injections was reported to be increased in men over 60 years [235].

Renal nerve activity in the aging may be altered by many nonrenal factors such as altered sympathetic function in other vascular beds, and neurogenic control mechanisms. In addition, extrapolating renal neural activity based on evidence obtained from other regional beds (arm, leg, etc.) is probably hazardous since there is accumulating evidence that regional vascular beds may respond differently to the same stimuli. This has been shown in the forearm and calf [236, 237], both for posture and stress. In addition, the data of Lawton *et al.* [203,204] in young borderline hypertensives suggest that there may also be differences in the neural response of the renal and calf vascular beds [203,204].

An additional factor may be the finding of age-related increased nerve terminal arborization in actively used muscle from mouse, rat, and humans [238]. Morphologic changes in nerves with aging is quite variable, which may well account in part for reported changes in catecholamine level and metabolism.

The effect of age on baroreflex activity and of the neurogenic control mechanisms

Studies in which lower body negative pressure (LBNP) was utilized to study reflex sympathetic responses in groups of older and younger subjects appeared to show that LBNP resulted in heightened total peripheral vascular resistance and forearm vascular resistance in older subjects [192,239]. Sowers & Mohanty report higher but proportionate increases of plasma norepinephrine concentration in response to LBNP, when older hypertensives were compared to younger hypertensives [192]. They also report greater responses in stimulated circulating norepinephrine, as well as in basal norepinephrine levels in older subjects (>55 years) as compared to younger individuals. The baroreflex activity of older hypertensive individuals was somewhat less than that of younger hypertensive subjects and greatly less than that of younger normotensive individuals. In addition, older hypertensive subjects showed a greater fall in systolic blood pressure in response to tilt and a greater rise in systolic blood pressure during dynamic exercise than young individuals [239]. The preponderance of evidence in humans, therefore, suggests that there is some impairment in baroreflex control of blood pressure and heart rate with age as well as in hypertension. Although there are no direct data, it seems likely that these abnormalities also would influence the neural control of renal circulation in humans. Since most, if not all, studies of renal function with clearance techniques have been done with subjects supine, the role that altered baroreflexes and renal nerves might play in the renal abnormalities noted above, has not been elucidated.

Clinical conditions

Although a number of changes in renal function occur with aging which may alter sodium balance, renin secretion, norepinephrine metabolism, and blood pressure, there is little experimental data at present to tie these changes to alterations in renal neural activity. The orthostatic hypotension which occurs in some older individuals certainly could be augmented by defects in postural-induced renin release secondary to loss of renal nerve activity, as in the patients reported by Bozovic et al. [240]. In one of the two patients over 70 years reported by this group, renin did increase subsequent to infusions of norepinephrine suggesting intact mechanisms for formation and release of renin, and supporting a lack of renal neural influence. Love et al. reported that the renin response to standing was probably primarily a function of the efferent autonomic system since afferent denervation did not influence renin release in two patients with Holmes—Adie syndrome [241]. This group of investigators suggest that renin release in these patients may also contribute to supine hypertension [241], sometimes noted with orthostatic hypotension. The lack of orthostatic-induced renin release and the inability of aged patients with orthostatic hypotension to maintain sodium balance may not be a function of age so much as a defect in sympathetic function, which also occurs in younger patients with orthostatic hypotension [242,243]. Certainly, substantial additional investigation is needed to sort out whether age-related deficits in postural blood pressure control are indeed due to age or are manifestations of other neurologic disease. To date, little has been done in this area.

A number of other clinical states sometimes associated with aging, such as sleep apnea syndrome and alterations in central nervous system function such as occur with stroke, central nervous system trauma, etc., are also associated with abnormalities in the renin—angiotensin system and catecholamine release. Whether alterations in renal nerve activity and renal function are also involved in these disorders is not known, but seems to be a reasonable probability.

Summary

There is substantial evidence in humans and animals for a role of the renal nerves in the control of renal function and, in all likelihood, blood pressure. Few studies are available to directly address the question of whether the aging process alters renal nerve activity. Indirect functional evidence certainly does not exclude aging as an influence on normal renal nerve activity control of certain aspects of renal function.

Acknowledgments

The work from the authors' laboratories was supported by NIH Grants DK 15843, HL 35163, HL 40222 and HL 14388, American Heart Association Grant-in-Aid 86063 and research grants from the Veterans Administration and the American Heart Association—Iowa Affiliate. The literature search was concluded November 1989.

References

1 Barajas L. Innervation of the renal cortex. Fed Proc 1978;37: 1192—1201.
2 Barajas L, Wang P, Powers KV, et al. Identification of renal neuroeffector junctions by electron microscopy of reembedded light microscopic autoradiograms of semithin sections. J Ultrastruct Mol Struct Res 1981;77:379—385.
3 Barajas L, Wang P. Localization of tritiated norepinephrine in the renal arteriolar nerves. Anat Res 1979;195:525—534.
4 Barajas L, Powers K, Wang P. Innervation of the renal cortical tubules: a quantitative study. Am J Physiol 1984; 247:F50—F60.
5 Barajas L, Powers KV. Innervation of the thick ascending limb of Henle. Am J Physiol 1988;255:F340—F346.
6 DiBona GF. Neurogenic regulation of renal tubular sodium reabsorption. Am J Physiol 1977;223:F73—F81.
7 Zimmerman HD. Electronenmikroskopische Befunde zur Innervation des Nephron nach Untersuchungen an der fetalen Nachniere des Menschen. Z Zellforschung 1972; 129:65—75.

8 Pang PKT, Uchiyama M, Sawyer WH. Endocrine and neural control of amphibian renal functions. Fed Proc 1972;41: 2365—2370.

9 Bell C, Lang WJ, Laska F. Dopamine-containing vasomotor nerves in the dog kidney. J Neurochem 1978;31:77—83.

10 Dienerstein RJ, Vannice J, Henderson RC, et al. Histo-fluorescence techniques provide evidence for dopamine-containing neuronal elements in canine kidney. Science 1979;204:497—499.

11 Oliver JA, Pinto J, Sciacca RR, et al. Basal norepine-phrine overflow into the renal vein: effect of renal nerve stimulation. Am J Physiol 1980;239:F371—F377.

12 Kopp U, Bradley T, Hjemdahl P. Renal venous outflow and urinary excretion of norepinephrine, epinephrine and dopamine during graded renal nerve stimulation. Am J Physiol 1983;244:E52—E60.

13 Bradley T, Hjemdahl P. Further studies on renal nerve stimulation induced release of noradrenaline and dopamine from the canine kidney in situ. Acta Physiol Scand 1984; 122:369—379.

14 Bradley T, Hjemdahl P. Renal overflow of noradrenaline and dopamine to plasma during hindquarter compression and thoracic inferior vena cava obstruction in the dog. Acta Physiol Scand 1986;127:305—312.

15 Bradley T, Hjemdahl P, DiBona GF. Increased release of norepinephrine and dopamine from canine kidney during bilateral carotid occlusion. Am J Physiol 1987;252: F240—F245.

16 Stephenson JA, Summers RJ. Autographic evidence for a heterogenous distribution of α-1 adrenoceptors labelled by [^{3}H] prazosin in rat, dog and human kidney. J Auton Pharmacol 1986;6:109—116.

17 Healy DP, Münzel PA, Insel PA. Localization of β-1 and β-2 adrenergic receptors in the rat kidney by autoradiography. Circ Res 1985;57:278-284.

18 Summers RJ, Stephenson JA, Kuhar MJ. Localization of beta adrenoceptor subtypes in rat kidney by light microscopic autoradiography. J Pharmacol Exp Ther 1985;232:561—569.

19 Pettinger WA, Umemura S, Smyth DD. Renal α-2 adreno-ceptors and the adenylate cyclase—camp system: Bio-chemical and physiological interactions. Am J Physiol 1987; 252:F119—F208.

20 Tamaki T, Hura CE, Kunai RT Jr. Dopamine stimulates cAMP production in canine arterioles via DA-1 receptors. Am J Physiol 1989;256:H626—H629.

21 Alkadhi KA, Sabouni MH, Ansari AF, et al. Activation of DA$_1$ receptors by dopamine or fenoldopam increases cyclic AMP levels in the renal artery but not in the superior cervical ganglion of the rat. J Pharmacol Exp Ther 1986;238: 547—553.

22 Sabouni MH, Alkadhi KA, Lokhandwala MF. Effect of dopamine receptor activation on ganglionic transmission and cyclic AMP levels in stellate ganglia and renal arteries on the dog. J Pharmacol Exp Ther 1987;240:93—98.

23 McPherson GA, Summers RJ. Evidence from binding studies for β-1 adrenoceptors associated with glomeruli isolated from rat kidney. Life Sci 1983;33:87—94.

24 Lew R, Summers RJ. Autoradiographic localization of β-adrenoceptor subtypes in guinea-pig kidney. Br J Pharmacol 1985;85:341—348.

25 Engel G, Maurer R, Perrot K, et al. β-Adrenoceptor sub-types in sections of rat and guinea pig kidney. Naunyn-Schmiedeberg's Arch Pharmacol 1985;328:354—357.

26 Sundaresan PR, Fortin TL, Kelvie SL. α- and β-Adrenergic receptors in proximal tubules of rat kidney. Am J Physiol 1987;253:F848—F856.

27 Summers RJ. Renal alpha-adrenoceptors. Fed Proc 1984;43: 2917—2922.

28 Matsushima Y, Akabane S, Ito K. Characterization of α-1 and α-2 adrenoceptors directly associated with basolateral membranes from rat kidney proximal tubules. Biochem Pharmacol 1986;35:2593—2600.

29 Umemura S, Marver D, Smyth DD, et al. α-2 Adrenoceptors and cellular cAMP levels in single nephron segments from the rat. Am J Physiol 1985;249:F28—F33.

30 Kusano E, Nakamura R, Asano Y, et al. Distribution of alpha-adrenergic receptors in the rabbit nephron. Tohoku J Exp Med 1984;142:275—284.

31 Murayama N, Ruggles BT, Gapstur S, et al. Evidence for beta adrenoceptors in proximal tubules. J Clin Invest 1985; 76:474—481.

32 Felder RA, Blecher M, Calcagno PL, et al. Dopamine receptors in the proximal tubule of the rabbit. Am J Physiol 1984;247:F499—F505.

33 Hagege J, Richet G. Proximal tubule dopamine histofluo-resence in renal slices incubated with L-DOPA. Kidney Int 1875;27:3—8.

34 Aperia A, Bertorello A, Seri I. Dopamine causes inhibition of Na$^+$−K$^+$−ATPase activity in rat proximal convoluted tubule segments. Am J Physiol 1987;253:F39—F45.

35 Morel FA, Doucet A. Hormonal control of kidney functions at cell level. Pharmacol Rev 1986;66:377—468.

36 Chabardes D, Montegut M, Imbert-Teboul M, et al. In-hibition of α-2 adrenergic agonists on AVP-induced cAMP accumulation in isolated collecting tubules of the rat kidney. Mol Cell Endocrinol 1984;37:263—275.

37 Teitelbaum I, Strasheim A, Berl T. Adrenergic control of cAMP generation in rat inner medullary collecting tubule cells. Kidney Int 1989;35:647—653.

38 Edwards RM, Gellai M. Inhibition of vasopressin-stimulated cyclic AMP accumulation by alpha-2 adrenoceptor agonists in isolated papillary collecting ducts. J Exp Pharmacol Ther 1988;244:526—530.

39 Kopp U, Aurell M, Nilsson I-M, et al. The role of beta-1 adrenoceptors in the renin release response to graded renal sympathetic nerve stimulation. Pflugers Arch 1980;387: 107—113.

40 DiBona GF, Sawin LL. Effect of renal nerve stimulation on

NaCl and H_2O transport in Henle's loop of the rat. Am J Physiol 1982;243:F576—F580.

41 Osborn JL, Kinstetter DD. Effects of altered NaCl intake on renal hemodynamic and renin release responses to renal nerve stimulation. Am J Physiol 1987;253:F976—F981.

42 Hollenberg NK, Adams DF, Solomon H, *et al*. Renal vascular tone in essential and secondary hypertension. Medicine 1975;54:29—44.

43 Sadowski J, Kurkus J, Gellert R. Denervated and intact kidney responses to saline load in awake and anesthetized dogs. Am J Physiol 1979;237:F262—F267.

44 DiBona GF. Influence of renal sympathetic nerve activity on autoregulation of renal blood flow. In Persson AEG, Boberg U, eds. *The Juxtaglomerular Apparatus*, vol. 11. Amsterdam: Elsevier, 1988:367—372.

45 Pelayo JC, Ziegler MG, Jose PA, *et al*. Renal denervation in the rat: analysis of glomerular and proximal tubular function. Am J Physiol 1983;244:F70—F77.

46 Kon V, Yared A, Ichikawa I. Role of sympathetic nerves in mediating hypoperfusion of renal cortical microcirculation in experimental congestive heart failure and acute extracellular fluid volume depletion. J Clin Invest 1985;76:1913—1920.

47 Tucker BJ, Mundy CA, Blantz RC. Adrenergic and angiotensin II influences on renal vascular tone in chronic sodium depletion. Am J Physiol 1987;252:F811—F817.

48 Kon V, Ichikawa I. Effector loci for renal nerve control of cortical microcirculation. Am J Physiol 1983;245:F545—F553.

49 Kon V. Neural control of circulation. Miner Electrolyte Metab 1989;15:33—44.

50 Edwards RM. Segmental effects of norepinephrine and angiotensin II on isolated microvessels. Am J Physiol 1983;244:F526—F534.

51 Wilson SK. The effects of angiotensin II and norepinephrine on afferent arterioles in the rat. Kidney Int 1986;30:895—905.

52 Wolff DW, Gesek FA, Strandhoy JW. *In vivo* assessment of rat renal alpha adrenoceptors. J Pharmacol Exp Ther 1987;241:472—476.

53 Holdaas H, DiBona GF. On the existence of renal vasodilator nerves. Proc Soc Exp Biol Med 1984;176:426—433.

54 Horn PT, Kohli JD, Listinsky JJ, *et al*. Regional variation in the alpha-adrenergic receptors in the canine resistance vessels. Naunyn-Schmiedeberg's Arch Pharmacol 1982;318:166—172.

55 Wolff DW, Buckalew VM, Strandhoy JW. Renal α-1 and α-2 adrenoceptor mediated vasoconstriction in dogs: comparison of phenylephrine, clonidine, and guanabenz. J Cardiovasc Pharmacol 1984;6(Suppl. 5):S793—S798.

56 Hesse IFA, Johns EJ. An *in vivo* study of the α-adrenoceptor subtypes on the renal vasculature of the anesthetized rabbit. J Auton Pharmacol 1984;4:145—152.

57 Bell C. Dopaminergic nerves. Proc Int Congr Pharmacol 1984;9:231—244.

58 Bell C. Dopamine release from sympathetic nerve terminals. Prog Neurobiol 1988;30:193—208.

59 Goldberg LI, Weder AB. Connections between endogenous dopamine, dopamine receptors and sodium excretion: evidences and hypothesis. Recent Adv Clin Pharmacol 1980;3:144—166.

60 Lee MR. Dopamine and the kidney. Clin Sci 1982;62:439—448.

61 Kopp UC, DiBona GF. Catecholamines and neurosympathetic control of renal function. In Fischer JW, ed. *Kidney Hormones*, vol. III. London: Academic Press, 1986:621—660.

62 Bell C, Lang WJ. Neural dopaminergic vasodilator control in the kidney. Nature 1973;246:27—29.

63 Hom GJ, Jandhyala BS. Effects of cerebroventricular administration of ouabain on renal hemodynamics in anesthetized dogs: evidence for participation of renal dopaminergic vasodilator fibers. J Pharmacol Exp Ther 1984;230:275—283.

64 Edwards RM. Response of isolated renal arterioles to acetylcholine, dopamine, and bradykinin. Am J Physiol 1985;248:F183—F189.

65 Seri I, Aperia A. Contribution of dopamine$_2$ receptors to dopamine-induced increase in glomerular filtration rate. Am J Physiol 1988;254:F196—F201.

66 Rogenes PR, Gottschalk CW. Renal function in conscious rats with chronic unilateral renal denervation. Am J Physiol 1982;242:F140—F148.

67 Szalay L, Colindres RE, Jackson R, *et al*. Effects of chronic renal denervation in conscious restrained rats. Int Urol Nephrol 1986;18:3—18.

68 Bencsáth P, Kottra G, Takács L. Intratubular and peritubular capillary hydrostatic and oncotic pressures after chronic renal sympathectomy in the anesthetized rat. Pflugers Arch 1983;398:60—63.

69 Bencsáth P, Szenasi G, Takács L, *et al*. Renal nerves and sodium conservation in conscious rats. Am J Physiol 1985;248:F616—F619.

70 DiBona GF. The functions of the renal nerves. Rev Physiol Biochem Pharmacol 1982;94:75—181.

71 Bello-Reuss E, Trevino DL, Gottschalk CW. Effect of renal sympathetic nerve stimulation on proximal water and sodium reabsorption. J Clin Invest 1976;57:1104—1107.

72 Abildgaard U, Holstein-Rathlou N-H, Leyssac PP. Effect of renal nerve activity on tubular sodium and water reabsorption in dog kidneys as determined by the lithium clearance method. Acta Physiol Scand 1986;126:251—257.

73 Göransson A, Ulfendahl HR. Increase in proximal tubular fluid reabsorption by renal nerve stimulation. A split oil droplet study. Acta Physiol Scand 1988;133:455—458.

74 DiBona GF. Neural mechanisms in body fluid homeostasis. Fed Proc 1986;45:2871—2877.

75 Prosnitz EH, DiBona GF. Effect of decreased renal sympathetic nerve activity on renal tubular sodium reabsorp-

tion. Am J Physiol 1978;235:F557—F563.

76 Kopp UC, DiBona GF. The neural control of renal function. In Seldin DW, Giebisch G, eds. The Kidney: Physiology and Pathophysiology. New York: Raven Press, 1992:1157—1204.

77 Epstein M. Renal effects of head-out water immersion in man: Implications for an understanding of volume homeostasis. Physiol Rev 1978;58:529—581.

78 Gilmore JP. Neural control of extracellular volume in the humane and nonhuman primate. In Shepherd JT, Abboud FM, eds. Handbook of Physiology. The cardiovascular system. Peripheral Circulation and oxygen blood flow, Part 3 Bethesda: American Physiology Society, 1983:885—915.

79 Miki K, Hayashida Y, Sagawa S, et al. Renal sympathetic nerve activity and natriuresis during water immersion in conscious dogs. Am J Physiol 1989;256: R299—R305.

80 Zimmerman RS, Edwards BS, Schwab TR, et al. Cardiorenal-endocrine dynamics during and following volume expansion. Am J Physiol 1987;252:R336—R340.

81 Morita H, Vatner SF. Effects of volume expansion on renal nerve activity, renal blood flow, and sodium and water excretion in conscious dogs. Am J Physiol 1985;249: F680—F687.

82 DiBona GF, Sawin LL. Renal nerve activity in conscious rats during volume expansion and depletion. Am J Physiol 1985;248:F15—F23.

83 DiBona GF, Sawin LL. High NaCl diet reduces cardiac vagal afferent nerve response to volume expansion. Am J Physiol 1987;252:R687—R692.

84 McMurray JJ, Seidelin PH, Balfour DJK, et al. Physiologic increases in circulating noradrenaline are anti-natriuretic in man. J Hypertens 1988;6:757—761.

85 Osborn JL, Holdaas H, Thames MD, et al. Renal adrenoceptor mediation of antinatriuretic and renin secretion responses to low frequency renal nerve stimulation in the dog. Circ Res 1983;53:298—305.

86 Hesse IFA, Johns EJ. The subtype of alpha-adrenoceptor involved in the neural control of renal tubular sodium reabsorption in the rabbit. J Physiol 1984;352:527—538.

87 Johns EJ, Manitius J. An investigation into the alpha-adrenoceptor mediating renal nerve induced calcium reabsorption by the rat kidney. Br J Pharmacol 1986;89: 91—97.

88 DiBona GF, Sawin LL. Role of renal alpha-2 adrenoceptors in spontaneously hypertensive rats. Hypertension 1987;9: 41—48.

89 Smyth DD, Umemura S, Pettinger WA. Renal nerve stimulation causes α-1 adrenoceptor-mediated sodium retention but not α-2 adrenoceptor antagonism of vasopressin. Circ Res 1985;57:304—311.

90 Krothapalli RK, Suki WN. Functional characterization of the alpha adrenergic receptor modulating the hydroosmotic effect of vasopressin on the rabbit cortical collecting tubule. J Clin Invest 1984;73:740—749.

91 Stanton B, Puglisi E, Gellai M. Localization of α-2 adrenoceptor-mediated increase in renal Na^+, K^+, and water excretion. Am J Physiol 1987;252:F1016—F1021.

92 Gellai M, Edwards RM. Mechanism of α-2 adrenoceptor agonist-induced diuresis. Am J Physiol 1988;255: F317—F323.

93 Bradley T, Frederickson ED, Goldberg LI. Effect of DA-1 receptor blockade with SCH 23390 on the renal response to electrical stimulation of the renal nerves. Proc Soc Exp Biol Med 1986;181:492—497.

94 Jose PA, Felder RA, Holloway RR, et al. Dopamine receptors modulate sodium excretion in denervated kidney. Am J Physiol 1986;250:F1033—F1038.

95 Smit AJ. Renal effects of exogenous and endogenous dopamine. PhD Thesis, The Netherlands: University of Groningen, 1988:1—158.

96 Bennett ED, Tighe D, Wegg D. Abolition by dopamine blockade of the natriuretic response produced by lower body positive pressure. Clin Sci 1982;63:361—366.

97 Coruzzi P, Musiari L, Biggi A, et al. Dopamine blockade abolishes the exaggerated natriuresis of essential hypertension. J Hypertens 1987;5:587—591.

98 Bertorello A, Hökfelt T, Goldstein M, et al. Proximal tubule $Na^+ - K^+ - ATPase$ activity is inhibited during high-salt diet: Evidence for DA-mediated effect. Am J Physiol 1988;254:F795—F801.

99 Baumbach L, Skøtt O. Renin release from different parts of rat afferent arterioles in vitro. Am J Physiol 1986;251: F12—F16.

100 Davis JO, Freeman RH. Mechanisms regulating renin release. Physiol Rev 1976;56:1—56.

101 Keeton TK, Campbell WB. The pharmacologic alteration of renin release. Pharmacol Rev 1980;32:81—227.

102 Thames MD. Renin release: reflex control and adrenergic mechanisms. J Hypertens 1984;2(Suppl.):57—66.

103 Kopp UC. Interaction of sympathetic nerves with baroreceptor and macula densa receptor mechanisms for renin secretion. In Persson AEG, Boberg U, eds. The Juxtaglomerular Apparatus, vol. 11. Amsterdam: Elsevier, 1988: 221—227.

104 Osborn JL, Johns EJ. Renal neurogenic control of renin and prostaglandin release. J Miner Electrolyte Metab 1989;15: 51—58.

105 Brosnihan KB, Bravo EL. Graded reductions of atrial pressure and renin release. Am J Physiol 1978;235: H175—H181.

106 Beers ET, Carroll RG, Young DB, et al. Effects of graded changes in reflex renal nerve activity on renal function. Am J Physiol 1986;250:F559—F565.

107 Bishop VS, Hasser EM. Artrial and cardiopulmonary reflexes in the regulation of the neurohumoral drive to the circulation. Fed Proc 1985;44:2377—2381.

108 Grandjean B, Annat G, Vincent M, et al. Influence of renal nerves on renin secretion in the conscious dog.

Pflugers Arch 1978;373:161−165.

109 Holdaas H, DiBona GF. The role of left atrial receptors in the regulation of renin release in anesthetized dogs. Acta Physiol Scand 1981;111:497−500.

110 Thames MD, Jarecki M, Donald DE. Neural control of renin secretion in anesthetized dogs. Interaction of cardiopulmonary and carotid baroreceptors. Circ Res 1978;42:237−245.

111 Gross R, Kirchheim H. Effects of bilateral carotid occlusion and auditory stimulation on renal blood flow and sympathetic nerve activity in the conscious dog. Pflugers Arch 1980;383:233−239.

112 Gross R, Hackenburg HM, Hackenthal E, et al. Interaction between perfusion pressure and sympathetic nerves in renin release by carotid baroreflex in conscious dogs. J Physiol 1981;313:237−250.

113 Gross R, Kirchheim H, Ruffman K. Effect of carotid occlusion and of perfusion pressure on renal function in conscious dogs. Circ Res 1981;48:774−784.

114 Carroll RG, Lohmeier TE, Brown AJ. Disparity between renal venous norepinephrine and renin responses to sodium depletion. Am J Physiol 1988;254:F754−F761.

115 Welch WJ, Ott CE, Lorenz JN, et al. Control of renin release by dietary NaCl in the rat. Am J Physiol 1987;253:F1051−F1057.

116 Esler MD, Willett I, Leonard PO, et al. Plasma norepinephrine kinetics in humans. J Auton Nerv Sys 1984;11:125−144.

117 Watson RDS, Esler MD, Leonard PO, et al. Influence of variation in dietary sodium intake on biochemical indices of sympathetic activity in normal man. Clin Exp Pharmacol Physiol 1984;11:163−170.

118 Pitcock J, Hartroft PH, Newmark LN. Increased renal pressor activity (renin) in sodium deficient rats and correlation with juxtaglomerular cell granulation. Proc Soc Exp Biol Med 1959;100:868−869.

119 Barajas L. Anatomy of the juxtaglomerular apparatus. Am J Physiol 1979;237:F333−F343.

120 Osborn JL, DiBona GF, Thames MD. Beta-1 receptor mediation of renin secretion elicited by low-frequency renal nerve stimulation. J Pharmacol Exp Ther 1981;216:265−269.

121 Kopp UC, DiBona GF. Interaction of renal β-1 adrenoceptors and prostaglandins in reflex renin release. Am J Physiol 1983;244:F418−F424.

122 Johns EJ. An investigation into the type of β-adrenoceptor mediating the sympathetically activated renin release in the cat. Br J Pharmacol 1981;73:749−754.

123 Kopp U, Aurell M, Sjölander M, et al. The role of prostaglandins in the alpha- and beta-adrenoceptor mediated renin release response to graded renal nerve stimulation. Pflugers Arch 1981;391:1−8.

124 Osborn JL, DiBona GF, Thames MD. Role of renal α-adrenoceptors mediating renin secretion. Am J Physiol 1982;242:F620−F626.

125 Hisa H, Hayashi Y, Satoh S. Effects of blockade of alpha and beta adrenoceptors and dopamine receptors on renal nerve stimulation-induced prostaglandin E_2 and renin release in anesthetized dogs. J Pharmacol Exp Ther 1985;235:481−486.

126 Blair ML. Inhibition of renin secretion by intrarenal α-adrenoceptor blockade. Am J Physiol. 1981;240:E682−E688.

127 Blair ML, Chen YH, Izzo JL. Influence of renal perfusion pressure on α- and β-adrenergic stimulation of renin release. Am J Physiol 1985;248:E317−E326.

128 Pfister SL, Keeton TK. The mechanism of yohimbine-induced renin release in the conscious rat. Naunyn-Schmiedeberg's Arch Pharmacol 1988;337:35−46.

129 Osborn JL, Kopp UC, Thames MD, et al. Interactions among renal nerves, prostaglandins, and renal arterial pressure in the regulation of renin release. Am J Physiol 1984;247:F706−F713.

130 Freeman RH, Davis JO, Villarreal D. Role of renal prostaglandins in the control of renin release. Circ Res 1984;54:1−9.

131 Gibbons GH, Dzau VJ, Farhi ER, et al. Interaction of signals influencing renin release. Annu Rev Physiol 1984;46:291−308.

132 Stella A, Calaresu F, Zanchetti A. Neural factors contributing to renin release during reduction in renal perfusion pressure and blood flow in cats. Clin Sci Mol Med 1976;51:453−461.

133 Stella A, Zanchetti A. Effects of renal denervation on renin release in response to tilting and furosemide. Am J Physiol 1977;232:H500−H507.

134 Thames MD, DiBona GF. Renal nerves modulate the secretion of renin mediated by nonneural mechanisms. Circ Res 1979;44:645−652.

135 Kopp UC, DiBona GF. Interaction between neural and nonneural mechanisms controlling renin secretion rate. Am J Physiol 1984;246:F620−F626.

136 Kirchheim HR, Finke R, Hackenthal E, et al. Baroreflex sympathetic activation increases threshold pressure for the pressure-dependent renin release in conscious dogs. Plugers Arch 1985;405:127−135.

137 Porter JP. Stress can enhance the renin response to reduced renal perfusion pressure. Am J Physiol 1989;256:R554−R559.

138 Guazzi MD, Barbier P, Loaldi A, et al. Intrarenal beta-receptor and renal baroreceptor interaction in the control of the renin response to transient reduction of the renal perfusion pressure in man. J Hypertens 1985;3:39−45.

139 Reis DJ, Morrison S, Ruggiero DA. The C1 area of the brainstem in tonic and reflex control of blood pressure. Hypertension 1988;11(Suppl. 1):I8−I13.

140 Ferrario CM. Neurogenic actions of angiotensin II. Hypertension 1983;5(Suppl. 5):V73−V79.

141 Böke T, Malik KU. Enhancement by locally generated angiotensin II of release of the adrenergic transmitter in the isolated rat kidney. J Pharmacol Exp Ther 1983;226: 900–907.

142 Handa RK, Johns EJ. Interaction of the renin–angiotensin system and the renal nerves in the regulation of rat kidney function. J Physiol 1985;369:311–321.

143 Johns EJ. The role of angiotensin II in the antidiuresis and antinatriuresis induced by stimulation of the sympathetic nerves to the rat kidney. J Auton Pharmacol 1987;7: 205–214.

144 Handa RK, Johns EJ. The role of angiotensin II in the renal responses to somatic nerve stimulation in the rat. J Physiol 1987;393:425–436.

145 Mizelle HL, Hall JE, Woods LL. Interactions between angiotensin II and renal nerves during chronic sodium deprivation. Am J Physiol 1988;255:F823–F827.

146 Ferrario CM, Gidenberg PL, McCubbin JW. Cardiovascular effects of angiotensin mediated by the central nervous system. Circ Res 1972;30:257–262.

147 Ferrario CM, Barnes KL, Szilagyi JE, et al. Physiologic and pharmacologic characterization of the area postrema pressor pathways in the normal dog. Hypertension 1979;1: 235–245.

148 Skoog KM, Mangiapane ML. Area postrema and cardiovascular regulation in rats. Am J Physiol 1988;254: H963–H969.

149 Koepke JP. Effect of environmental stress on neural control of renal function. J Miner Electrolyte Metab 1989;15:83–87.

150 Katholi RE. Renal nerves and hypertension: An update. Fed Proc 1985;44:2846–2850.

151 Kopp UC. Renorenal reflexes: Neural and functional responses. Fed Proc 1985;44:2834–2839.

152 Katholi RE, Woods WT. Afferent renal nerves and hypertension. Clin Exp Hypertens 1987;A(Suppl. 1):211–226.

153 Winternitz SR, Oparil S. Importance of the renal nerves in the pathogenesis of experimental hypertension. Hypertension 1982;4(Suppl. 3):III108–III115.

154 Janssen BJA, van Essen H, Vervoort-Peters LHTM, et al. Role of afferent renal nerves in spontaneous hypertension in rats. Hypertension 1989;13:327–333.

155 Wyss JM, Aboukarsh A, Oparil S. Sensory denervation of the kidney attenuates renovascular hypertension in the rat. Am J Physiol 1986;250:H82–H86.

156 Pickering G. Arterial pressure in populations. In High Blood Pressure. New York: Grune & Stratton, 1968:203–228.

157 Epstein FH, Eckoff RD. The epidemiology of high blood pressure—geographic distributions and etiological factors. In Stamler J, Stamler R, Pullman T, eds. The Epidemiology of Hypertension. New York: Grune & Stratton, 1967: 155–166.

158 Takahaski E. Discussion (Lovell paper). In Stamler J, Stamler R, Pullman T, eds. The Epidemiology of Hypertension. New York: Grune & Stratton, 1967:133–138.

159 Shaper AG. Blood pressure studies in East Africa. In Stamler J, Stamler R, Pullman T, eds. The Epidemiology of Hypertension. New York: Grune & Stratton, 1967: 139–145.

160 White PD. Hypertension and atherosclerosis in the Congo and in the Gabon. In Stamler J, Stamler R, Pullman T, eds. The Epidemiology of Hypertension. New York: Grune & Stratton, 1967:150–154.

161 Lovell RRH. Race and blood pressure, with special reference to Oceania. In Stamler J, Stamler R, Pullman T, eds. The Epidemiology of Hypertension. New York: Grune & Stratton, 1967:122–129.

162 Khaw K-T, Barrett-Connor E. The association between blood pressure, age, and dietary sodium and potassium: a population study. Circulation 1988;77:53–61.

163 Umeda T, Iwaoka T, Miura F, et al. Is salt sensitivity in essential hypertension affected by ageing? J Hypertens 1988;6:S205–S208.

164 Zemel MB, Sowers JR. Salt sensitivity and systemic hypertension in the elderly. Am J Cardiol 1988;61:H7–H12.

165 Svardsudd K, Tibblin G. A longitudinal blood pressure study. Change of blood pressure during 10 years in relation to initial values. The study of men born in 1913. J Chron Dis 1980;33:627–636.

166 Rabkin SW, Mathewson MB, Tate RB. Relationship of blood pressure in 20–39 year old men to subsequent blood pressure and incidence of hypertension over a 30-year observation period. Circulation 1982;65:291–300.

167 Timio M, Verdecchia P, Venanzi S, et al. Age and blood pressure changes: a 20-year follow-up study in nuns in a secluded order. Hypertension 1988;12:457–461.

168 Lindeman RD, Goldman R. Anatomic and physiologic age changes in the kidney. Exp Gerontol 1986;21:379–406.

169 Brown WW, Davis BB, Spry LA, et al. Aging and the kidney. Arch Intern Med 1986;146:1790–1796.

170 Tauchi H, Tsuboi K, Okutomi J. Age changes in the human kidney of the different races. Gerontologia 1971;17:87–97.

171 Anderson S, Brenner BM. Effects of aging on the renal glomerulus. Am J Med 1986;80:435–442.

172 McLachlair MSF. The ageing kidney. Lancet 1978;11: 143–146.

173 Goyal VK. Changes with age in the human kidney. Exp Gerontol 1982;17:321–331.

174 Takazakura E, Sawabu N, Handa A, et al. Intrarenal vascular changes with age and disease. Kidney Int 1972;2:224–230.

175 Scott EB. Modification to the basal architecture of renal tubule cells in aged rats. Proc Soc Exp Biol Med 1964;117: 586–590.

176 Darmady EM, Offer J, Woodhouse MD. The parameters of the aging kidney. J Pathol 1973;109:195–207.

177 Hollenberg NK, Adams DF, Solomon HS, et al. Senescence and the renal vasculature in normal man. Circ Res 1974;34: 309–316.

178 Ljungqvist A, Ungerstedt U. Sympathetic innervation of the

juxtaglomerular cells of the kidney in rats with renal hypertension. Acta Pathol Microbiol Scand 1972;80:38–46.

179 Galbusera M, Garattini S, Remuzzi G, et al. Catecholamine receptor binding in rat kidney: effect of aging. Kidney Int 1988;33:1073–1077.

180 Kopp UC, Smith LA. Renorenal reflexes present in young and Captopril-treated adult spontaneously hypertensive rats. Hypertension 1989;13:430–439.

181 Gehreg JJ Jr, Jamison RL, Boylis C, et al. Effect of intermittent feeding on renal hemodynamics in conscious rats. Am J Physiol 1986;250:F566–F572.

182 Corman B, Pratz J, Poujeol P. Changes in anatomy, glomerular filtration, and solute excretion in aging rat kidney. Am J Physiol 1985;248:R282–R287.

183 Lewis WH Jr, Alving AS. Changes with age in the renal function in adult men. I. Clearance of urea. II. Amount of urea nitrogen in the blood. III. Concentrating ability of the kidneys. Am J Physiol 1938;123:500–515.

184 Davies DF, Shock NW. Age changes in glomerular filtration rate, effective renal plasma flow, and tubular excretory capacity in adult males. Age changes in renal function. J Clin Invest 1950;29:496–507.

185 Wesson LG Jr. Renal hemodynamics in physiological states. In Wesson LG Jr, ed. Physiology of the Human Kidney. New York: Grune & Stratton, 1969:98–100.

186 Rowe JWA, Andres R, Tobin JD, et al. The effect of age on creatinine clearance in men: A cross-sectional and longitudinal study. J Gerontol 1976;31:155–163.

187 Lindeman RD, Tobin JD, Shock NW. Association between blood pressure and the rate of decline in renal function with age. Kidney Int 1984;26:861–868.

188 Lindeman RD, Tobin JD, Shock NW. Longitudinal studies on the rate of decline in renal function with age. J Am Geriatr Soc 1985;33:278.

189 Miller JH, McDonald RK, Shock NW. The renal extraction of P-aminohippurate in the aged individual. J Gerontol 1961;6:213–216.

190 McDonald RK, Solomon DH, Shock NW. Aging as a factor in the renal hemodynamic changes induced by a standardized pyrogen. J Clin Invest 1951;5:457–462.

191 Ebert TJ, Hughes CV, Tristani FE, et al. Effect of age and coronary heart disease on the circulatory responses to graded lower body negative pressure. Cardiovasc Res 1982;16:663–669.

192 Sowers JR, Mohanty PK. Effect of advancing age on cardiopulmonary baroreceptor function in hypertensive men. Hypertension 1987;10:274–279.

193 Landowne M, Stanley J. Aging of the cardiovascular system. In Shock NW, ed. Aging—Some Social and Biological Aspects. New York: American Association for the Advancement of Science, 1960.

194 Bender AD. The effect of increasing age on the distribution of peripheral blood flow in man. J Am Geriat Soc 1965;13:192–198.

195 Yamada Y, Miyajima E, Tochikubo O, et al. Age-related changes in muscle sympathetic nerve activity in essential hypertension. Hypertension 1989;13:870–877.

196 Luft FC, Fineberg NS, Miller JZ, et al. The effects of age, race and heredity on glomerular filtration rate following volume expansion and contraction in normal man. Am J Med Sci 1980;279:15–24.

197 Beers ET, Carroll RG, Young DB, et al. Effects of graded changes in reflex renal nerve activity on renal function. Am J Physiol 1986;250:F559–F565.

198 Epstein M, Hollenberg NK. Age as a determinant of renal sodium conservation in normal man. J Lab Clin Med 1976;87:411–417.

199 Mizelle HL, Hall JE, Woods LL, et al. Role of renal nerves in compensatory adaptation to chronic reductions in sodium intake. Am J Physiol 1987;252:F291–F298.

200 Weidmann P, De Myttenaere-Bursztein S, Maxwell MH, et al. Effect of aging on plasma renin and aldosterone in normal man. Kidney Int 1975;8:325–333.

201 Tajima F, Sagawa S, Iwamoto J, et al. Renal and endocrine responses in the elderly during head-out water immersion. Am J Physiol 1988;254:R977–R983.

202 Ohashi M, Fujio N, Nawata H, et al. High plasma concentrations of human atrial natriuretic polypeptide in aged men. J Clin Endocrinol Metab 1987;64:81–85.

203 Lawton WJ, Sinkey CA, Fitz AE, et al. Dietary salt produces abnormal renal vasoconstrictor responses to upright posture in borderline hypertensive subjects. Hypertension 1988; 11:529–536.

204 Lawton WJ, Sinkey C, Floras J, et al. The effect of dietary sodium loading and restriction on microneurographic measurement of sympathetic nervous system activity and renal sodium handling. Clin Res 1985;33:A868.

205 Campese VM, Romoff MS, Levitan D, et al. Abnormal relationship between sodium intake and sympathetic nervous system activity in salt-sensitive patients with essential hypertension. Kidney Int 1982;21:371–378.

206 Lake CR, Ziegler MG, Coleman MD, et al. Age-adjusted plasma norepinephrine levels are similar in normotensive and hypertensive subjects. New Engl J Med 1977;296:208–209.

207 Esler M, Skews H, Leonard P, et al. Age-dependence of noradrenaline kinetics in normal subjects. Clin Sci 1981;60:217–219.

208 Linares OA, Halter JB. Sympathochromaffin system activity in the elderly. J Am Geriatr Soc 1987;35:448–453.

209 Crane MG, Harris JJ. Effect of aging on renin activity and aldosterone excretion. J Lab Clin Med 1976;87:947–959.

210 Skott P, Giese J. Age and the renin–angiotensin system. Acta Med Scand Suppl 1983;676:45–51.

211 Cleland JGF, Dargie HJ, Robertson JIS, et al. Renin and angiotensin responses to posture and exercise in elderly patients with heart failure. Eur Heart J 1984;5(Suppl. E):9–11.

212 Sequeira SJ, Loughlin T, Cunningham S, *et al.* Evaluation of an aldosterone radioimmunoassay: The renin−angiotensin−aldosterone axis as a function of sex and age. Ann Clin Biochem 1986;23:65−75.

213 Chebotarev DF, Korkushko OV, Asinova MI, *et al.* The state of the renin−angiotensin−aldosterone system in various clinical forms of hypertension in aging. Arch Gerontol Geriatr 1985;4:21−28.

214 Prinz PN, Halter JB, Benedette C, *et al.* Circadian variation in plasma catecholamines in young and old men: relationship to eye movement and slow wave sleep. J Clin Endocrinol Metab 1979;49:300.

215 Aoi W, Weinberger MH. The effect of age and norepinephrine on renin release by rat kidney slices *in vitro.* Proc Soc Exp Biol Med 1976;151:47−52.

216 Ikemoto F, Itoh S, Tanaka M, *et al.* Detection and possible mechanism of formation of renal high molecular weight renin in aged stroke-prone spontaneously hypertensive rats. J Hypertens 1986;4(Suppl. 3):S359−S360.

217 Ferris JB, Sullivan PA, Gonggrejp H, *et al.* Plasma angiotensin II and aldosterone in unselected diabetic patients. Clin Endocrinol 1982;17:261−269.

218 Skott P, Ingerslev J, Damkjaer M, *et al.* The renin−angiotensin−aldosterone system in normal 85-year-old people. Scand J Clin Lab Invest 1987;47:69−74.

219 Meier A, Gubelin U, Weidmann P, *et al.* Age-related profile of cardiovascular reactivity to norepinephrine and angiotensin II in normal and hypertensive man. Klin Wochenschr 1980;58:1183−1188.

220 Thomas D, Harris PJ, Morgan TO. Age-related changes in angiotensin II-stimulated proximal tubule fluid reabsorption in the spontaneously hypertensive rat. J Hypertens 1988;6(Suppl 4):S449−S451.

221 Annat G, Vincent A, Tourniaire A, *et al.* Relationships between blood pressure and plasma renin, aldosterone, and dopamine-b-hydroxylase in the elderly. Gerontology 1981; 27:266−270.

222 Young JB, Rowe JWA, Pallotta JA, *et al.* Enhanced plasma norepinephrine response to upright posture and oral glucose administration in elderly human subjects. Metabolism 1980;29:532−539.

223 Esler M, Jennings G, Korner P, *et al.* Assessment of human sympathetic nervous system activity from measurement of norepinephrine turnover. Hypertension 1988;11:3−20.

224 Esler M, Jennings G, Lambert G. Noradrenaline release and the pathophysiology of primary human hypertension. Am J Hypertens 1989;2:S140−S146.

225 Linares OA, Supiano MA, Marrow LA, *et al.* Norepinephrine (NE) release and metabolism in the elderly by compartmental analysis: Relation to dietary salt intake. Clin Res 1986;34:A950.

226 Elliott HL, Sumner DJ, McLean K, *et al.* Effect of age on vascular α-adrenoceptor responsiveness in man. Clin Sci 1982;63:S305−S308.

227 Amann FW, Bolli P, Kiowski W, *et al.* Enhanced α-adrenoceptor mediated vasoconstriction in essential hypertension. Hypertension 1981;3:I119−I123.

228 Feldman RD, Limbird LE, Nadeau J, *et al.* Alterations in leukocyte b-receptor affinity with aging. A potential explanation for altered b-adrenergic sensitivity in the elderly. New Engl J Med 1984;310:815−819.

229 Feldman RD. Physiologic and molecular correlates of age-related changes in the human β-adrenergic receptor system. Fed Proc 1986;45:48−50.

230 Van Brummelen P, Buhler FR, Kiowski W, *et al.* Age-related decrease in cardiac and peripheral vascular responsiveness to isoprenaline: Studies in normal subjects. Clin Sci 1981;60:571−577.

231 Vestal RE, Wood AJJ, Shand DG. Reduced β-adrenoceptor sensitivity in the elderly. Clin Pharmacol Ther 1979;26: 181−186.

232 Pan HYM, Hoffman BB, Peshe RA, *et al.* Decline in beta adrenergic receptor-mediated vascular relaxation with aging in man. J Pharmacol Exp Ther 1986;239:802−807.

233 Cimino M, Vantini G, Algeri S, *et al.* Age-related modification of dopaminergic and b-adrenergic receptor system: Restoration to normal activity by modifying fluidity with s-adenosylmethionine. Life Sci 1984;34:2029−2039.

234 Bucher B, Heitz C, Stoclet J-C. Age-related changes of *in vivo* β-adrenergic responsiveness in normotensive and spontaneously hypertensive rats. Eur J Pharmacol 1984; 102:31−37.

235 Korkushko OV, Asinova MI. The renin−angiotensin−aldosterone system and adaptation to stress in old age. Hum Physiol 1985;10:300−303.

236 Anderson EA, Wallin BG, Mark AL. Dissociation of sympathetic nerve activity in arm and leg muscle during mental stress. Hypertension 1987;9(Suppl. 3):III114−III119.

237 Duprez D, Essandoh LK, Shepherd JT. Postural cardiovascular reflexes involve forearm but not calf resistance vessels. J Hypertens 1987;5(Suppl. 5):S331−S332.

238 Smith DO. Cellular and molecular correlates of aging in the nervous system. Exp Gerontol 1988;23:399−412.

239 Rowlands DB, Stollard TJ, Littler WA. Comparison of ambulatory blood pressure and cardiovascular reflexes in elderly hypertensives, elderly normotensives, and young hypertensives. J Hypertens 1983;1(Suppl. 2):71−73.

240 Bozovic L, Castenfors J, Oro L. Plasma renin activity in patients with disturbed sympathetic vasomotor control (postural hypotension). Acta Med Scand 1970;188: 385−388.

241 Love DR, Brown JJ, Chinn RH, *et al.* Plasma renin in idiopathic orthostatic hypotension: differential response in subjects with probably afferent and efferent autonomic

failure. Clin Sci 1971;41:289–299.

242 Gordon RD, Kuchel O, Liddle GW, *et al*. Role of the sympathetic nervous system in regulating renin and aldosterone production in man. J Clin Invest 1967;46:599–605.

243 Shear L. Renal function and sodium metabolism in idiopathic orthostatic hypotension. New Engl J Med 1963;268: 347–352.

Influence of age on baroreceptor reflexes

Alberto U. Ferrari

Introduction

It has long been known that aging is accompanied by a reduced effectiveness of cardiovascular regulatory mechanisms. This has been suggested clinically by the propensity of elderly subjects to experience postural hypotension [1,2] and experimentally by the demonstration that with advancing age the ability of arterial baroreceptors to modulate heart rate is partially lost, the impairment occurring not only in hypertensive subjects but also in normotensive subjects [3,4]. Based on these observations it was believed to be well established that the circulatory lability typical of the elderly individual depends upon a dysfunction of arterial baroreceptor reflexes. A growing body of evidence, however, although largely confirming the classic findings mentioned above, indicates that the effects of aging on cardiovascular homeostasis are multifold, involving alterations in reflex as well as nonreflex control mechanisms. This is therefore a complex and difficult area of research on which much more experimental work is needed [5,6].

The major biologic and methodologic problems in the study of aging and cardiovascular control can be summarized as follows.

1 Similarly to various normal (exercise, emotion) or abnormal (heart failure, hypertension) conditions, aging may produce nonuniform alterations of reflex cardiovascular control, i.e. different functions may be differentially affected. This entails that no extrapolations can be safely made and any conclusions on the age-related changes of a given reflex function (and even more so on their possible clinical implications) must be based upon direct experimental evidence on that function in humans and/or in animal models.

2 As pointed out in a recent National Institute of Health Symposium [6], the effects of aging on many factors crucially involved in cardiovascular regulation, such as central and efferent neural mechanisms, membrane and ion transport systems, endothelial function, etc., which are still largely unexplored.

3 Any age-related alterations, especially when human subjects are studied, may not be solely due to aging but also to the coexistence of disease independently affecting reflex cardiovascular regulation [7,8]. This may be particularly intriguing for disorders such as heart failure, atherosclerosis, and diabetes whose prevalence (in an overt or subclinical form) is particularly high in aged populations.

Despite the above-mentioned difficulties, new findings are rapidly accumulating in the area and a review of the currently available evidence is worthwhile. This chapter initially focuses on the effects of aging on arterial baroreceptor reflexes in animals and on arterial and cardiopulmonary baroreceptor reflexes in humans. It then discusses current knowledge about the mechanisms of the age-related reflex alterations and eventually describes some age-dependent modifications of the cardiovascular adjustments to various stimuli in which baroreflexes are known to play a role.

Aging and arterial baroreflexes in experimental animals

Wei *et al.* [9] reported that the blood pressure fall accompanying a ramp pressure increase in the isolated carotid sinus from 20 to 200 mmHg is not smaller in old as compared to young rats. This suggests that baroreceptor control of the peripheral circulation is not impaired by the aging process, although the same authors had previously observed that old animals did show altered responses to tilting [10] (Fig. 4.1). Thus abnormal homeostatic adjustments may be present in aged animals free of obvious baroreflex dysfunction. It is also to be considered, however, that the above-mentioned experiments were conducted in anesthetized animals. To avoid this potentially confounding factor we then set up to examine the effects of age on arterial baroreceptor reflexes in conscious animals. The vasoactive drug technique and the common carotid occlusion technique were employed to evaluate respectively baroreceptor control of heart rate and of blood pressure in chronically instrumented normotensive rats whose age ranged from 5 to 90 weeks [11]. As to the former function, both the bradycardic response to a phenylephrine-induced baroreceptor stimulation and the tachycardic response to a nitroprusside-induced baroreceptor deactivation were found to be markedly attenuated in the old as compared to the younger animals. As to the latter function the peak blood pressure rise accompanying carotid occlusion was of a similar magnitude irrespective of age. This would validate the observations from anesthetized animals [9]; however, old rats could not be said to have an entirely normal response inasmuch the peak blood pressure rise induced by the occluding maneuver occurred significantly later in old as compared to young or adult rats (Fig. 4.2). Taken together these

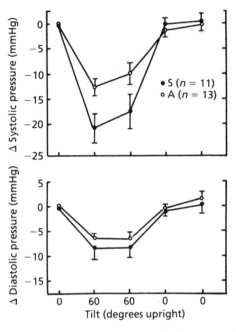

Fig. 4.1 Systolic (upper panel) and diastolic (lower panel) blood pressure response to 60° upright tilt in adult (A) and senescent (S) rats. The latter animals had significantly ($P < 0.02$) larger falls in systolic pressure. It is noteworthy that in this same study as well as in separate experiments the afferent and the overall reflex functions of carotid sinus baroreceptors was unimpaired in the aged as compared to the control animals [9]. (From Wei *et al.* [10].)

observations suggest that in normotensive rats aging may differentially affect the cardiac and vascular target of the baroreflex, the former undergoing a clearcut impairment but the latter being much better preserved and only becoming slower in time course.

Aging and cardiovascular reflexes in humans

Arterial baroreceptor reflexes

In the early 1970s, Gribbin *et al.* [3] evaluated the bradycardic responses to a phenylephrine-induced baroreceptor stimulation in a large group of subjects aged 19–66 years and observed that baroreflex sensitivity progressively declined with age. As shown in Figure 4.3, the authors could also demonstrate that the age-related effect was present irrespective of the existence of chronic hypertension—a condition they had previously shown to also adversely affect the reflex [12].

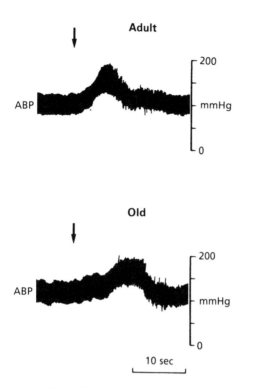

Adult

ABP

200

mmHg

0

Old

ABP

200

mmHg

0

10 sec

Fig. 4.2 Original recordings from one adult and one old unanesthetized normotensive rat showing the arterial blood pressure (ABP) responses to a 12-s bilateral common carotid artery occlusion obtained via chronically implanted bilateral balloon-in-cuff occluding devices. Arrows indicate the onset of the occlusion. The peak increase in blood pressure was the same in the two animals, but the time course of the response was much slower in the old as compared to the adult rat. (From Ferrari *et al.* [11].)

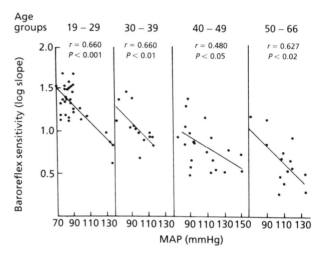

Fig. 4.3 Independent effects of age and of baseline mean arterial pressure (MAP) on baroreceptor control of heart rate. Baroreflex sensitivity was calculated from the bradycardic response to baroreceptor stimulation produced by intravenous bolus injections of phenylephrine. Data are presented in four separate panels comprising progressively older subjects (age ranges indicated on top of each panel). Within each panel baroreflex sensitivity is plotted as a function of baseline blood pressure. The negative effect of either factor on baroreflex sensitivity is readily apparent. (From Gribbin *et al.* [3].)

Subsequent studies confirmed these findings and additionally showed that aging attenuates not only the cardioinhibitory but also the cardioexcitatory influence of baroreceptors [2,5], that the attentuation may be extreme at very advanced age [14] but may be sizeable even in the middle-age range [2], and that it is evident with rapid bolus injections of the vasoactive drugs as well as with slower administrations of these substances, indicating that the age-related impairment involves the fast as well as the more delayed cardiac influences of the reflex [2]. Since the baroreceptor-mediated bradycardia largely depends on the parasympathetic system whereas the baroreceptor-mediated tachycardia also engages the sympathetics [15], it is likely that both the vagal and the sympathetic components of the reflex are adversely affected by the aging process.

Although one can hold as well established that in humans aging progressively impairs baroreceptor control of heart rate, much less evidence has been obtained on the effects of age on arterial baroreflex control of blood pressure. One of the main reasons for this is that the techniques to examine this function are complex and by no means free of limitations. The only accepted approach consists of the neck chamber technique, which requires enclosing the neck (in a way such as to encompass the area of the carotid bifurcation) in an isolated atmosphere whose pressure may be increased or reduced at will by a pneumatic pump, thereby increasing or reducing carotid sinus transmural pressure and baroreceptor activity [16,17].

Few authors employed this method to evaluate the effects of aging on the carotid baroreceptor control of circulation. In a recent study [17] the cardiovascular responses to a sustained (3 min) neck suction were assessed in 45 apparently healthy subjects divided into four groups of progressively increasing age. The neck suction-induced decreases in heart rate, cardiac index, and systolic blood pressure (sphygmomanometric measurements) tended to be attenuated in the older groups. However, most of the age-related differences were observed between the 19–35 and the 36–50 year age groups, the further changes in the 51–66 and 66–80 year age groups being nonsignificant. Therefore this study suggests, in agreement with previous evidence [18], that carotid baroreceptor control of circulation is slightly reduced from the young adult to the mature age range, but does not support the idea that any major adverse effects on this control occur when the truly advanced age range is entered.

In our laboratory negative and positive neck chamber pressures (accompanied by reflex reductions and increases of arterial blood pressure, respectively) were applied to a large number of subjects of a wide age range. Repeated tests were performed in every subject, different degrees of positive and negative neck chamber pressure being randomly applied. Each test lasted 2 min allowing the reflex changes in blood pressure—measured intra-arterially—to be evaluated in an "early" (within 15 s) as well as in a late or "steady-state" (final 30 s) phase of the response [19]. The results are summarized in Figure 4.4; when carotid baroreceptor activity was increased by negative neck pressure application no age-related differences were observed in the reflex depressor responses. In contrast, when carotid baroreceptor activity was reduced by positive neck pressure application the older subjects had smaller reflex pressor responses as compared to the younger are groups, this being only the case, however, during the "early" and not during the "steady-state" phase of the test.

It is interesting to note that this pattern reproduces the results of the rat experiments mentioned in the previous section [11] and allows to outline an overall view of the age-induced changes in arterial baroreflexes, the control they exert on heart rate definitely losing part of its effectiveness but their vascular influences being much better preserved. Indeed, the available evidence suggests that in advanced age the blood pressure influences of arterial baroreceptors are qualitatively altered, their time course being delayed, but quantitatively normal, their amplitude being largely unmodified. As a consequence, the original concept of an overall impairment of arterial

Fig. 4.4 Carotid baroreceptor control of blood pressure as evaluated by the neck chamber technique in four groups of subjects of progressively increasing age. In each subject several negative and positive neck pressure (NTP) applications of variable intensity and constant duration (2 min) were performed to respectively stimulate and deactivate carotid sinus baroreceptors thus obtaining reflex decreases and increases in blood pressure (MAP). The reflex responses were quantitated from the relationship between the changes in NTP induced by the neck chamber and the attendant changes in MAP, separately considering the early (left panels) and steady-state (right panels) phases of the baroreceptor deactivations (upper panels) and stimulations (lower panels). Among all the responses tested, only the early blood pressure rise in response to baroreceptor deactivation showed an age-related decline. For further explanations see text. (From Mancia *et al.* [19].)

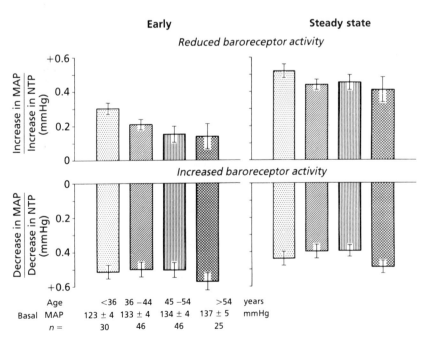

baroreflexes with aging has to be updated by taking into account the more subtle age-related changes in the various components of the reflex, along with their possible (and as yet unknown) clinical implications.

Cardiopulmonary receptor reflexes

Beside the sinoaortic baroreceptor area, a further major reflexogenic area in the cardiovascular system, is the cardiopulmonary region. Receptors located in the atria, ventricles, pulmonary vessels, and lung parenchima reach the central nervous system via nonmedullated and, to a lesser extent, medullated fibers traveling in the vagi or in afferent sympathetic branches [20]. Only the former will be considered in this discussion, however, because no information is as yet available about the physiologic role of the latter in young as well as elderly individuals. Vagal cardiopulmonary receptors are activated by the mechanical stretch of the cardiac and vascular walls in which they are located. Distension of these structures due to an increased or centralized blood volume will then increase receptor discharge, reflexly inhibiting sympathetic outflow and lowering the circulating level of humoral factors such as renin, noradrenaline, and vasopressin [21,22].

These features make the cardiopulmonary reflex system an important contributor to the control of sodium and water excretion and body fluid balance. Considering that elderly individuals have a reduced ability to cope with volume-depleting conditions such as low salt intake and diuretic treatment [23], knowledge of cardiopulmonary reflex function in advanced age is of great interest. Only a few studies, however, have addressed this issue. In a report on middle-aged and elderly subjects no age-dependent alterations in cardiopulmonary reflex control of forearm vascular resistance were observed [24]. The independent effects of age may not have been fully appreciated in this series, however, because the patients had high blood pressure which can by itself alter the cardiopulmonary reflex [25,26].

Recently, Cleroux et al. [27] evaluated the cardiopulmonary reflex in young, middle-aged, and elderly subjects all with normal and comparable blood pressure levels. The activity of the receptors was reduced and increased by lower body negative pressure and leg raising, respectively. During either maneuver the vascular (arterial blood pressure, forearm blood flow, and forearm vascular resistance) as well as the humoral influences of the reflex

(plasma renin and noradrenaline levels) were measured. Although the changes in central venous pressure induced by lower body negative pressure and leg raising were similar in the three groups, the reflex responses were clearly blunted in elderly as compared to middle-aged and young subjects, this being the case for both the vascular and the humoral components of the reflex (Fig. 4.5). Although the number of subjects in this study was not large, the remarkable magnitude of the age-related differences in the various reflex responses tested strongly supports the conclusion that in humans cardiopulmonary reflexes are impaired by aging.

Mechanisms of age-induced alterations in reflex control

Arterial baroreceptor reflexes

Information in this area is largely incomplete. Evidence obtained in rats using an isolated aortic arch—aortic nerve preparation suggests that aging reduces the afferent signal from arterial baroreceptors [28]. An age-dependent reduction in afferent baroreceptor firing would be consistent with the known dependency of baroreceptor discharge sensitivity upon arterial compliance which is reduced by aging [29]. However, other authors [10] recorded carotid sinus nerve activity in vivo and found that various blood pressure-altering stimuli produced similar baroreceptor responses in young and old rats. The evidence on the effect of aging on afferent baroreceptor function is therefore far from being definitive and awaits new and hopefully conclusive experimental evidence.

Virtually no data are available about the effects of aging on the central processing of the baroreceptor signal. On the other hand we have some information on the age-related changes of the efferent pathways of the arterial baroreflex; there is good evidence that sympathetic activity increases with age [30], whereas indirect evidence suggests that the efferent cardiac vagal activity undergoes an age-dependent reduction [31—33].

A final factor possibly contributing to the age-related alterations of the various baroreflex responses reviewed above is the ability of the effector organs to respond to neural stimuli. The cardiac and vascular targets of the baroreflex need to be separately considered.

The aging heart is hyporesponsive to sympathetic stimuli [34,35] possibly because of a down-regulation of

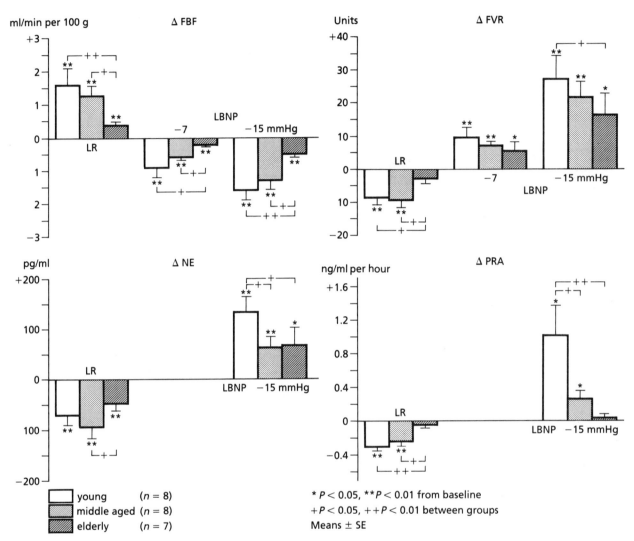

Fig. 4.5 Effects of age on the responses to cardiopulmonary receptor stimulation by leg raising (LR) and deactivation by lower body negative pressure (LBNP) at −7 and −15 mmHg. Each panel shows the changes from control in forearm blood flow (FBF, pletysmography; FVR, forearm vascular resistance; NE, plasma norepinephrine; and PRA, plasma renin activity). Data are means SE of three groups (symbols at foot of the Figure) whose ages were, respectively 24 ± 2, 41 ± 1, and 69 ± 2 years. (From Cleroux *et al.* [27].)

β-adrenergic receptors secondary to the augmented sympathetic outflow, but is probably hyperresponsive to parasympathetic stimuli. Indeed, we recently observed [36] that in normotensive rats the bradycardic effect of intravenously injected acetylcholine is three times as large in old as compared to young animals (Fig. 4.6). This would be consistent with an age-dependent up-regulation of cardiac muscarinic receptors secondary to a diminished vagal outflow. The evidence concerning vascular sympathetic responsiveness in advanced age is not univocal. Elliott *et al.* [37] observed an age-dependent reduction in vascular α-adrenoreceptor responsiveness in humans, whereas other investigators failed to observe age-related differences in the vasoconstrictor response to α-adrenergic agonists in animals [38] and humans [39]. For a summary on the available evidence concerning this

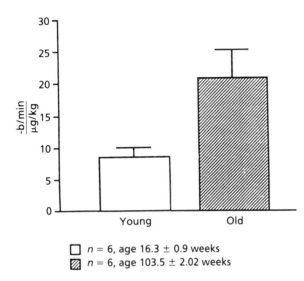

□ n = 6, age 16.3 ± 0.9 weeks
▨ n = 6, age 103.5 ± 2.02 weeks

Fig. 4.6 Bradycardic responses to rapid intravenous injections of acetylcholine (2, 4, and 8 µg/kg) in six young and six old anesthetized, vagotomized rats. Histograms indicate the regression coefficients of the relationship between the injected dose and the atttendant reduction in heart rate. See text for further explanations. (From Ferrari *et al.* [36].)

controversial issue the reader is referred to an excellent brief review by Vanhoutte [40].

Cardiopulmonary reflexes

No direct experimental work has so far attempted to locate the defective portion(s) of the reflex arch responsible for the age-dependent impairment of the cardiopulmonary reflex. However, some indirect insight may come from the experiments by Cleroux *et al.* [27]. In their series the hemodynamic responses to cold pressor test were similar in the elderly and in the younger age groups, suggesting that the efferent neural pathways and the vascular effector were not impaired by aging. Therefore, the defect is most likely due to a reduced afferent signal and/or to an alteration in its central integration. No information is available on the latter possibility, similarly to what applies to the central integration of arterial baroreceptor input in advanced age (see above). Indeed, the input from both reflexogenic areas projects largely on the same central nucleus, namely on the nucleus tractus solitarii [21].

On the other hand, there are reasons to believe that aging decreases the afferent activity of cardiopulmonary

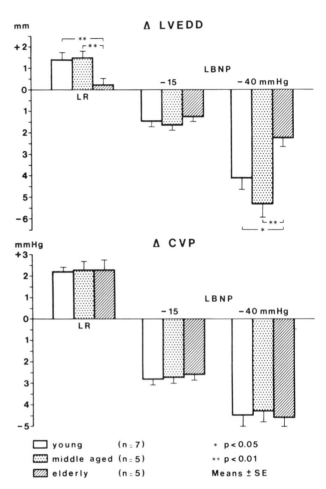

□ young (n = 7)   * p < 0.05
▨ middle aged (n = 5)   ** p < 0.01
▨ elderly (n = 5)   Means ± SE

Fig. 4.7 Effects of leg raising (LR, left) and of lower body negative pressure (LBNP) at −15 and −40 mmHg (center and right) on left ventricular and diastolic dimension (LVEDD, upper panel) and central venous pressure (CVP, lower panel) in young, middle-aged, and elderly subjects (numbers in each group at bottom of Figure). The attenuated changes in LVEDD of aged subjects (despite changes in CVP similar to the younger groups) suggest an age-related reduction in cardiac compliance. For further explanations see text. (From Cleroux *et al.* [27].)

receptors. In the study by Cleroux *et al.* [27] echocardiographic measurements of left ventricular mass and of the changes in left ventricular dimension accompanying lower body suction and leg raising were performed. These measurements allowed respectively to evaluate left ventricular anatomy and to estimate the actual stimulus to the receptors (i.e., wall strain) during either maneuver better than it could be done by simply monitoring central venous pressure. The results showed that elderly subjects had slightly hypertrophied and less compliant hearts as compared to the younger age groups (Fig. 4.7). Since cardiac hypertrophy can impair cardiopulmonary reflex responses (and regression of the hypertrophy can restore them) [26], these findings suggest that one contributing factor to the age-dependent impairment of cardiopulmonary reflexes may be a reduced ability of central blood volume shifts to alter cardiac volume and cardiopulmonary receptor activity. Caution is to be exerted, however, before drawing definitive conclusions from these observations, considering that they were performed in a limited number of subjects, were necessarily based on indirect measurements, and were confined to the characteristics of the left ventricle, which may not be representative of other areas of the cardiopulmonary region. Clearly, our knowledge of the age-dependent changes in cardiopulmonary reflexes and of their underlying mechanisms needs to be expanded by additional and more direct studies in humans as well as in animal models.

Aging and cardiovascular adjustment to various stimuli

Elderly subjects often display altered cardiovascular responses to common laboratory or naturally occurring circumstances such as the Valsalva maneuver, food ingestion, orthostasis, and many others. In all cases baroreceptor reflexes as well as nonbaroreflex mechanisms participate to the homeostatic response and the relative role of each factor may be difficult to establish. Due to their pathophysiologic and clinical relevance, however,

the age-dependent alterations in some of these responses will be briefly commented upon.

The heart rate changes accompanying the various phases of the Valsalva maneuver, as well as those associated to normal breathing [41], cough [32], head-up tilt, and standing [42,43] are progressively reduced with advancing age (Fig. 4.8). On the other hand, the blood pressure changes induced by some of these maneuvers and by food ingestion [44] are clearly larger in elderly as compared to young subjects. All of these age-dependent phenomena may be at least partly accounted for by an impaired ability of arterial and cardiopulmonary receptors to adjust cardiovascular function in time and offset the hemodynamic consequences of a given disturbance. As far as digestion is concerned for example, postprandial hypotension has been recently recognized as a relatively common occurrence in elderly subjects (Fig. 4.9). The underlying mechanism may relate to failure of appropriate reflex vasoconstriction to compensate for blood pooling in the splanchnic region. If confirmed on larger populations, this might prove to be a new important clinical entity possibly implicated in the genesis of syncopal episodes in this age group [44]. Recent experiments also brought new insight into the orthostatic hypotensive syndrome typically affecting the elderly. Impairment of rapid cardiovascular adjustments by baroreflexes may not be the only involved mechanism. Indeed, Shannon *et al.* [45] recently described a group of elderly subjects in whom assumption of the upright posture had no adverse effects under baseline conditions but produced substantial blood pressure falls after moderate sodium depletion (Fig. 4.10). Therefore, not only the short-term neurally mediated mechanisms but also the longer-acting humoral and volume mechanisms (no matter how far the

Fig. 4.8 Changes in heart rate observed in the 30 s following standing (continuous lines) and head-up tilt (dashed lines) in young and progressively older age groups (age ranges on top of Figure). Both the very marked and the more moderate response to the respectively active and passive postural change were age-dependently attenuated. The solid black symbols indicate the time of the postural maneuver. (From Dambrink & Wieling [43].)

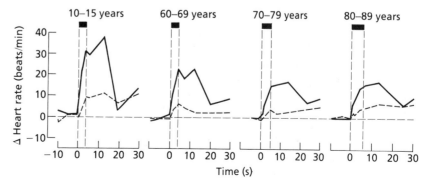

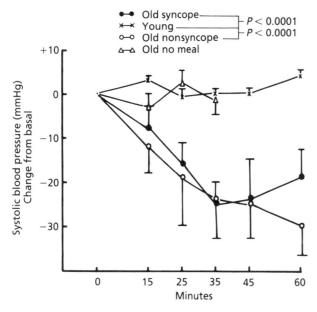

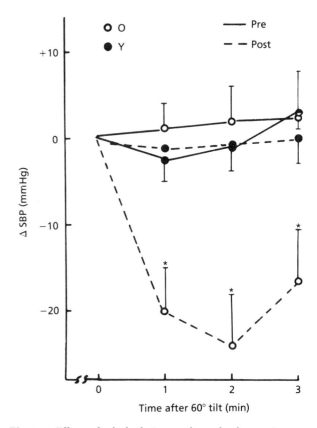

Fig. 4.9 Systolic blood pressure values observed in the 60 min following food ingestion in 10 elderly subjects with syncope (solid circles), 10 elderly subjects without syncope (open circles, mean age for both groups 87 ± 1 years), and 11 healthy young subjects (crosses, mean age 27 ± 1 years). In nine additional elderly subjects (triangles) no food was given. Postprandial changes in blood pressure for elderly subjects were similar irrespective of the occurrence of syncope but differed significantly from those in young ($P < 0.0001$) and fasting elderly ($P < 0.0001$) subjects. (From Lipsitz [44].)

Fig. 4.10 Effects of salt depletion on the early changes in systolic blood pressure (SBP) accompanying 60° upright tilt in six young (Y) and six old (O) subjects. Continuous (PRE) and dashed (POST) lines indicate the SBP values observed before and after a 2-day oral treatment with hydrochlorothiazide, 100 mg/day. Asterisks indicate significant changes from prediuresis values ($P < 0.02$).

latter are intermingled with the former) may contribute to the age-dependent propensity to postural hypotension.

In addition to separately analyzing the cardiovascular responses to individual stimuli, the effects of aging can also be evaluated by a complimentary and more integrated approach, that is, by measuring the variability of heart rate and of blood pressure as it occurs "spontaneously" during a 24-hour continuous recording of intraarterial blood pressure by the Oxford portable recorder. The findings obtained by this technique in a fairly large group of subjects studied in our laboratory are shown in Figure 4.11. As compared to subjects less than 38 years old, the subjects aged 48 or more had greater blood pressure variability and smaller heart rate variability [46]. It is interesting to note that this matches the general trend outlined by examining the responses to individual stimuli, i.e. it indicates that the aging cardiovascular system

has a reduced heart rate-modulating ability associated with an impaired blood pressure-buffering function. The two alterations may well be linked through a causal relationship also involving arterial baroreceptor reflexes. Indeed, studies on large numbers of hypertensive human subjects showed that baroreflex sensitivity correlates positively with heart rate variability and negatively with blood pressure variability [47,48]. Furthermore in unanesthetized rats administration of atropine almost completely suppresses baroreceptor control of heart rate and produces variability effects similar to those brought about by aging and hypertension in humans, i.e., it respectively reduces and increases the variabilities of heart rate and of blood pressure [49] (Fig. 4.12).

Fig. 4.11 Effects of age on blood pressure and heart rate variabilities. Histograms indicate short-term (within) and long-term (among) variabilities of mean arterial pressure (MAP, left panel) and heart rate (HR, right panel) calculated from beat-to-beat computer analysis of 24-hour intraarterial blood pressure recording in subjects younger than 38 years ($n = 31$) and older than 48 years ($n = 26$) with similar 24-hour blood pressure values. Note lower heart rate variability and short-term (but not long-term) blood pressure variability in older subjects. For further explanation see text. (From Ferrari *et al.* [5].)

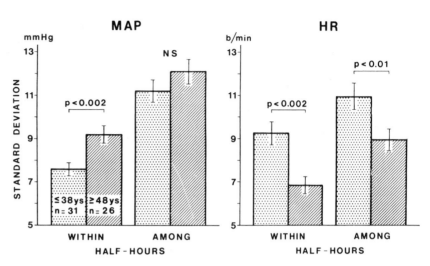

These observations support the concept that part of the moment-to-moment blood pressure oscillations can be normally buffered by changes in heart rate. For example, the blood pressure rise (or fall) associated to a transient peripheral vasoconstriction (or vasodilation) would be made less pronounced if a prompt reduction (or increase) in heart rate, and hence in cardiac output, occurs. Since the cardiac vagal limb of the baroreflex seems to be the principal factor involved in this compensatory adjustment, an impairment of its effectiveness with aging is not unexpected and may contribute to the altered variability profile observed in elderly subjects.

Fig. 4.12 Original recording of arterial blood pressure (ABP, femoral catheter) and heart rate (HR) in an unanesthetized, unrestrained, normotensive rat showing the effects of cholinergic blockade by intravenous atropine. Following the injection (arrow), the variabilities of heart rate and of blood pressure undergo opposite changes, the former being greatly diminished and the latter greatly augmented. (From Ferrari *et al.* [49].)

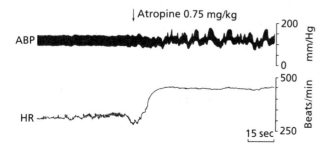

Acknowledgments

The author gratefully acknowledges the teaching, encouragement, intellectual stimulus, and material support from Drs Alberto Zanchetti and Giuseppe Mancia, without whom this work would not have been possible.

References

1 Caird FI, Andrews GR, Kennedy RD. Effect of posture on blood pressure in the elderly. Br Heart J 1973;35:527–530.
2 MacLennan WJ, Hall MRP, Timothy JI. Postural hypotension in old age: is it a disorder of the nervous system or of blood vessels? Age Ageing 1980;9:25–32.
3 Gribbin B, Pickering TG, Sleight P, *et al.* Effect of age and high blood pressure on baroreflex sensitivity in man. Circ Res 1971;29:424–431.
4 Korner PI, West MJ, Shaw J, *et al.* Steady-state properties of the baroreceptor-heart rate reflex in essential hypertension in man. Clin Exp Pharmacol Physiol 1974;1:65–76.
5 Ferrari AU, Grassi G, Mancia G. Alterations in reflex control of the circulation associated with aging. In Amery A, Staessen J, eds. *Handbook of Hypertension*, vol. 12. Hypertension in the elderly. Amsterdam: Elsevier, 1989:39–50.
6 Horan MJ, Steinberg GM, Dunbar JB, *et al.* Summary of NIH Symposium on blood pressure regulation and aging. Hypertension 1986;8:178–180.
7 Bennett T, Gardiner SM. Physiological aspects of the aging cardiovascular system. J Cardiovasc Pharmacol 1988; 12(Suppl. 8):S1–S7.
8 Cristofalo VJ. The biology of aging—an overview. In Horan MJ, Steinberg GM, Dunbar JB, *et al.*, eds. *Blood Pressure*

Regulation and Aging. New York: Biomedical Info. Corp., 1986:31–40.

9 Wei JY, Mendlowitz D, Anastasi N, *et al.* Maintenance of carotid baroreflex function in advanced age in the rat. Am J Physiol 1986;250:R1047–R1051.

10 Wei YJ, Mendelowitz D, Anastasi N, *et al.* Influence of age on cardiovascular reflex response in anesthetized rats. Am J Physiol 1985;249:R31–R38.

11 Ferrari AU, Daffonchio A, Albergati F, *et al.* Differential effects of aging on the heart rate and blood pressure influences of arterial baroreceptors in awake rats. J Hypertens 1991;9:615–621.

12 Bristow JD, Honour AJ, Pickering GW, *et al.* Diminished baroreflex sensitivity in high blood pressure. Circulation 1969;39:48–54.

13 Rowlands DB, Stallard TJ, Littler WA. Continuous ambulatory monitoring of blood pressure and assessment of cardiovascular reflexes in the elderly hypertensive. J Hypertens 1984;2:615–622.

14 Mancia G, Mark AL. Arterial baroreflexes in humans. In Shepherd JT, Abboud FM, eds. *Handbook of Physiology*, Sect. 2, The Cardiovascular System, vol. III, Peripheral Circulation and Organ Blood Flow, part 2. American Physiological Society, Washington DC. Baltimore: Williams & Wilkins, 1983:755–794.

15 Ernsting J, Parry DJ. Some observations on the effects of stimulating the stretch receptors in the carotid artery in man (abstr.). J Physiol 1957;137:P45–P46.

16 Ludbrook J, Mancia G, Ferrari A, *et al.* The variable-pressure neck chamber method for studying the carotid baroreflexes in man. Clin Sci Mol Med 1977;53:165–171.

17 Hainsworth R, Al-Shamma YMH. Cardiovascular responses to stimulation of carotid baroreceptors in healthy subjects. Clin Sci 1988;75:159–165.

18 Linblad LE. Influence of age on sensitivity and effector mechanisms of the carotid baroreflex. Acta Physiol Scand 1977;101:43–49.

19 Mancia G, Grassi G, Bertinieri G, *et al.* Arterial baroreceptor control of blood pressure in man. J Auton Nerv Syst 1984;11:115–124.

20 Malliani A. Cardiovascular sympathetic afferent fibers. Rev Physiol Biochem Pharmacol 1982;94:11–74.

21 Mark AL, Mancia G. Cardiopulmonary baroreflexes in humans. In Shepherd JT, Abboud FM, eds. *Handbook of Physiology*, 2 The cardiovascular system, vol. III, Peripheral circulation and organ blood flow, part 2. American Physiological Society: Washington DC. Baltimore: Williams & Wilkins, 1983:795–813.

22 Ferrari AU, Grassi G, Mancia G. The cardiopulmonary reflex in hypertension. In Laragh JH, Brenner BM, eds. *Hypertension: Pathophysiology, Diagnosis and Management.* New York: Raven Press, 1990:349–357.

23 Shannon RP, Minaker KL, Rowe JW. The influence of age on water balance in man. Semin Nephrol 1984:4:346–352.

24 Sowers JR, Mohanty PK. Effect of advancing age on cardiopulmonary baroreflex control of forearm vascular resistance in borderline hypertension. Hypertension 1987;10:274–279.

25 Mark AL, Kerber RE. Augmentation of cardiopulmonary baroreflex control of forearm vascular resistance in borderline hypertension. Hypertension 1982;4:39–46.

26 Grassi G, Giannattasio C, Cleroux J, *et al.* Cardiopulmonary reflex before and after regression of left ventricular hypertrophy in essential hypertension. Hypertension 1988;12:227–237.

27 Cleroux J, Giannattasio C, Bolla GB, *et al.* Decreased cardiopulmonary reflexes with aging in normotensive humans. Am J Physiol 1989;257:H961–H968.

28 Andresen MC. Short- and long-term determinants of baroreceptor function in aged normotensive and spontaneously hypertensive rats. Circ Res 1984;54:750–759.

29 Learoyd BM, Taylor MG. Alterations with age of the viscoelastic properties of human arterial walls. Circ Res 1966;18:278–292.

30 Wallin BG, Sundlof G. A quantitative study of muscle nerve sympathetic activity in resting normotensive and hypertensive subjects. Hypertension 1979;1:67–77.

31 Alicandri C, Boni E, Fariello R, *et al.* Parasympathetic control of heart rate and age in essential hypertensive patients. J Hypertens 1987;5(Suppl. 5):S345–S347.

32 Wei JY, Rowe JW, Kestenbaum AD, *et al.* Post-cough heart rate response: influence of age, sex, and basal blood pressure. Am J Physiol 1983;245:R18–R24.

33 Dauchot P, Gravenstein JS. Effects of atropine on the electrocardiogram in different age groups. Clin Pharmacol Ther 1971;12:274–280.

34 van Brummelen P, Buhler FR, Kiowski W, *et al.* Age-related decrease in cardiac and peripheral vascular responsiveness to isoprenaline: studies in normal subjects. Clin Sci 1981;60:571–577.

35 Feldmann RD, Limbird LE, Nadeau J. Alterations in leukocyte beta-receptor affinity with aging. A potential explanation for altered beta-adrenergic sensitivity in the elderly. N Engl J Med 1984;310:815–819.

36 Ferrari AU, Daffonchio A, Gerosa S, *et al.* Effects of aging on parasympathetic function in rats (abstr.). *Fourth European Meeting on Hypertension.* Milan, 1989:257.

37 Elliott HL, Summer DJ, McLean K, *et al.* Effect of age on the responsiveness of vascular alfa-adrenergic receptors in man. J Cardioavasc Pharmacol 1982;4:388–392.

38 Duckles SP, Carter B, Williams CL. Vascular adrenergic neuroeffector function does not decline in aged rats. Circ Res 1985;56:109–116.

39 Buhler FR, Kiowski W, van Brummelen P, *et al.* Plasma catecholamines and cardiac renal and peripheral vascular adrenoceptor mediated responses in different age groups in normal and hypertensive subjects. Clin Exp Hypertens 1980;2:409–426.

40 Vanhoutte PM. Aging and vascular responsiveness. J Cardiovasc Pharmacol 1988;12(Suppl. 8):S11−S18.

41 Hellmann JB, Stacy RW. Variation of respiratory sinus arrhythmia with age. J Appl Physiol 1976;41:734−738.

42 Kalbfleisch JH, Reinke JA, Porth CJ, et al. Effect of age on circulatory response to postural and Valsalva tests. Proc Soc Exp Biol Med 1977;156:100−103.

43 Dambrink JHA, Wieling W. Circulatory response to postural change in healthy male subjects in relation to age. Clin Sci 1987;72:335−341.

44 Lipsitz LA. Abnormalities in blood pressure homeostasis associated with aging and hypertension. In Horan MJ, Steinberg GM, Dunbar JB, et al., eds. Blood Pressure Regulation and Aging. New York: Biomedical Info. Corp., 1986: 201−211.

45 Shannon RP, Wei JY, Rosa RM, et al. The effect of age and sodium depletion on cardiovascular response to orthostasis. Hypertension 1986;8:438−443.

46 Mancia G, Ferrari A, Gregorini L, et al. Blood pressure and heart rate variabilities in normotensive and hypertensive human beings. Circ Res 1983;53:96−104.

47 Mancia G, Parati G, Pomidossi G, et al. Arterial baroreflexes and blood pressure and heart rate variabilities in humans. Hypertension 1986;8:147−153.

48 Conway J, Boon N, Davies C, et al. Neural and humoral mechanisms involved in blood pressure variability. J Hypertens 1984;2:203−208.

49 Ferrari AU, Daffonchio A, Albergati F, et al. Inverse relationship between heart rate and blood pressure variabilities in rats. Hypertension 1987;10:533−537.

5

Pathophysiology of hypertension in the elderly

Harriet P. Dustan

Introduction

In industrialized societies blood pressure rises with age and the prevalence of hypertension increases. Until relatively recently this was considered a natural consequence of aging; however, in the last 30 years there has been a growing awareness that these pressure increases are associated with risks for cardiovascular complications, particularly strokes and heart attacks. Furthermore, since many elderly people are normotensive, there is increasing interest in the pathophysiology of hypertension in the elderly because understanding it could lead to prevention or, failing that, better methods of control either through dietary modifications or use of drug therapy.

Types of hypertension in the elderly are, for the most part, no different from those found in younger people. Thus, the most common is essential hypertension which, for the elderly in the last decade of this century, means survival from a previously fatal condition through therapy that has resulted in striking decreases in deaths directly related to hypertension: cardiac failure, hemorrhagic strokes, and renal failure.

In contrast with essential hypertension, isolated systolic hypertension (systolic ≥160; diastolic <90 mmHg) is almost exclusively a problem of the elderly. Although it occurs in young people as a hallmark of aortic coarctation or hyperdynamic circulation, its prevalence is insignificant compared to that found in elderly people.

Renovascular hypertension due to atherosclerotic renal artery stenosis is the most frequent secondary hypertension found in the older population. It can develop *de novo* in previously normotensive individuals or can intensify long-standing essential hypertension. Although the true prevalence of renovascular hypertension is not known, this type is well recognized and is of particular concern in the elderly. It is usually severe and can present as malignant hypertension, a condition inappropriate for essential hypertension in elderly people [1].

These are the issues related to hypertension in the elderly. Although the focus of this chapter is on pathophysiology it will provide a background as to prevalence, normal arterial control mechanisms, and cardiovascular consequences of aging in order to give perspective to pathophysiology.

Definition and prevalence

Definition

Arterial blood pressure in a population is distributed normally in a bell-shaped curve so it is not the case of one curve for normotension and one for hypertension [2]. This characteristic has made the definition of hypertension difficult. Current definitions for systolic and diastolic pressure used in the United States are derived from actuarial data that have shown the beginnings of excess hypertension-related mortality at systolic pressures of 140 mmHg and diastolic pressures of 90 mmHg. As these pressures increase so too does mortality but this increase is not linear and rises sharply at the upper end of the pressure range [3].

Definitions on which the prevalence data are based were formulated in 1984 by the National High Blood Pressure Education Program (NHBPEP) of the National Heart, Lung and Blood Institute (NHLBI) [4]. Table 5.1 defines systolic and diastolic pressures separately thus acknowledging that elevation in either pressure carries risk of cardiovascular complications. For the first time also, diastolic pressures of 85−89 mmHg were listed as

"high normal" because such levels often presage development of persistent diastolic hypertension. As for higher levels of diastolic pressure 90−104 mmHg is termed "mild", 105−114 mmHg "moderate", and ≥115 mmHg, "severe." As noted below about 10% of the population has elevated systolic pressure but with normal diastolic pressure, i.e. less than 90 mmHg. This is termed "isolated systolic hypertension": 140−159 mmHg is considered "borderline" while pressures of 160 mmHg or greater, definite "isolated systolic hypertension."

Prevalence

Until about 25 years ago there was no comprehensive information about the prevalence of hypertension in the United States. Prior to that time, fragmentary information had come from insurance companies beginning in 1925 with the Society of Actuaries first report on over a half million men [5]. Reports from that source continued, the most recent being the Blood Pressure Study 1979 [6], but as helpful as these were they concerned only insured people so had limited value for the country as a whole.

In 1956 the United States Congress established The National Center for Health Statistics (NCHS) to determine the prevalences of chronic diseases in this country. The Center has conducted two surveys of large population samples designed to be representative of the entire country with the exception of military personnel, institutionalized people, children, and people aged 75 years and older. Data from the most recent study, The National Health and Nutrition Examination Survey (NHANES II) carried out between 1976 and 1980, provide the information about hypertension prevalence in use today [7]. The data presented here concern the civilian, noninstitutionalized population aged 18−74 years. Some additional hypertension prevalence data in the elderly comes from The Systolic Hypertension in the Elderly Program (SHEP) of NHLBI [8].

The overall prevalence of hypertension according to age is shown in Table 5.2 which establishes the progressive increase in arterial pressure with age and shows that blacks have more tendency towards hypertension than whites.

Table 5.3 presents interesting data about the prevalence of the blood pressure categories noted above. Again we see that hypertension is more common in blacks than in whites and not only that, but it is also more severe. These

Table 5.1 Definition of diastolic and systolic blood pressures. (From Subcommittee on Definition and Prevalence of the 1984 Joint National Committee [7])

Diastolic blood pressure (DBP) (mmHg)	Category
<85	Normal blood pressure
85−89	High normal blood pressure
90−104	Mild hypertension
105−114	Moderate hypertension
≥115	Severe hypertension
Systolic blood pressure (SBP) (mmHg) when DBP <90 mmHg	Category
<140	Normal blood pressure
140−159	Borderline isolated systolic hypertension
≥160	Isolated systolic hypertension

Table 5.2 Hypertension* prevalence rates by sex, race, and age. Civilian, noninstitutionalized population (ages 18–74 years) 1976–80. (From Subcommittee on Definition and Prevalence of the 1984 Joint National Committee [7])

Age (years)	Males			Females			Total		
	Whites (%)	Blacks (%)	All races (%)	Whites (%)	Blacks (%)	All races (%)	Whites (%)	Blacks (%)·	All races (%)
18–74	32.6	37.9	33.0	25.3	38.6	26.8	28.8	38.2	29.8
18–24	16.2	10.9	15.2	2.3	9.6	3.5	9.1	10.2	9.2
25–34	21.1	23.2	20.9	5.7	15.3	6.9	13.3	18.8	13.7
35–44	26.4	44.2	28.4	16.6	37.0	19.3	21.3	40.1	23.7
45–54	42.6	55.2	43.7	36.3	67.4	39.1	39.4	61.7	41.3
55–64	51.4	66.3	52.6	50.0	74.3	52.6	50.6	70.7	52.6
65–74	59.2	67.1	60.2	66.2	82.9	67.5	63.1	76.1	64.3

Source: NHANES II.
* Defined as the average of three blood pressure measurements ≥140/90 mmHg on a single occasion or reported taking of antihypertensive medication.

Table 5.3 Frequency distribution by blood pressure level regardless of medication status. Civilian, noninstitutionalized population (ages 18–74 years) 1976–80. (From Subcommittee on Definition and Prevalence of the 1984 Joint National Committee [7])

Blood pressure level	Males			Females			Total		
	Whites (%)	Blacks (%)	All races (%)	Whites (%)	Blacks (%)	All races (%)	Whites (%)	Blacks (%)	All races (%)
Normal blood pressure*	60.5	54.8	60.0	73.3	62.9	72.1	67.1	59.3	66.3
High normal blood pressure*	8.9	9.5	9.0	5.6	5.9	5.6	7.2	7.6	7.2
Mild high blood pressure	18.4	20.6	18.7	10.8	17.9	11.7	14.5	19.1	15.0
Moderate high blood pressure	1.9	3.0	2.0	1.1	3.1	1.3	1.5	3.1	1.6
Severe high blood pressure	0.5	2.2	0.7	0.4	0.8	0.5	0.5	1.4	0.6
Borderline isolated systolic hypertension	8.5	8.8	8.4	7.2	6.9	7.1	7.8	7.7	7.7
Isolated systolic hypertension	1.3	1.2	1.3	1.7	2.4	1.8	1.5	1.9	1.5
Total	100	100	100	100	100	100	100	100	100

Source: NHANES II.
* Includes those hypertensives who are controlling their blood pressures.

differences concern diastolic hypertension but borderline isolated systolic hypertension and isolated systolic hypertension are not more severe in blacks than in whites. Whatever may be the mechanism of this type of hypertension, it does not seem to have racial determinants.

Normal arterial control mechanisms

Hemodynamics
In the simplest of terms, arterial pressure is a function of cardiac output and vascular resistance. It can be concep-

tualized by the equation MAP = CO × TPR where MAP stands for mean arterial pressure, CO for cardiac output and TPR for total peripheral resistance. Thus, cardiac output, or the flow of blood, and the resistance to that flow, vascular resistance or TPR, are two of the direct determinants of arterial pressure (Table 5.4). There are two others: one is aortic impedance which is resistance to phasic blood flow and the other is diastolic arterial volume. The heart provides the energy for the circulation of blood. With each contraction, it delivers a small volume (about 70 ml at rest) into a system that is distensible and elastic, it already contains a substantial volume from previous ejections and has an outflow that, in comparison with inflow, is somewhat restricted. This results in a pressure pulse. The height of that pressure pulse, which we measure as systolic pressure, depends upon the speed of ejection, the force of ejection, the amount ejected (stroke volume), diastolic arterial volume, and elasticity of the aorta and its proximal large branches. The level to which the pressure falls when the heart is not contracting (diastolic pressure) depends primarily on outflow resistance.

The elasticity of the aorta is important in any discussion of hypertension in elderly people. A normally elastic aorta dampens the pulse by dilating during systole then during diastole it recoils creating diastolic flow (Fig. 5.1). When elasticity decreases, as it does with aging, the arterial wall does not "give" during ejection and the full force of ejection pressure is expressed as an elevated systolic pressure. As will be discussed later, loss of elasticity of the aorta and large vessels with advancing age, sets the stage for an elevated systolic pressure.

Diastolic arterial volume is a theoretical construct because it cannot now be measured but it must be import-

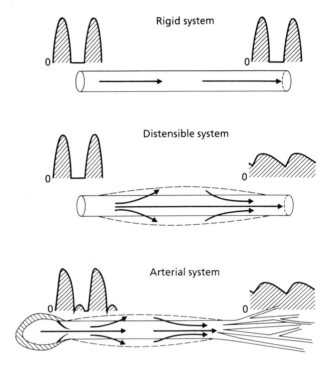

Fig. 5.1 Schematic illustration of the Windkessel effect of a distensible tube system: a rhythmic fluid ejection is transformed into a fairly uniform flow with reduced pressure oscillations. (From Folkow & Neil [22].)

ant because it distends the arteries during diastole. Since flow out of the aorta and large vessels is governed mostly by the arterioles and precapillary sphincters, the volume remaining in the arterial system and distending it at the end of diastole must influence arterial pressure. Hyperthyroidism is a good example of the importance of vascular resistance in determining the effect of diastolic arterial volume on diastolic pressure. This condition is characterized by elevated systolic pressure because of a hyperkinetic heart, and a low diastolic pressure because of vasodilation. The low-diastolic pressure means a facilitated run-off during diastole and a relatively low end-diastolic arterial volume.

Normally, arterial pressure is maintained within fairly narrow limits. This is the result of close integration of a variety of indirect determinants that influence cardiac output, vascular resistance, the capacity of the aorta and large vessels, and end-diastolic arterial volume (Table 5.4). There are exceptions to this generalization because during sleep arterial pressure may fall as low as

Table 5.4 Determinants of arterial pressure

Direct
Cardiac output
Vascular resistance
Aortic impedance
Diastolic arterial volume

Indirect
Activity of the autonomic nervous system
Body sodium stores and/or extracellular fluid volume
The renin–angiotensin system
Salt-active steroids

60/40 mmHg and during exercise can rise markedly, particularly the systolic pressure. This control of arterial pressure is due to the interaction of the indirect determinants. These are the activity of the autonomic nervous system, particularly its sympathetic component, total body sodium stores, and/or the extracellular fluid volume (ECF), the renin–angiotensin system, and salt-active steroids. Although prostaglandins and the kallikrein-kinin system may influence arterial pressure, there is as yet no clear picture of their roles. The same can be said for vasopressin and atrial natriuretic peptides.

The dominant systems controlling arterial pressure are intimately interrelated. For example, activity of the nervous system influences renin release and the angiotensin II produced not only causes vasoconstriction but controls aldosterone production which in turn, affects fluid and electrolyte balance as well as possibly having a independent effect on vascular smooth muscle. Angiotensin II also affects the renal excretion of salt and water.

These direct and indirect determinants of arterial pressure are important to any consideration of the pathophysiology of hypertension. With regard to hypertension in the elderly not all the roles for each of the indirect determinants have been defined so we do not have a clear picture as to how they function in each circumstance.

The primacy of blood flow and resistance to flow in the control of arterial pressure is indicated by the formula $MAP = CO \times TPR$. It is obvious then that in the presence of an increased cardiac output arterial pressure is controlled within the normal range only if vascular resistance falls and the elasticity of the aorta and its large branches is normal. A good case in point is the hyperdynamic heart syndrome described by Gorlin [9] because the patients he studied were normotensive. In contrast, the patients reported by Frohlich et al. [10] were mildly hypertensive because vascular resistance were either inappropriately normal or slightly elevated.

Cardiac output becomes elevated through two mechanisms [11]. One is an increase in myocardial contractility with a rise in ejection fraction, while the other is an elevated central blood volume associated with either hypervolemia or decreased capacity of venous reservoirs. Obesity with its expanded blood volume is an example of the former [12] while the latter, which leads to a central translocation of blood and an increased ratio of cardiopulmonary volume to total blood volume is found primarily in young hypertensives [13].

Peripheral resistance is controlled by neural, humoral, and local factors. The neural influence is supplied by adrenergic nerves that provide for vasoconstriction and this has been implicated in hypertension of the elderly, as will be discussed later. The renal pressor system, i.e., renin and angiotensin released from the kidney, is a possible humoral factor but since renin falls with age [14] this seems to be a less likely candidate affecting hypertension in the elderly than the renin–angiotensin system now known to occur in the blood vessel walls [15]. However, as yet, we have no direct information as to the role of the vascular renin–angiotensin system in any form of hypertension. Other local factors are coming under increased investigation. One possibility is an abnormality of the vascular smooth muscle contractile mechanism [16,17]. The focus is on the control of intracellular sodium, potassium, and calcium because their concentrations determine membrane potential and vascular smooth muscle contractility. In the elderly, the possibility of insulin resistance as a hallmark of deficient metabolic control is under investigation [18–21]. Other local factors, such as prostaglandins and kinins may play a role in peripheral resistance but as yet there is no clear evidence of their importance in hypertension at any age.

Neural mechanisms

The autonomic nervous system, primarily its sympathetic component, is important for normal circulatory control. It is particularly concerned with rapid adjustments to a variety of stimuli such as changes in posture, intrathoracic pressure, and temperature. Also a growing body of evidence links abnormalities of central vasomotor centers to the genesis and maintenance of hypertension.

The nervous system influences arterial pressure in two ways. One mechanism is through neural reflexes and the other is through an on-going maintenance of sympathetic vasomotor tone [22]. The Valsalva maneuver allows us to see an example of reflex operations. The increase in intrathoracic pressure diminishes venous return so that cardiac output and arterial pressure fall. The decrease in venous return is sensed by the low pressure intrathoracic mechanoreceptors and the fall in arterial pressure, by baroreceptors in the aorta and carotid sinus. This leads to a disinhibition of central vasomotor centers so that sympathetic outflow increases, thus raising heart rate and causing arteriolar constriction. When straining stops, blood rapidly returns to the thorax and the sudden increase in cardiac output is delivered into a vasoconstricted arteriolar bed so pressure rises abruptly. This pressure rise is felt by the baroreceptors of the carotid sinus and aortic arch; they send impulses to the central vasomotor centers resulting in sympathetic inhibition which slows heart rate and reduces pressure.

The maintenance of pressure in the standing position or with a head-up tilt is an example of reflex circulatory control that is relevant for a discussion of hypertension in the elderly. It is similar to the Valsalva maneuver in that there is a decrease in venous return in the upright position leading to a decreased cardiac output and arterial pressure. Sympathetic outflow along the cardiac and vasomotor nerves increases heart rate and causes venous and arteriolar vasoconstriction. The venoconstriction helps to maintain venous return and arteriolar constriction helps to maintain blood pressure. These reflexes sometimes fail in the elderly [23].

One way to look at reflex control of the circulation is that normally it serves to elevate pressure when it falls and reduce it when it rises. Obviously the mechanism is not completely effective in hypertension and, as will be detailed below, this failure may be important in hypertension in the elderly. We do know that there is an upward resetting of aortic and carotid baroreceptor sensitivity with advancing age [24] so that pressure rises are inadequately sensed resulting, potentially, in less inhibition of sympathetic vasomotor centers. However, such a role has not been completely defined in the on-going control of arterial pressure of hypertension at any age.

There is a growing body of evidence pointing to the possibility that sympathetic vasomotor tone is not normal in elderly people [25,26]. All vessels are richly supplied with sympathetic vasomotor nerves which not only function during reflex operations but also in the maintenance of varying degrees of vasomotor tone. Both reflex and tonic control of the circulation is carried out through the noradrenergic neuroeffector system through the production and release of norepinephrine. All sympathetic nerves make and store norepinephrine which is released from nerve endings by impulses passing down them. Norepinephrine synthesis begins with the amino acid tyrosine which is taken up by brain, peripheral neurons, and chromaffin tissue in the adrenal medulla. In the nerve mitochondria, tyrosine is acted upon by tyrosine hydroxylase to form L-dopa, which migrates to the cytoplasm where it is decarboxylated to dopamine. Dopa-

mine, in turn, moves into vesicles where, through the action of dopamine β-oxidase, it becomes norepinephrine. Epinephrine is formed from the methylation of norepinephrine by the enzyme, phenylethanolamine-N-methyl-transferase. The largest amounts of this enzyme are in the adrenal medulla which is the major source of epinephrine.

The amount of norepinephrine released by nerve impulses is far greater than that needed to produce a response and the excess is handled in several ways. Some escapes into the circulation, some is transformed into normetanephrine by the enzyme, catechol-O-methyltransferase (COMT), and is excreted as such in the urine. Some is deaminated by monoamine oxidase and then methylated by COMT to form vanillmandelic acid (VMA) and methoxyhydroxyphenylglycol (MHPG) which are excreted in the urine. One final mechanism, reuptake by nerve endings, represents the major pathway whereby the released norepinephrine is disposed of.

Extracellular fluid volumes

As indicated in Table 5.4, ECF and/or body sodium stores are important in hypertension but the reasons for that importance have not been defined. Extracellular fluid volume is made up of interstitial fluid and plasma volume and these two compartments are separated by capillary endothelium through which nutrients, gases, electrolyte, and water are exchanged. Sodium is the major cation of the ECF and most of it is freely exchangeable so that its amount can be measured. Sodium does get into cells and here our major interest is in vascular smooth muscle. Because potassium is the major cation of the vascular smooth muscle, sodium has to be extruded by active enzyme systems so as to maintain the membrane potential normally. This extrusion is through the enzyme, sodium–potassium adenosine triphosphatase (Na–K–ATPase). Calcium concentration is also affected. Intracellular sodium of VSM is the focus of much current interest because its effects on potassium and calcium are considered likely to be a factor in the increased vascular resistance that characterizes hypertension.

Plasma volume (PV) is the intravascular component of ECF and it plays a significant hemodynamic role [27]. Plasma volume and red cell mass comprise the total blood volume (TBV) which fills the vascular bed. The bulk of TBV is contained on the venous side of the circulation and the capacity of venous reservoirs below heart level is a determinant of pulmonary blood volume and therefore an important factor in cardiac output. As will be discussed later, blood volume is often reduced in elderly people [28], perhaps because of inactivity, and this may play a role in the age-related decrease in cardiac output that is sometimes found.

In middle-aged hypertensives, PV is characteristically diminished except for primary aldosteronism, in which it is often elevated [29]. This decrease of PV probably reflects the effects of high arterial pressure and diminished venous capacity as well because the veins contain about 75% of the TBV, the arteries 20% and the capillaries only 5% [30]. Plasma volume is determined by sodium balance so that when sodium balance is negative, ECF and PV fall and when positive, they increase. The increase in PV is limited in hypertensives because of pressure natriuresis. Sodium balance is determined not only by sodium intake but also by the ability of the kidney to excrete sodium. With regard to hypertension of the elderly, this may be important because there are age-related decreases in glomerular filtration rate (GFR) and because there is evidence that salt sensitive hypertension is more frequent in the elderly hypertensive than in those younger [31].

The renin−angiotensin system

Until recently the kidney was considered to be the sole source of the renin−angiotensin system. About 50 years ago it was found that the kidney produces a proteolytic enzyme, renin, that splits off a 10-amino acid peptide, angiotensin I, from a plasma protein substrate. This then is acted upon by converting enzyme to produce an eight-amino acid peptide, angiotensin II. This peptide is a powerful vasoconstrictor; it provides the main stimulus for aldosterone release and in some circumstances it seems to have a direct inhibiting effect on sodium excretion.

We recently have learned that the renin−angiotensin system is also present in the brain and blood vessel walls thus providing other possible mechanisms for blood pressure control [15].

The importance of the renin−angiotensin system in elderly hypertensives has not been explored fully. The antihypertensive effectiveness of converting enzyme inhibitors in young hypertensives suggest that it plays an important role in the early stages of hypertension, and the relative ineffectiveness of these drugs in elderly hypertensives suggests that later on the system is not so important. It is, however, the primary mechanism for renovascular hypertension and the renin-dependent hypertension of end-stage kidney disease.

Aldosterone

The zona glonerulosa of the adrenal cortex synthesizes and releases aldosterone, the major salt-active steroid. This synthesis is predominantly controlled by angiotensin II so that aldosterone levels in the blood or urine are positively correlated with factors that influence the renin−angiotensin system, at least that of the kidney. Thus, whereas plasma aldosterone concentrations are positively correlated with plasma renin activity or angiotensin II levels, they are negatively correlated with urinary sodium excretion [32].

Aldosterone increases sodium reabsorption and facilitates potassium excretion by the distal nephron. Not only is it the major steroid influencing potassium homeostasis but furthermore its production is influenced by potassium intake. Thus a high potassium intake increases aldosterone and hormone levels fall with potassium depletion. The importance of the relation of aldosterone and potassium is well exemplified by the rare circumstance of hyporeninemia, hypoaldosteronism, and hyperkalemia, which is occasionally found in older people [33].

Primary aldosteronism, which occasionally occurs in the elderly, is due to increased production of aldosterone and is accompanied by increases of ECF, PV, and total exchangeable sodium. Until recently aldosterone was not thought to be pressor by itself but rather causing a salt-dependent hypertension, because it produced a positive sodium balance [34]. However, a recent report suggests that it may play a direct role in salt-dependent hypertension independent of its effect on sodium balance [35]. Severe renovascular hypertension, an important hypertensive syndrome in the elderly, is characterized by hyperreninemia which, in turn, increases aldosterone release and this is responsible for the hypokalemia often found. Also in young and middle-aged essential hypertensives, there is an exaggerated production of aldosterone in response to infusions of angiotensin II, yet responses to upright posture and sodium depletion are diminished [36]. Suffice to say that, for the most part, the role of aldosterone in hypertension is yet to be completely elucidated.

Aging, arterial pressure, and its control mechanisms

Cardiovascular

Changes in cardiovascular structure

There are a variety of age-related changes that occur in blood vessels both large and small. Those that affect the aorta and its large branches have the potential for influencing systolic pressure in a major way and those that occur in small arteries and arterioles can affect peripheral resistance and, in the case of the kidney, renal excretory function.

The arterial system is divided into three segments:

1 the aorta and its large branches, called conduit or elastic arteries;

2 large and medium-sized arteries or muscular arteries; and

3 arterioles [37].

The morphology of the wall of the aorta and its large branches is distinctly different from other segments because these vessels serve a reservoir function for each stroke volume. The wall of these elastic arteries has three components: the intima, the media, and the adventitia. The intima is composed of endothelium which lies on a thin layer of connective tissue containing collagen and glycosaminoglycans, underneath which is the internal elastic membrane. The media is made up of smooth-muscle cells, layers of elastic tissue, and some collagen, while the adventitia is composed of connective tissue. The elastic fibers provide for distensibility and the collagen for strength while the smooth-muscle cells permit some dynamic change in diameter [22]. With aging there is increased production of collagen while the elastic tissue becomes frayed and fragmented. The result is a loss of elasticity and a diminution in the reservoir function of the aorta and its large branches. The importance of the elastic element of these vessels can be seen by the fact that elastic fibers make up 30% of the aortic wall while smooth muscle comprises 40% and collagen 30% [22].

Under normal circumstances, i.e., in youth or young adulthood, with each cardiac contraction the aorta and its large branches are distended by the stroke volume, thus permitting temporary storage of at least part of it and dampening the pressure rise. During diastole the vessels return to their resting diameter and in so doing discharge blood into the peripheral circulation.

With advancing age the distensibility of the aorta and its large branches diminishes and the full force of ejection is expressed (Fig. 5.1). This results in a high systolic pressure, a major amount of flow during systole, and a lesser amount during diastole.

This decrease in elasticity with advancing years is accompanied by an increase in pulse wave velocity and diminished compliance. These functions have been investigated intermittently during much of this century. In the 1920s Bramwell *et al.* [38] showed that pulse wave velocity increased with increasing age indicating a decrease in the elasticity of the arteries. Hallock & Benson studied the elastic properties of aortas obtained at autopsy [39,40]. They measured the volume—elasticity characteristics of 18 aortic segments taken from the descending aorta just beyond the arch. They found that young aortas had greater elasticity than old ones so that they could accommodate much larger volumes of blood without a change in pressure. They concluded

> The aorta as well as its main branches constitute an important dynamic unit of the cardiovascular apparatus. Thus, as a result of its elastic retraction during the phase of cardiac diastole, the aortic chamber functions in the capacity of a buffer system converting a cardiac outflow which would otherwise be intermittent into one which is continuous in the capillaries. In addition to its influence on the peripheral circulation the aorta tends to minimize the work of the heart by facilitating the discharge of blood from the left ventricle.

We have plenty of evidence that the latter conclusion is an important feature in isolated systolic hypertension and its risk for cardiac failure but we have no information that continuous flow into capillaries as provided by the elastic aorta has physiologic advantages.

Abboud & Huston [41,42], using a technique for estimating large artery rigidity developed by Conway & Smith [43] confirmed the findings of Hallock & Benson, that aortic rigidity increases with age. Other efforts to measure this change with advancing years have employed measurement of pulse wave velocity [44,45,46] because it is a direct function of arterial rigidity. The original demonstration by Bramwell *et al.* [38] of increasing pulse velocity with advancing age was confirmed by these studies [44,45,46]. Perhaps the most recent was that of

Avolio *et al.* [47] who used this measurement to study the effects of aging on arterial distensibility in an urban and a rural community in China with a high and low prevalence of hypertension, respectively. They confirmed that the increase in pulse wave velocity with age was independent of arterial pressure, although they found, as have others, that hypertension itself increases arterial rigidity.

These *in vitro* and *in vivo* studies have shown clearly that the compliance of the aorta and large vessels decreases with advancing age and, although this has been used as an explanation for systolic hypertension in the elderly, it seems clear that these changes occur in the absence of hypertension as well as in its presence.

Aging also affects small arteries independent of hypertension. Bell [48] studied the distribution of disease in small renal arteries and arterioles of 741 people of all ages, whose blood pressures prior to death were never higher than 140/90 mmHg. Of these, 534 were over the age of 50. He reported that about 31% of the latter group had evidence of intimal thickening of small arteries while 13.5% had evidence of arteriolosclerosis as shown by a subendothelial deposit of hyaline. Intimal thickening of small arteries increased with age and was most marked in the kidney. Arteriolosclerosis was very rare before the age of 40 and increased to 13.5% in those over 50 years. Bell concluded that the lesions of small renal arteries and arterioles are age changes occurring independent of hypertension.

Moritz & Oldt [49] did a similar autopsy study comparing the prevalence of lesions in small arteries and arterioles of normotensives and hypertensives. They found, as had Bell, that intimal hyalinization of these vessels was the most common change in nonhypertensives. Occasionally, medial hypertrophy was found as was endothelial hyperplasia. Lesions were not localized to the kidneys but found in the spleen, pancreas, adrenal, gastrointestinal tract, skeletal muscle, and liver in descending order of occurrence. Renal arteriolosclerosis was observed in 12% of normotensive individuals but this occurrence was substantially less than that reported by Bell. There were no sex or race differences in the frequency of renal arteriolar changes in normal people. They were struck by the differences between normotensives and hypertensives with regard to the frequency of renal lesions. Of the 200 autopsies examined, 109 had evidences of renal arteriolosclerosis and of these, 97

proved to be cases of chronic hypertension. This led them to conclude that renal arteriolosclerosis was a cause of chronic hypertension.

Since GFR is known to decrease with age, it becomes important to look for evidences of renal senescence other than in the arterioles and small arteries of the kidney. Kaplan *et al.* [50] examined kidneys obtained at autopsy from 122 patients ranging in age from 1 to 89 years who had no clinical evidence of renal disease or hypertension. They counted the percentage of sclerotic glomeruli as a function of age. This was found to range from less than 1% in ages up to 30, to 13.4% in ages 70−79, and 10.2% for ages 80−89. This increase in the number of sclerotic glomeruli with advancing age may, in part, be the reason for the decreases in renal blood flow (RBF) and glomerular filtration found with advancing years [51].

Hemodynamic changes

Systemic hemodynamic changes in response to age have been a focus of many studies since measurement of cardiac output became possible. Most of these showed a gradual reduction in the ability to sustain strenuous physical exercise and a lowered cardiac output, even at rest [52−55]. More recently it has become apparent that these changes do not totally reflect the effects of aging but rather relate significantly to the physical fitness of the subjects under study [56].

An example of one of the earlier studies is that of Julius *et al.* [55] which reported measurements of cardiac output and oxygen consumption of 54 sedentary subjects at rest and during progressive exercise up to the point of maximal voluntary effort. The subjects, who ranged in age from 18 to 68 years, were divided into three groups according to age: Group 1, 18−34 years; Group 2, 35−49 years; and Group 3, 50−69 years. The oldest subjects (Group 3) had a lower cardiac output at rest than the youngest ($P < 0.05$), but the change with exercise was similar to that of Groups 1 and 2. They also had the lowest maximum tolerated exercise level and, with exercise, a slower heart rate. Systolic pressure was slightly higher at rest in Group 3 than in Group 1 but this difference was not significant. However, during exercise it was significantly higher with an average of 203 mmHg as opposed to 173 mmHg for Group 1.

In 1985 investigators of the Baltimore Longitudinal Study on Aging clearly defined the importance of physical activity on cardiovascular performance during exercise [56]. Their study included 61 participants who ranged in age from 25 to 79 years and had no cardiac disease as far as stress electrocardiographic and thallium scintigraphic studies could determine. In this exercise study, left ventricular volume was determined by use of gated cardiac blood pool scans. The subjects carried out vigorous exercise on a bicycle ergometer. The study showed that resting cardiac output, end-systolic or end-diastolic volumes, and ejection fraction were not related to age. Similarly, during vigorous exercise cardiac output was not related to age but the age influence was seen in an increase in end-diastolic volume and stroke volume as well as a decrease in heart rate. Thus, the older subjects were able to maintain their cardiac output by a higher stroke volume, compensating for the decrease in heart rate. This increase in stroke volume was made possible by a larger end-diastolic volume. Positive correlations with age were found for systolic pressure at rest and, during exercise, with end-systolic and end-diastolic volumes. Heart rate during exercise was inversely correlated with age.

Another study showing the importance of physical activity in the maintenance of cardiovascular function is that of Parizkova et al. [57]. They investigated the influence of body composition and capillary density on aerobic capacity of young and elderly men. The young group averaged 21 years in age and although in good physical condition, they were not top athletes; mean age of the elderly men was 73 years. Lean body mass was significantly greater in the young than in the elderly men. Similarly, maximum oxygen uptake was greater in the young men but heart rate was slower. Examination of muscle biopsies from the quadriceps revealed that the number of muscle fibers per square millimeter was significantly higher in the elderly men whereas the number of capillaries was similar in both groups. Thus the capillary/fiber ratio was significantly higher in the young men and this was interpreted as representing a more favorable condition for the supply of oxygen and nutrients to working muscles.

Effects of age on renal hemodynamics have also been studied [58−60]. All have shown an age-related decline in RBF and GFR. In addition, Hollenberg et al. [60] have reported a smaller vasodilation of the renovascular bed following administration of acetylcholine or a sodium load. Lindeman et al. [51] studied subjects during water diuresis and found decreases of osmolar clearance and excretion rates of sodium, potassium, and chloride with age. In addition, free water clearance was affected less by a vasopressin infusion in older people than in younger. Epstein & Hollenberg examined the effects of age on renal sodium conservation during a 10 mmol sodium diet in 89 normal subjects who ranged in age from 18 to 76 years [61]. The half-time of the reduction in urinary sodium was 17.6 hours in subjects younger than 30 years, 23.5 for those aged 30 to 59, and 30.9 for those over 60 years of age.

Thus it can be seen that the renovascular bed is affected by age physiologically as well as anatomically. No one, however, has reported the effect of physical fitness on renal function as has been reported for cardiovascular performance. If the renal changes occur independently of systemic flow this would mean that there is a progressive decrease in the renal fraction of cardiac output [28] and this could be significant for a variety of kidney functions related to control of blood pressure.

Neural control mechanisms

Plasma norepinephrine concentration rises with age and this has been interpreted as indicating that there is a "constant hyperadrenergic state in the elderly" [25,26]. The evidence in support of this "hyperadrenergic state" has been summarized by Rowe et al. [26]. They note that not only is norepinephrine concentration increased with age but so also are the responses of plasma norepinephrine to stimuli that raise it such as standing and isometric exercise. Plasma norepinephrine has been reported to rise more in older people following an oral glucose load than in younger people. Levels of serum-free fatty acids taken as an indirect index of sympathoadrenal activity have been used in studies of the effects of serial learning tasks. It has been found that elderly men manifested significantly higher levels of free fatty acids during the task than did younger men and levels remained elevated for a longer time. Sleep studies have shown the relationship between plasma norepinephrine levels and sleep/wake stages. Older subjects were more wakeful than younger ones and had less Stage 4 and rapid-eye movement (REM) sleep. Plasma norepinephrine was found to be positively correlated with the percentage of wakefulness and negatively correlated with the percentage of Stage 4 sleep.

Review of the available literature suggests that whereas there may be abnormalities of the autonomic nervous system with aging, these are not consistent with a hyper-adrenergic state. Esler *et al.* [62] have demonstrated a reduced clearance of norepinephrine from the circulation with advancing age. Since this was not accompanied by an increased norepinephrine spillover rate into the circulation, the decreased clearance could be responsible for the higher norepinephrine levels found with advancing years. Not only is the clearance rate diminished but so also is the sensitivity of β-adrenoceptors as shown by Vestal *et al.* [63]. These investigators studied heart rate responses to intravenously administered isoproterenol and propranolol and found diminished sensitivity to both which was positively correlated with age. Further, Schocken & Roth [64] have reported a reduced number of β-receptors on human lymphocytes with advancing age although there was no change in affinity.

It is now well established that baroreflex sensitivity is diminished with advancing years [24] and this could account for the frequent occurrence of orthostatic hypotension in elderly people. In fact, this can be rather striking. Caird *et al.* [23] have reported the effect of 1 min of quiet standing in 494 people 65 years or older who were studied at home. They found that 24% of this population had a drop in systolic pressure of 20 mmHg or more on standing, 9% had a decrease of 30 mmHg or more, and in 5% the fall was 40 mmHg or greater. The frequency of orthostatic hypotension increased with age.

This discussion will not resolve the question whether the elevated plasma norepinephrine levels with advancing age represent a hyperadrenergic state or merely a diminished clearance with failure of the elevated levels to have physiologic significance because of reduced adrenergic receptor responsiveness. Since the sympathetic nervous system plays such an important role in hypertension, we will return to the subject in discussing the pathophysiology of hypertension in the elderly.

Renin–angiotensin–aldosterone system

This system has great importance in the control of pressure under normal circumstances. Angiotensin is the primary regulator of aldosterone secretion. Both renin–angiotensin and aldosterone have found to be influenced by age. Crane & Harris [14] studied patients aged 20–80 years with 20 or more in each decade—all normal subjects and none was hypertensive. Measurements were made on an unrestricted sodium intake and on the third day of a low-sodium diet (<10 mmol/day). Renin was measured on blood samples taken after 2 hours of ambulation. Both during the unrestricted sodium intake and the low-sodium diet, plasma renin activity was found to decline with increasing age so that values of subjects in the seventh decade was about 60% of those in younger age groups. In addition the response of renin activity to sodium restriction and standing was less in older subjects than in those younger. Aldosterone excretion rates also declined with increasing age so values for subjects in the eighth decade were 46% lower than those in the third decade. Similar decreases in aldosterone with advancing age were found on the low-sodium diet as well. These investigators noted, as had others [61], that there was a diminished ability to conserve sodium on a low-sodium diet with advancing years.

Glucose homeostasis

Aging impairs glucose metabolism and, like the control of arterial pressure, limits glucose homeostasis. As the United States' population's average blood pressure rises with age so too does fasting blood sugar. As the prevalence of hypertension increases with each decade from the second on (Table 5.2) so does the prevalence of diabetes mellitus (Table 5.5) and most of that increase is in the noninsulin dependent type. The reason for discussing

Table 5.5 Prevalence (percentage of population) of various classes of glucose intolerance, United States, 1976–1980. (From Minaker [66])

	Age (years)				
	20–74	20–44	45–54	55–64	65–74
Diagnosed diabetes	3.4	1.1	4.3	6.6	9.3
Undiagnosed diabetes	3.3	1.0	4.4	6.5	8.6
Impaired glucose tolerance	11.3	6.5	14.9	15.2	22.9
Total	18.0	8.6	23.6	28.3	40.8

the age-related impairment of glucose homeostasis in this chapter is because hypertension prevalence is increased by diabetes (Table 5.6) and this is widely believed to be related to insulin resistance. Two excellent reviews, one by Davidson [65] and the other by Minaker [66], succinctly describe the effect of aging on glucose metabolism. Those effects will be summarized briefly here and in a later chapter the relationship of hyperinsulinemia and insulin resistance to hypertension will be discussed.

In nondiabetics, fasting blood glucose levels rise with age at the rate of about 1 mg/dl per decade [65]. This seemingly insignificant change, which is not influenced by sex, fails to reveal the true situation and that becomes manifest under the influence of a glucose load. Thus Davidson reports that 1 hour values are increased on the average by 9.5 mg/dl per decade and for 2 hour values the average is 11 mg/dl per decade. Again these increases are the same in men as in women. The distribution of blood glucose levels after a glucose load is unimodel, as was found years ago by Pickering for blood pressure [2] and not bimodel indicating that there are not two separate populations, one diabetic and one normal. This effect is not due to an abnormality in glucose absorption since this has been found to be unaffected by age. It is well known that physical inactivity and low-carbohydrate diets can affect the results of glucose tolerance curves but when these factors are either taken into account or eliminated, the age effects are still seen although they have less impact [66]. Glucose absorption from the gastrointestinal tract is not affected by age because intravenous glucose tolerance tests show the same results as oral glucose loading.

Plasma insulin levels measured after oral or intravenous glucose tolerance tests have revealed slightly elevated levels in older people than in younger subjects. Using the hyperglycemic glucose clamp technique with steady-state plasma glucose levels maintained at 140, 180, 220, and 300 mg/dl, Andres & Tobin were able to study insulin release in subjects of varying ages [67]. They found that insulin secretory capacity decreased with age at all but the highest blood glucose level. Part of the increase has been shown to result from a progressive decline in insulin clearance [68,69]. This decrease makes possible slightly elevated insulin levels in the face of declining insulin release.

As mentioned before, there is much interest in decreased sensitivity of peripheral tissues to insulin (insulin resistance) as a possible mechanism in hypertension. Techniques used to measure this have involved insulin injection, euglycemic insulin infusions, i.e. by the insulin clamp technique, and forearm glucose uptake during varying degrees of hyperinsulinemia. The results have shown a reduction in glucose uptake in response to injections of insulin with advancing age and, with the euglycemic glucose clamp technique, age-related impairment of glucose disposal [70,71]. Even nonobese healthy men with normal glucose tolerance tests, eating normally and being physically active, showed marked insulin resistance. This appears to be due to a decrease in insulin-mediated glucose uptake that is not because of a change in insulin-receptor number or affinity.

Since the prevalence of diabetes mellitus, of the non-insulin-dependent type, increases with advancing years, as does glucose intolerance, it is important to realize that

Table 5.6 Changes in carbohydrate economy in aging and diabetes mellitus. (From Minaker [66])

	Aging	Diabetes mellitus
Fasting hyperglycemia	−	+++
Fasting hypoinsulinemia	−	++
Increased basal hepatic glucose production	−	+++
Decreased insulin release	+	+++
Impaired insulin clearance	+	±
Peripheral insulin resistance	+	+++
Decreased insulin receptors	−	++
Postreceptor defects	+	++
Obesity	+	++

Table 5.7 Percentage of diabetic and nondiabetic patients reporting a medical history of high blood pressure, United States, 1976−1980. (From Minaker [66])

Glucose tolerance status	Age (years)				
	20−74	20−44	45−54	55−64	65−74
Diagnosed diabetes	56.2	40.0	54.7	62.9	62.9
Undiagnosed diabetes*	50.0	31.2	51.4	50.5	58.9
Impaired glucose tolerance*	42.4	18.8	36.7	58.7	56.8
Normal glucose tolerance*	21.4	14.1	27.0	31.7	40.4
Ratio of diabetic patients/normal subjects	2.6	2.8	2.0	2.0	1.6

* National Diabetes Data Group criteria applied to the results of a 2-hour, 75 g oral glucose tolerance test.

these two situations are qualitatively and quantitatively different (Table 5.7).

Nondiabetic older subjects have no fasting hyperglycemia or hyperinsulinemia, no increased hepatic glucose production, or decreased insulin receptors. These characteristics are present in frankly diabetic individuals who also have decreased numbers of insulin receptors, greater postreceptor defects, and much greater prevalence of obesity, but the insulin clearance is not so impaired in the frankly diabetic as it is in the nondiabetic elderly. Since obesity is so common in people with Type II diabetes and much more prevalent than in the nondiabetic older subjects, it is tempting to suggest that the differences between the two groups is a function of obesity since the distribution of blood glucose levels is unimodel and not bimodel, which would suggest that the diabetes of the elderly is distinctly different from that of the glucose-impaired individuals.

Pathophysiology

Hemodynamics and volume factors

Essential hypertension
No clear qualitative differences between isolated systolic and systolic/diastolic hypertension have been defined. For this reason, the discussion of them is combined in this section. This absence of differences is probably not surprising since long-standing systolic/diastolic hypertension is associated with the same structural changes in the vascular system as occurs with aging. Three studies exemplify the abnormalities found in hypertensive

elderly people and the differences between systolic hypertension in young people and those older.

Messerli *et al.* [28] reported hemodynamics, plasma volume, plasma renin activity, and plasma catecholamine levels in 30 individuals older than 65 years comparing the results with those obtained in 30 individuals who were younger than 42 years. All patients were considered to have essential hypertension and all had diastolic pressures >90 mmHg when measured in the outpatient clinic. If patients had been under treatment, drugs were discontinued for at least 4 weeks before the study. The older and the younger subjects were matched for MAP. This meant that both systolic and diastolic pressures obtained at the time of the hemodynamic measurements were considerably different in the elderly as opposed to the young. The former group had an average systolic pressure of 182 and diastolic pressure of 81 mmHg while in the younger, the pressure averaged 153/93 mmHg. Mean arterial pressures were 114 and 113, respectively. Table 5.8 gives some of the results of the study. In the elderly group the following functions were significantly lower than those of the younger: cardiac index, stroke volume, mean rate of left ventricular ejection, central blood volume, total blood volume, RBF, and plasma renin activity; the following were significantly higher: TPR, ejection time, and renal vascular resistance. Echocardiography showed that the elderly group had significantly thicker left ventricular walls, more septal thickness, and greater left ventricular mass indices. As had been previously found for younger hypertensives, TPR was negatively correlated with total blood volume and these correlations held for both the elderly and the young group.

Table 5.8 Comparison of hemodynamic, volume, and humoral factors in old and young hypertensives. (From Messerli *et al.* [28])

	Old	Young	P
Age	73 ± 7	32 ± 7	
Systolic blood pressure	182 ± 32	153 ± 23	<0.001
Diastolic blood pressure	81 ± 11	93 ± 14	<0.001
Mean blood pressure	114 ± 17	113 ± 16	NS
Cardiac index (l/min per m²)	2.6 ± 0.48	3.4 ± 0.5	<0.001
Mean left ventricular ejection rate (ml/s)	214 ± 54	292 ± 55	<0.001
Total peripheral resistance (units)	26 ± 7	19 ± 4	<0.001
Ejection time (ms)	332 ± 30	295 ± 26	<0.001
Central blood volume (l)	2.4 ± 0.65	2.8 ± 0.58	<0.050
Total blood volume (l)	4.1 ± 0.80	4.6 ± 1.01	<0.032
Renal blood flow (ml/min)	674 ± 92	1110 ± 296	<0.001
Renal vascular resistance (units)	1691 ± 153	1012 ± 33	<0.001
Plasma renin activity (μg/ml per min)	0.45 ± 0.38	1.15 ± 0.87	<0.047

* Reprinted with modifications.
NS, not significant.

Adamopoulos *et al.* [72] studied systolic hypertension in 13 subjects <35 years of age and 13 subjects >35 years of age. Age of the young group averaged 27 years and that of the older, 49 years. Each group of hypertensives was age-matched with normotensive subjects. The younger hypertensives were distinguished from their age-matched normotensive controls by having higher pressures, faster heart rates, and a higher left ventricular ejection rate indices; TPR was the same in both groups. In contrast, the older hypertensives were distinguished from their control group by having not only higher pressures but also a diminished cardiac index, slower mean rate of left ventricular ejection, and higher TPR. Since the age of the older group was only given as >35 years, one could question including these results here. However, these were subjects with isolated systolic hypertension, all having diastolic pressures <90 mmHg and systolic pressures >140 mmHg. Furthermore, their hemodynamic features were the same as those reported by Messerli *et al.* for older hypertensives with isolated systolic hypertension at the time of study [28]. These investigators also reported that in two larger groups of older and younger hypertensives (31 and 29 men, respectively) plasma volume was significantly reduced in the older group. They concluded that systolic hypertension in the young has significantly different pathophysiologic characteristics in comparison to those older. The younger patients had a hyperkinetic circulation shown by an increased

heart rate, a rapid left ventricular ejection rate, slightly elevated cardiac index, and normal TPR. In contrast, the older patients had reduced cardiac output and left ventricular ejection rate with increased systemic vascular resistance.

Simon *et al.* [44] studied 27 men with systolic hypertension and compared findings with those obtained in 24 normotensive controls. Systolic hypertension was defined as a systolic pressure of ≥160 mmHg when diastolic pressure was always <95 mmHg. All subjects were matched with normotensives so that diastolic pressure was within 10 mmHg and age within 5 years. They estimated systemic arterial compliance by analyzing the diastolic phase of the arterial pressure curve. Patients were separated into those older than 35 years and those younger than 35 years. In contrast to the findings of Adamopoulos *et al.*, the older subjects did not have an increase in systemic vascular resistance when compared with control subjects, nor did they have a lower cardiac output. The difference was a decrease in arterial compliance.

Tarazi *et al.* [73] estimated aortic rigidity from the pulse pressure/stroke volume ratio and by measurement of pulse transmission time, i.e. from the onset of the second aortic sound to the nadir of the dicrotic wave recorded from the carotid artery. They reported that the pulse pressure/stroke volume ratio was significantly influenced not only by age but by diastolic pressure and

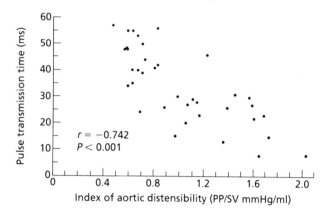

Fig. 5.2 Inverse relationship between pulse transmission time measured by a noninvasive technique and the index of aortic rigidity defined as PPISV; the greater the rigidity of the larger arteries the shorter the time for pulse transmission from the aorta to the carotid artery. (From Tarazi *et al.* [73].)

heart rate (Fig. 5.2). Pulse transmission time and the pulse pressure/stroke volume ratio were significantly correlated at a *P* of <0.001. Normotensives were found to have a pulse pressure/stroke volume of 0.56 and essential hypertensives (average age 40 years, average diastolic pressure 112 mmHg) a pulse pressure/stroke volume of 0.92. In an attempt to estimate aortic impedance clinically, they used the ratio of mean systolic pressure/ systolic flow. In 36 normal subjects with an average pressure of 121/73 and TPR of 29 μ/m^2, the systolic blood pressure/stroke volume was 754. In 40 patients with moderately severe hypertension (178/112 mmHg), TPR was 41 and systolic blood pressure/stroke volume was 1052. In contrast, in 23 patients with systolic hypertension (170/85), TPR was less than that of diastolic hypertensives at 35 μ/m^2 but systolic blood pressure/ stroke volume was 1052. Forty-five patients with much higher pressures were studied (205/128); TPR, as would be expected, was markedly elevated at 47 μ/m^2 up 63% from the normal value, while systolic blood pressure/ stroke volume was 1280 up 70% from the control value.

In summary, hemodynamic studies have shown that both essential hypertension and isolated systolic hypertension are usually associated with an increase in TPR. There does not seem to be any qualitative difference in the hemodynamic characteristics of these two types of hypertension; the difference is quantitative and relates to the magnitude of the TPR.

Renovascular hypertension

This discussion of the hemodynamics of renovascular hypertension in the elderly is limited by the fact that studies have not been restricted to older subjects with atherosclerotic stenosis and have included younger patients with fibrous dysplasia [74]. Regardless of pathology, this type of hypertension covers the broad spectrum seen in other types and can be classified as borderline, mild, moderate, severe, or accelerated. Regardless of type, the underlying cause is stimulation of the renin– angiotensin system of the kidney.

Cardiac output is often modestly elevated although it can be normal or decreased; peripheral resistance is elevated [74]. There is also evidence for stimulation of the nervous system, as shown in some cases by increased mean rate of left ventricular ejection, elevation of heart rate, and increase of the ratio of central blood volume/ total blood volume which indicated a decreased capacity of venous reservoirs [75]. In addition, orthostatic hypertension can be demonstrated as well as an exaggerated Valsalva overshoot. Plasma volume is characteristically decreased and correlates negatively with plasma renin activity [76].

Renin–angiotensin–aldosterone

Essential hypertension

As shown in the previous section, Crane & Harris [14] reported that plasma renin activity and aldosterone excretion rates fall with age. To determine the affect of elevated blood pressure on these functions, Tuck *et al.* [77] examined responses to 5 days of a low-sodium diet (10 mmol/day) in 100 patients with essential hypertension ranging in age from 20 to 65 years and compared results with those found in 50 normotensive subjects, 20–60 years of age. Plasma renin activity in response to the low-sodium diet and upright posture fell progressively with age from 20 ng/ml per 3 hours in the essential hypertensive group age 20–30 to 9.5 ng/ml per 3 hours in the patients aged 51–65. Aldosterone secretory rate similarly decreased from the youngest to the oldest age groups. This resulted in a significant increase in the incidence of low-renin hypertension with advancing years. With increasing levels of diastolic blood pressure there was also a significant increase in the incidence of suppressed renin activity and a fall in aldosterone secretory rate.

Known duration of hypertension did not appear to be a factor in determining plasma renin activity or aldosterone secretory rates.

Renovascular hypertension

Although the renin−angiotensin system of the kidney is responsible for renovascular hypertension, hyper-reninemia is not a constant finding. We found that plasma renin activity and arterial pressure were positively correlated so that hyperreninemia occurred only when arterial pressure was moderately to severely elevated [76]. Others reported that plasma angiotensin II levels correlated positively with arterial pressure in this type of hypertension [36]. Hypokalemia can occur in patients with severe renovascular hypertension and this is due to angiotensin-induced secondary aldosteronism. Brown et al. [36] reported finding a positive correlation of plasma angiotensin II and plasma aldosterone levels as well as evidence for inappropriate stimulation of aldosterone production because plasma aldosterone levels were higher for any given angiotensin II levels than found in normal subjects given angiotensin infusions.

Neural factors

As discussed in the previous section, aging has multiple effects on the sympathetic nervous system which could play a role in hypertension of the elderly. The increased plasma catecholamine levels, when taken as an index of increased sympathetic activity [26], may have little physiologic effect because of decreased responsiveness of receptors. However, the only receptor sensitivity decrease that has been associated with age is that of the β-adrenergic type and there has been no evidence for a decrease in α-receptor sensitivity. This could mean that stimulation of the latter is more effective because it is not counterbalanced by stimulation of the former.

The elevation of plasma norepinephrine and exaggerated responses to stimuli in the elderly could play a role in hypertension as a reflection of the decreased baroreflex sensitivity. The effectiveness of centrally acting α-agonists in the treatment of elevated pressure in such patients certainly indicates the importance of a neural component. However, great care must be taken in the use of these drugs because of the possibility of exaggerating already-present orthostatic hypotension [78].

There is, however, the possibility that adrenergic activity is different in older hypertensives than in older normotensives. Stern et al. found that 24-hour plasma catecholamine levels were lower in older subjects with essential hypertension than in age-matched controls, both groups being matched for body weight [79]. Goldstein et al. [80] observed that the age-effect on plasma norepine-phrine levels was obscured in hypertensives because of elevated values in those younger than in the elderly subjects.

Salt sensitivity

There are two lines of evidence suggesting that hypertension in the elderly is more apt to be of the salt-dependent type than that in younger individuals. The first comes from the SHEP of NHLBI which showed a surprising antihypertensive effectiveness of the diuretic chlorthalidone in people with isolated systolic hypertension [8]. The second line of evidence concerns the arterial pressure responses to rapid volume expansion followed by volume contraction as carried out by investigators at Indiana University [31,81]. These studies involved 378 normotensive subjects who ranged in age from 15 to 72 years and 198 essential hypertensives, 18−79 years. All subjects received 2 liters of normal saline over a 4-hour period from 8 am to 12 pm on the first day followed by a second day in which sodium and volume depletion were accomplished by a 10 mmol/sodium diet and three doses of furosemide (40 mg) given at 4-hour intervals. The arterial pressure measured at the end of the saline infusion was compared to that found the morning after the sodium and volume depletion. Subjects were divided according to age into groups less than 40 years and greater than 40 years. Those individuals who had a fall in blood pressure of more than 10 mmHg from salt loading to salt depletion were considered to have salt sensitive blood pressures whereas those having less than 5 mmHg or an increase in MAP were considered salt-resistant. Of the normotensives, 33% of those less than 40 years were found to have salt sensitive blood pressure and that percentage increased to 56% in those older than 40 years. The situation was different in the hypertensives because 52% of those less than 40 years had MAP responsive to volume expansion and contraction and that characteristic increased to 67% in those greater than 40 years. In both the normotensive and hypertensive groups, arterial pressure responses of the older subjects were significantly different from those of the younger. These findings have led to the recent recommendation [82] that hypertension in the elderly be treated routinely with moderate sodium restriction.

A role for insulin

One of the areas of great contemporary interest concerning the pathogenesis of hypertension is a role for insulin in increased vascular resistance. As discussed above, aging is associated with a progressive decline in carbohydrate tolerance and exaggerated glucose and insulin responses to a variety of stimuli. Insulin has also been demonstrated to have an acute effect on sodium metabolism by enhancing tubular reabsorption [18]. However, there is as yet no evidence that it can influence sodium balance in the long-run.

Hypertensives are more often obese than normotensives and obese individuals are well known to have glucose intolerance [19,83]. The current interest concerns linking hypertension to hyperinsulinemia or, in the case of non-obese young people [21], to insulin resistance. Modan et al. [83] concluded that membrane transport abnormalities and increased red cell sodium concentrations are characteristic of both hypertension and diabetes and that there is evidence for insulin involvement in potassium balance by affecting its uptake by liver and muscle. Their study showed significantly increased sodium concentrations in red blood cells and reduced erythrocyte potassium in both hypertension and obesity associated with abnormal glucose tolerance. Varricchio et al. [84] postulate that hyperinsulinemia plays a major role in the increased vascular resistance of essential hypertensives not only through its effect on intracellular cation concentrations but also overall on sodium balance and body sodium stores as well as being a growth factor for vascular smooth-muscle.

Reaven, in a masterly summary of the role of insulin resistance in human disease, suggests that hyperinsulinemia is related to hypertension, in part, through activation of the sympathetic nervous system [85]. Hwang I-S et al. found that fructose feeding to rats produced hyperinsulinemia, insulin resistance, and hypertension [86]. All abnormalities remitted when fructose feeding was stopped and they also could be attenuated if the fructose-fed rats were not caged but were allowed to exercise spontaneously [87]. In man, exercise reduced mildly elevated blood pressures in those individuals whose plasma catecholamine levels fell as well [88]. Furthermore, administration of clonidine prevented the hypertension of fructose feedings [87].

These are exceptionally interesting observations because not only do they provide new insights into possible mechanisms of hypertension but also hold promise for explaining the hypertension of obesity and, possibly, hypertension in the elderly.

References

1 Wilson LL, Dustan HP, Page IH, et al. Diagnosis of renal arterial lesions. Arch Intern Med 1963;27:1018–1027.

2 Pickering TG. The inheritance of arterial pressure. In Pickering TG, ed. High Blood Pressure, 2nd edn. New York: Grune & Stratton, 1968.

3 Pickering TG. Is there a dividing line between normal and raised arterial pressure? In Pickering G, ed. High Blood Pressure, 2nd edn. New York: Grune & Stratton, 1968.

4 The 1984 Report of the Joint National Committee on Detection, Evaluation, and Treatment of High Blood Pressure. Arch Intern Med 1984;144:1045–1057.

5 Blood Pressure Study. Acturial Society of America and Association of Life Insurance Medical Directors. New York, 1925.

6 Blood Pressure Study 1979. Association of Life Insurance Medical Directors and the Society of Actuaries, 1980.

7 Subcommittee on Definition and Prevalence of the 1984 Joint National Committee. Hypertension prevalence and the status of awareness, treatment and control in the United States. Hypertension 1985;7:457–468.

8 Hulley SB, Furberg CD, Gurland B, et al. Systolic Hypertension in the Elderly Program (SHEP): Anti-hypertensive efficacy of chlorthalidone. Am J Cardiol 1985;56:913–920.

9 Gorlin R. The hyperkinetic heart syndrome. J Am Med Assoc 1962;182:823–829.

10 Frohlich ED, Tarazi RC, Dustan HP. Hyperdynamic beta-adrenergic circulatory state. Arch Intern Med 1966;117:614–619.

11 Dustan HP, Tarazi RC, Hinshaw LB. Mechanisms controlling arterial pressure. In Frohlich ED, ed. Pathophysiology: Altered Regulatory Mechanisms in Disease, 2nd edn. Philadelphia: Lippincott, 1976.

12 Frohlich ED, Messerli FH, Reisin E, et al. The problem of obesity and hypertension. Hypertension 1983;5:III71–III77.

13 Ulrych M, Frohlich ED, Tarazi RC, et al. Cardiac output and distribution of blood volume in central and peripheral circulations in hypertensive and normotensive man. Brit Heart J 1969;31:570–574.

14 Crane MG, Harris JJ. Effect of aging on renin activity and aldosterone excretion. J Lab Clin Med 1987;87:947–959.

15 Dzau VJ. Significance of the vascular renin–angiotensin pathway. Hypertension 1986;8:553–559.

16 Overbeck HW, Derifield RS, Pamnani MB, et al. Attenu-

ated vasodilator responses to K[+] in essential hypertensive man. J Clin Invest 1974;53:678–686.

17 Meyer P, Garay RP, De Mendonca M. Ion transport systems in hypertension. In Genest J, Kuchel O, Hamet P, et al., eds. Hypertension, 2nd edn. New York: McGraw-Hill, 1983.

18 DeFronzo RA. The effect of insulin on renal sodium metabolism. Diabetologia 1981;21:165–171.

19 Drury PL. Diabetes and arterial hypertension. Diabetologia 1983;24:1–9.

20 Fournier AM, Gadia MT, Kubrusly DB, et al. Blood pressure, insulin, and glycemia in nondiabetic subjects. Am J Med 1986;80:861–704.

21 Ferrannini E, Buzzigoli G, Bonadonna R, et al. Insulin resistance in essential hypertension. N Engl J Med 1987;317:350–357.

22 Folkow B, Neil E. Chap. 16. The principles of vascular control. In Folkow B, Neil E, eds. Circulation. New York: Oxford University Press, 1971.

23 Caird FI, Andrews GR, Kennedy RD. Effect of posture on blood pressure in the elderly. Br Heart J 1973;35:527–530.

24 Gribbin B, Pickering TG, Sleight P, et al. Effect of age and high blood pressure on baroreflex sensitivity in man. Circ Res 1971;29:424–431.

25 Sowers JR. Hypertension in the elderly. Am J Med 1987;82:1–8.

26 Rowe JW, Minaker KL, Pallotta JA, et al. Characterization of the insulin resistance of aging. J Clin Invest 1983;71:1581–1587.

27 Tarazi RC. Hemodynamic role of extracellular fluid. Circ Res 1976;38:II73–II83.

28 Messerli FH, Sundgaard-Ruse K, Ventura HO, et al. Essential hypertension in the elderly: haemodynamics, intravascular, volume, plasma renin activity, and circulating cathecholamine levels. Lancet 1983;2:983–985.

29 Tarazi RC, Dustan HP, Frohlich ED, et al. Plasma volume and chronic hypertension. Arch Intern Med 1970;125:835–842.

30 Rushmer RF. Properties of the vascular system. In Rushmer RF, ed. Cardiovascular Dynamics. Philadelphia: WB Saunders Co., 1970.

31 Luft FC, Weinberger MH, Fineberg NS, et al. Effects of age on renal sodium homeostasis and its relevance to sodium sensitivity. Am J Med 1987;82:9–15.

32 Laragh JH, Sealey JE, Sommers SC. Patterns of adrenal secretion and urinary excretion of aldosterone and plasma renin activity in normal and hypertensive subjects. Circ Res 1966;19:158–174.

33 Hudson JB, Chobanian AV, Relman AS. Hypoaldosteronism. N Engl J Med 1957;257:529–536.

34 Bravo EL, Dustan HP, Tarazi RC. Spironolactone as a nonspecific treatment for primary aldosteronism. Circulation 1973;48:491–498.

35 Dustan HP, Kirk KA. The case for or against salt in hypertension. Hypertension 1989;13:696–705.

36 Brown J, Casals-Stenzel J, Cumming AMM, et al. Angiotensin II, aldosterone and arterial pressure: a quantitative approach. Hypertension 1979;1:159–178.

37 Titus JL, Kim HS. Blood vessels and lymphutics. In Kissane JM, ed. Anderson's Pathology, 8th edn. St. Louis: CV Mosby Co., 1985.

38 Bramwell JC, Hill AV, McSwiney BA. The velocity of the pulse wave in man in relation to age as measured by the hot-wire sphygmograph. Heart 1923;10:233–255.

39 Hallock P. Arterial elasticity in man in relation to age as evaluated by the pulse wave velocity method. Arch Intern Med 1934;54:770–797.

40 Hallock P, Benson IC. Studies on the elastic properties of human isolated aorta. J Clin Invest 1937;16:595–602.

41 Abboud FM, Huston JH. The effects of aging and degenerative vascular disease on the measurement of arterial rigidity in man. J Clin Invest 1961;40:933–939.

42 Abboud FM, Huston JH. Measurement of arterial aging in hypertensive patients. J Clin Invest 1961;40:1913–1921.

43 Conway J, Smith KS. A clinical method of studying the elasticity of large arteries. Br Heart J 1956;18:467–474.

44 Simon AC, Safar ME, Levenson JA, et al. An evaluation of large arteries compliance in man. Am J Physiol 1979;237:H550–H554.

45 Eliakim M, Sapoznikov D, Weinman J. Pulse wave velocity in healthy subjects and in patients with various disease states. Am Heart J 1971;82:448–457.

46 Avolio AP, Chen SG, Wang RP, et al. Effects of aging on changing arterial compliance and left ventricular load in a northern Chinese urban community. Circulation 1983;68:50–58.

47 Avolio AP, Quan DF, Qiang LW. Effects of aging on arterial distensibility in populations with high and low prevalence of hypertension: comparison between urban and rural communities in China. Circulation 1985;71:202–210.

48 Bell ET. The pathological anatomy in primary hypertension. In Bell ET, Clawson BJ, Fahr GE, eds. Hypertension, A Symposium. Minneapolis: University of Minnesota Press, 1951.

49 Moritz AR, Oldt MR. Arteriolar sclerosis in hypertensive and nonhypertensive individuals. Am J Pathol 1937;13:679–735.

50 Kaplan C, Pasternack B, Shah H, et al. Age-related incidence of sclerotic glomeruli in human kidneys. Am J Pathol 1975;80:227–234.

51 Lindeman RD, Lee TD Jr, Yiengst MJ, et al. Influence of age, renal disease, hypertension, diuretics, and calcium on the antidiuretic responses to suboptimal infusions of vasopressin. J Lab Clin Med 1966;68:206–223.

52 Brandfonbrener M, Landowne M, Shock NW. Changes in cardiac output with age. Circulation 1955;12:557–566.

53 Strandell T. Circulatory studies on healthy old men. Acta Med Scand 1964;175(Suppl.414):1–44.

54 Granath A, Jonsson B, Strandell T. Circulation in healthy old men studied by right heart catheterization at rest and during exercise in supine and sitting position. Acta Med Scand

1964;176:425−446.

55 Julius S, Amery A, Whitlock LS, *et al.* Influence of age on the hemodynamic response to exercise. Circulation 1967;36:222−230.

56 Rodeheffer RJ, Gerstenblith G, Becker LC, *et al.* Exercise cardiac output is maintained with advancing age in healthy human subjects: cardiac dilatation and increased stroke volume compensate for a diminished heart rate. Circulation 1984;69:203−213.

57 Parizkova J, Eiselt E, Sprynarova S, *et al.* Body composition, aerobic capacity, and density of muscle capillaries in young and old men. J Appl Physiol 1971;31:323−325.

58 Papper S. The effects of age in reducing renal function. Geriatrics 1973;28:83−87.

59 Davies DF, Shock NW. Age changes in glomerular filtration rate, effective renal plasma flow and tubular excretory capacity in adult males. J Clin Invest 1950;29:496−507.

60 Hollenberg NK, Adams DF, Solomon HS, *et al.* Senescence and the renal vasculature in normal man. Circ Res 1974;34:309−316.

61 Epstein M, Hollenberg NK. Age as a determinant of renal sodium conservation in normal man. J Lab Clin Med 1976;87:411−417.

62 Esler M, Skews H, Leonard P, *et al.* Age-dependence of noradrenaline kinetics in normal subjects. Clin Sci 1981;60:217−219.

63 Vestal RE, Wood AJJ, Shand DG. Reduced β-adrenoceptor sensitivity in the elderly. Clin Pharmacol 1979;26:181−186.

64 Schocken D, Roth G. Reduced β-adrenergic receptor concentrations in aging man. Nature 1977;267:856−858.

65 Davidson MB. The effect of aging on carbohydrate metabolism: a review of the english literature and a practical approach to the diagnosis of diabetes mellitus in the elderly. Metabolism 1979;28:688−705.

66 Minaker KL. Aging and diabetes mellitus as risk factors for vascular disease. Am J Med 1987;82:47−53.

67 Andres R, Tobin JD. Aging and the disposition of glucose. Adv Exp Med Biol 1975;61:239−249.

68 Minaker KL, Rowe JW, Tonino RB. Influence of age on clearance of insulin in man. Diabetes 1982;31:851−855.

69 Chen M, Bergman RN, Pacini G, *et al.* Pathogenesis of age-related glucose intolerance in man: insulin resistance and decreased b-cell function. J Clin Endocrinol Metab 1985;60:13−20.

70 Fink RI, Kolterman OG, Griffin J, *et al.* Mechanisms of insulin resistance in aging. J Clin Invest 1983;71:1523−1535.

71 Rowe JW, Minaker KL, Pallotta JA, *et al.* Characterization of the insulin resistance of aging. J Clin Invest 1983;71:1581−1587.

72 Adamopoulos PH, Chrysanthakopoulis SG, Frohlich ED. Systolic hypertension: nonhomogeneous diseases. Am J Cardiol 1975;36:697−701.

73 Tarazi RC, Magrini F, Dustan HP. The role of aortic distensibility in hypertension. In Milliez P, Safar M, eds. *Recent Advances in Hypertension.* Laboratoires Boehringer Ingelheim 1975;2:133−141.

74 Tarazi RC, Frohlich ED, Dustan HP. Contribution of cardiac output to renovascular hypertension: relation to surgical treatment. Am J Cardiol 1973;31:600−605.

75 Frohlich ED, Tarazi RC, Dustan HP. Hemodynamic and functional mechanisms in two renal hypertensions: arterial and pyelonephritis. Am J Med Sci 1971;261:189−195.

76 Dustan HP, Tarazi RC, Frohlich ED. Functional correlates of plasma renin activity in hypertensive patients. Circulation 1970;41:555−567.

77 Tuck ML, Williams GH, Cain JP, *et al.* Relation of age, diastolic pressure, and known duration of hypertension to presence of low renin essential hypertension. Am J Cardiol 1973;32:637−642.

78 Gifford RW. Isolated systolic hypertension in the elderly. J Am Med Assoc 1982;247:781−785.

79 Stern N, Buhm E, McGinty D. Dissociation of 24 hour catecholamine levels from blood pressure in older men. Hypertension 1985;7:1023−1029.

80 Goldstein DS, Lake CR, Chernow B. Age-dependence of hypertensive−normotensive differences in plasma norepinephrine. Hypertension 1983;5:100−104.

81 Weinberger MH, Miller JZ, Luft FC. Sodium sensitivity and resistance of blood pressure: definitions and characteristics. Hypertension 1986;8:127−134.

82 The 1988 Report of the Joint National Committee on Detection, Evaluation, and Treatment of High Blood Pressure. Arch Intern Med 1988;148:1023−1038.

83 Modan M, Halkin H, Almog S, *et al.* Hyperinsulinemia: a link between hypertension obesity and glucose intolerance. J Clin Invest 1985;75:809−817.

84 Varricchio M, Paolisso G, Torella R, *et al.* Diabetes and hypertension in the elderly. J Hypertens 1988;6:S41−S44.

85 Reaven GM. Banting Lecture 1988. Role of insulin resistance in human disease. Diabetes 1988;37:1595−1607.

86 Hwang I-S, Ho H, Hoffman BB, *et al.* Fructose-induced insulin resistance and hypertension in rats. Hypertension 1987;10:512−516.

87 Reaven GM, Ho H, Hoffman BB. Attenuation of fructose-induced hypertension in rats by exercise training. Hypertension 1988;12:129−132.

88 Duncan JJ, Farr JE, Upton SJ, *et al.* The effects of aerobic exercise on plasma catecholamines and blood pressure in patients with mild essential hypertension. J Am Med Assoc 1985;254:2609−2613.

6

Isolated systolic hypertension in the elderly

José L. Cangiano
Manuel Martinez-Maldonado

Introduction

In most western societies systolic blood pressure (SBP) and diastolic blood pressures (DBP) begin to increase in adolescence. This trend is continued until the age of 45−59 years when DBP reaches a plateau and SBP gradually increases in disproportion to the DBP [1]. As age advances SBP may continue to increase. This progressive increase in SBP without elevation of DBP may then give rise to isolated systolic hypertension (ISH).

Isolated systolic hypertension was ignored for many years, but as clinical studies began to demonstrate an increased cardiovascular risk in systemic hypertension, close attention was given to the elevation of the SBP and DBP. Initially, particular emphasis was focused on DBP as a cardiovascular risk factor [2−5] and the relevance of increased levels of SBP was not critically examined. Nonetheless, a growing body of epidemiologic data documented an increase in morbidity and mortality in people over 65 years of age with elevation of SBP alone [6]. Moreover, it became apparent that systolic hypertension may be a more significant contributor to the development of cardiovascular disease than is diastolic hypertension [7−10].

In view of this strong epidemiologic evidence, it was of particular importance to ascertain the benefits or risks of lowering SBP in elderly patients in whom systolic hypertension is common. Preliminary reports in small groups of patients emphasized that antihypertensive medications may lower SBP without major deleterious effects [11,12]. In recent years a large multiclinic, controlled study, The Systolic Hypertension in the Elderly Program (SHEP), was designed in an attempt to establish a definitive approach for the management of ISH [13]. The final results of the study were recently published.

It is the intention of this chapter to review the definition, epidemiology, and pathophysiologic mechanisms of ISH. Data from SHEP are reviewed and the risks involved in the management of ISH are discussed. Finally, some practical suggestions about therapeutic interventions are made.

Definition

In middle-aged individuals systemic hypertension is defined as a SBP above 150 mmHg and a DBP above 90 mmHg. In this age group pure diastolic hypertension may occur, but most individuals have a systolic/diastolic hypertension. In contrast to the younger group, pure diastolic hypertension is very rare in the elderly and most patients have systolic/diastolic hypertension or purely systolic hypertension. In the elderly individual an accepted definition of diastolic hypertension is a level of DBP above 90 mmHg. However, a precise definition of systolic hypertension in the elderly has been lacking for many years. Different investigators used arbitrary cut-off values to define systolic hypertension suggesting levels of 150, 160, or even 180 mmHg. For this reason, various reports in the elderly are difficult to reconcile and a great deal of caution must be used to make final interpretations. Nonetheless, recent reports have attempted to standardize the definitions of hypertensive states in the elderly.

Table 6.1 shows that hypertension in the elderly can be classified into two general categories: systolic/diastolic hypertension and pure systolic hypertension.

Systolic/diastolic hypertension is further subdivided into proportionate and disproportionate. Proportionate or classical hypertension is the form of hypertension which most clinical trials have addressed and is the most prevalent in middle-aged individuals. It is defined as an increase in DBP over 90 mmHg with a proportionate elevation of SBP. Disproportionate systolic hypertension is mostly observed in elderly individuals and has been arbitrarily defined as SBP exceeding twice the DBP minus 15 mmHg [14].

The 1984 Report of the Joint National Committee on Detection, Evaluation and Treatment of High Blood Pressure divided pure systolic hypertension into borderline ISH and ISH [15]. Borderline ISH was defined as a SBP of 140–159 mmHg with a DBP of 90 mmHg or less. On the other hand, ISH was defined as a SBP over 160 mmHg with a DBP of 90 mmHg or less.

Epidemiology

It is not a universal observation that as people get older, elevation of SBP generally predominates over DBP. For example, in primitive societies SBP and DBP maintain a low level throughout their lifetime [16]. A lesser increase in blood pressure has also been observed in certain rural communities [17,18]. Nutritional, environmental, and/or behavioral changes may be responsible for this observation. In contrast, it is a common finding in the individuals of industrialized nations to present a rise in SBP and pulse pressure with age.

Several studies have been able to determine the prevalence of ISH in different populations. The National Health Examination Survey for 1960–1962 obtained blood pressure readings at a single visit [19,20]. An average of three consecutive readings were obtained. Isolated systolic hypertension was defined as a SBP greater than 160 mmHg with a DBP less than 95 mmHg. The prevalence was virtually nonexistent before age 44 years, but progressively increased after this age. It was higher in women and blacks as compared to men and whites. In this study white men aged 65–74 exhibit a prevalence of 15% and prevalence was 42% in black women aged 75–79.

The Framingham Study has reported a similar increase in SBP with age [21]. This study started in 1948 with a cohort population of 5209 individuals between the ages of 30–62. Blood pressure was recorded in a standardized manner, the second of three sitting left arm measurements. Isolated systolic hypertension was uncommon below the age of 45 years; the prevalence rose after the age of 55 years in both sexes but most steeply in women.

In 1982 Wing *et al.* [22] reported the prevalence of ISH in 3102 residents of Evans County, Georgia. This biracial population was screened in 1960 and re-examined in

Table 6.1 Classification and definition of hypertension in the elderly

Classification	Definition

Systolic/diastolic hypertension
    Proportionate (classical) — increase
    in DBP over 90 mmHg with a
    proportionate elevation of SBP
    Disproportionate — SBP exceeding
    twice the DBP minus 15 mmHg
	Pure systolic hypertension
	    Borderline isolated — SBP of
	    140–159 mmHg with a DBP of
	    90 mmHg or less
	    Isolated — SBP over 160 mmHg with a
	    DBP of 90 mmHg or less

1967–1969. The mean of the second and third readings of blood pressure was determined. As in the previous studies, ISH was rare below age 50 years. The prevalence increased with age for all sex/race groups.

The Hypertension Detection and Follow-Up Program [23] reported the prevalence of ISH in 160 000 patients aged 60–69 yeas in 14 communities. The definition of ISH used in this study was different from other studies. Isolated systolic hypertension was defined as a SBP greater than 160 mmHg with a DBP less than 90 mmHg. The prevalence of ISH was higher in women than men and higher in blacks than whites. It was reported as 8.3% for black women and 7.4% for white women, and 6.4% for black men and 5.7% for white men. A prospective report of this study showed a prevalence of 3.3% in patients 60–64 years and 10.9% in those 75 years of age and over [24].

After 30 years of follow-up in the Framingham Study [25] the age-adjusted prevalence of ISH was 14.4% of the males over age 65 years, whereas 22.8% of females over age 65 years had this condition. Of interest, the increased prevalence and incidence was not exclusive to the elderly, but a sharp increase was observed from ages 35 to 64 years. The peak of the incidence in women is reported from 55 to 64 years, whereas in men the incidence continues to rise from ages 65 to 74 years. Isolated systolic hypertension accounted for 57.4% of all hypertensive conditions in men 65 years or older and 65.1% in women older than 65 years.

In addition, the SHEP pilot study revealed a prevalence of 10% in people more than 70 years of age and 20% in people more than 80 years of age [26].

As can be observed, most studies have shown an increased prevalence of ISH in the elderly. However, variations can be expected in reporting prevalence of ISH, especially when using different definitions, different numbers of readings, and times of obtaining blood pressure [8,23]. Other factors may also be important in explaining these variations. McClellan et al. [27] conducted a population-based survey on 4672 adult residents of Georgia in 1981. Prevalence rates in this community were considerably below those reported in the above studies. These investigators concluded that the decrease in prevalence of the population in Georgia may represent an overall trend for early and more aggressive treatment of hypertension in the adult and in the elderly.

Risk of systolic hypertension

The pathogenic significance of systolic hypertension has been a controversial issue. Some clinicians downplay the importance of systolic hypertension claiming that diastolic hypertension produces an increased number of cardiovascular complications. This notwithstanding, epidemiologic data unequivocally supports that when compared to diastolic hypertension, systolic hypertension is associated with a greater increase in cardiovascular morbidity and mortality.

The 1959 Build and Blood Pressure study [28] provided ample evidence to support the increased cardiovascular risk with systolic hypertension. This study obtained the pooled experience of 26 insurance companies in the United States and Canada with 3.9 million policy holders between the ages of 15–69 years. The results suggest that, at any level of DBP, mortality increases in proportion to the levels of systolic pressure up to 158–167 mmHg over a follow-up average period close to 9 years. More recent data in this study demonstrates a reduction in mortality for a subgroup of 20 000 men receiving antihypertensive treatment [29].

The Chicago People Gas Company Study made a longitudinal assessment of the natural history of cardiovascular disease in white men between the ages of 40–59 years [30]. After a 15-year follow-up period patients with ISH at the time of enrollment had nearly two-fold increase in the expected death rate.

The Chicago Stroke Study [31] included 2772 black and white people between the ages of 65–74 years. A subgroup with entry DBP less than 95 mmHg showed no changes in mortality until systolic pressure was over 180 mmHg, at which point mortality increased by 59%. This group had twice the risk of death from cardiovascular and renal involvement and a 2.5 times greater incidence of stroke.

In the Framingham Study the level of SBP rather than DBP, was strongly associated to coronary heart disease, cerebrovascular disease, congestive heart failure, and left ventricular hypertrophy [32–35]. Although age is an important factor in cardiovascular mortality, this study has shown a high correlation between stroke and the level of systolic pressure which appeared to be independent of age [36].

A prospective study in 2632 residents of Rancho

Bernardo, California [24], analyzed the mortality rate associated with ISH. During an average follow-up period of 6.3 years, men had a higher mortality rate despite the fact that women had a higher prevalence of ISH.

In the Leisure World Retirement Community at Seal Beach, California, [8] 72 patients with ISH, mean age 65–74 years, were matched for age, sex, and DBP with patients whose blood pressure were below 140/90 mmHg. During a 4-year follow-up period patients with ISH had a higher cardiovascular mortality. A trend for an increase in coronary heart disease and stroke was observed, although the increase did not attain statistical significance.

It can be argued that SBP elevation is a manifestation of decreased arterial compliance which in turn, may be a consequence of atherosclerosis. As a result, an increase in cardiovascular morbidity and mortality can be expected. However, the Framingham Study further demonstrates that SBP is a risk factor independent of arterial rigidity and atherosclerosis [21].

It has been known for several years that left ventricular hypertrophy is an independent cardiovascular risk factor [37]. It is also recognized that left ventricular hypertrophy is more prevalent in the elderly and is highly correlated to SBP [38]. Therefore, the presence of left ventricular hypertrophy on systolic hypertension confers an increased risk for overall cardiovascular mortality, which makes the treatment of ISH of greater importance in patients with left ventricular hypertrophy. Other risk factors such as increased total cholesterol and decreased high-density lipoprotein may compound the risk for elderly patients with ISH.

Determinants of SBP and DBP

The arterial pressure is given by two variables: mean arterial pressure (MAP) and pulse pressure. Mean arterial pressure is the average pressure in the arterial system during a cardiac cycle. It can be approximated by the equation $MAP = 1/3 \ (2 \times DBP + SBP)$. In the cardiovascular system, MAP is directly proportional to cardiac output and total peripheral resistance. An increase in cardiac output or total peripheral resistance results in an increase in MAP, with an increase in SBP and DBP. It is predominantly determined by the arterial distensibility or compliance and by the stroke volume. Arterial distensibility is the change in volume produced by a unit change in pressure in the arterial tree. Arterial distensibility has no effect on MAP as long as cardiac output and total peripheral resistance remain constant.

Stroke volume also determines pulse pressure. If heart rate remains constant an increase in stroke volume may result in an increase in cardiac output and, therefore, MAP. Both SBP and DBP increase but SBP will rise to a much greater extent. It is also evident that as stroke volume increases the pulse pressure also increases. In addition, a rise in SBP occurs as the arterial wall becomes stiffer when stretched rapidly and as the velocity of ejection increase.

Figure 6.1 shows the principal determinants of SBP and DBP. Systolic blood pressure is influenced or modified by the arterial distensibility, stroke volume, and the velocity of ejection or the rate at which blood is pumped into the elastic reservoir. On the other hand, DBP is determined by the height of the SBP and the rate at which blood leaves the aorta. The latter is influenced by the peripheral resistance and the duration of diastole.

Pathophysiologic characteristics

Structural changes

Advancing age affects the anatomy and physiology of the cardiovascular system. Structural and functional changes are observed in the arteries and cerebrocardiorenal parenchymas. The aorta and large vessels normally possess viscoelastic properties which relate to the presence of

Systolic determinants		Diastolic determinants
Systolic ejection velocity,	Systolic Diastolic	Starting systolic pressure
Stroke volume	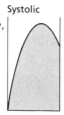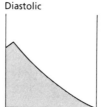	Aortic compliance
Aortic compliance		Heart rate
Volume leaving aorta during systole		Peripheral resistance

Fig. 6.1 The principal determinants of systolic and diastolic blood pressures.

elastic and smooth-muscle fibers. With senescence there is arterial intimal thickening [39]. The endothelial surface appears irregular with an increased number and accummulation of subendothelial cells [40]. In the arterial media, collagen content increases and elastin is replaced by lipid infiltration, followed by thickening and atheromatous formation with vascular wall calcification [41]. Other changes may occur such as waterlogging and redesign of elastic lamellar units and interlamellar space [42]. There is loss of elasticity and compliance with elongation, tortuosity, and obstruction of arteries. These abnormalities together with an increased prevalence of atherosclerosis make the vessels become like rigid tubes and may result in increased peripheral vascular resistance and aortic impedance [43].

Blood flow and pressure increase during systole and fall during diastole. However, the elastic recoil (Windkessel effect) of the aorta and large vessels maintain pressure and flow during diastole. In addition, aortic distensibility reduces the workload of the left ventricle on ejection of the stroke volume. It is then clear that a decrease in aortic distensibility does not sustain forward flow in diastole, requiring that the left ventricle adapts to maintain forward flow. In due time this functional maladaptation results in left ventricular hypertrophy.

Functional changes

In addition to the above mentioned changes in vascular structure, age-related changes in vascular function have been described. The α- and β-adrenergic responsiveness of vascular smooth muscle has been extensively studied in the elderly. Although many conflicting results have been published, the α-adrenergic responsiveness appears to be unchanged with age [44]. Beta-adrenergic responsiveness of vascular smooth muscle is reduced with age [45,46]. This abnormality may decrease the relaxation of vascular smooth muscle and contribute to the increased peripheral resistance. In fact, Abrass [44] has postulated that the increase in peripheral resistance in elderly hypertensives is a result of diminished β-adrenergic mediated vasodilation with unopposed α-adrenergic mediated vasoconstriction. If this abnormality is critical for the increased peripheral resistance in the elderly hypertensive, it makes α-adrenergic inhibitors very attractive for treatment.

In recent years, distinct abnormalities in ion transport across cellular membranes have been identified in hyper-

tensive patients. There is ample evidence to support a critical role of the calcium ion in vascular smooth muscle contraction and increased peripheral vascular resistance. Perturbations of Na−K cotransport, Na−Li countertransport, ouabain sensitive Na−K−ATPase activity, and intracellular calcium have been described in middle-aged hypertensives. Similar abnormalities have not been demonstrated with age, except for the experimental studies of Cohen & Berkowitz [47] who showed that senile rat aortic strips were dependent on extracellular calcium for norepenephrine-induced contraction. More studies concerning intracellular calcium abnormalities in the elderly are needed. However, the important role of increased intracellular calcium in sustaining blood pressure in the elderly is favored by the salutary response of elderly hypertensives to calcium channel blockers [48].

Endocrine and renal involvement

Advancing age displays major changes in the endocrine and renal function. Systems which control blood pressure such as the renin−angiotensin−aldosterone system, prostaglandin system, and atrial natriuretic peptide are clearly affected. Other systems, such as the kallikrein−kinin system, may also be affected but these have not been studied in depth with aging.

A persistent decline of plasma renin, aldosterone, plasma and angiotensin II levels is observed with age [49]. In addition to a low-renin state, the capacity to increase renin and aldosterone secretion following sodium restriction or furosemide administration is markedly impaired in elderly subjects [50]. This abnormal response to volume contraction makes the elderly more vulnerable to hypovolemia and hypotension.

As already mentioned, the prostaglandin system can also be affected. A diminution of prostaglandin excretion has been reported in old age [51]. Although the importance of this finding is not clear, it is well accepted that a reduction of prostaglandins could diminish sodium excretion.

Atrial natriuretic peptide has also been studied in the hypertensive elderly. Genest et al. [52] reported an increasing level of atrial natriuretic with age. Again, the relevance of this peptide to hypertensive disease in the elderly has not been clearly elucidated.

The kidneys are also affected by old age. Longitudinal studies have established a decline in glomerular filtration rate (GFR) even in the absence of renal disease [53]. Also, there is impairment of the capacity to retain or excrete sodium. Elderly people take longer to excrete a saline load but true retention of sodium is not usually observed. At present, renal mechanisms do not appear to be involved in the pathophysiology of ISH in the elderly. However, further studies of the role of endocrine and renal function in elderly patients with ISH should be undertaken.

Aortic distensibility

Several studies have documented that aortic distensibility decreases with age. Hallock & Benson [54] measured the changes in aortic volume and aortic pressure of 18 autopsied subjects between the ages of 20 and 78 years. Aortic distensibility decreased with age, beginning with the third decade of life. In another study with autopsy material in 13 subjects, Ho et al. [55] related the distensibility characteristics to the histologic findings. They investigated the relationship between changes in wall tension and aortic circumference. A progressive loss of aortic distensibility was observed with age, which appeared to be accelerated by the presence of atherosclerosis.

Clinical studies have also demonstrated a significant correlation between age and aortic rigidity. Abboud & Huston [56] showed that hypertensive patients had evidence of increased aortic rigidity with higher systolic pressures and pulse pressures. In their study, the individuals mostly affected were women (59%), diabetics (30%), and patients with aortic calcifications on chest X-ray studies.

Little is known about the regulating factors of aortic distensibility. Using lower body negative pressure, which modifies preload and adrenergic activity, Aziz Madkour et al. [57] reported modulation of arterial compliance in normal individuals but not in hypertensive patients. This study gives support to the early observation of Tarazi & Dustan [58] that an increased sympathetic tone might diminish distensibility of the aortic and large arteries.

Hemodynamic changes

Isolated systolic hypertension in the young patient is generally attributed to increased sympathetic tone, resulting in an increased cardiac output, increased heart rate, and a rapid ejection period. Total peripheral resistance is normal or diminished. In the elderly with systolic/diastolic hypertension cardiac output decreases, heart rate remains constant, and stroke volume is reduced. The hemodynamic derangement in ISH in the elderly, however, has been the subject of numerous studies. Simon et al. [59] have proposed that the main abnormality is a reduced arterial distensibility without a rise in total peripheral resistance. This observation has been challenged by the results of Smulyan et al. [60] who suggested that the decrease in aortic distensibility is the result rather than the cause of an increased SBP. Moreover, Adamopoulos et al. [61] showed a greater total peripheral resistance in elderly patients with ISH compared to normotensive individuals in the same age group. These results have been supported by the studies of Vardan et al. [62] who lowered total peripheral resistance by the use of thiazide therapy. In addition, Berger & Li [63], using a computer simulation of the modified Windkessel model, concluded that ISH is the result of a greatly reduced arterial compliance along with a smaller but significant increase in peripheral resistance.

Patients with ISH usually show no changes in resting systolic left ventricular performance but have a reduced left ventricular diastolic performance [64]. Left ventricular hypertrophy, as detected by echocardiography, is a common finding in ISH [65]. The association of left ventricular hypertrophy and ISH carry an increased cardiovascular morbidity and mortality.

Pulse wave reflection

Another important aspect of the investigation of the mechanism involved in the production of ISH is based on the observation of the pressure contour in systemic arteries. The amplitude of systolic pressure is largely determined by the arterial distensibility, vascular impedance, pulse wave velocity, and pulse wave reflection. Recent work has shown that systolic pressure in the central aorta is markedly increased in hypertension [66]. O'Rourke [67,68] has proposed that early wave reflection due to arterial stiffening and degeneration may augment systolic pressure in the aorta. Superimposition in systole of forward and reflected waves may, therefore, explain the marked elevation of the systolic peak pressure. This phenomenon has been implicated in pathologic conditions which affect the blood vessels. For instance, systolic hypertension occurs frequently in coarctation of the aorta, traumatic amputation of lower limbs, and atherosclerosis obliterans of lower limbs. In such patients early wave reflections arise from those abnormalities.

Possible mechanisms and a basis for therapeutic intervention

It has been proposed that the fundamental pathophysiologic abnormality responsible for ISH is a decrease in aortic distensibility, an increased total peripheral resistance, and early wave reflections arising from the periphery. Figure 6.2 shows the possible pathophysiologic mechanisms involved in the production of ISH.

The therapeutic strategy in decreasing blood pressure in hypertensive patients must be targeted to correct the existent hemodynamic abnormalities. In order to decrease MAP, either cardiac output or peripheral resistance must be reduced. A rational approach would be to lower total peripheral resistance without altering cardiac output. On the other hand, to decrease pulse pressure, one must decrease stroke volume, increase the arterial distensibility, decrease the systolic ejection velocity, or decrease the total peripheral resistance (allowing a larger fraction of stroke volume to leave the elastic reservoir during systole). The main problem in treating patients with disproportionate systolic/diastolic hypertension or ISH is that on lowering MAP in these patients the DBP will be lowered still further. Theoretically, a low DBP may impair perfusion of vital organs, especially the heart where coronary blood flow occurs mainly in diastole. Therefore, low DBP may limit the use of current antihypertensive therapy in ISH. In the future, however, therapeutic agents which increase arterial distensibility, diminish early wave reflections, and/or decrease total peripheral resistance could be of help in controlling SBP.

Evaluation of patients with ISH

Patients with suspected ISH should have their blood pressure measured on different days for several times before the diagnosis is established. Blood pressure should be measured in the supine, sitting, and standing positions. After the diagnosis of ISH is established, secondary and potentially curable causes of systolic hypertension should be excluded. The differential diagnosis of ISH in the elderly include aortic insufficiency, arteriovenous fistula, thyrotoxicosis, Paget's Disease, beriberi, and severe anemia. Pseudohypertension should be suspected in patients with severe ISH who do not have signs of end-organ damage. This diagnosis can be suspected with the aid of a bedside technique, the Osler's maneuver [69]. Palpation of a calcified radial or brachial artery which does not collapse after raising the sphygmomanometer mercury above the SBP is a positive Osler's maneuver. It is felt that pseudohypertension is not a prevalent condition and is indeed a rare entity. However, clinicians must be alert to an occasional patient with rigid or calcified vessels in whom the indirect method of blood pressure measurement may overestimate the actual blood pressure.

The diagnostic evaluation of the elderly patient with ISH should include a thorough history and physical examination (including auscultation for carotid, aortic, and renal bruits), complete blood count, serum potassium, blood urea nitrogen, creatinine and cholesterol levels, a chest radiograph, and an electrocardiogram. Further evaluation of possible underlying causes for systolic hypertension may include thyroid function tests and bone survey for Paget's disease if a high index of suspicion is present.

Efficacy of therapy reducing mortality in ISH

The few isolated reports alluding to the effects of therapy on ISH in the elderly have given little information regarding the morbidity and mortality [70]. One of these studies compared the morbidity and mortality rates of 54 elderly

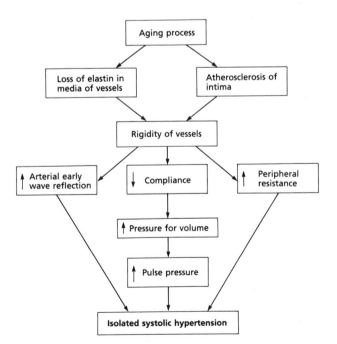

Fig. 6.2 Pathogenesis of isolated systolic hypertension.

patients with untreated ISH with those of 18 patients who received treatment for a 4-year period [8]. Morbid events and mortality rates were lower in the treated group (33% vs. 27.7% in morbid events and 13% vs. 5.6% in mortality rates). However, the major difficulty in the interpretation of this study was that patients had no randomization and therapy was not standardized. In another trial, Ikeda [71] studied the effects of diuretics on the survival of hypertensive patients of a geriatric home in Tokyo. All patients were studied for 5 years and most of them had ISH but a few had a mild diastolic hypertension. Of the 112 patients studied, 63 were on diuretics, and 49 received placebo. In patients with a SBP of 160–180 mmHg the incidence of cardiovascular attacks was 8.3% in the treated group vs. 28% in the placebo group. For those patients with a SBP of 180 mmHg or more the incidence of "cardiovascular attacks" was 7.2% in the treated group and 44% in the placebo group. Exact pretreatment blood pressure and extent of blood pressure reduction were not reported. The data suggests, however, that diuretic therapy is useful in reducing morbidity and mortality rates in elderly patients with systolic hypertension. A recent report by the European Working Party on High Blood Pressure in the Elderly [72] which examined 247 patients with ISH demonstrated a beneficial trend for active treatment (diuretics, methyldopa) but no statistical significance could be achieved between active and placebo groups. To date, the effect on mortality of other forms of therapy have not been reported.

Indications and selection of treatment

Therapeutic intervention should be considered in ISH when the level of SBP exceeds 160 mmHg. The goals of therapy should be directed to careful and individualized treatment programs. Safety, convenience, and simplicity are important aspects of treatment. One must be certain that the patient understands and accepts the rationale of treatment.

Two forms of therapy are available, nonpharmacologic and pharmacologic. Nonpharmacologic therapy including weight reduction, sodium restriction, decreased alcohol intake, aerobic exercise, and relaxation therapy may be useful. Nonetheless, alterations in lifelong style habits may be difficult and may have limited success in the elderly. Yet, most clinicians place a high priority in modifications of lifestyle, rather than in medical therapy, for the initial approach of treatment of ISH in this age group. Unfortunately, the efficacy of a nonpharmacologic approach has not been established in ISH. Niarchos et al. [73] showed no significant effect on SBP or DBP with a low-sodium diet in 10 patients with ISH. No large-scale studies are currently available on the effect of the already mentioned nonpharmacologic modalities of treatment in ISH.

If nonpharmacologic treatment proves inappropriate for adequate control of blood pressure, the clinician must rely on pharmacologic therapy. Considering the pathophysiology of ISH which includes decreased arterial distensibility, increased peripheral resistance, early wave reflections, and a tendency to low-cardiac output, patients with ISH are predictably favored by the use of drugs which modify these abnormalities. At present, medications which lower peripheral resistance, such as some diuretics, vasodilators, calcium channel blockers, and angiotensin-converting enzyme inhibitors may be recommended in the elderly.

A review of the use of antihypertensive agents in the elderly hypertensive has been published elsewhere [74]. In this chapter we discuss the data related to the use of antihypertensive agents in patients with ISH. Although there are no major differences among the currently available antihypertensive agents in their relative effects on systolic and diastolic pressures, some agents are better suited for a particular individual.

Diuretics

The efficacy, safety, tolerance, and low cost of diuretics as well as the longer experience with their use have influenced clinicians to select them as best initial drug in the treatment of hypertension. Thiazide diuretics have shown to be effective in lowering both systolic and diastolic pressure in the elderly [75]. In patients with ISH low-dose diuretics have been efficacious in decreasing SBP without a major drop in DBP [76]. Morledge et al. [77] studied 171 elderly patients with ISH. They were randomly assigned to receive chlorthalidone in doses of 12.5, 25, and 50 mg or placebo once daily for 12 weeks. The success rates with chlorthalidone ranged from 63% to 81%; whereas with placebo it was 22%. The 50 mg dose enhanced efficacy only minimally; side effects with this dose were more prevalent than with the 12.5 mg dose. Therapeutic success was observed in 637 patients with no clinically significant biochemical alterations or side effects.

The present recommendation is to use diuretics in a low dose (equivalent to 12.5−25 mg of hydrochlorothiazide) and slowly titrate up to 50 mg daily. Two major side effects of diuretics can be observed in patients with ISH, hypokalemia, and orthostasis. It is advisable that diuretics be avoided as first line therapy in elderly patients with significant baseline electrocardiographic abnormalities.

Beta-blockers

Several investigators have reported that β-blockers are less effective in the elderly hypertensive [78,79]. However, two large randomized trials [80,81] and data from the Veterans Administration [82] infer that β-blockers may be as efficacious as diuretics in the elderly. They may be indicated in the subgroup of hypertensive elderly patients described by Topol et al. [83] who exhibit concentric hypertrophy, congestive heart failure, and higher ejection fraction than other hypertensives. In addition, the combination of β- and α1-adrenoreceptor blockade, as with labetalol, may exert a salutary effect on the hemodynamic abnormality in ISH. Alpha-1-blockade may reduce peripheral resistance and β-blockade decreases stroke volume and the rate of ventricular ejection. A recent study revealed adequate control of blood pressure in 16 patients with ISH treated with labetalol [84]. Furthermore, 24-hour blood pressure monitoring in these patients demonstrated blunting of the early morning surge in blood pressure and heart rate, an event which has been associated with increased incidence of stroke, sudden death, and myocardial infarction [85].

Nonetheless, β-blockers might be a poor choice in elderly hypertensive patients with diabetes, chronic obstructive pulmonary disease, peripheral vascular disease, and with compromised cardiac function and sick sinus syndrome.

Calcium channel blockers

A few small studies suggest that calcium channel blockers may be more effective in the elderly than in young people with hypertension [86,87]. However, large, randomized, well-controlled, comparative studies are lacking in the elderly hypertensive. Moreover, calcium channel blockers have not been carefully studied in ISH. Their main problem in this age group has been the tendency of these patients to develop peripheral edema and postural hypotension. In addition, these agents, particularly verapamil, can make the elderly greatly suscep-

tible to cardiac conduction abnormalities and impairment of myocardial contractility [88].

Angiotensin-converting enzyme inhibitors

Angiotensin-converting enzyme inhibitors have been used with greater frequency in the treatment of hypertension and congestive heart failure in the elderly. Of interest is that elderly patients may show a blood pressure lowering effect despite a low renin state. Their hemodynamic action include a decrease in total peripheral resistance without changes in cardiac output [89], conservation of cerebral blood flow [90,91], and preservation or improvement of renal function [92]. They also increase large artery compliance [93] and have the potential to be effective in ISH. Although recent studies report their use in the elderly [94−96], no controlled trials have been reported in ISH.

Vasodilators and alpha-blockers

Hydralazine effectively lowers systolic and diastolic pressures in the elderly. It does not cause reflex tachycardia as in the younger patient [97]. In patients with ISH, sustained release isosorbide dinitrate produced a significant lowering of SBP without tolerance and a low incidence of adverse effects [98]. Alpha-blockers such as labetalol and prazosin are also effective in the elderly but these agents are more likely to cause postural hypotension. In patients with a spontaneous postural blood pressure drop of 15 mmHg or more these agents should not be used.

Central adrenergic inhibitors

Central adrenergic inhibitors, such as α-methyldopa, clonidine, and guanabenz lower blood pressure by reducing α-mediated sympathetic output. They also lower total peripheral resistance. Low-dose α-methyldopa was found to be effective in the EPWHE trial. In patients with ISH two reports show a salutary effect on SBP with the use of guanabenz, 8−64 mg daily [99] and clonidine, 0.1−2 mg daily [101]. Lethargy and dry mouth were prominent side effects of these agents.

Complications of antihypertensive therapy

Elderly hypertensive patients are prone to serious complications from the use of antihypertensive medication. Overzealous use of drugs and poor selection of the available agents are the most common causes of these complications. The major effects observed are postural hypotension and neurologic sequelae. Goldberg & Raferty [101] studied 11 hypertensive patients, seven of whom were between the ages of 60 and 68 years. Patients were treated with guanethidine, bethanidine, and debrisoquin. Marked postural reduction of blood pressure was detected by continuous ambulatory monitoring of intraarterial pressure. Three patients developed electrocardiographic evidence of ischemia during hypotension and one patient experienced a transient episode of weakness during exercise. Similarly, Jackson *et al.* [102] observed severe reduction in blood pressure resulting in orthostatic hypotension and unconsciousness in six elderly hypertensive patients treated with sympatholytic agents. Taken together, these reports point to the fact that drugs which are associated with orthostasis should be avoided in the elderly.

A similar experience has occurred with the use of potent vasodilators. Their use has been associated with worsening of angina and even myocardial infarction. These complications have been observed after the use of hydralazine [103], nifedipine [104], and minoxidil [105]. Of course, if therapy with these agents is necessary, low doses should be initially given to avoid such complications.

Effect on coronary heart disease

A large number of well-controlled multiclinic trials on the treatment of diastolic hypertension have shown no effect on the rate of coronary heart disease [106–108]. In some reports, treatment even increased the risk of coronary heart disease [109–111]. A clear explanation for this paradoxical finding has not been given but several theories have been raised to account for this. In the first instance, a J-shaped relation between treated levels of diastolic pressure and mortality from myocardial infarction has been described [112]. Patients with the greatest lowering of DBP had higher rates of myocardial infarction than those with less lowering of DBP [113,114]. In an elderly group of patients, Coope & Warrender [115] further analyzed this relationship. They found the J-shaped relation, but it was present both in the treatment and placebo groups, perhaps raising the question that both groups of patients had severe occult coronary heart disease. Nonetheless, the higher mortality in some studies can be due to overzealous treatment and a profound lowering of DBP. In ISH this relationship is most important since patients having a normal DBP could be adversely affected. It is then prudent that a close scrutiny of symptoms and signs of coronary heart disease should be monitored in these patients. Again, the use of antihypertensive agents should be given in low doses to avoid this problem.

Another possibility to explain the lack of effect of treatment in coronary heart disease is the alteration of lipid, electrolyte, and glucose homeostasis. The beneficial impact of lowering the blood pressure might be offset by lipid, electrolyte, and glucose alterations induced by treatment, particularly diuretic therapy and β-blockers. Thiazides and loop diuretics may increase total cholesterol, low-density lipoprotein, and triglycerides without affecting high-density lipoprotein [116]. Patients with these abnormalities may be at increased risk of developing atherosclerotic vascular disease. A reduction of blood pressure that is not accompanied by a reduction in cholesterol has less impact on the risk for coronary heart disease [113]. Studies of lipid profile in the elderly hypertensive indicate that diuretic treatment only has a transient effect on serum lipids [117]. However, these studies used lower dose of diuretics. Nevertheless, thiazides do not seem a reasonable choice as first-line therapy in hyperlipidemic patients with hypertension profile.

Hypokalemia is not uncommon in patients receiving diuretics. It is usually a function of the dose and the duration of action of the diuretic. Hypokalemia has been reported to increase the incidence of ventricular ectopy at rest and during exercise [118]. In addition, it increases the risk of sudden death after acute myocardial infarction [119]. Alternatively, untreated hypertensive patients with left ventricular hypertrophy demonstrate increased ventricular ectopy [120] and increased cardiovascular mortality [121]. Taken together these observations underscore the potential danger of hypokalemia and left ventricular hypertrophy in patients treated with diuretics. Based on these facts, the studies of the Multiple Risk Factor Intervention Trial (MRFIT) and the Oslo trial raised the possibility of increased coronary mortality in patients receiving thiazides when compared to the control group. These studies inferred that metabolic electrolyte perturbations had induced malignant arrhythmias such as ventricular tachycardia and/or ventricular fibrillation. In recent years, these implications have met considerable criticism since adequate proof was not provided that sudden death was indeed the result of hypokalemia. In fact, analysis of the MRFIT data shows no relation between the potassium level and mortality from coronary heart disease [122] but a correlation existed between serum potassium levels and rates of ventricular premature contractions [123]. Further analysis of the Oslo trial demonstrated that participants with baseline electrocardiographic abnormalities had higher incidence of coronary heart disease events [124]. Of great concern was the report of the Hypertension Detection and Follow-up Group. In a subset of white men with electocardiographic abnormalities, they found a higher rate of death from coronary heart disease [125]. Although these studies have not exclusively analyzed data from an elderly group, the risks of coronary heart disease are obviously greater with age. Celentano *et al.* [126] reported that age increased the severity of arrhythmias. Therefore, low doses of diuretics should be given to elderly individuals and even mild degrees of hypokalemia should be treated with potassium replacement or a potassium-sparing diuretic. Diuretics should be avoided in elderly men with substantial electrocardiographic abnormalities.

Alterations of carbohydrate metabolism can occur in hypertensive and elderly patients. Glucose intolerance, insulin resistance, and hyperinsulinemia have been associated to hypertension [127]. Abnormal glucose tolerance has been reported in the elderly [128]. These abnormalities provide for an increased risk for coronary heart disease [129]. This interesting finding needs more investigation to assess the importance of carbohydrate metabolism especially in the elderly hypertensives.

Quality of life
The justification for a specific antihypertensive agent should include maintenance or improvement of quality of life. Levine & Croog [130] defined seven major aspects of quality of life:
1 general well being;
2 intellectual performance;
3 psychologic and emotional state;
4 physiologic state;
5 family role;
6 work role; and
7 community role.

The effect of antihypertensive agents on quality of life aspects have been assessed in several clinical trials. Studies in the elderly hypertensive have been rather scarce and no attempts have been made to describe qualitatively or quantitatively the degree of impact of drug treatment on physical, emotional, cognitive, or behavioral aspects. However, the SHEP trial addresses the quality of life in ISH.

The SHEP trial
The SHEP trial was designed to determine, for a period of 5 years, the effects of therapy on ISH. The details of design, recruitment procedure, selection, and other characteristics of the sample population have been described elsewhere [26,131]. Basically, subjects who were accepted had to be 60 years of age or older and have a SBP of 160 mmHg or greater and a DBP less than 90 mmHg. Exclusion criteria included several specific illnesses, a chronic condition within the past 6 months, stroke, cancer, chronic obstructive pulmonary disease, and presence of dementia. Recruitment began in 1985 and extended until 1988. The minimum follow-up was to be 4 years and the maximum 6 years.

The early report of this study involved random assignment of 551 volunteers to treatment and placebo groups in a double-blind fashion. The treatment group consisted of 443 individuals and the placebo group of 108 subjects. Active treatment was initially started with chlorthalidone followed, if needed, by a Step 2 drug (reserpine, metoprolol, or hydralazine). The initial results have been reported by Hulley *et al.* [132]. Seventy-five percent of patients in the treatment group attained goal SBP with the diuretic alone. No undue decline in DBP occurred. Mean systolic and diastolic pressures were reduced 30/7 mmHg in the treatment group and 11/4 mmHg in the placebo group. Twelve percent of those completing 1 year of treatment required another drug, whereas 16% of those on a diuretic no longer required it, and another 16% were not compliant with the prescribed regime.

The final results of the SHEP study were published in 1991 [133]. A population of 4736 elderly people (age over 60 years) were randomized (2365 to active treatment and 2371 to placebo). The range of SBP was from 160 to 219 mmHg and the DBP was less than 90 mmHg. The average SBP was 170 mmHg and the average DBP was 77 mgHg. The mean age was 72 years, 57% were women, and 14% were black. The participants were stratified by clinical center and by antihypertensive medication status. The Step 1 of the trial was divided in 2 doses of chlorthalidone; dose 1 was 12.5 mg/day, and dose 2 was 25 mg/day. Step 2 dose 1 was atenolol 25 mg/day or placebo, dose 2 was 50 mg/day of atenolol. The average follow up was 4.5 years. The results showed a decrease in mean SBP for the active treatment group of about 26 mmHg and mean DBP of about 9 mmHg.

The 5 year average SBP was 155 mmHg for the placebo group and 143 mmHg for the active treatment group. The 5-year average DBP was 72 and 68 mmHg, respectively. The incidence of stroke was less in the actively treated group, 5.2 for 100 participants for active treatment and 8.2 per 100 for placebo. Nonfatal and fatal cardiovascular events were consistently lower for active treatment.

The SHEP study demonstrated significant efficacy of stepped care treatment with low-dose chlorthalidone in preventing stroke and major cardiovascular events. It reduced the incidence of stroke by 36% and major cardiovascular events with 5-year absolute benefit of 55 events per 1000. The regimen of drug therapy was associated with an infrequent report of side-effects.

Gurland *et al.* [134] reported the effects of treatment on ISH on cognitive state and depression in the SHEP trial. After 1 year of treatment behavioral assessment showed no beneficial effects in cognitive function or level of depression. However, the treatment regime was highly successful in controlling ISH with a relatively safe profile in behavioral function. The recent final report concludes that there was "no excess incidence of depression or dementia."

Our final conclusion is that diuretics are efficacious and safe for ISH in the elderly. Other drugs must show similar or advantageous results in well-controlled studies in order to be recommendable in this special group of patients.

References

1 Stamler J, Stamler R, Riedlinger W, *et al.* Hypertension screening of 1 million Americans: Community hypertension evaluation clinic (CHEC) program 1973–1975. J Am Med Assoc 1976;235:2299–2306.

2 Kannel WB. Some lessons in cardiovascular epidemiology from Framingham. Am J Cardiol 1974;37:269–282.

3 Kannel WB, Gordon T. Evaluation of cardiovascular risk in the elderly. Bull NY Acad Med 1978;54:573–591.

4 Kannel WB, Wolf P, Dawber TR. Hypertension and cardiac impairments increase stroke risk. Geriatrics 1978;33:71–83.

5 Kannel WB, Castelli WP, McNamara P, *et al.* Role of blood pressure in the development of congestive heart failure. The Framingham Study. N Engl J Med 1972;287:781–787.

6 Tarazi RC. Clinical importance of systolic hypertension. Ann Intern Med 1978;88:426–427.

7 Kannel WB. Status of risk factors and their consideration in antihypertensive therapy. Am J Cardiol 1987;59:A80–A90.

8 Colandrea MA, Friedman GD, Nichaman MZ, *et al.* Systolic hypertension in the elderly. Circulation 1970;41:239–245.

9 Kannel WB, Dawber TR, Sorlie P, *et al.* Systolic versus diastolic blood pressure and risk of coronary heart disease. Am J Cardiol 1971;27:335–346.

10 Birkenhager WH, Deleeuw PW. Impact of systolic blood pressure on cardiovascular prognosis. J Hypertens 1988;6 (Suppl. 1):S21–S24.

11 European Working Party on High Blood Pressure in the Elderly (EWPHE). Antihypertensive therapy in patients above age 60. Acta Cardiológica 1978;33:113–134.

12 Hall W, Wollam G. Systolic hypertension. Curr Probl Cardiol 1982;7:7–40.

13 Hulley SB, Feigal D, Ireland C, *et al.* Systolic hypertension in the elderly program (SHEP). The first three months. J Am Ger Soc 1986;34:101–105.

14 Koch-Weser J. Correlation of pathophysiology and pharmacotherapy in primary hypertension. Am J Cardiol 1973; 32:499–510.

15 The Joint National Committee on Detection, Evaluation and Treatment of Hypertension. Report of 1984. Arch Intern Med 1984;144:1045–1057.

16 Page LB, Sidd JJ. Medical management of arterial hypertension. N Engl J Med 1977;287:960–963.

17 García-Palmieri MR, Cortés R Jr, Cruz-Vidal M, *et al.* Milk consumption, calcium intake and decreased hypertension in Puerto Rico. Hypertension 1984;6:329–335.

18 Sever PS, Peart WS, Gordon D, *et al.* Blood pressure in urban and tribal Africa. Lancet 1980;2:58–64.

19 Blood pressure of adults by race and area US. 1960–62 National Health Survey, National Center for Health Statistics, United States Department of Health, Education and Welfare, Series 11, No. 4, 1964.

20 Blood pressure of adults by age and sex, US 1960–62 National Health Survey, National Center for Health Statistics, United States Department of Health, Education and Welfare, Series 11, No. 5, 1964.

21 Kannel WB, Dawber T, McGee D. Perspectives on systolic hypertension. The Framingham Study. Circulation 1980; 61:1179–1182.

22 Wing S, Aubert R, Hansen J, *et al.* Isolated systolic hypertension in Evans County 1. Prevalence and screening considerations. J Chron Dis 1982;35:735–742.

23 Curb JD, Borhani NO, Entwisle G, *et al.* Isolated systolic hypertension in 14 communities. Am J Epidemiol 1985; 121:362–370.

24 Garland C, Barret-Connor E, Suárez L, *et al.* Isolated systolic hypertension and mortality after 60 years: A prospective population-based study. Am J Epidemiol 1983;118: 365–376.

25 Wilking SVB, Belanger A, Kannel WB, *et al.* Determinants

of isolated systolic hypertension. J Am Med Assoc 1988; 260:3451–3455.

26 Vogt TM, Ireland CC, Black D, et al. Recruitment of elderly volunteers for multicenter trial: The SHEP pilot study. Controlled Clin Trials 1986;7:118–133.

27 McClellan W, Hall WD, Brogan D, et al. Isolated systolic hypertension: Declining prevalence in the elderly. Prev Med 1987;16:686–695.

28 Gubner R. Systolic hypertension: A pathogenetic entity. Significance and therapeutic considerations. Am J Cardiol 1962;9:773–776.

29 Ad Hoc Committee of the 1979 Build and Blood Pressure study (press release). Association of Life Insurance Medical Directors and the Society of Actuaries, Chicago, Society of Actuaries, 1978.

30 Stamler J, Berkson DM, Dyer A, et al. Relationship of multiple variable to blood pressure-findings from Chicago Epidemiologic Studies. In Paul O, ed. Epidemiology and Control of Hypertension. New York: Stratton Intercontinental Medical Book Corp., 1975:307–356.

31 Shevelle R, Ostfeld A, Klawans H. Hypertension and the risk of stroke in an elderly population. Stroke 1974;5: 71–75.

32 Kannel WB. Hypertension and other risks factors in coronary heart disease. Am Heart J 1987;114:918–925.

33 Kannel WB, Castelli W, McNamara P, et al. Role of blood pressure in the development of congestive heart failure. The Framingham Study. N Engl J Med 1972;287:781–787.

34 Kannel WB, Gordon T, Schwartz M. Systolic versus diastolic blood pressure and risk of coronary disease. Am J Cardiol 1971;27:335–346.

35 Vokonas PS, Kannel WB, Cupples LA. Epidemiology and risk of hypertension in the elderly. The Framingham Study 1988;6(Suppl. 1):S3–S9.

36 Kannel WB, Wolf PA, McGee DL, et al. Systolic blood pressure, arterial rigidity, and risk of stroke. The Framingham Study. J Am Med Assoc 1981;245:1225–1229.

37 Kannel WB, Gordon T, Castelli WB, et al. Electrocardiographic left ventricular hypertrophy and risk of coronary heart disease. The Framingham Study. Ann Intern Med 1970;72:813–818.

38 Savage DD, Garrison RJ, Kannel WB, et al. The spectrum of left ventricular hypertrophy in a general population sample. The Framingham Study. Circulation 1987;75(Suppl. 1): I26–I33.

39 French JE, Jennings MP, Paoli JCF, et al. Intimal changes in the arteries of the aging swine. Proc Roy Soc Biol 1963;158: 24–25.

40 Haudenschild CC, Prescott MF, Chobanian AV. Aortic endothelial and subendothelial cells in experimental hypertension and aging. Hypertension 1981;3:148–153.

41 Lakatta EG, Mitchell JH, Pomerance A, et al. Human aging: Change in structure and function. J Am Coll Cardiol 1987; 10:A42–A47.

42 Wolinsky H. Long-term effects of hypertension on the rat aortic wall and their relation to concurrent aging changes. Circ Res 1972;30:301–309.

43 Chobanian AV. Pathophysiologic considerations in the treatment of the elderly hypertension patients. Am J Cardiol 1983;16:595–602.

44 Abrass IB. Catecholamine levels and vascular responsiveness in aging. In Horan MJ, Steinberg GM, Dunbar JB, et al., eds. Blood Pressure Regulation and Aging, an NIH Symposium. New York: Biomedical Info. Corp., 1986: 123–130.

45 Fleisch JH, Maling HM, Brodie BB. Beta-receptor activity in aorta: variations with age and species. Circ Res 1970;26: 151–162.

46 Fleisch JH, Hooker CS. The relationship between age and relaxation of vascular smooth muscle in the rabbit and rat. Circ Res 1976;38:243–249.

47 Cohen ML, Berkowitz BA. Vascular contraction: Effect of age and extracellular calcium. Blood Vessels 1976;13: 139–154.

48 Abernethy DR, Schwartz JB, Todd EL, et al. Verapamil pharmacodynamics and disposition in young and elderly hypertensive patients: altered electrocardiographic and hypotensive responses. Ann Intern Med 1986;105:329–366.

49 Crane MG, Harris JJ. Effect of aging on renin activity and aldosterone excretion. J Lab Clin Med 1976;87:947–959.

50 Weidmann P, De-Myttenaere-Bursztein S, Maxwell MH, et al. Effect of aging on plasma renin and aldosterone in normal man. Kidney Int 1975;8:325–333.

51 Sowers JR, Zawada EF. Hypertension in the aged. In Zawada EJ, Sica DA, eds. Geriatric Nephrology and Urology. Littleton: PSG Publications, 1985:265–281.

52 Genest J, Larochelle P, Cussan JR, et al. The atrial natriuretic factor in hypertension. Hypertension 1988;11(Suppl. 1): 1–3.

53 Rowe JW, Andrés R, Tobin JD, et al. The effect of age on creatinine clearance in men: a cross-sectional and longitudinal study. J Gerontol 1976;31:155–163.

54 Hallock P, Benson I. Studies on the elastic properties of human isolated aorta. J Clin Invest 1937;16:595–602.

55 Ho J, Lin L, Galysh F. Aortic compliance: Studies on its relationship to aortic constituents in man. Arch Pathol 1972;94:537–546.

56 Abboud FM, Huston JH. The effects of aging and degenerative vascular disase on the measurement of arterial rigidity in man. J Clin Invest 1973;16:595–602.

57 Aziz Madkour M, Levenson J, Bravo EL, et al. Preload, adrenergic activity and aortic compliance is normal and hypertensive patients. Am Heart J 1989;118:1243–1248.

58 Tarazi RC, Dustan HP. The hemodynamics of labile hypertension in adolescents. In Strauss J, ed. Pediatric Nephrology, vol. 3. New York: Plenum Publishing Co., 1976: 97–106.

59 Simon AC, Safar ME, Levenson JA, et al. Systolic hyper-

tension: hemodynamic mechanism and choice of anti-hypertensive treatment. Am J Cardiol 1979;44:505−511.

60 Smulyan H, Vardan S, Griffiths A, et al. Forearm arterial distensibility in systolic hypertension. J Am Coll Cardiol 1984;3:387−393.

61 Adamopoulos PN, Chrysanthakapoulis SG, Frohlich EDD. Systolic hypertension: nonhomogeneous diseases. Am J Cardiol 1975;36:697−708.

62 Vardan S, Dunsky MH, Hill E, et al. Systemic systolic hypertension in the elderly: correlation of hemodynamics, plasma volume, renin, aldosterone, urinary metanephrine, and response to thiazide therapy. Am J Cardiol 1986;58: 1030−1034.

63 Berger DS, Li JKJ. Concurrent compliance reduction and increased peripheral resistance in the manifestation of isolated systolic hypertension. Am J Cardiol 1990;65:67−71.

64 Giles TD, Campeau RJ, Roffidal LE, et al. Isolated systolic hypertension is associated with similar abnormalities in left ventricular function as is diastolic hypertension. Am J Hypertens 1988;1:A10.

65 Pearson AC, Gudipati R, Cohen G, et al. Prevalence of left ventricular hypertrophy and diastolic filling abnormalities in elderly patients with isolated systolic hypertension. J Am Coll Cardiol 1987;9:A244.

66 Kelly R, Daley J, Avolio A, et al. Arterial dilation and reduced wave reflection: Benefit of dilevalol in hypertension. Hypertension 1989;14:14−21.

67 O'Rourke MF. Basic concept for the understanding of large arteries in hypertension. J Cardiovasc Pharmacol 1985;7: S14−S21.

68 O'Rourke MF. Arterial stiffness, systolic blood pressure and logical treatment of arterial hypertension. Hypertension 1990;15:339−347.

69 Messerli FH, Ventura HO, Anrodeo C. Osler's maneuver and pseudohypertension. N Engl J Med 1985;312: 1548−1551.

70 Gray D, Weber M, Drayer J. Effects of low dose antihypertensive therapy in elderly patients with predominant systolic hypertension. J Gerontol 1983;38:302−306.

71 Ikeda M. Prognosis and pathology of mild hypertension and stroke control in one community. Geneva World Health Organization 1976;77:248−257.

72 European Working Party on High Blood Pressure in the Elderly: Mortality and morbidity results from the European Working Party on High Blood Pressure in the Elderly Trial. Lancet 1985;1:1349.

73 Niarchos AP, Laragh JH. Renin dependency of blood pressure in isolated hypertension. Am J Med 1984;77:407−414.

74 Cangiano JL, Martinez-Maldonado M. Hypertension in the elderly: Pathophysiology and its implications for treatment. In Macias-Nunez JF, Stewart Cameron J, eds. *Renal Function and Disease in the Elderly*. London: Butterworths, 1987:94.

75 Myers MG. Hydrochlorothiazide with or without amiloride for hypertension in the elderly. Arch Intern Med 1987;147: 1026−1030.

76 Vardan S, Mookherjee S, Warner R, et al. Systolic hypertension in the elderly: Hemodynamic response to long-term thiazide diuretic therapy and its side effects. J Am Med Assoc 1983;250:2807−2813.

77 Morledge JH, Eltinger B, Aranda J, et al. Isolated systolic hypertension in the elderly. A placebo-controlled, dose response evaluation of chlorthalidone. J Am Geriatr Soc 1986;34:199−206.

78 Buhler FR, Boli P, Kiowski W, et al. Renin profiling to select antihypertensive baseline drugs. Am J Med 1984;77: 36−42.

79 Berter O, Buhler FR, Kiowski W, et al. Decreased beta-adrenoreceptor responsiveness as related to age, blood pressure, and plasma catecholamine in patients with essential hypertension. Hypertension 1980;2:130−138.

80 Andersen GS. Atenolol vs. bendroflumethiazide in middle aged and elderly hypertensives. Acta Med Scand 1985;218: 165−172.

81 Wikstrand J, Westergren G, Berglund G, et al. Antihypertensive treatment with metoprolol or hydrochlorothiazide in patients aged 60−75 years. J Am Med Assoc 1986;255: 1304−1310.

82 Veterans Administration Cooperative Study group on antihypertensive agents. Efficacy of nadolol alone and combined with bendromethiazide and hydralazine for systemic hypertension. Am J Cardiol 1983;52:1230−1237.

83 Topol EJ, Traill TA, Fortuin NJ. Hypertensive hypertrophic cardiomyopathy of the elderly. N Engl J Med 1985;312: 1277−1283.

84 De Quattro V, Lee DD, Allen J, et al. Labetalol blunts morning pressor surge in systolic hypertension. Hypertension 1988;11(Suppl. 1):198−201.

85 Muller JE, Ludmer PL, Wallich SN, et al. Cardiac variation in the frequency of sudden cardiac death. Circulation 1987; 75:131−138.

86 Buhler FR, Kiowski W. Age and antihypertensive response to calcium antagonists. J Hypertens 1987;5(Suppl. 4): S11−S114.

87 Stessman J, Leibel B, Yagil Y, et al. Nifedipine in the treatment of hypertension in the elderly. J Clin Pharm 1985;125:193−196.

88 Massie BM, Hirsch AT, Inouye IK, et al. Calcium channel blockers as antihypertensive agents. Am J Med 1984;77:135−142.

89 Fouad FM, Tarazi RC, Bravo EL. Cardiac and hemodynamic effects of enalapril. J Hypertens 1983;1(Suppl. 1):135−142.

90 Frei A, Muller-Brand J. Cerebral blood flow and antihypertensive treatment with enalapril. J Hypertens 1986;4: 305−368.

91 Paulson OB, Jordan JO, Goptfredsen J, et al. Cerebral blood flow in patients with congestive heart failure in

treatment with captopril. Am J Med 1984;76:91.

92 Hollenberg NK. Angiotensin-converting enzyme inhibitor: renal aspects. J Cardiovasc Pharmacol 1985;7(Suppl. 1): 40–44.

93 Simon AC, Levenson JA, Safar AM, et al. ACE inhibition and brachial artery haemodynamics in hypertension. Br J Clin Pharmacol 1984;18(Suppl. 2):243–246.

94 Di Veralli C, Pastorelli R. Acute captopril treatment in elderly hypertensive patients: a controlled study. J Hypertens 1988;6(Suppl. 1):S95–S96.

95 Veterans Administration Cooperative Study group on antihypertensive agents. Low dose captopril for treatment of mild to moderate hypertension. Hypertension 1983;5: III139–III144.

96 Verqa M, Cacciapuoti F, Spiezia R, et al. Effects of angiotensin-converting enzyme inhibitor enalapril compared with diuretic therapy in elderly hypertensive patients. J Hypertens 1988;6(Suppl. 1):S97–S99.

97 Efficacy of nadolol alone and combined with bendromethiazide and hydrolazine for systemic hypertension. Veterans Administration Cooperative Study Group on antihypertensive agents. Am J Cardiol 1983;52:1230–1237.

98 Duchier J, Imnascoli F, Safar M. Antihypertensive effect of sustained-release isosorbide dinitrate for isolated systolic hypertension in the elderly. Am J Cardiol 1987;60:99–102.

99 Weber MA, Drayer J. Treatment of hypertension in the elderly. South Med J 1986;79:323–326.

100 Gray D, Weber MA, Drayer J. Effects of low dose antihypertensive therapy in elderly patients with predominant systolic hypertension. J Gerontol 1983;38:302–306.

101 Goldberg AD, Raferty EB. Patterns of blood pressure during chronic administration of post gangionic sympathetic blocking drugs for hypertension. Lancet 1976;2:1052–1054.

102 Jackson G, Pierscianowski TA, Mahon W, et al. Inappropriate antihypertensive therapy in the elderly. Lancet 1976;2: 1317–1318.

103 Moyer JH. Hydrallazine (Apresoline) hydrochloride: Pharmacologic observations and clinical results in the therapy of hypertension. Arch Intern Med 1953;91:419–439.

104 O'Mailia JJ, Sander GE, Giles TD. Nifedipine associated myocardial ischemia or infarction in the treatment of hypertensive urgencies. Ann Intern Med 1987;107:185–186.

105 Traub YM, Aygen MM, Rosenfeld JB. Hazards in treatment of systolic hypertension. Am Heart J 1979;97:174–177.

106 Effects of morbidity in hypertension I. Results in patients with diastolic blood pressure averaging 90 through 114 mmHg. Veterans Administration Cooperative Study group on anti-hypertensive agents. J Am Med Assoc 1970; 213:1143–1152.

107 United States Public Health Hospital Cooperative Study Group. Morbidity and mortality in mild hypertension. Circ Res 1972;30:110.

108 Australian National Blood Pressure Study Management Committee. The Australian therapeutic trial in mild hypertension. Lancet 1980;1:1261.

109 Multiple Risk Factor Intervention Trial: Multiple Risk Factor Intervention Trial Research Group. J Am Med Assoc 1982;248:1465–1472.

110 MRC trial of treatment of mild hypertension principal results: Medical Research Council Working Party. Br Med J 1985;291:97–104.

111 Helgeland A. Treatment of mild hypertension. A fine controlled drug trial. The Oslo Study. Am J Med 1980;60: 725–732.

112 Cruickshank JM, Thorp JM, Zacharias FJ. Benefits and potential harm of lowering high blood pressure. Lancet 1987;2:658–661.

113 Samuelsson O, Wilhelmsen L, Anderson OK, et al. Cardiovascular morbidity in relation to change in blood pressure and serum cholesterol levels and treated hypertension. J Am Med Assoc 1987;258:1768–1776.

114 Berglund G, Samuelsson O. Lowering blood pressure and the J-shaped curve. Lancet 1987;1:1154–1155.

115 Coope J, Warrender TS. Lowering blood pressure. Lancet 1987;11:518.

116 Joos C, Kervits H, Reinhold-Kourniati D. Effects of diuretics on plasma lipoprotein in healthy men. Eur J Clin Pharmacol 1980;17:251–258.

117 Amery A, Birkenhager W, Bulpitt C. Influence of antihypertensive therapy on serum cholesterol in elderly hypertensive patients. Acta Cardiol 1982;37:235–244.

118 Holland OB, Nixon NV, Hubert LK. Diuretic induced ventricular ectopic activity. Am J Med 1981;70:761–762.

119 Nordrehaug JE, Vander Lippe G. Hypokalemia and ventricular fibrillation in acute myocardial infarction. Br Heart J 1983;50:525–529.

120 Messerli FA, Ventura HO, Elizardi DJ, et al. Hypertension and sudden death in left ventricular hypertrophy. Am J Med 1984;77:18–22.

121 Kannel WB. Prevalence and natural history of electrocardiographic left ventricular hypertrophy. Am J Med 1983;75: 4–11.

122 Kuller LH, Hulley SB, Cohen JD, Neaton J. Unexpected effects of treating hypertension in men with electrocardiographic abnormalities: A critical analysis. Circulation 1987; 73:114–123.

123 Cohen JD, Neaton JD, Prineas RJ, et al. Diuretics, serum potassium and ventricular arrhythmias in the Multiple Risk Factor Intervention Trial. Am J Cardiol 1987;60: 548–554.

124 Holme I, Helgeland A, Hjermann I, et al. Treatment of mild hypertension with diuretics: The importance of ECG abnormalities in the Oslo studies and in MRFIT. J Am Med Assoc 1984;251:1298–1299.

125 The effect of antihypertensive drug treatment on mortality in the presence of resting electrocardiographic abnormal-

ities at baseline: The Hypertension Detection and Follow-up Cooperative Research Group. Circulation 1984;70: 996–1003.

126 Celentano A, Galderisi M, Mureddu GF, *et al.* Arrhythmias, hypertension and the elderly: Holter evaluation. J Hypertens 1988;6(Suppl. 1):S29–S32.

127 Ferranini E, De Fianzo RA. The Association of Hypertension, Diabetes and Obesity: A review. J Nephrol 1989;1: 3–15.

128 Davidson MB. The effect of aging on carbohydrate metabolism. Metabolism 1979;28:688–705.

129 Pollare T, Lithell H, Berne C. A comparison of the effects of hydrochlorotiazide and captopril on glucose and lipid metabolism in patients with hypertension. N Engl J Med 1989;321:868–873.

130 Levine S, Croog SA. Quality of life and patient's response to treatment. J Cardiovasc Pharmacol 1985;7:S312–316.

131 Furberg CD, Black DM. The systolic hypertension in the elderly pilot program: Methodological issues. Eur Heart J 1988;9:223–227.

132 Hulley SB, Furberg CD, Gurland B, *et al.* Systolic Hypertension in the Elderly Program (SHEP): Antihypertensive efficacy of chlorthalidone. Am J Cardiol 1985;56:913–920.

133 SHEP Co-operative Research Group. Prevention of stroke by antihypertensive drug treatment in older persons with isolated systolic hypertension. J Am Med Assoc 1991;265: 3255–3264.

134 Gurland BJ, Teresi J, Smith WM, *et al.* Effects of treatment for isolated systolic hypertension on cognitive status and depression in the elderly. J Am Geriatr Soc 1988;36: 1015–1022.

7

Atrial natriuretic factor in hypertension and congestive heart failure: implications in the elderly

Patricia G. Cavero
John C. Burnett Jr

Introduction

Cardiovascular disease, including congestive heart failure and hypertension, continues to be a leading cause of morbidity and mortality in the elderly [1]. Both of these states are characterized by derangements in sodium homeostasis, activation of the renin–angiotensin–aldosterone system, and alterations in blood pressure. The atrial peptide system is an important hormonal system of cardiac origin which participates in the regulation of volume homeostasis [2,3]. Atrial natriuretic factor (ANF) enhances sodium excretion, inhibits the renin–angiotensin–aldosterone system, and has potent vasorelaxant properties (Fig. 7.1). The physiologic actions of ANF on the cardiovascular, renal, and endocrine systems thus serve to defend the circulation from volume and/or pressure overload. Thus a potential role has emerged for ANF in the pathophysiology of congestive heart failure and hypertension. This chapter focuses upon our current understanding of the atrial peptide system in the regulation of body fluid homeostasis and the potential role of ANF in the etiology and treatment of congestive heart failure and hypertension with an emphasis on implications in the elderly.

Fig. 7.1 Flow diagram demonstrating the mechanism of ANF secretion by atrial stretch. Effector sites include the kidney (promotion of sodium and water excretion and inhibition of renin), adrenal gland (inhibition of aldosterone), and systemic vasculature (decrease in venous return). Net actions combine to control extracellular fluid (ECF) and prevent extracellular volume overload.

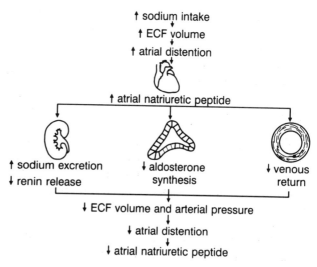

Physiologic actions of ANF

Effects on cardiovascular function

Atrial nutriuretic factor may serve in an important regulatory capacity to maintain cardiac function. The administration of synthetic ANF reduces blood pressure independent of its natriuretic action. Several studies have demonstrated this hypotensive response to exogenous ANF in both animals and humans [4,5]. Furthermore, the administration of ANF reduces arterial pressure in pathophysiologic states. In studies in rats with spontaneous hypertension or in animals made hypertensive with angiotensin II, the infusion of exogenous ANF has been demonstrated to decrease arterial pressure [6,7]. More than one mechanism may mediate this arterial pressure response to ANF.

A potential mechanism is supported by studies from several laboratories in which a potent vasorelaxant action of ANF has been reported. *In vitro* studies have demonstrated that ANF produces smooth-muscle relaxation in isolated aortic strips [8]. This ANF-induced vasodilatation appears to be endothelium independent like nitroprusside and associated with increases in cyclic guanosine monophosphate (cGMP) [9]. Recent *in vivo* studies further support the vasorelaxant action of ANF [10]. In human subjects using an intra-arterial bolus of ANF in an isolated forearm preparation, ANF significantly decreased forearm vascular resistance in the absence of any systemic effects.

However, in both animal and human studies, the decrease in arterial pressure in response to synthetic ANF infusions is mediated by a fall in cardiac filling pressures and cardiac output rather than by a decrease in total peripheral resistance [11,12]. The decrease in cardiac preload does not appear to be due to venodilation as ANF *in vitro* has a minimal venodilator action [13]. The mechanism by which ANF decreases cardiac preload is most likely due to an ANF-induced shift of volume from the intravascular to the extravascular space [14]. Atrial natriuretic factor mediates this shift by either increasing capillary permeability or by increasing resistance to venous return by increasing postcapillary resistance as suggested by Trippodo *et al.* [15]. Thus the reduction in cardiac output in response to ANF appears to be due to a decrease in venous return.

Studies by Wangler *et al.* [16] have suggested another mechanism for the hypotensive effect of ANF. These investigators suggested that the reduction in cardiac output in response to the administration of ANF may result from an ischemia-induced decrease in cardiac function. In an isolated perfused heart preparation, these investigators demonstrated a coronary vasoconstrictor response to pharmacologic doses of ANF. However, studies from our laboratory and others both *in vivo* and *in vitro* utilizing both pharmacologic and physiologic concentrations of ANF have not demonstrated any coronary vasoconstrictor or negative inotropic affect [17,18]. A transient coronary vasodilatory action of ANF was actually observed.

While an initial infusion of ANF may decrease arterial pressure by decreasing venous return and cardiac output with no change in peripheral resistance, recent studies have suggested that the long-term administration of ANF results in a differential response [19]. In elegant studies by Parkes *et al.* [19] the 5-day administration of low-dose ANF to conscious sheep resulted in a decrease in arterial pressure mediated by arterial vasodilatation with a decrease in systemic vascular resistance. Initially, the acute administration of ANF in these studies resulted in a characteristic decrease in arterial pressure and cardiac output mediated by a reduction in venous return (Fig. 7.2). This was associated with an increase in the total peripheral resistance observed on the first day. However, with the continued administration of ANF a reduction in arterial pressure was maintained due to a decrease in systemic vascular resistance with a return of cardiac output to baseline. The mechanism of this response is unclear but suggests a differential vascular response to long-term infusions of ANF.

The chronic administration of ANF may also modulate cardiac reflexes by blunting the initial reflex increase in sympathetic activity in response to ANF-mediated hypotension [20]. Thus the reduction of arterial pressure with the short-term administration of ANF appears to be mediated by an initial decrease in venous return and cardiac output, but the long-term reduction of arterial pressure appears to be mediated by an arterial vasodilatory action of ANF.

Renal and endocrine effects of ANF

Studies from our laboratory and others have demonstrated that the administration of synthetic ANF results in a marked increase in urine volume and sodium excretion [3,21]. This diuresis and natriuresis is associated with an

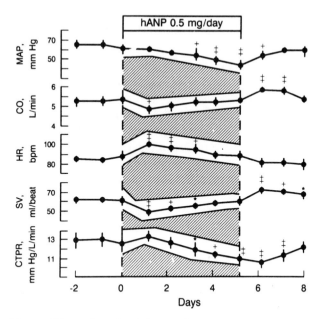

Fig. 7.2 Effects of a 5-day infusion of ANF (99–126) at 0.5 mg/day in five conscious sheep on mean arterial pressure (MAP), cardiac output (CO), heart rate (HR), stroke volume (SV), and calculated total peripheral resistance (CTPR). Results are as means ± SE. * $P \le 0.05$, † $P \le 0.001$ comparable with experimental days. (From Parkes *et al.* [19].)

A unique renal blood flow (RBF) response is observed with the intrarenal administration of ANF [21]. The RBF increases transiently and then returns to control values despite the continued infusion of ANF. The mechanism of this biphasic RBF response is unclear and may be due to the modulation of preglomerular arteriolar resistance by an intrarenal vasoconstrictor released in response to increases in sodium delivery to the macula densa. Despite the transient decrease in RBF, GFR remains increased suggesting that the postglomerular resistance is increased with exogenous ANF [21,22]. By altering both pre-glomerular and postglomerular resistance, ANF increases the glomerular hydrostatic pressure with a resultant increase in the GFR [23]. Atrial natriuretic factor may also increase the ultrafiltration coefficient K_f to directly increase the GFR [24]. These studies taken together suggest that the natriuresis observed with the administration of ANF is mediated by an enhancement of renal hemodynamics. However, if the increase in GFR is prevented in response to exogenous ANF, a natriuresis is still observed although it is attenuated supporting a renal tubular action of ANF [25].

In response to the administration of exogenous ANF the fractional excretion of sodium increases indicating that ANF decreases the tubular reabsorption of sodium [21,23]. The site of action of ANF may be at multiple nephron segments. Recent studies support an action of ANF at the proximal tubule [21,26]. The mechanism by which ANF decreases proximal tubule sodium reabsorption is unclear as the proximal tubule does not appear to

increase in the fractional excretion of sodium and a decrease in proximal tubule reabsorption of sodium, as measured by lithium clearance (Fig. 7.3). Plasma renin is also suppressed despite a decrease in arterial pressure [3].

Fig. 7.3 Effects of ANF infusion on renal function. Abbreviations: ANF, atrial natriuretic factor; V, urine flow; GFR, glomerular filtration rate; $U_{Na}V$, absolute sodium excretion; FE_{Na}, fraction excretion of sodium; U_kV, absolute potassium excretion; FE_k, fractional excretion of potassium; RBF, renal blood flow; RVR, renal vascular resistance; FE_{Li}, fractional excretion of lithium; U_{osm}, urine osmolality. * $P \le 0.05$ compared to control. (From Zimmerman *et al.* [21].)

ANF dose, μg/kg/min	$\dot{V}$, ml/min	GFR, ml/min	$U_{Na}\dot{V}$, μEq/min	FE_{Na}, %	$U_k\dot{V}$, μEq/min	FE_k, %	RBF, ml/min	RVR, mm Hg/ml/ min	FE_{Li}, %	UOsm, mOsm/ kg H$_2$O
Control	0.16 ± 0.02	37.6 ± 1.4	22 ± 6	0.41 ± 0.11	29 ± 3	20 ± 2	147 ± 12	0.90 ± 0.08	0.21 ± 0.02	1,292 ± 136
0.0025	0.38 ± 0.08*	34.5 ± 2.5	66 ± 15*	1.30 ± 0.33*	32 ± 3	27 ± 4	144 ± 9	0.90 ± 0.05	0.32 ± 0.03*	994 ± 137*
0.005	0.72 ± 0.15*	36.3 ± 2.9	131 ± 26*	2.61 ± 0.55*	39 ± 4*	30 ± 2*	148 ± 7	0.88 ± 0.05	0.43 ± 0.06*	741 ± 86*
0.01	0.94 ± 0.14*	31.7 ± 1.5	171 ± 26*	3.76 ± 0.54*	37 ± 2*	34 ± 2*	143 ± 9	0.91 ± 0.07	0.50 ± 0.09*	608 ± 52*
0.3	2.66 ± 0.46*	38.2 ± 3.9	397 ± 151*	6.81 ± 0.60*	56 ± 6*	42 ± 4*	166 ± 11	0.70 ± 0.06*	0.67 ± 0.18*	431 ± 30*
Recovery	0.40 ± 0.06*	38.2 ± 4.0	70 ± 9*	1.31 ± 0.41*	29 ± 3	22 ± 3	136 ± 14	1.01 ± 0.11	0.32 ± 0.08	743 ± 50*

have receptors for ANF. Recent studies by Schwab *et al.* [27] have suggested that the mechanism of action of ANF at the proximal tubule may be due to changes in the renal interstitial pressure, an intrarenal physical factor, by ANF. Another potential mechanism as suggested by Winaver *et al.* [28] is that dopamine may act as a secondary messenger for ANF at the proximal tubule. Atrial natriuretic factor may stimulate the generation of intrarenal dopamine and thus act indirectly at the proximal tubule.

Studies have also demonstrated an action of ANF at other nephron segments such as the collecting duct [29]. The action of ANF at the medullary collecting duct may be via a direct effect of ANF receptor-mediated alterations in tubular reabsorption and linked to the cGMP second messenger system. Thus, in summary, the natriuretic action of ANF appears to be mediated by both an increase in the GFR and decrease in tubular reabsorption at and beyond the proximal tubule.

Atrial natriuretic factor, in addition to its natriuretic actions, exerts effects on the renin–angiotensin–aldosterone system and vasopressin. Atrial natriuretic factor inhibits renin secretion despite observed decreases in arterial pressure [4,30]. Studies by Opgenorth *et al.* [30] demonstrated that the ANF-induced reduction in renin release is mediated by an increase in solute delivery to the macula densa. In the nonfiltering kidney model in which there is no functional macula densa, ANF was unable to inhibit renin release. However, renin release was inhibited in response to ANF administration in a filtering kidney possibly mediated by the increased solute delivery to the macula densa. These investigators thus concluded that the inhibition of renin release by ANF is mediated by increased solute delivery to the macula densa rather than by a direct action of ANF upon renin release. However, other investigators employing pharmacologic doses of ANF have demonstrated a direct inhibitory action of ANF on renin release from isolated juxtaglomerular cells [31]. Aldosterone secretion is also inhibited by ANF both directly, by inhibiting the release of aldosterone from zona glomerulosa cells, and by inhibiting angiotensin II-stimulated aldosterone release [32,33]. Thus, these studies suggest an opposing action of ANF on the renin–angiotensin–aldosterone system.

Evidence for a physiologic role for ANF

As reviewed above, ANF regulates cardiovascular, renal, and endocrine functions. The physiologic role of ANF in regulating body fluid homeostasis, however, continues to emerge. Many studies investigating the actions of ANF utilized pharmacologic concentrations of ANF which may not elucidate the physiologic actions of this peptide hormone. However, recent investigations employing more physiologic concentrations of ANF as seen in response to volume expansion, have sought to elucidate the physiologic role of ANF in volume homeostasis. In studies by Richards *et al.* [34], the administration of exogenous ANF, which increased ANF concentrations within the normal range (mean increase of 8 pmol/liter), resulted in a significant natriuresis and suppression of plasma renin activity as well as aldosterone. Systolic blood pressure also decreased by approximately 7 mmHg as compared to placebo controls although the GFR and RBF did not increase with the exogenous ANF. Other investigators utilizing a dose of exogenous ANF which mimicked circulating concentrations of ANF observed in volume expansion, reported an increase in total urinary sodium excretion, fractional excretion of sodium, and fractional excretion of lithium [35]. A greater increase in plasma ANF with an ANF infusion was required to decrease atrial pressures and cardiac output. Studies by Hirth *et al.* [36] also support a physiologic role for ANF. These investigators employing monoclonal antibodies to ANF were able to block the natriuretic response to volume expansion in the rat. In additional studies these investigators also abolished the natriuretic and hypotensive response to exogenous ANF by infusing monoclonal antibodies to ANF.

Other studies have investigated the role of ANF in volume homeostasis in response to daily alterations in sodium intake. Weidmann *et al.* [37] reported that a change in sodium consumption from 10 to 310 mmol/day in normal human subjects resulted in a significant increase in sodium excretion despite no elevation in plasma ANF concentrations. Although ANF was not increased, plasma renin and aldosterone were suppressed. These studies would thus suggest that ANF may not be an important factor in the regulation of body fluid homeostasis in response to dietary alterations in sodium intake.

Atrial natriuretic factor may, however, play a role in the response to acute changes in intravascular volume to physiologic maneuvers such as volume expansion [38,39]. Recent studies by Schwab *et al.* [38] demonstrated in rats with and without intact right atrial appendages that the natriuretic response to volume expansion was dependent on increases in circulating ANF. A right atrialectomy attenuated the natriuretic response to volume expansion as compared to the rats with intact right atriums. This response was associated with a blunted increase in plasma ANF. Similar studies by Veress & Sonnenberg [39] reported an attenuated natriuretic response to volume expansion in the rat after resection of the right atrium. Thus, current studies support the physiologic role of ANF in modulating acute changes in body fluid homeostasis through its actions on cardiovascular, renal, and endocrine functions.

Plasma and cardiac ANF in congestive heart failure and hypertension

Congestive heart failure

Congestive heart failure is a syndrome characterized by sodium retention and edema in association with the activation of the renin−angiotensin−aldosterone system. Thus investigators initially hypothesized that the edema formation and fluid retention in congestive heart failure may be secondary to a deficiency in ANF. Initial studies by Chimoskey *et al.* [40] employing immunohisto-chemical techniques observed a decrease in the atrial content of ANF in the cardiomyopathic hamster.

Edwards *et al.* [41] also reported a decrease of immuno-reactive ANF within the atria of the cardiomyopathic Syrian hamster. However, the decrease in atrial granularity was associated with elevated circulating concentrations of plasma ANF. The decrease in atrial granules in congestive heart failure in the presence of elevated plasma ANF concentrations as suggested by these investigators would be consistent with an increased synthesis and release of ANF into the circulation. Sub-sequent studies from our laboratory have since reported that circulating concentrations of ANF are elevated in the human with both acute and chronic congestive heart failure [42,43]. Furthermore, elevations in plasma ANF levels correlate with the severity of heart failure with the highest levels seen in patients with NYHA Class IV congestive heart failure.

Congestive heart failure is therefore not characterized by an absolute deficiency of ANF but by a compensatory increase in peptide synthesis and release. Yet congestive heart failure is characterized by sodium retention and activation of the renin−angiotensin−aldosterone system despite increased plasma levels of ANF. The mechanism of this blunted response to both endogenous and exo-genous ANF is not entirely clear and will be discussed below. Furthermore, while the action of ANF may be blunted, recent studies suggest that endogenous ANF in congestive heart failure may nevertheless still play a role in opposing the activated vasoconstrictor systems.

Hypertension

Investigators have postulated a role for ANF in the pathogenesis of essential hypertension, a syndrome characterized by alterations in arterial pressure and volume regulation. Yet the circulating plasma concen-trations of ANF in hypertension remain unclear. Sagnella *et al.* [44] have reported elevations in plasma ANF in humans with essential hypertension. These studies, however, involved few patients, some with long-standing hypertension who may have had either hypertension-induced ventricular hypertrophy or reductions in ven-tricular function. However, these reports would be consistent with other studies in the spontaneously hyper-tensive rat model of hypertension in which plasma ANF is elevated [45].

In contrast, studies by Zachariah *et al.* [46] have reported that plasma ANF concentrations in patients with uncomplicated essential hypertension were not elevated. These patients demonstrated no evidence of left ventricular hypertrophy or congestive heart failure. Furthermore, plasma ANF levels decreased in response to therapy possibly due to an improvement in cardiac hemodynamics. While ANF levels were not increased in these patients with uncomplicated hypertension, these investigators postulated that an alteration for stimulus−release in ANF secretion may exist in the hypertensive patient. This speculation was based on previous studies demonstrating evidence of increased atrial pressures in humans with essential hypertension, even in the absence of left ventricular hypertrophy or systolic dysfunction, due to either a decrease in the compliance of the venous bed or left ventricle [47]. Thus, the release of ANF from the atria in early essential hypertension may be attenuated in response to increased atrial pressures and stretch without evidence of ventricular hypertrophy. An altered atrial pressure–volume relationship in hypertension may thus contribute to alterations in pressure and volume regulation which characterize hypertension.

Recent animal and human studies support such a hypothesis. Ferrier *et al.* [48] reported that with acute volume expansion, an attenuated increase in plasma ANF levels was present in the spontaneously hypertensive rat as compared to normal controls. These investigators also reported a similar attenuated response in ANF secretion to increases in cardiac volume in the offspring of hypertensive parents as compared to offspring of normotensive parents (Fig. 7.4). Hypertensive offspring in response to a high-sodium diet failed to increase plasma levels of ANF in contrast to the significant elevation in ANF observed in the offspring of normotensive parents [49]. Taken together these studies suggest an altered stimulus–release relationship of ANF from the atria in essential hypertension.

Recent studies have, however, reported conflicting results in patients with essential hypertension in response to volume expansion. Studies by Mimran *et al.* [50] in patients with uncomplicated essential hypertension reported similar increases in ANF levels with volume expansion as compared to controls. Yet other studies [51] reported an exaggerated increase in plasma ANF levels with volume expansion in hypertensives as compared to controls. However, these patients at baseline already demonstrated increased plasma ANF levels. One possible explanation for an exaggerated increase in ANF is that these patients had ventricular hypertrophy which may have altered their response to volume expansion. Studies by Sudhir *et al.* [52] support this hypothesis. Hypertensive patients with exercise demonstrated a greater increase in plasma ANF as compared to normal controls with a positive correlation present between left ventricular mass and the percentage rise in ANF.

Ventricular ANF in congestive heart failure and hypertension

Studies have demonstrated the presence of ventricular ANF in congestive heart failure and in hypertension associated with left ventricular hypertrophy in both humans and animal models. In congestive heart failure, Edwards *et al.* [53] demonstrated the presence of immunoreactive ANF in the ventricular myocardium of both the cardiomyopathic hamster and in the human. In the normal myocardium no immuno-reactive ANF was present in the ventricle. In congestive heart failure, the ANF granules in the ventricle were found primarily within the subendocardium. Studies have demonstrated that intramural tension appears to be the greatest in the subendocardium [54]. This observation suggests that in congestive heart failure production of ANF by the ventricle may be stimulated by the presence of pressure and/or volume overload. Furthermore, atrial ANF in patients with congestive heart failure was significantly decreased consistent with prior studies by Chimoskey [40] in which atrial ANF content was assessed by immunohistochemical techniques.

Recent elegant studies in humans by Yasue *et al.* (55) have investigated further the contribution of ventricular ANF to plasma levels of ANF in patients with congestive heart failure as compared to control subjects. These investigators cannulated the coronary sinus and advanced a catheter into the anterior interventricular vein which almost exclusively drains the left ventricle and not the atria. They were thus able to obtain samples from the anterior interventricular vein, coronary sinus, and aorta (Fig. 7.5). In the control subjects, plasma ANF from the aorta and anterior interventricular vein were not elevated. However, coronary sinus ANF concentrations were significantly increased, reflecting release of ANF from the

Fig. 7.4 Plasma immunoreactive ANF (irANF) concentrations and urinary sodium excretion with various levels of sodium intake in normotensive parents and normotensive sons of parents with essential hypertension (Mean ± SEM) (From Ferrier *et al.* [48].)

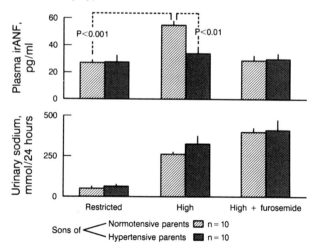

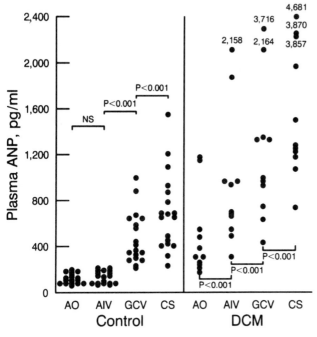

Fig. 7.5 Plasma atrial natriuretic peptide (ANP) levels in the AO (aorta), AIV (anterior interventricular vein), GCV (greater cardiac vein), and CS (coronary sinus) in the control subjects and the patients with DCM. There was no significant difference in the plasma ANP levels between the AO and the AIV, but there were highly significant differences between the AIV and the GCV and between the GCV and the CS in the control subjects. On the other hand, there was a significant step-up in the plasma ANP levels between the AO and the AIV in the patients with DCM (dilated cardiomyopathy). (From Yasue *et al.* [55].)

atria. In contrast, the patients with congestive heart failure demonstrated significantly increased concentrations of ANF in the aorta and coronary sinus as well as from the anterior interventricular vein. Thus this study demonstrates that ANF in congestive heart failure is secreted from the ventricle. Furthermore, the highest concentrations of ANF were observed in the coronary sinus in congestive heart failure even when compared to coronary sinus ANF levels in normals, reflecting increased release of ANF from the heart as a whole in patients with congestive heart failure. This study supports a role for the ventricle in the release of ANF into the circulation in congestive heart failure. The ventricle with the atria may participate in the regulation of volume homeostasis in

states characterized by volume overload such as congestive heart failure.

Several studies have also reported the presence of ventricular ANF in animal models of spontaneous hypertension and during chronic pressure and/or volume overload in association with ventricular hypertrophy [45,56,57]. Arai *et al.* [45] reported that tissue levels of ANF and ANF mRNA were markedly increased in the ventricles of spontaneously hypertensive rats at the stage of established hypertension and ventricular hypertrophy. The presence of increased concentrations of ventricular ANF was also reported by Lattion *et al.* [56] in the hypertensive DOCA-salt rat.

Insight into the mechanism and time course of ventricular ANF gene expression in pressure overload and hypertrophy was gained in studies by Mercardier *et al.* [57]. In the hypertensive rat model produced by suprarenal acute coarctation of the abdominal aorta, these investigators measured cardiovascular hemodynamics, left ventricular hypertrophy, and left ventricular ANF mRNA in this rat model of hypertension at 5 and 8 hours and every 2 days up to a total of 30 days. A biphasic accumulation of left ventricular ANF mRNA was observed with a peak at 4 days. Of interest, ventricular ANF mRNA was present before the development of hypertrophy. The initial increase in ANF mRNA was associated with a marked increase in left ventricular end-diastolic pressure rather than an increase in left ventricular mass or thickness. Atrial natriuretic factor mRNA then decreased transiently at 10 days followed by a subsequent rise which stabilized to levels about 10 times greater than control. These investigators thus suggested that the increase in left ventricular end-diastolic pressure resulted in a marked increase in wall stress with the subsequent activation of ventricular ANF gene expression. With continued hypertension, left ventricular end-diastolic pressure decreased and left ventricular mass increased with evidence for mild ventricular dilatation. This may have continued to stimulate ventricular ANF mRNA due to an increase in end-diastolic wall stress in association with sustained hypertension.

Recent studies in the spontaneously hypertensive rat model investigated the mechanism of ventricular ANF release. Ruskoaho *et al.* [58] reported the response to exercise in the spontaneously hypertensive rat with left ventricular hypertrophy and increased concentrations of ventricular ANF mRNA as compared to the normotensive

Wistar Kyoto (WKY) control rats. With exercise, increases in ANF secretion were associated with a depletion of ventricular ANF mRNA in the spontaneously hypertensive rat. Evidence of depletion of endocardial stores of ANF as determined by immunohistochemical studies was also present. Furthermore, the degree of left ventricular hypertrophy correlated in the spontaneously hypertensive rat with the amount of ANF released. No reduction in the atrial content of ANF with exercise was reported in the spontaneously hypertensive rat or WKY rats. Furthermore, no evidence of ventricular ANF in the WKY rat was noted.

Additional experiments by these investigators in an isolated perfused spontaneously hypertensive rat heart after atrialectomy, demonstrated that the release of ANF from the ventricle appeared to be in a constitutive manner. Phorbol ester, known to increase ANF secretion from intact perfused hearts, had only a limited effect on ANF release in the spontaneously hypertensive rat heart after atrialectomy.

In summary, ventricular ANF both in hypertension associated with hypertrophy and in congestive heart failure appears to be increased in response to increases in volume and/or pressure overload. Furthermore, ventricular ANF is released into the circulation in both congestive heart failure and hypertension. The role of ventricular ANF may be to regulate ventricular preload and sodium excretion in congestive heart failure and hypertension.

Functional significance of ANF in congestive heart failure and hypertension

Congestive heart failure

As congestive heart failure is characterized by sodium retention and activation of the renin−angiotensin−aldosterone system, the functional significance of elevated plasma concentrations of ANF in congestive heart failure is unclear. Recent studies have advanced our understanding of the potential role of ANF in both acute and chronic congestive heart failure.

The role of endogenous ANF in acute congestive heart failure was examined by Lee *et al.* [59] in recent studies in the canine model of congestive heart failure produced by rapid ventricular pacing. This model is characterized by a decrease in cardiac output and arterial pressure with an increase in atrial pressures and circulating levels of

ANF. Although arterial pressure decreased significantly with the induction of acute congestive heart failure, diuresis and sodium excretion were maintained and renin and aldosterone were not stimulated. In contrast, in a low-output model of congestive heart failure produced by thoracic inferior vena caval obstruction with no elevation in atrial pressures and plasma ANF, sodium retention and activation of the renin−angiotensin−aldosterone system were observed despite similar reductions in arterial pressures. Subsequently, with the exogenous administration of ANF in the low-output model of congestive heart failure in concentrations calculated to mimic the levels observed in the high-ANF congestive heart failure model, no sodium retention or activation of the renin−angiotensin−aldosterone system was observed. Thus, this study supports a role for ANF in acute congestive heart failure to maintain sodium excretion and suppress the activation of the renin−angiotensin−aldosterone system despite a significant reduction in arterial pressure.

Drexler *et al.* [60] investigated the role of ANF in chronic congestive heart failure by administering monoclonal ANF antibodies in a rat model of congestive heart failure produced by myocardial infarction. In response to the administration of ANF antibodies a further increase in systemic vascular resistance, decrease in cardiac output, and increase in atrial pressures were observed. This study suggests that endogenous ANF in chronic congestive heart failure may thus serve as an endogenous vasodilator. In a similar rat model of myocardial infarction, Awazu *et al.* [61] reported the renal response in congestive heart failure in the presence of ANF monoclonal antibodies. With the administration of ANF antibodies a marked decrease in sodium excretion was observed in the absence of a further reduction in the GFR or RBF. These two studies taken together thus support a role for ANF in chronic congestive heart failure both as an endogenous vasodilator and modulator of sodium and water excretion.

Studies by Hodsman *et al.* [62] further support the modulating action of ANF in congestive heart failure. These investigators examined the plasma hormonal response and changes in myocardial ANF mRNA content in the rat model of congestive heart failure after myocardial infarction. At 2 months after induction, plasma ANF as well as atrial and ventricular ANF mRNA were increased. However, plasma aldosterone was not elevated despite an increase in plasma renin activity in this model of congestive heart failure. As ANF can inhibit aldosterone release directly [63], these investigators suggested that ANF in this model of congestive heart failure may serve to decrease aldosterone secretion. Furthermore, while ANF was not able to inhibit an increase in renin, ANF could have limited this release of renin in response to reductions in arterial pressure. The role of ANF both in acute and chronic congestive heart failure may be to modulate the activation of vaso-constrictor and antinatriuretic hormones so as to defend the system against volume and/or pressure overload.

Despite the potential beneficial role of ANF in congestive heart failure, the renal natriuretic response to exogenous ANF is attenuated in congestive heart failure [64]. Scriven & Burnett [64] reported that the intrarenal infusion of ANF in both normal dogs and those with low-output congestive heart failure resulted in a significant increase in GFR and decrease in proximal tubule re-absorption of sodium as measured by the lithium clearance technique. However, the congestive heart failure group was characterized by a significantly blunted diuretic and natriuretic response as compared to controls.

The mechanism of the blunted response to exogenous ANF observed in congestive heart failure may be multifactorial. Receptor down-regulation as suggested by Schiffrin et al. [65] with evidence of down-regulation of ANF receptors in platelets in patients with congestive heart failure is one potential mechanism. Tsundo et al. [66] in the rat myocardial infarction model of congestive heart failure reported a reduction in renal medullary ANF receptors in association with increased ANF plasma levels. These two studies suggest that the blunted natriuretic response in congestive heart failure may be in part secondary to a down-regulation of ANF receptors in association with increased circulating levels of ANF.

Another potential mechanism for the attenuated renal response in congestive heart failure to synthetic ANF may be the antagonizing action of the renin−angiotensin−aldosterone system which is activated in congestive heart failure. While exogenous ANF may decrease plasma renin in congestive heart failure [67], it may not be suppressed adequately and intrarenal angio-tensin II activity may remain increased. Studies by Schowalter et al. [68] investigated the role of intrarenal angiotensin II in modulating the renal response to exogenous ANF in the anesthetized dog. A significant

attenuation of the natriuretic response to ANF was observed in association with a blunted action of ANF on the GFR. Extending these studies to congestive heart failure would suggest that the renin−angiotensin−aldosterone system in congestive heart failure may be an important opposing modulator of ANF. Furthermore, the activation of renal sympathetic activity in congestive heart failure in the presence of lowered renal perfusion pressure may also contribute to the sodium retention and blunted renal response to ANF by stimulating intrarenal angiotensin II.

Recent studies have also demonstrated that renal perfusion pressure is an important modulator of the renal response to ANF. Furthermore, renal perfusion pressure may play a dominant role over other potential mechanisms. Studies by Redfield et al. [63] in a canine acute low-output model of congestive heart failure reported the restoration of the natriuretic response to ANF when renal perfusion pressure was restored with the administration of intrarenal angiotensin II. However, blockade of the renin−angiotensin−aldosterone system with saralasin, a partial antagonist of angiotensin II, only partially restored the natriuretic response to ANF. Thus these studies suggest that the attenuated natriuretic response to exogenous ANF in congestive heart failure may be due to multiple mechanisms.

Investigators have recently suggested that while ANF release is increased in congestive heart failure, a "relative" deficiency of ANF for any given increase in atrial or ventricular filling pressures may exist. The release of ANF from the heart in congestive heart failure in response to an increase in atrial pressure may be attenuated as suggested in studies by Raine et al. [69]. These investigators reported that in patients with heart failure the increase in plasma concentrations of ANF in response to increases in atrial pressures was attenuated compared to normal subjects. Recent studies by Redfield et al. [70] have extended this observation. In the canine model of congestive heart failure produced by rapid ventricular pacing, these investigators demonstrated a "maximal" release of ANF in response to volume expansion. Thus while congestive heart failure is characterized by an elevation in plasma ANF, the secretory capacity of the heart may not meet the demands of the system creating a "relative" deficiency of ANF in congestive heart failure.

Hypertension

The functional role of ANF in both uncomplicated essential hypertension and hypertension in the presence of hypertrophy or congestive heart failure is unclear. Recent studies by Itoh *et al.* [71] support a functional role for ANF in hypertension especially in the presence of elevated circulating ANF. These investigators employed ANF monoclonal antibodies in the spontaneously hypertensive stroke-prone rat and DOCA-salt rats. The acute administration of ANF monoclonal antibodies in the spontaneously hypertensive stroke-prone rat resulted in a significant elevation of arterial pressure with a concomitant reduction in plasma cGMP. The chronic administration of ANF antibodies in this rat model also resulted in a significant increase in the arterial pressure as compared to controls.

In the DOCA-salt rat, a similar response was observed, with a significant acceleration in the development of hypertension with the chronic administration of ANF monoclonal antibodies, as compared to controls. Taken together, these studies suggest that in hypertension associated with ventricular hypertrophy in which plasma ANF levels are elevated, ANF may act as an endogenous vasodilator to defend the system against pressure overload.

Studies by Schiffrin *et al.* [72] recently reported that in patients with hypertension with elevated concentrations of plasma ANF and evidence of left ventricular hypertrophy, down-regulation of platelet ANF receptors was observed. In patients with mild essential hypertension, however, no reduction in platelet ANF receptors was reported. These results may explain why patients with hypertension in the presence of elevated concentrations of ANF appear to have a decreased hypotensive response to exogenous ANF [73]. This hypothesis is further supported by studies in the DOCA-salt hypertensive rat model in the presence of elevated plasma ANF levels in which the development of hypertension is associated with a down-regulation of vascular ANF receptors and glomerular cGMP production [74,75]. Yet, studies in both patients with essential hypertension and in the spontaneously hypertensive rat model of hypertension are associated with a normal or enhanced natriuretic response to exogenous ANF.

Therapeutic implications for ANF in congestive heart failure and hypertension

A role for ANF as a therapeutic agent in congestive heart failure and hypertension is supported, as reviewed in this chapter due to ANF's cardiovascular, renal, and endocrine actions. The effects of ANF resemble those of several pharmacologic agents currently used in the treatment of both congestive heart failure and hypertension. Atrial natriuretic factor like other vasodilators, in states characterized by volume and/or pressure overload, can decrease preload, and potentially decrease peripheral vascular resistance due to its vasorelaxant properties. It is also a diuretic with an antialdosterone action like spironolactone and ANF inhibits the renin–angiotensin–aldosterone system thus resembling the action of converting enzyme inhibitors. Based on these actions a potential therapeutic role for ANF in congestive heart failure and in hypertension has been suggested.

ANF in the treatment of congestive heart failure

Several studies have investigated the functional response of the cardiovascular, renal, and endocrine systems to the exogenous administration of ANF in congestive heart failure. Both the effect of bolus and short-term infusions of ANF has been reported. Studies by Cody *et al.* [67] reported the effect of the infusion of synthetic ANF in patients with congestive heart failure and in normal subjects. A short-term infusion of ANF in normals induced a natriuresis with suppression of renin and aldosterone despite a decrease in systolic pressure. The subjects with congestive heart failure demonstrated an increase in cardiac index, decrease in systemic vascular resistance, and left atrial pressure. However, no significant diuresis or natriuresis was observed. Although plasma renin was not suppressed aldosterone concentrations decreased.

Saito *et al.* [76] reported similar observations with the administration of exogenous ANF in patients with congestive heart failure. Cardiac output increased in association with a decrease in arterial pressure and systemic vascular resistance. While aldosterone was suppressed, no renal action to increase sodium excretion was observed. Thus ANF infusions in congestive heart failure exert a beneficial cardiovascular hemodynamic response with an increase in cardiac output, decrease in peripheral resistance, and a reduction in atrial pressures.

However, no effect of ANF on natriuresis or renin was observed with these infusions of synthetic ANF.

In contrast to the infusion studies in congestive heart failure, studies by Reigger *et al.* [77], with the bolus administration of ANF, reported a significant natriuretic and diuretic response in patients with congestive heart failure. Additionally, a similar beneficial cardiovascular response was demonstrated in response to the bolus administration of ANF with an increase in cardiac output and decrease in peripheral resistance. The mechanism of the differential response in congestive heart failure to the bolus vs. infusion administration of ANF is unclear. In preliminary studies from our laboratory, employing a low-dose infusion of ANF in patients with congestive heart failure a selective renal response was observed in the absence of any reduction in arterial pressure, atrial pressures, or peripheral resistance [78]. In contrast to prior studies which employed higher concentrations of ANF, low-dose ANF increased RBF, GFR, and decreased renal vascular resistance. This was associated with a decrease in both renin and aldosterone. A significant increase in the fractional excretion of sodium was also observed with a decrease in the fractional reabsorption of lithium supporting an action of ANF on the proximal tubule.

Based on these previous studies, the therapeutic role for exogenous ANF in congestive heart failure begins to emerge. The favorable vasodilating action of high-dose ANF could be employed to improve cardiac output and decrease systemic vascular resistance. Furthermore, plasma aldosterone is suppressed in these studies. Yet, renin is not inhibited with high-dose exogenous ANF. However, the lack of an increase in renin despite a reduction in arterial pressure with ANF suggests a relative inhibition of renin release by ANF. This relative inhibition of renin activation by ANF is in contrast to other vasodilators used in the treatment of congestive heart failure, which may stimulate renin release. While no beneficial renal response is observed with high-dose ANF, low-dose ANF could be employed for selective renal vasodilatation and inhibition of both renin and aldosterone.

Recent studies by Abbassi *et al.* [79] have suggested another potential therapeutic scenario for exogenous ANF in congestive heart failure. Previous studies in congestive heart failure have demonstrated that the attenuated response to exogenous ANF may be due to the antagonizing activation of the renin−angiotensin−aldosterone system in congestive heart failure. Based on these observations, these investigators hypothesized that inhibition of the renin−angiotensin−aldosterone system with angiotensin-converting enzyme inhibition may restore the attenuated natriuretic response to ANF. In the arteriovenous fistula rat model of congestive heart failure, these investigators reported the modulating effect of chronic angiotensin-converting enzyme inhibition on the cardiorenal response to exogenous ANF. The infusion of exogenous ANF in the sodium retaining rats in the absence of chronic angiotensin-converting enzyme inhibition with enalapril resulted in a markedly attenuated diuretic and natriuretic response (Fig. 7.6). However, in the sodium-retaining rats treated with enalapril a dramatic improvement in the diuretic and natriuretic response to ANF

Fig. 7.6 Effects of incremental doses of ANF on fractional excretion of sodium (FE_{Na}; A), glomerular filtration rate (GFR; B), and mean arterial blood pressure (BP; C) in sham controls and sodium-retaining rats with arteriovenous (AV) fistula in presence and absence of enalapril treatment. + Statistically significant difference ($P \leq 0.05$) between sham controls and sodium-retaining rats without enalapril treatment. * Statistically significant difference ($P \leq 0.05$) between enalapril-treated and nontreated rats with AV fistula. (From Abbassi *et al.* [79].)

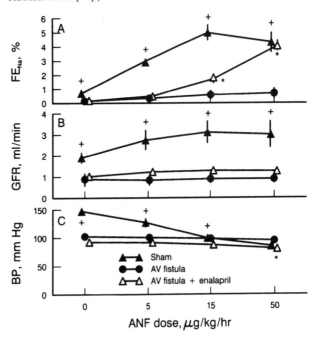

administration was observed. The increase observed in the fractional excretion of sodium in response to ANF at 50 µg/kg per hour in the congestive heart failure rats was actually similar to the response observed in the sham control rats. Furthermore, the enhanced natriuretic response to ANF in the enalapril treated group occurred despite a significant reduction in the mean arterial pressure. Similar studies by Villarreal and Freeman [80] in the atriovenous fistula dog model of congestive heart failure also demonstrated a restoration of the renal responsiveness to synthetic ANF with chronic captopril treatment. These two studies thus suggest a potential therapeutic role for ANF, possibly in association with angiotensin-converting enzyme inhibition.

In contrast to the above studies utilizing infusions of exogenous ANF, recent interest has centered on the use of specific inhibitors of ANF degradation [81]. Studies have demonstrated that a major pathway for degradation of ANF is by neutral endopeptidase 24.11 [82]. This enzyme is located principally within the proximal tubule brush border of the kidney. A specific inhibitor of neutral endopeptidase could thus have a potential therapeutic role in congestive heart failure by increasing the endogenous ANF concentrations.

Investigators employing a specific neutral endopeptidase inhibitor (NEP-I) recently reported a natriuretic and diuretic action in normal animals in association with increased concentrations of plasma ANF. In elegant studies by Margulies et al. [83], the natriuretic action of NEP-I SQ(28603) was potentiated with the intrarenal administration of pathophysiologic concentrations of ANF. These studies would thus suggest a potential therapeutic role for neutral endopeptidase inhibitors in congestive heart failure in the presence of elevated plasma ANF concentrations.

Recent studies from our laboratory as well as others have investigated the actions of specific neutral endopeptidase inhibitors in congestive heart failure [84,85]. The effect of NEP-I administered in 2 incremental doses was compared to an infusion of exogenous ANF (100 ng/kg per min) in two groups of dogs with severe congestive heart failure produced by rapid ventricular pacing [84]. As in previous studies in congestive heart failure, an attenuated natriuretic response was observed with exogenous ANF despite an increase in the GFR. However, with the administration of NEP-I a dose-dependent diuresis and natriuresis was observed with increases in both the fractional excretion of sodium and fractional excretion of lithium, the latter a marker for whole kidney proximal tubule sodium reabsorption. The marked natriuretic response was not associated with an increase in the GFR or RBF supporting a tubular action of NEP-I (Fig. 7.7). Furthermore, the natriuretic action of NEP-I did not parallel observed increases in plasma ANF.

In a separate group with congestive heart failure the administration of exogenous ANF to mimic plasma levels achieved with NEP-I failed to increase sodium or water excretion despite similar increases in the circulating concentrations of ANF (Fig. 7.8). This would suggest that the natriuretic response to NEP-I in congestive heart

Fig. 7.7 Renal hemodynamics and excretory response to NEP-I or ANF infusion in congestive heart failure. Values are given as mean ± SEM. * $P \leq 0.05$ compared with baseline; † $P \leq 0.05$ NEP-I 60 mg/kg compared with NEP-I 30 mg/kg. Atrial natriuretic factor infusion rate, 100 ng/kg per min.

	GFR, ml/min	RBF, ml/min	$U_{Na}\dot{V}$, µcq/min	FE_{Na}, %	FE_{Li}, %	$\dot{V}$, ml/min	ANF, pg/ml
NEP-I (group 1; n = 5)							
Baseline	36 ± 6	168 ± 22	14.87 ± 7.81	0.44 ± 0.3	28.4 ± 7.1	0.23 ± 0.11	372 ± 81
NEP-I 30 mg/kg	40 ± 7	168 ± 26	57.18 ± 14.54*	1.18 ± 0.32*	46.3 ± 11.8*	0.68 ± 0.21*	518 ± 73*
NEP-I 60 mg/kg	38 ± 5	190 ± 35	125.62 ± 29.77*†	2.23 ± 0.28*†	49.5 ± 5.7*	1.07 ± 0.43*†	489 ± 76
ANF (100 ng/kg/min) (group 2; n = 5)							
Baseline	27 ± 3	130 ± 18	14.37 ± 9.76	0.43 ± 0.17	24.5 ± 6.0	0.15 ± 0.05	372 ± 76
ANF	36 ± 3*	126 ± 18	50.63 ± 25.8	0.91 ± 0.47	31.5 ± 5.0	0.37 ± 0.11	638 ± 41*

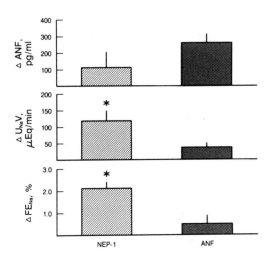

Fig. 7.8 Bar graphs of peak changes in plasma ANF, $U_{Na}V$, urinary sodium excretion and FE_{Na}, fraction excretion of sodium in congestive heart failure with neutral endopeptidase inhibitor (NEP-I) 30 mg/kg followed by NEP-I (60 mg/kg) or with exogenous ANF (100 ng/kg per min). * $P \leq 0.05$ NEP-I group vs. ANF group. (From Cavero et al. [84].)

failure may not be associated with changes in renal hemodynamics or elevations in circulating levels of ANF, but rather supports a local renal tubular action of NEP-I in congestive heart failure.

In studies by Northridge et al. [85] employing NEP-I (UK 69578) in human subjects with mild congestive heart failure, a similar diuretic and natriuretic response was observed in association with an elevation in plasma ANF and decrease in renin. A decrease in the right atrial pressure was also observed suggesting a beneficial action of NEP-I on preload. Taken together these studies support a potential therapeutic role for NEP-inhibition in congestive heart failure. Furthermore, studies by Parkes et al. [19] have reported a beneficial renal and cardiovascular action of ANF with the long-term infusion of ANF in sheep. Therefore the response to chronic elevations of circulating ANF with either NEP-I or synthetic ANF may be significantly different than that observed with acute elevations in ANF and suggest a potential therapeutic role for ANF in congestive heart failure.

ANF in the treatment of hypertension

Several groups have investigated the effect of ANF administration in patients with hypertension as well as in various animal models of hypertension. Lappe et al. [86] in the spontaneously hypertensive rat compared the hemodynamic response to bolus vs. sustained infusions of ANF. A dose-dependent decrease in mean arterial pressure was observed with bolus ANF in association with transient decreases in renal, mesenteric, and hindquarter vascular resistances. The renal excretory response was not investigated. Similarly, with incremental infusions of ANF a reduction in the mean arterial pressure was observed. However, an increase in regional vascular resistance in all three vascular beds was noted. These data suggest that in hypertension the bolus administration of ANF may result in an acute vasodilatory action not observed with a steady-state infusion. The mechanism of this differential hypotensive response to the bolus administration vs. infusion of ANF is unclear. This antihypertensive effect with ANF infusions has also been observed in other animal models with norepinephrine or angiotensin II-induced hypertension [86,87].

Studies with exogenous ANF administration in humans with hypertension have, however, shown conflicting results. In studies employing high-dose bolus administration of ANF in subjects with mild essential hypertension, Richards et al. [88] reported an enhanced natriuretic action of ANF compared to normotensive controls. However, no decrease in arterial pressure was observed in the hypertensive patients in contrast to the significant fall in pressure observed in the normal volunteers. Other investigators have also reported similar results in hypertensive patients with either enhanced or similar natriuretic and diuretic response to ANF infusions as in controls with a minimal effect on arterial pressure observed. In contrast, a study by Weidmann et al. [89] employing a bolus followed by an infusion of 0.1 µg/kg per min of ANF in hypertensive patients showed an enhanced natriuresis and diuresis as well as a reduction in arterial pressure. Data from these studies suggest that while the natriuretic response appears to be enhanced in hypertension, the vasodepressor effects of bolus or short-term ANF may be attenuated in essential hypertension.

In contrast, recent studies employing low-dose and/or more chronic infusions of ANF have reported not only a natriuretic response but a reduction in arterial pressure in hypertension. Garcia et al. [90] in a renin-dependent two-kidney, one-clip rat model of hypertension chronically infused synthetic ANF (1 µg/hour per rat) for 7 days. A gradual decrease in arterial pressure and natriuresis was observed with a subsequent reduction in the initial pressure natriuresis and maintenance of the hypotensive effect. Normalization of the plasma renin activity with ANF infusion suggests that the mechanism of the hypotensive response in this model of hypertension may be through the inhibition of angiotensin II mediated increase in vascular resistance. However, in the volume dependent one-kidney one-clip hypertensive model the observed ANF-induced reduction in arterial pressure may be secondary to volume depletion. Thus different mechanisms may be responsible for the hypotensive action of ANF in different animal models of hypertension.

Recent human studies have investigated the action of either low-dose and/or chronic infusions of ANF in patients with essential hypertension [91,92]. Tonolo *et al.* [91] in a placebo-controlled crossover study in mild hypertensives serial low doses of ANF at 1 and 2 pmol/kg per min were each infused for 2 hours. A significant dose-related fall in arterial pressure was observed which was sustained for 2 hours after the infusion. This hypotensive response appeared to be mediated by plasma volume contraction with a decrease in preload and cardiac output rather than by a reduction in peripheral resistance. In another study, with a very low-dose ANF infusion (0.75 pmol/kg per min) to raise the plasma level of ANF by approximately 8 pmol, no significant change in arterial pressure was observed as compared to normal controls [92]. Although no hypotensive effect was observed, an enhanced natriuresis and suppression of renin was reported. These studies again suggest a possible attenuated depressor response to ANF in patients with hypertension despite a normal or enhanced natriuretic effect.

As suggested in studies by Parkes *et al.* [19], however, long-term infusions with low-dose ANF may be needed in order to observe the vasodilatory as well as natriuretic actions of ANF. This temporal cardiovascular and renal action of ANF may be especially important in hypertension if indeed an attenuated response to ANF is present. More prolonged elevations in circulating ANF may be required as the onset of the vasodilatory response to ANF in hypertension may be delayed.

A recent report by Janssen *et al.* [93] lends support to this concept. A chronic 5-day infusion of ANF (0.2 μg/min) in hypertensive patients resulted in a decrease in mean arterial pressure. However, this response was seen only after 12 hours of ANF administration with a progressive decline in arterial pressure which leveled off after 40 hours. Furthermore, the 10% reduction in arterial pressure observed with the ANF infusion was sustained during the recovery period. Atrial natriuretic factor administration also resulted in an immediate natriuretic response which was attenuated after 2 days, possibly secondary to the decline in arterial pressure and/or activation of counterregulatory systems. This observed differential vasodilatory response pattern is consistent with previous studies in the hypertensive rat in which a 5-day chronic ANF infusion was required to reduce arterial pressure to normal [90]. These studies suggest that the actions of small but chronically sustained elevations in plasma ANF should not be inferred from acute studies. Additional studies are thus required to investigate further the effects of chronic elevations of ANF in hypertension.

As in congestive heart failure, another potential therapeutic scenario for ANF in hypertension is in association with angiotensin-converting enzyme inhibition. Studies in the spontaneously hypertensive rat with left ventricular hypertrophy recently reported the effects of chronic therapy with angiotensin-converting enzyme inhibition or hydralazine on plasma ANF concentrations and renal ANF receptors [94]. In this renin-dependent hypertensive model, while both captopril and hydralazine decreased the arterial pressure to a similar degree, regression of cardiac hypertrophy was only observed in the captopril treated group. Angiotensin-converting enzyme inhibitor therapy was also associated with a decrease in plasma ANF concentrations and evidence of an increase in the binding affinity and capacity of renal ANF receptors. This study would thus suggest that in patients with essential hypertension, especially those with left ventricular hypertrophy, and evidence of increased circulating levels of ANF, angiotensin-converting enzyme inhibitor therapy may modulate and enhance the depressor and renal actions of ANF.

As increased wall stress and ventricular volumes in the spontaneously hypertensive rat may lead to the stimulation of ventricular ANF mRNA, these studies by Fukui *et al.* [94] suggest that treatment with captopril may suppress ANF gene expression. Treatment of hypertension in the spontaneously hypertensive rat with captopril resulted in a significant reduction (62%) in ventricular ANF mRNA concentration in association with regression of hypertrophy. However, despite similar reductions in arterial pressure in the hydralazine-treated spontaneously hypertensive rat no significant reduction in left ventricular hypertrophy was noted with a decrease in ANF mRNA of approximately 30%. These studies would thus also suggest treatment with captopril in hypertension may modulate the expression of ANF mRNA by decreasing left ventricular wall stress and hypertrophy.

Recent studies have also addressed the potential therapeutic action of NEP-I in hypertension. In preliminary studies by Samuels et al. [95], the depressor action of NEP-I in the one-kidney DOCA-salt rat model of hypertension was reported. The bolus administration of a specific NEP-I significantly reduced blood pressure by 30 mmHg. This depressor action of NEP-I was sustained for 4 hours. Furthermore, the chronic administration of NEP-I in this model of hypertension, first administered 24 hours after surgery, reduced the rate of development of hypertension compared to the control vehicle treated group. The antihypertensive effect of NEP-I in these studies was associated with an increase in plasma ANF concentrations. Thus neutral endopeptidase inhibitors may have potential benefit in patients with hypertension.

In summary, these studies support a therapeutic potential for ANF in hypertension possibly in association with angiotensin-converting enzyme inhibition. However, additional studies are required to investigate the modulating action and potential therapeutic role of chronic elevations of plasma ANF, either with NEP-I or via ANF infusion, on volume and pressure regulation in hypertension.

ANF: implications in the elderly

With age, alterations in cardiovascular, renal, and hormonal function occur [96]. Cardiovascular changes associated with aging include evidence of increased peripheral vascular resistance, increased vascular stiffness, cardiac hypertrophy, and reduced left ventricular compliance. An age-related reduction in RBF and GFR, perhaps due to the progressive loss of nephrons, is also observed. Furthermore, in the elderly plasma renin and aldosterone are often suppressed with an age-related increase in plasma catecholamines. Atrial natriuretic

factor due to its renal, endocrine, and cardiovascular actions may thus have a physiologic role in the elderly normotensive subject as well as in the elderly patients with hypertension or congestive heart failure.

Several investigators have reported plasma ANF concentrations in the elderly. McKnight et al. [97] examined the correlation between age, arterial pressure, and plasma ANF concentrations in healthy normotensive patients. An independent positive correlation was present between age and ANF levels. In studies employing echocardiography to assess left atrial dimensions as well as degree of left ventricular hypertrophy, Ezaki et al. [98] reported similar observations with increased plasma concentrations of ANF in the elderly subjects in the absence of echocardiographic abnormalities. Taken together these studies suggest that an age-related increase in plasma ANF may be present.

Several factors could account for the observed increase in plasma ANF levels in the elderly. Jamieson & Palade [99] reported that the frequency of atrial granules appeared to increase with age in the rat. Studies by Akimoto et al. [100] have also reported an age-related increase in atrial ANF. Thus, increased production and release of ANF in the elderly may contribute to elevations in plasma ANF. The release of ANF may also be stimulated by plasma norepinephrine which appears to increase with age and has been shown in vitro to enhance the release of ANF [101].

Another potential explanation for the elevation in plasma ANF in the elderly is based on studies which have suggested that the atrial volume and/or pressure may increase with age independent of hypertrophy [96]. The increase in atrial stretch could then stimulate the increased release of ANF. In addition, the increased incidence of left ventricular hypertrophy in the elderly, with the subsequent stimulation of ventricular ANF as seen in hypertension, may also contribute to elevations in plasma ANF. However, additional studies are required in elderly patients with simultaneous measurements of central hemodynamics and plasma ANF levels. Age-related decreases in renal function may also alter the clearance of ANF and result in elevated plasma levels of ANF as suggested by Ohashi et al. [102].

The functional significance of elevated concentrations of ANF in the elderly is unclear. To date no studies have addressed this issue. Atrial natriuretic factor in the

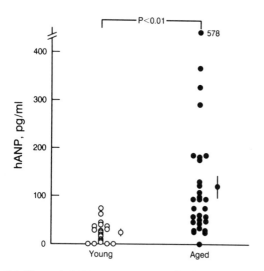

Fig. 7.9 Plasma h ANP concentrations in healthy young ($n = 19$) and aged men ($n = 31$). (From Ohashi *et al.* [102].)

normotensive elderly patient, as in the patient with congestive heart failure or hypertension, may serve as an endogenous vasodilator to defend the system against volume and/or pressure overload in the presence of age-related increases in peripheral resistance, and decreases in renal function. Furthermore, age-related suppression of the renin—angiotensin—aldosterone system may be due to a modulating action of ANF on renin and aldosterone release.

The potential role of ANF in the treatment of hypertension or congestive heart failure as it pertains to the elderly is now emerging. To date, only one study has specifically investigated the hemodynamic and renal response to ANF in the elderly population although many studies have included elderly patients as part of their study subjects [102] (Fig. 7.9). In this study, older patients with baseline elevations in plasma ANF demonstrated a greater incremental increase in plasma ANF concentration with the administration of exogenous ANF than in controls. However, no difference in sodium excretion between the two groups was observed. This study thus suggests that in the elderly as compared to controls a "relative" renal resistance to physiologic concentrations of ANF may be present. This resistance may be due to the down-regulation of renal receptors in the presence of elevated concentrations of plasma ANF or due to age-related decreases in renal function.

In theory, the actions of ANF to maintain volume and pressure homeostasis through increased sodium excretion, inhibition of the renin—angiotensin—aldosterone system, and reductions in peripheral resistance and preload suggest a therapeutic role for ANF in elderly patients with congestive heart failure or hypertension. Atrial natriuretic factor as a therapeutic agent in the elderly has several advantages. Like angiotensin-converting enzyme inhibitors which have been found to be well tolerated in the elderly, ANF further suppresses the renin—angiotensin—aldosterone system. Furthermore, with chronic elevations in plasma ANF, a vasodilatory action of ANF may occur and would serve to decrease peripheral resistance. Atrial natriuretic factor, unlike furosemide, could also enhance natriuresis without a kaliuresis or activation of the renin—angiotensin—aldosterone system. Based on these observations a potential role for the treatment of congestive heart failure and hypertension in the elderly with NEP-I or infusions of ANF possibly in association with angiotensin-converting enzyme inhibition emerges as a rational therapeutic approach in this population.

References

1 Brody JA, Brock DB, Williams TF. Trends in the health of the elderly population. Annu Rev Public Health 1987; 8:211—234.

2 de Bold AJ, Borenstein HB, Veress AT, *et al.* A rapid and potent natriuretic response to intravenous injection of atrial myocardial extract in rats. Life Sci 1981;28:89—94.

3 Burnett JC Jr, Granger JP, Opgenorth TJ. Effects of synthetic atrial natriuretic factor on renal function and renin release. Am J Physiol 1984;247:F863—F866.

4 Maack T, Marion DN, Camargo MJ, *et al.* Effects of auriculin (atrial natriuretic factor) on blood pressure, renal function, and the renin—aldosterone system in dogs. Am J Med 1984;77:1069—1075.

5 Bussien JP, Biollaz J, Waeber B, *et al.* Dose-dependent effect of atrial natriuretic peptide on blood pressure, heart rate, and skin blood flow of normal volunteers. J Cardiol Pharm 1986;8:216—220.

6 Debinski W, Kuchel O, Garcia R, *et al.* Atrial natriuretic factor inhibits the sympathetic nervous activity in one-kidney, one-clip hypertension in the rat. Proc Soc Exp Biol Med 1986;181:173—176.

7 Edwards BS, Schwab TB, Zimmerman RS, *et al.* Cardiovascular, renal, and endocrine response to atrial natriuretic peptide in angiotensin II mediated hypertension. Circ Res 1986;59:663−667.

8 Garcia R, Thibault G, Cantin M, *et al.* Effect of a purified atrial natriuretic factor on rat and rabbit vascular strips and vascular beds. Am J Physiol 1984;247:R34−R38.

9 Windquist RJ, Faison EP, Waldman SA, *et al.* Atrial natriuretic factor elicits an endothelium-independent relaxation and activates particulate guanylate cyclase in vascular smooth muscle. Proc Nat Acad Sci 1984;81:7661.

10 Fujita T, Ito Y, Noda H, *et al.* Vasodilatory actions of alpha-human atrial natriuretic peptide and high effects in normal man. J Clin Invest 1987;80:832−835.

11 Bie P, Wang BC, Leadley RJ, *et al.* Hemodynamic and renal effects of low dose infusions of atrial peptide in awake dogs. Am J Physiol 1988;254:R161−R169.

12 Breuhaus BA, Saneii HH, Brandt MA, *et al.* Atriopeptin II lowers cardiac output in conscious sheep. Am J Physiol 1985;249:R776−R780.

13 Holtz J, Stewart DJ, Elsner D, *et al. In vivo* atrial peptide venodilatation: minimal potency relative to nitroglycerin in dogs. Life Sci 1986;39:2177−2184.

14 Fluckinger JP, Waeber B, Matsueda G, *et al.* Effect of atriopeptin III on hematocrit and volemia of nephrectomized rats. Am J Physiol 1986;251:H880−H883.

15 Trippodo N, Chien Y, Frohlich E. Atrial natriuretic peptide increases resistance to venous return. Am J Physiol 1987;252:H894−H897.

16 Wangler RD, Breuhaus BA, Otero HO, *et al.* Coronary vasoconstrictor effects of atriopeptin II. Science 1985;230:558−560.

17 Burnett JC Jr, Rubanyi GM, Edwards BS, *et al.* Atrial natriuretic peptide decreases arterial pressure in the absence of coronary vasoconstriction. Proc Soc Exp Biol Med 1987;186:313−317.

18 Chu A, Cobb FR. Effects of atrial natriuretic peptide on proximal epicardial coronary arteries and coronary blood flow in conscious dogs. Circ Res 1987;61:485−488.

19 Parkes DG, Coghlan JP, McDougall JG, *et al.* Long-term hemodynamic actions of atrial natriuretic factor (99−126) in conscious sheep. Am J Physiol 1988;254:H811−H815.

20 Thoren P, Mark A, Morgan D, *et al.* Activation of vasodepressor reflexes by atriopeptins inhibits renal sympathetic nerve activity. Am J Physiol 1986;251:H1252−H1257.

21 Zimmerman RS, Schirger J, Edwards BS, *et al.* Cardiorenal endocrine dynamics during step-wise infusion of physiologic and pharmacologic concentrations of atrial natriuretic factor in the dog. Circ Res 1987;61:63−69.

22 Tikkanen I, Metsarinne K, Fyhrquist F, *et al.* Plasma atrial natriuretic peptide in cardiac disease and during infusion in healthy volunteers. Lancet 1985;2:66−69.

23 Freid TJ, Stein J. Effect of atrial natriuretic factor on glomerular function. Am J Physiol 1986;250:F119−F122.

24 Ichikawa S, Dunn BR, Troy GL, *et al.* Influence of atrial natriuretic peptide on glomerular microcirculation *in vivo.* Clin Res 1985;33:A487.

25 Burnett JC Jr, Opgenorth TJ, Granger JP. The renal actions of atrial natriuretic peptide during control of glomerular filtration. Kidney Int 1986;30:16−19.

26 Hammond T, Yusufi A, Knox F, *et al.* Administration of atrial natriuretic factor inhibits sodium transport in proximal tubules. J Clin Invest 1985;75:1983−1989.

27 Schwab TR, Edwards BS, Zimmerman RS, *et al.* Renal interstitial hydrostatic pressure dynamics during atrial natriuretic peptide administration. In Brenner B, Laragh J, eds. *Proceedings of the First World Congress of Biologically Active Atrial Peptides.* New York: Raven Press, 1988.

28 Winaver J, Burnett JC Jr, Tyce JM, *et al.* Inhibition of Na^+−H^+ antiport in renal brush border membrane elicited by ANF *in vivo* is mediated by dopamine (abstr.). ASN 1989;A155.

29 Ichikawa S, Saito T, Okada K, *et al.* Atrial natriuretic factor increases cyclic GMP and inhibits cyclic AMP in rat renal papillary collecting tubule cells in culture. Biochem Biophys Res Comm 1985;130:1147−1153.

30 Opgenorth TJ, Burnett JC Jr, Granger JP, *et al.* Effects of atrial natriuretic peptide on renin secretion in non-filtering kidney. Am J Physiol 1986;250:F798−F801.

31 Dunn BR, Ichikawa I, Troy JL. Effect of atrial natriuretic peptide (ANP) on hydraulic pressures in the rat renal papilla: Implications for ANP-induced natriuresis (abstr.). Kidney Int 1986;29:382.

32 Atarashi K, Mulrow PJ, Franco-Saenz R. Inhibition of aldosterone production by atrial extract. Science 1984;224:992−993.

33 Campbell WB, Currie MC, Needleman P. Inhibition of aldosterone biosynthesis by atriopeptins in rat adrenal cells. Circ Res 1985;57:113−118.

34 Richards AM, Ikram H, Yandle TG, *et al.* Renal, hemodynamic, and hormonal effects of alpha atrial natriuretic peptide in healthy volunteers. Lancet 1985;1:545−548.

35 Anderson JV, Donckier J, Payne N, *et al.* Atrial natriuretic hormone at physiologic plasma concentrations in man. Clin Sci 1987;72:305−312.

36 Hirth C, Stasch J-P, Kazda S, *et al.* The renal response to acute hypervolemia is caused by atrial natriuretic peptides. J Cardiovasc Pharm 1986;8:268−275.

37 Weidmann P, Hellmueller B, Uehlinger DE, *et al.* Plasma levels and cardiovascular, endocrine, and excretory effects of atrial natriuretic peptide during different sodium intakes in man. J Clin Endocrinol Metab 1986;62:1026−1027.

38 Schwab TR, Edwards BS, Heublein DM, *et al.* The role of atrial natriuretic peptide in volume expansion natriuresis. Am J Physiol 1986;251:R310−R313.

39 Veress AT, Sonnenberg H. Right atrial appendectomy

reduces the renal response to acute hypervolemia in the rat. Am J Physiol 1984;247:R610–R613.

40 Chimoskey JE, Spielman WS, Brandt MA, et al. Cardiac atria of bio 14.6 hamsters are deficient in natriuretic factor. Science 1984;223:820–822.

41 Edwards BS, Ackermann DM, Schwab TR, et al. The relationship between atrial granularity and circulating atrial natriuretic peptide in hamsters with congestive heart failure. Mayo Clin Proc 1986;61:517–522.

42 Burnett J, Kao PC, Hu DC, et al. Atrial natriuretic peptide elevation in congestive heart failure in the human. Science 1986;231:1145–1147.

43 Shenker Y, Sider RS, Ostafin EA, et al. Plasma levels of immunoreactive atrial natriuretic factor in healthy subjects and in patients with edema. J Clin Invest 1985;76:1684–1687.

44 Sagnella GA, Markandu ND, Shore AC, et al. Raised circulating levels of atrial natriuretic peptides in essential hypertension. Lancet 1986;1:179–181.

45 Arai H, Nakao K, Saito Y, et al. Augmented expression of atrial natriuretic polypeptide gene in ventricles of spontaneously hypertensive rats (SHR) and SHR-stroke prone. Circ Res 1988;62:926–930.

46 Zachariah PK, Burnett JC Jr, Ritter S, et al. Atrial natriuretic peptide in essential hypertension. Mayo Clin Proc 1987;62:782–786.

47 London GM, Safar ME, Safar AL, et al. Blood pressure in the "low-pressure system" and cardiac performance in essential hypertension. J Hypertens 1985;3:337–342.

48 Ferrier C, Weidmann P, Hollman R, et al. Impaired response of atrial natriuretic factor to high salt intake in persons prone to hypertension. N Engl J Med 1988;319:1224–1225.

49 Van Hooft I, Grobbee DE, Hofman A, et al. Atrial natriuretic factor and sodium intake in off-spring of hypertensive and normotensive parents. N Engl J Med 1989;320:867–868.

50 Mimran A, Nussberger J, Ribstein J, et al. Response of atrial natriuretic peptide to acute saline loading in essential hypertension. Am J Physiol 1988;241:F1085–F1090.

51 Saito Y, Nakao K, Sugawara A, et al. Clinical application of atrial natriuretic polypeptide in patients with congestive heart failure: beneficial effects on left ventricular function. Am Heart J 1988;116:1053–1057.

52 Sudhir K, Woods RL, Jennings GL, et al. Exaggerated atrial natriuretic peptide release during acute exercise in essential hypertension. J Hum 1988;1:299–304.

53 Edwards BS, Ackermann DM, Lee ME, et al. Hypertens identification of atrial natriuretic factor within ventricular tissue in hamsters and humans with congestive heart failure. J Clin Invest 1988;81:82–86.

54 Ritman EL, Pao YC. Finite element analysis of myocardial diastolic stress and strain relationship in the intact heart. Eur J Cardiol 1978;7:S105–S119.

55 Yasue H, Obata K, Okumura K, et al. Increased secretion of

atrial natriuretic polypeptide from the left ventricle in patients with dilated cardiomyopathy. J Clin Invest 1989;83:46–51.

56 Lattion AL, Michel JB, Arnauld E, et al. Myocardial recruitment during ANF mRNA increases with volume overload in the rat. Am J Physiol 1986;251:H890–H896.

57 Mercardier JJ, Samuel JL, Michel JB, et al. Atrial natriuretic factor gene expression in rat ventricle during experimental hypertension. Am J Physiol 1989;257:H979–H987.

58 Ruskoaho H, Kinnunen P, Taskinen T, et al. Regulation of ventricular atrial natriuretic peptide release in hypertrophied rat myocardium. Circulation 1989:390–400.

59 Lee ME, Edwards BS, Miller W, et al. Role of endogenous atrial natriuretic factor in acute congestive heart failure. J Clin Invest 1989;84:1962–1966.

60 Drexler H, Hirth C, Morich F, et al. Vasodilatory action of endogenous ANP in chronic congestive heart failure as determined by monoclonal ANP-antibodies. Circulation 1987;76:A532.

61 Awazu M, Imada H, Kon V, et al. Assessment of the functional role of endogenous atrial natriuretic peptide by purified anti-ANP antibody: study in rat model of congestive heart failure. Kidney Int 1988;33:253–261.

62 Hodsman GP, Kohzuki M, Howes LG, et al. Neurohormonal responses to chronic myocardial infarction in rats. Circulation 1988;78:376–381.

63 Redfield MM, Edwards BS, Heublein DM, et al. Restoration of renal response to ANF in experimental low-output heart failure. Am J Physiol 1989;257:R917–R923.

64 Scriven TA, Burnett JC Jr. Effects of synthetic atrial natriuretic peptide on renal function and renin release on acute experimental congestive heart failure. Circulation 1985;72:892–897.

65 Schiffrin E, Des Longchamps T, Thibaut G. Platelet binding for atrial natriuretic factor in humans. Hypertension 1986;11:64–66.

66 Tsundo K, Mendelsohn F, Sexton P, et al. Decreased atrial natriuretic peptide binding in renal medulla in rats with chronic congestive heart failure. Circ Res 1988;62:155–161.

67 Cody RJ, Atlas SA, Laragh JH, et al. Atrial natriuretic factor in normal subjects and heart failure patients: plasma levels and renal, hormonal, and hemodynamic responses to peptide infusion. J Clin Invest 1986;78:1362–1374.

68 Schowalter CJ, Zimmerman RS, Schwab TR, et al. Renal response to atrial natriuretic factor is modulated by intrarenal angiotensin II. Am J Physiol 1988;254:R453–R456.

69 Raine A, Burgisser E, Muller F, et al. Atrial natriuretic peptide and atrial pressure in patients with congestive heart failure. N Engl J Med 1986;315:533–537.

70 Redfield MM, Edwards BS, McGoon MD, et al. Failure of ANF to increase with volume expansion in acute and chronic congestive heart failure in the dog. Circulation 1989;80:651–657.

71 Itoh H, Nakao K, Mukoyama M, *et al.* Chronic blockade of endogenous atrial natriuretic peptide (ANP) by monoclonal antibodies against ANP accelerates the development of hypertension in spontaneously hypertensive and deoxycorticosterone acetate-salt hypertensive rats. J Clin Invest 1989;84: 145–154.

72 Schiffrin E, St-Louis J, Essiambre R. Platelet binding sites and plasma concentration of atrial natriuretic factor in patients with essential hypertension. J Hypertens 1988;6: 565–572.

73 Schiffrin E, St-Louis J. Decreased density of vascular receptors for atrial natriuretic factor in DOCA-salt sensitive rats. Hypertension 1987;9:504–512.

74 Gauquelin G, Schiffrin E, Cantin M, *et al.* Specific binding of atrial natriuretic factor to renal glomeruli in DOCA-salt sensitive rats. Biochem Biophys Res Comm 1987;145:522–531.

75 Richards AM, Nicholls MG, Espiner EA, *et al.* Effects of a human natriuretic peptide in essential hypertension. Hypertension 1985;7:812–817.

76 Saito Y, Nakao K, Nishimura K, *et al.* Clinical application of atrial natriuretic polypeptide in patients with congestive heart failure: beneficial effects on left ventricular function. Circulation 1987;76:115–124.

77 Reigger GA, Kromer EP, Kochsiek K. Human atrial natriuretic peptide: plasma levels, hemodynamic, hormonal, and renal effects in patients with severe congestive heart failure. J Cardiovasc Pharmacol 1986;8:1107–1112.

78 Burnett JC Jr, Edwards BS, Zimmerman RS. Renal–cardiovascular–endocrine response to atrial natriuretic factor in congestive heart failure (abstr.). Clin Res 1986;34:A972.

79 Abbassi Z, Haramati A, Hoffman A, *et al.* Effect of converting enzyme inhibition on the renal response to ANF in rats with experimental heart failure. Am J Physiol 1990;259: R84–R89

80 Villarreal D, Freeman RH. Captopril restores the renal responsiveness to synthetic atrial natriuretic factor in dogs with heart failure. Circulation 1989;80(Suppl. II):112.

81 Berg JA, Hayashi M, Fujii Y, *et al.* Renal metabolism of atrial natriuretic peptide in the rat. Am J Physiol 1988;255: F466–F473.

82 Kenny AJ, Stephenson SL. Role of endopeptidase-24.11 in the inactivation of atrial natriuretic peptide. FEBS Letter 1988;232:1–8.

83 Margulies KB, Cavero PG, Seymour AA, *et al.* Neutral endopeptidase inhibition potentiates the renal actions of ANF. Kidney Int 1990;38:67–72.

84 Cavero PG, Margulies KB, Winaver J, *et al.* Cardiorenal actions of neutral endopeptidase inhibition in experimental congestive heart failure. Circulation 1990;82:196–201.

85 Northridge DB, Jardine AG, Alabaster CT, *et al.* Effects of UK 69578: a novel atriopeptidase inhibitor. Lancet 1989; 591–595.

86 Lappe RW, Todt JA, Wendt RL. Hemodynamic effects with infusion versus bolus administration of atrial natriuretic factor. Hypertension 1986;8:866–871.

87 Edwards BS, Schwab TR, Zimmerman RS, *et al.* Cardiovascular, renal, and endocrine response to atrial natriuretic peptide in angiotensin II mediated hypertension. Circ Res 1986;59:663–666.

88 Richards AM, Nicholls G, Espiner E, *et al.* Effects of a human atrial natriuretic peptide in essential hypertension. Hypertension 1985;7:812–817.

89 Weidmann P, Gnadinger MP, Ziswiler H, *et al.* Cardiovascular, endocrine, and renal effects of atrial natriuretic peptide in essential hypertension. J Hypertens 1986 (Suppl. 2);S71–S83.

90 Garcia R, Thibault G, Gutkowska J, *et al.* Effect of chronic infusion of synthetic atrial natriuretic factor (ANF 8–33) in conscious two-kidney, one-clip hypertensive rats. Proc Soc Exp Biol Med 1985;178:155–159.

91 Tonolo G, Richards AM, Manunta P, *et al.* Low-dose infusion of atrial natriuretic factor in mild essential hypertension. Circulation 1989;80:893–902.

92 Cusson JR, Thibault G, Kuchel O, *et al.* Cardiovascular, renal, and endocrine responses to low doses of atrial natriuretic factor in mild essential hypertension. J Hum Hypertens 1989;3:89–96.

93 Janssen WM, de Zeeuw D, van der Hem GK, *et al.* Antihypertensive effect of a 5-day infusion of atrial natriuretic factor in humans. Hypertension 1989;13:640–646.

94 Fukui K, Iwao H, Nakamura A, *et al.* Captopril and hydralazine suppress atrial natriuretic peptide (ANP) gene expression in the ventricle of spontaneously hypertensive rat. Biochem Biophys Res Comm 1989;160:310–316.

95 Samuels GMR, Barclay PL, Shepperson NB, *et al.* The acute and chronic antihypertensive efficacy of atriopeptidase inhibition in rats (abstr.). JACC 1989;13:A276.

96 Messerli FH, ed. *Cardiovascular Disease in the Elderly.* Boston: Martinus Nijhoff Publishing, 1985.

97 McKnight JA, Roberts G, Sheridan B, *et al.* Relationship between basal and sodium-stimulated plasma atrial natriuretic factor, age, sex, and blood pressure in normal man. J Hum Hypertens 1989;3:157–163.

98 Ezaki H, Matsushita S, Shiraki M, *et al.* Clinical evaluation of the plasma levels of immunoreactive atrial natriuretic peptide in elderly patients with heart disease. J Am Geriatr Soc 1988;36:537–541.

99 Jamieson JD, Palade GE. Specific granules in atrial muscle cells. J Cell Biol 1964;23:151–172.

100 Akimoto K, Miyata A, Kangawa K, *et al.* Molecular forms of atrial natriuretic peptide in the atrium of patients with cardiovascular disease. J Clin Endocrinol Metab 1988;67: 93–97.

101 Shimamoto K, Nakagawa M, Fukuyama S, *et al.* Effects of

norepinephrine and angiotensin II on plasma atrial natriuretic peptide concentrations in humans. J Cardiovasc
Pharmacol 1989;13(Suppl. 6):559–562.

102 Ohashi M, Fujio N, Nawata H, *et al.* Pharmacokinetics of
synthetic (beta)-human atrial natriuretic polypeptide in
normal men; effect of aging. Regul Pept 1987;19:265–272.

8

Pharmacokinetics of renal and antihypertensive drugs in the elderly

D. Craig Brater

Introduction

The disposition of and response to a number of drugs is changing in elderly patients. This chapter will first review physiologic changes of aging that influence drug disposition and response. A more detailed assessment of response to diuretics and antihypertensive agents will follow. This section will focus on not only the disposition of such agents in elderly patients but also changes in response (both efficacious and toxic). Lastly, in tabular form will be presented known data for drugs with which there is changed disposition in elderly patients. These data can be used to guide dosing changes of drugs in patients who require dose alterations.

Physiologic changes of aging: effects on drug disposition

The aging process results in a number of physiologic changes which can influence drug disposition (Table 8.1) (for review see [1–6]).

Changes in gastrointestinal function

On average, gastric pH increases with age and the prevalence of achlorhydria increases in elderly patients to as high as 20% of patients [7–9]. This decrease in acidity of gastric contents is probably of negligible importance for most drugs; on the other hand, a drug such as ketoconazole clearly requires intact gastric acidification to be absorbed [10] though the closely related azole antifungal compounds fluconazole and itraconazole do not have similar requirements. One would expect at least some elderly patients to malabsorb ketoconazole and perhaps other drugs, but there are no data to allow adequate conclusions. Clinicians should be aware that changes in gastric acidity occur in elderly patients and that this effect may potentially influence absorption of some drugs.

Most drugs are absorbed from the small intestine; thus the rate of gastric emptying influences access to sites of absorption and how quickly a drug is absorbed. Elderly patients have slowed gastric emptying which can cause a delay in and diminished rate of absorption without affecting the extent of absorption (bioavailability) [7,8,11].

Other age-related changes have been documented in the gastrointestinal tract including decreased absorptive surface area and decreased splanchnic blood flow [3,7,8]. It seems doubtful that these alterations importantly influ-

Table 8.1 Physiologic changes of aging that may influence drug disposition

Physiologic change	Potential effect on drug disposition
Changes in gastrointestinal function	
↑ Gastric pH; ↑ prevalence of achlorhydria	↓ Absorption of acid-soluble drugs (e.g., ketoconazole)
Delayed gastric emptying	Delay in absorption and/or ↓ rate of absorption
↓ Absorptive surface	?
↓ Splanchnic blood flow	?
Changes in body composition	
↓ Lean body mass; ↑ adipose mass	↑ Vd of lipid-soluble drugs (e.g., diazepam)
↓ Total body water	↓ Vd of water-soluble drugs (e.g., ethanol)
Changes in protein binding	
↓ Serum albumin concentrations	↑ Vd and ↑ Clearance of total drug; no change in unbound drug
Changes in hepatic function	
↓ Hepatic size	?
↓ Hepatic blood flow	↓ Clearance and first pass metabolism of highly extracted (flow-dependent) drugs (e.g., propranolol)
↓ Hepatic metabolism	↓ Clearance of capacity-limited drugs
Changes in renal function	
↓ Glomerular filtration rate and blood flow	↓ Clearance of drugs and metabolites excreted by the kidney

Vd, volume of distribution.

ence drug absorption in elderly patients since studies to date have shown no clinically important changes in quantitative drug absorption with age [12–14]. It must be acknowledged, however, that the absorption of relatively few drugs has been studied in elderly patients and clin-icians must be alert to possible differences from younger counterparts.

In summary, the diminished acidity of gastric contents may decrease absorption of ketoconazole and related compounds. In addition, slowed gastric emptying may delay absorption and decrease its rate, which would manifest as a later time of peak concentration and a diminished peak concentration, respectively. This effect is unlikely to be clinically important. To date most potential permutors of drug absorption in elderly patients are theoretical.

Changes in body composition

The aging process entails changes in body composition that can influence the distribution of drugs (Table 8.1). Lean body mass diminishes while that of adipose tissue increases with age. In men the percentage of body weight that is fat increases from 18 to 36%, and in women from 33 to 45% as age exceeds 65 years [15]. In addition, total body water decreases from 10 to 15% between ages 20 and 80 [1]. These changes can affect distribution of drugs among tissues. Thus, drugs such as ethanol which are restricted in their distribution to total body water have a smaller volume in which to distribute and thereby attain a higher blood concentration relative to dose in elderly patients [16]. Conversely, highly lipid-soluble drugs such as diazepam have relatively more adipose tissue in which to distribute, resulting in larger volumes of distribution in elderly patients [17,18].

Such changes in volume of distribution would affect the size of a loading dose if one were administered and would also influence the half-life, since half-life = $0.693\,Vd/Cl$ where Vd = volume of distribution and Cl = clearance. The half-life influences the time needed to reach steady state. For example, for a drug like diazepam in which a loading dose is not usually given, the only clinically important manifestation of the increased Vd in elderly patients is the greater time needed to attain steady state when dosing is commenced or changed. It is important to emphasize that such changes in Vd or half-life do not affect the maintenance dose administered which is only influenced by clearance.

Changes in protein binding

Many drugs are bound to circulating proteins, acidic compounds binding predominantly to albumin and basic drugs binding predominantly to α1-acid glycoprotein. If in excess of about 90% of a drug is bound, it is subject to displacement from binding by other compounds or by diminished protein concentrations.

Even healthy elderly people have diminished serum albumin concentrations compared to their young counterparts, and elderly patients with concomitant clinical conditions are more likely to have decreased albumin values [1–6,19,20]. On average, elderly patients have albumin concentrations about 20% lower than young patients. This magnitude of decrease is sufficient to decrease the protein binding of highly bound drugs and can thereby result in an increase in the percentage of unbound or free drug which is pharmacologically active.

It is frequently presumed that this phenomenon always results in increased unbound drug concentrations and increased effect. In truth, this does not always occur, for the unbound drug concentration can remain unchanged while the total concentration of drug in the circulation (bound plus unbound) is diminished. Thus, while the percentage of unbound drug is increased relative to total drug, the actual concentration of unbound drug is the same. This phenomenon can lead to considerable confusion in the medical literature when disposition parameters are expressed relative to total rather than unbound drug. More specifically, the lower total drug concentration results in a calculated Vd and Cl that are higher in the patient with diminished protein binding compared to normal; such values are misleading since the same parameters calculated relative to unbound, pharmacologically active drug would be unchanged. An example of a drug that behaves in this fashion is phenytoin.

An extension of this scenario could result in a different misinterpretation. If binding diminished yet the ability to clear the unbound drug was diminished, then the unbound drug would accumulate and thereby increase the total drug concentration. In this case, of which naproxen is an example [21] the clearance of unbound drug is diminished in elderly patients, an effect that would mandate dose adjustment. Parameters calculated relative to total drug are unchanged in elderly patients. Thus, if data were assessed only in terms of total drug concentration, an inappropriate conclusion would be reached that drug disposition was unchanged in the elderly patient with no need for dose adjustment, whereas when assessed as unbound drug, an opposite conclusion is reached.

The lesson from these examples is that for drugs highly bound to albumin, one needs data assessing the disposition of unbound drug in elderly patients. If data are offered for total drug only, the clinician should realize that such information may be misleading.

A number of basic drugs are highly bound to α1-acid glycoprotein (e.g., propranolol). This protein is an acute phase reactant and its concentration may be altered in disease states; age *per se* does not affect its concentration. As a consequence, there is little need for concern about protein binding of basic drugs in elderly patients.

Changes in hepatic function

A number of changes in hepatic physiology occur with aging (Table 8.1). Absolute liver size and weight as a proportion of body weight decrease with age. Whereas in younger patients liver weight is about 2.5% of total body weight, in elderly patients this value declines to about 1.6% [1,8]. Since hepatic size *per se* is probably not a limiting factor in drug metabolism, it is doubtful that this change is an important determinant of altered drug metabolism in elderly patients.

On the other hand, age-related decrements in hepatic blood flow and in the intrinsic capacity of the liver to metabolize drugs have a major impact on drug metabolism. At age 65, hepatic blood flow is reduced from 40 to 45% compared to younger patients [1,5,8]. Such decrements can theoretically diminish the elimination of drugs having a high extraction rate, so-called flow-limited drugs, the elimination of which is dependent on hepatic blood flow [22–24]. Examples of such drugs are presented in Table 8.2. Though not all such drugs have been studied in elderly patients, convincing data have been generated for propranolol [25–27] and for lidocaine [28] and for a number of other agents in patients with hepatic dysfunction of other causes; all these data support the hypothesis that the decrease in hepatic blood flow with aging will diminish the metabolism of drugs with high hepatic extraction. Thus, clinicians should realize that any such drug may need dose modification in elderly patients.

Drugs of this type are not only subject to diminished clearance but also to increased bioavailability if administered by mouth. Flow-limited drugs not only have decreased elimination after intravenous administration, but after oral dosing first-pass elimination is also diminished causing an increase in bioavailability [24]. Thus, for

Table 8.2 Examples of drugs for which metabolism is affected by diminished hepatic metabolizing capacity associated with aging. (From Williams & Mamelok [22] and Williams [23])

Drugs with high extraction ratios (flow-limited drugs)	Drugs with low extraction ratios (capacity-limited)
Chlormethiazole	Amobarbital
Labetalol	Antipyrine
Lidocaine	Chloramphenicol
Meperidine	Chlordiazepoxide
Metoprolol	Cimetidine
Morphine	Diazepam
Lidocaine	Lorazepam
Nortriptyline	Naproxen
Pentazocine	Oxazepam
Propoxyphene	Phenytoin
Propranolol	Quinidine
Verapamil	Theophylline
	Tolbutamide
	Warfarin

drugs such as labetalol, metoprolol, and propranolol, two changes in disposition occur with decreased hepatic blood flow, the effects of which are additive. The net effect is that dosing modification must account for both effects; in other words, a decrease in clearance alone requires a lower dose as does an increase in bioavailability. If a drug is administered intravenously, only the effect of diminished clearance must be accommodated; if administered by mouth changes in both clearance and bioavailability mandate an even greater dosage modification.

Elderly patients also seem to have a diminished ability to metabolize drugs over and above any change in blood flow [1–6]. This effect in general is restricted to metabolic pathways of hydroxylation, N-dealkylation, sulfoxidation, reduction, and hydrolysis; so-called Phase I reactions [5]. In contrast, conjugation or Phase II pathways seem to be spared of an effect [5]. These pathways include glucuronidation, acetylation, and sulfation. As a consequence, a priori prediction of whether a capacity-limited drug may have diminished clearance in an elderly patient requires knowledge of its metabolic pathway. For such drugs, clinicians should anticipate decreased clearance in elderly patients and be prepared to administer lower doses. If one is uncertain, it is best to administer low doses with subsequent increases based on response

of the patient. It is always easy to administer additional drug; on the other hand, if one initially gives too large a dose, iatrogenic adverse effects may result that could have been avoided.

Changes in renal function

A widely held axiom in medicine is that renal function inexorably declines with age such that glomerular filtration rate (GFR) and renal blood flow (RBF) in elderly patients are about two-thirds those of younger patients [1–6,29,30]. Paradoxically, this decline in renal function does not manifest itself by an increase in concentration of serum creatinine, because there appears to be a parallel decrease in muscle mass and thereby creatinine production with age. As a consequence, though an elderly patient may have diminished renal function, a determination of serum creatinine concentration may be within the "normal" range and thereby be misleading. This phenomenon has spurred the derivation of algorithms and nomograms to allow estimation of renal function based on age and serum creatinine concentrations [31,32]. A reliable and often used method is that of Crockcroft & Gault [31] wherein:

$$\text{creatinine clearance corrected to 72 kg body weight} = \frac{140 - \text{age}}{\text{serum creatinine}}$$

where age is expressed in years and the serum creatinine concentration is expressed in mg/dl or mg%. To account for the smaller muscle mass in women, this value should be multiplied by 0.85.

This algorithm or similar methods allow clinicians to approximate renal function in elderly patients. However, one should realize that not all elderly patients suffer decrements in renal function. In fact, recent data indicate that many healthy elderly patients have normal renal function and decrements with age may be more limited to elderly patients with concomitant disease [33]. Thus, algorithms and nomograms may be most relevant to sicker patients and not as accurate in healthy elderly patients.

To decide whether a dose of a drug needs altering because of a decline in renal function, one must know approximately how much of the drug is eliminated by renal excretion in subjects with normal renal function. If 30–40% of a dose is excreted as unchanged drug in the urine, dosage modification in elderly patients is usually necessary. If less than this amount is eliminated by renal routes, renal function is unlikely to affect clearance to a clinically important extent. As with hepatic metabolism, if one is uncertain, it is best to begin therapy with low doses and escalate cautiously.

Some drugs are converted to active metabolites which depend on the kidney for excretion. Classical examples include *N*-acetylprocainamide and normeperidine, the metabolites of procainamide and meperidine, respectively. The former has activity as an antiarrhythmic but can be cardiotoxic in high concentrations; the latter has no analgesic effect like the parent drug but instead is toxic to the central nervous system and can cause seizures. Patients with diminished renal function, including elderly patients, can selectively accumulate such metabolites and suffer adverse effects [34]. Clinicians should be alert to this possibility.

Changes in response

Over and above changes in disposition of drugs in elderly patients, many examples are cited in the medical literature of altered response. Unfortunately, many of these reports are anecdotal and few such instances have been explored in detail. Table 8.3 offers a listing of some changes in response that have been observed, most of which need to be studied in greater detail [1,3–6]. Such changes may occur through alterations in receptor number or affinity, in secondary messengers, in cellular or subcellular effect, etc., and are fruitful areas for further research. Clinicians must recognize the possibility, if not probability, of altered response in elderly patients even if doses are altered to account for changes in drug disposition. As a result, patients must be followed closely for

Table 8.3 Examples of altered response to drugs in elderly patients

---

↓ Response to sympathomimetics and adrenergic antagonists

↓ Baroreceptor reflex with ↑ effects of venodilators and ↑ risk of postural hypotension

↑ Sedation from analgesics, sedative/hypnotics, antipsychotics, antidepressants, etc.

Paradoxical response to sedative/hypnotics

↑ Anticholinergic effects of antipsychotics and antidepressants

↑ Effects of some anesthetic agents

↑ Response to oral anticoagulants

---

clinical endpoints of efficacy and toxicity with further dosage modifications as dictated by response of each individual patient.

Clinical pharmacology of diuretics in elderly patients

Diuretics are frequently used in elderly patients for treatment of edematous disorders and hypertension. Few studies have assessed the influence of age on disposition and response to diuretics, the exception being the loop diuretic furosemide [35–39]. It is likely, however, that findings with furosemide can be extrapolated to other diuretics, excluding spironolactone. All diuretics except spironolactone inhibit renal tubular sodium reabsorption from the lumen, or urine, side of the nephron rather than the peritubular, or blood, side. Therefore, they must gain access to the urine to have an effect. In turn, all of these diuretics but mannitol reach the urine by active secretion from blood to urine at the straight segment of the proximal tubule. In contrast, mannitol passes through the glomerulus. Two different secretory pathways are used to transport diuretics into the urine; that for organic acids secretes acetazolamide, loop diuretics, and thiazide diuretics; that for organic bases secretes triamterene and amiloride.

The capacity of the nephron to secrete diuretics to their intraluminal sites of action is a function of the amount of drug reaching the transport sites at the nephron which, in turn, is a function of RBF. Thus, clinical conditions in which renal perfusion is decreased are associated with diminished delivery of diuretics to their sites of action and diminished response. One would predict, therefore, that patients with diminished renal function of any cause, but including that associated with the aging process, would have diminished delivery of diuretic to the urine causing decreased response. This prediction is shown to be true in elderly patients in Table 8.4, using furosemide as a prototype [35–38]. This diminished delivery of furosemide to its site of action is indeed associated with a decreased response [39].

Thus, it is clear that elderly patients on average deliver about half as much diuretic into the urine as do younger patients. Relative to amounts of diuretic reaching the urine, it is also important to address whether response is normal or whether other renal changes associated with aging alter response over and above these changes in disposition. When diuretic-induced sodium excretion is

Table 8.4 Effect of age on renal excretion of furosemide

Young	Elderly	Reference number
Creatinine clearance (ml/min)		
135 ± 11	95 ± 8	[35]
125 ± 11	95 ± 9	[38]
Renal clearance of furosemide (ml/min)		
114 ± 33	75 ± 9	[35]
$95 - 135$	$20 - 65$	[36]
	40 ± 18	[37]

assessed as a function of furosemide in the urine, it is clear that elderly patients follow the same relationship as do young patients with normal renal function [36–38]. In other words, if sufficient doses of diuretic are administered to attain "normal" amounts in the urine, a normal response will ensue. It is a reasonable presumption that the findings with furosemide extrapolate to all other diuretics but spironolactone, since the same principles apply. On average, elderly patients require twice the dose of a diuretic that would be used in younger patients with normal renal function. Such a dose will induce a normal response, but it is important to note that this will occur at the expense of a higher blood concentration of the diuretic. Because of the wide therapeutic margin of this class of drugs, this cost is usually negligible.

It is important to emphasize that the strategy to be employed with these diuretics (namely, doubling the usual dose) is diametrically opposite to usual recommendations for dosing of drugs in elderly patients. The usual admonition is to always use lower doses of any drug in elderly patients because of the risk of diminished clearance caused by changes in hepatic and renal function with age. Diuretics represent a special and unique exception simply because their mechanism of action requires a urinary site of effect. To my knowledge, these drugs represent the only exception to the general rule of using smaller doses in elderly patients.

Antihypertensive agents in elderly patients

All of the considerations discussed previously related to changed disposition of drugs in elderly patients apply to antihypertensive agents and will not be recapitulated here. Moreover, in the last section of this chapter, guidelines will be presented for dosing changes in elderly patients based on alterations in disposition. Over and above these considerations, however, one must also consider unique characteristics of elderly hypertensive patients which may alter response to these drugs. Table 8.5 presents examples of responses in elderly patients that differ from their younger counterparts and must be considered when selecting among a variety of possible drug choices and in guiding dosing [40,41].

Elderly patients have diminished baroreflex activity and thus are more likely to have postural hypotension [42]. In turn, if given antihypertensives that themselves can cause postural hypotension, the risk of such events becomes much greater in elderly patients. As a consequence, agents with such effects may be relegated to secondary importance.

Some evidence indicates that elderly patients may respond less well to β-adrenergic antagonists [41]. In addition, these agents (excepting those with intrinsic sympathomimetic activity) diminish cardiac output

Table 8.5 Examples of altered response to antihypertensive agents in elderly patients

Drug	Response
Diuretics	↑ Prevalence and risk of electrolyte abnormalities ↑ Postural hypotension
β-adrenergic antagonists	Diminished efficacy ? ↑ CNS effects ↓ Cardiac output (excepting those with ISA)
α-adrenergic antagonists	
α1-selective	↑ Postural hypotension
nonselective	Prohibitive postural hypotension (guanidinium agents) ↑ CNS effects (reserpine)
Central α2-agonists	↑ CNS effects
Calcium antagonists	? ↑ Risk of conduction abnormalities (excepting dihydropyridines)

CNS, central nervous system; ISA, intrinsic sympathomimetic activity.

which could be detrimental in some elderly patients. It seems reasonable to relegate these agents to patients needing blockade of reflex tachycardia.

The α1-selective antagonists prazosin, terazosin, and doxazosin can all cause venodilation and worsen postural hypotension. At least with prazosin this appears to occur mainly with the initiation of therapy, but it should be realized that there is some risk at any time with this class of drugs.

Guanidinium agents (guanethidine and guanadrel) should not be used in elderly patients because of their postural effects. Similarly, reserpine should be relegated to historical interest because of its long duration of action, postural effects, and central nervous system depression.

Central α2-agonists (methyldopa, clonidine, guanabenz, and guanfacine) represent a paradox in that their central nervous system effects of sleepiness and dry mouth may be worse in elderly patients. On the other hand, elderly patients have elevated concentrations of circulating catecholamines which can be suppressed by these agents [40]. Thus, if efficacious in sufficiently low doses that side effects are avoided, these drugs are quite useful in elderly patients with hypertension. On the other hand, if adverse effects occur at low doses, then other agents should be tried.

Calcium channel antagonists seem to be particularly effective in elderly patients [43,44] and are being advocated as first-line agents in them. However, it is important to note that verapamil in particular and diltiazem to a lesser extent have negative inotropic effects and slow cardiac conduction. Elderly patients are probably more susceptible to adverse effects related to such pharmacology. In addition, the constipating effects of verapamil may be more pronounced in elderly patients. The dihydropyridine calcium antagonists are relatively free of these effects; on the other hand, they are potent vasodilators and may have greater effects than desired in some elderly patients.

Inhibitors of converting enzyme (captopril, enalapril, etc.) have not been specifically studied in elderly patients but should be useful agents.

Overall, specific characteristics of elderly patients exemplified in Table 8.5 result in a different prioritization of antihypertensive agents for elderly patients compared to their younger counterparts. Clinicians should realize, however, that response to such drugs is highly individual

and an agent that works well in one patient may not in another. Thus, one should attempt to tailor therapy to the individual patient and should not be reluctant to discontinue a drug with less than adequate effects or with toxicity and try a different agent with the goal of finding the antihypertensive that is best for each individual patient.

When some elderly patients are treated for elevated blood pressures, concomitant with blood pressure lowering are adverse symptoms that occur with virtually any agent utilized. Such patients may have so-called "pseudohypertension" in which the blood pressure measured by cuff overestimates intraarterial pressure. This discrepancy seems to be a particular problem in elderly patients [45–48] whose diastolic pressure may frequently be overestimated by 15 mmHg or more. Clinicians should be alert to the possibility of pseudohypertension. Unfortunately, the only certain method for diagnosing this entity is by obtaining a measurement of intra-arterial pressure through a positive "Osler's maneuver" which may provide a clue as to its presence [47]. Osler's maneuver refers to the presence of a palpable radial or brachial artery when the blood pressure cuff is inflated to a level sufficient to occlude blood flow. If Osler's maneuver is positive, a high level of suspicion of pseudohypertension is warranted. This may influence the aggressiveness with which treatment of the hypertension is pursued.

Drug dose adjustment in elderly patients

Though data are not available for all drugs, in fact not even for a majority, considerable information has been published assessing changes in drug disposition in elderly patients [49]. Such data allow derivation of dosing recommendations as presented in Tables 8.6 and 8.7. These guidelines can serve as a reasonable starting point for use of the listed drugs in elderly patients. However, the recommendations are best viewed as approximations and further dosage adjustment may be needed in individual patients. With drugs in Table 8.7, if patients have diminished renal function but the drug has a wide therapeutic margin, dose adjustment is probably not needed. On the other hand, if dose adjustment is required, published guidelines based on renal function should be used [49]. For drugs not included in Tables 8.6 and 8.7, the principles discussed earlier in this chapter apply. Excepting diuretics, the admonition of "start low and go slow" is best; in other words, underestimate rather than overestimate the dose needed and increase doses slowly and in small increments. Basing this on individual patient response should allow one to optimize therapy in elderly patients.

Table 8.6 Drug dosing recommendations in elderly patients

Drug	Dosing adjustment
Analgesics	
Meperidine	Avoid: active metabolite (normeperidine) accumulates and causes CNS toxicity
Morphine	Active metabolite (morphine glucuronide) may accumulate if ↓ renal function
Antianxiety agents, sedatives, and hypnotics	
Bromazepam	One-half usual dose
Brotizolam	One-half usual dose
Quazepam	Avoid: active metabolite accumulates
Anticholinergics and cholinergics	
Cisapride	↓ Elimination; quantitative guidelines are not available; use cautiously or avoid
Anticonvulsants	
Primidone	One-half usual dose to adjust for accumulation of active metabolite
Valproic acid	One-third usual dose
Antihistamines	
Hydroxyzine	One-half usual dose
Antiinflammatory agents	
Naproxen	One-half usual dose
Bronchodilators	
Theophylline	One-half to three-quarters usual dose

Table 8.6 (*cont.*)

Drug	Dosing adjustment
Cardiovascular agents	
Antianginal agents	
Amlodipine	One-half usual dose
Felodipine	One-half usual dose
Isradipine	One-third to one-half usual dose
Verapamil	Three-quarters usual dose
Antiarrhythmic agents	
Quinidine	One-half usual dose
Antihypertensives	
α_1-adrenergic antagonists	
Terazosin	One-half usual dose
Urapidil	One-half usual dose
β-adrenergic antagonists	
Acebutolol	One-half usual dose to account for accumulation of active metabolite
Betaxolol	One-half usual dose
Labetalol	One-half usual dose
Converting-enzyme inhibitors	
Perindopril	One-half usual dose
Vasodilators	
Nitroprusside	Toxic metabolite (thiocyanate) may accumulate
Hypoglycemic agents	
Acetohexamide	Avoid: active metabolite (hydroxyhexamide) accumulates
Hypouricemic agents	
Allopurinol	One-third to one-half usual dose to account for accumulation of active metabolite (oxipurinol)
Psychotherapeutic agents	
Trazodone	One-half to two-thirds usual dose
Miscellaneous agents	
Buflomedil	Two-thirds usual dose
Terodiline	One-third usual dose

CNS, central nervous system.

Table 8.7 Drugs with substantial renal elimination requiring dose adjustment in elderly patients (if renal function is diminished)

Analgesics

Codeine

Anesthetics

Alcuronium
4-Aminopyridine
Gallamine
Metocurine
Pancuronium
D-tubucurarine
Vecuronium

Antianxiety agents, sedatives, and hypnotics

Barbital
Phenobarbital

Anticholinergics and cholinergics

Metoclopramide
Neostigmine
Pyridostigmine

Anticoagulants, antifibrinolytics, and antiplatelet agents

Epsilon aminocaproic acid
Tranexamic acid

Anticonvulsants

Vigabatrin

Antihistamines

Cimetidine
Etintidine
Famotidine
Nizatidine
Ranitidine
Roxatidine

Anti-inflammatory agents

Azapropazone
Penicillamine

Antimicrobials

Aminoglycosides
 Aminoglycoside antibiotics
 Spectinomycin

Table 8.7 (*cont.*)

Carbapenems
 Imipenem
Cephalosporins
 Cefaclor
 Cefadroxil
 Cefamandole
 Cefatrizine
 Cefazolin
 Cefmenoxime
 Cefonicid
 Ceforanide
 Cefotaxime
 Cefotetan
 Cefotiam
 Cefoxitin
 Cefroxadine
 Cefsulodin
 Ceftazidime
 Ceftizoxime
 Ceftriaxone
 Cefuroxime
 Cephacetrile
 Cephalexin
 Cephalothin
 Cephapirin
 Cephradine
Chloramphenicol and thiamphenicol
 Thiamphenicol
Macrolide antibiotics
 Roxithromycin
Monobactams
 Aztreonam
 Carumonam
 Moxalactam
Penicillins
 Amdinocillin
 Amoxicillin
 Ampicillin
 Azlocillin
 Carbenicillin
 Cloxacillin
 Dicloxacillin
 Mecillinam
 Methicillin
 Mezlocillin
 Penicillin
 Piperacillin
 Temocillin
 Ticarcillin

Table 8.7 (*cont.*)

Polymyxins
  Colistin
  Polymyxin B
Quinolones
  Ciprofloxacin
  Enoxacin
  Fleroxacin
  Lomefloxacin
  Ofloxacin
  Pipemidic acid
Sulfonamides
  Sulfadiazine
  Sulfisoxazole
  Trimethoprim
Vancomycin
  Vancomycin
  Teicoplanin

Antifungals

Flucytosine

Antimalarials

Chloroquine
Proguanil

Antiparasitics

Pentamidine

Antituberculous agents

Ethambutol

Antiviral agents

Acyclovir
Amantadine
Foscarnet
Ganciclovir

Antineoplastic agents

Bleomycin
Carboplatin
Cis-platinum
Methotrexate
Pentostatin

Antispasticity agents

Baclofen

Table 8.7 (*cont.*)

Bronchodilators

Dyphylline
Enprofylline
Nedocromil
Prenalterol
Terbutaline

Cardiovascular agents

Antiarrhythmic agents
  N-acetylprocainamide
  Bretylium
  Cibenzoline
  Disopyramide
  Procainamide
  Sotalol
  Tocainide

Antihypertensives

β-adrenergic antagonists
  Atenolol
  Bisoprolol
  Carteolol
  Cetamolol
  Nadolol
Central α2-stimulants
  Clonidine
Converting-enzyme inhibitors
  Captopril
  Enalapril
  Lisinopril
  Pentopril
Inotropic agents
  Digoxin
  Milrinone
Lipid-lowering agents
  Bezafibrate
  Clofibrate

Hypoglycemic agents

Chlorpropamide
Glibenclamide (glyburide)
Metformin
Phenformin

Psychotherapeutic agents

Lithium
Sulpiride

Table 8.7 (*cont.*)

Sympathomimetics

Phenylpropanolamine
Xamoterol

Miscellaneous agents

L-Carnitine
Clodronate

References

1 Vestal RE. Drug use in the elderly: A review of problems and special considerations. Drugs 1978;16:358−382.

2 Schmucker DL. Age-related changes in drug disposition. Pharmacol Rev 1979;30:445−456.

3 Ouslander JG. Drug therapy in the elderly. Ann Intern Med 1981;95:711−722.

4 Everitt DE, Avorn J. Drug prescribing for the elderly. Arch Intern Med 1986;146:2393−2396.

5 Greenblatt DJ, Sellers EM, Shader RI. Drug disposition in old age. N Engl J Med 1982;306:1081−1088.

6 Beers MH, Ouslander JG. Risk factors in geriatric drug prescribing: a practical guide to avoiding problems. Drugs 1989;37:105−112.

7 Bender AD. Effect of aging on intestinal absorption: implications for drug absorption in the elderly. J Am Geriatr Soc 1968;16:1331−1339.

8 Geokas MC, Haverback BJ. The aging gastrointestinal tract. Am J Surg 1969;117:881−892.

9 Montgomery RD, Haeny MR, Ross IN, et al. The aging gut: a study of intestinal absorption in relation to nutrition in the elderly. Q J Med 1978;47:197−211.

10 Lake-Bakaar G, Tom W, Lake-Bakaar D, et al. Gastropathy and ketoconazole malabsorption in the acquired immunodeficiency syndrome (AIDS). Ann Intern Med 1988;109:471−473.

11 Evans MA, Triggs EJ, Cheung M, et al. Gastric emptying rate in the elderly: implications for drug therapy. J Am Geriatr Soc 1981;29:201−205.

12 Kramer PA, Chapron DJ, Benson J, et al. Tetracycline absorption in elderly patients with achlorhydria. Clin Pharmacol Ther 1978;23:467−472.

13 Ochs HR, Greenblatt DJ, Allen MD, et al. Effect of age and Billroth gastrectomy on absorption of desmethyldiazepam from clorazepate. Clin Pharmacol Ther 1979;26:449−456.

14 Ochs HR, Otten H, Greenblatt DJ, et al. Diazepam absorption: effects of age, sex, and Billroth gastrectomy. Dig Dis Sci 1982;27:225−230.

15 Novak LP. Aging, total body potassium, fat-free mass, and cell mass in males and females between ages 18 and 35 years. J Gerontol 1972;27:438−443.

16 Vestal RE, McGuire EA, Tobin JD, et al. Aging and ethanol metabolism. Clin Pharmacol Ther 1977;21:343−354.

17 Macklon AF, Barton M, James O, et al. The effect of age on pharmacokinetics of diazepam. Clin Sci 1980;59:479−483.

18 Ochs HR, Greenblatt DJ, Divoll M, et al. Diazepam kinetics in relation to age and sex. Pharmacology 1981;23:24−30.

19 Woodford-Williams E, Alvarez AS, Webster D, et al. Serum protein patterns in "normal" and pathological aging. Gerontologia. 1964/1965;10:86−99.

20 Wallace SM, Verbeeck RK. Plasma protein binding of drugs in the elderly. Clin Pharmacokinet 1987;12:41−72.

21 Upton RA, Williams RL, Kelly J, et al. Naproxen pharmacokinetics in the elderly. Br J Clin Pharmacol 1984;18:207−214.

22 Williams RL, Mamelok RD. Hepatic disease and drug pharmacokinetics. Clin Pharmacokinet 1980;5:528−547.

23 Williams RL. Drug administration in hepatic disease. N Engl J Med 1983;309:1616−1622.

24 Wilkinson GR. Clearance approaches in pharmacology. Pharmacol Rev 1987;39:1−47.

25 Vestal RE, Wood AJJ, Branch RA, et al. Effects of age and cigarette smoking on propranolol disposition. Clin Pharmacol Ther 1979;26:8−15.

26 Castleden CM, George CF. The effect of ageing on the hepatic clearance of propranolol. Br J Clin Pharmacol 1979;7:49−54.

27 Feely J, Crooks J, Stevenson IH. The influence of age, smoking, and hyperthyroidism on plasma propranolol steady state concentration. Br J Clin Pharmacol 1981;12:73−78.

28 Nation RL, Triggs EJ, Selig M. Lignocaine kinetics in cardiac patients and aged subjects. Br J Clin Pharmacol 1977;4:439−448.

29 Friedman SA, Raizner AE, Rosen H, et al. Functional defects in the aging kidney. Ann Intern Med 1972;76:41−45.

30 Rowe JW, Andres R, Tobin JD, et al. The effects of age on creatinine clearance in man: a cross-sectional longitudinal study. J Gerontol 1976;31:155−163.

31 Crockcroft DW, Gault MH. Prediction of creatinine clearance from serum creatinine. Nephron 1976;16:31−41.

32 Bjornsson TD. Use of serum creatinine concentrations to determine renal function. Clin Pharmacokinet 1979;4:200−222.

33 Lindeman RD, Tobin JD, Shock NW. Longitudinal studies on the rate of decline in renal function with age. J Am Geriatr Soc 1985;33:278−285.

34 Verbeeck RK, Branch RA, Wilkinson GR. Drug metabolites in renal failure: pharmacokinetic and clinical implications. Clin Pharmacokinet 1981;6:329−345.

35 Andreasen F, Hansen U, Husted SE, et al. The pharmacokinetics of frusemide are influenced by age. Br J Clin Pharmacol 1983;16:391−397.

36 Kerremans ALM, Gribnau FWJ. Changes in pharmacokinetics and in effect of furosemide in the elderly. Clin Exp Hypertens 1983;A5:271−284.

37 Kerremans ALM, Tan Y, van Baars H, *et al*. Furosemide kinetics and dynamics in aged patients. Clin Pharmacol Ther 1983;34:181–189.

38 Andreasen F, Hansen U, Husted SE, *et al*. The influence of age on renal and extrarenal effects of frusemide. Br J Clin Pharmacol 1984;18:5–74.

39 Chaudhry AY, Bing RF, Castleden CM, *et al*. The effect of ageing on the response to frusemide in normal subjects. Eur J Clin Pharmacol 1984;27:303–306.

40 Sowers JR. Hypertension in the elderly. Am J Med 1987;82(Suppl. 1B):1–8.

41 O'Malley K, O'Brien E. Management of hypertension in the elderly. N Engl J Med 1980;302:1397–1401.

42 Gribbin B, Pickering TG, Sleight P, *et al*. Effect of age and high blood pressure on baroreflex sensitivity in man. Circ Res 1971;29:424–429.

43 Kiowski W, Buhler FR, Fadayomi MO, *et al*. Age, race, blood pressure, and renin: predictors for antihypertensive treat-ment with calcium antagonists. Am J Cardiol 1985;56:H81–H85.

44 Massie B, MacCarthy EP, Ramanathan KB, *et al*. Diltiazem and propranolol in mild to moderate essential hypertension as monotherapy or with hydrochlorothiazide. Ann Intern Med 1987;107:150–157.

45 Spence JD, Sibbald WJ, Cape RD. Pseudohypertension in the elderly. Clin Sci Mol Med 1978;55:S399–S402.

46 Vardan S, Mookherjee S, Warner R, *et al*. Systolic hypertension: direct and indirect BP measurements. Arch Intern Med 1983;143:935–938.

47 Messerli FH, Ventura HO, Amodeo C. Osler's maneuver and pseudohypertension. N Engl J Med 1985;312:1548–1551.

48 Hla KM, Feussner JR. Screening for pseudohypertension. A quantitative, noninvasive approach. Arch Intern Med 1988;148:673–676.

49 Brater DC. *Pocket Manual of Drug Use in Clinical Medicine*, 3rd edn. Toronto: B.C. Decker, Inc., 1987.

9

Hypertension in the elderly: rationale for therapy

George L. Bakris
Edward D. Frohlich

Introduction

Aging is a process associated with physiologic alterations in cardiovascular, renal, and neural regulatory functions [1–4]. One consequence of these changes includes a failure to maintain arterial pressure within acceptable limits [1]. A recent study compared the cardiovascular regulatory functions of elderly normotensive subjects with young normotensive subjects [5]. Elderly subjects (age ≥66 years) had a lower baroreceptor reflex sensitivity, renin–aldosterone axis, β-adrenoreceptor responsiveness, resting vagal activity, and a blunted response to heart rate secondary to increased blood pressure [1,5–8]. Plasma norepinephrine levels were significantly increased in the elderly as were total peripheral resistance and vascular stiffness [1,5–8]. Furthermore, circadian variation in blood pressure was maintained in the elderly. However, younger subjects had a much greater drop in blood pressure during sleep when compared to elderly subjects [5,9]. Thus, these altered homeostatic responses in blood pressure regulation that occur with the aging process contribute to elevated arterial pressures in the elderly.

Thirty percent of individuals between the ages of 60–65 years are hypertensive and 40% of those over the age of 65 years as defined by a diastolic pressure of ≥96 mmHg or a systolic pressure of ≥160 mmHg [10]. Hence, hypertension is a common malady in the elderly population, and is distinguished from hypertension in young individuals by its low renin, high vascular resistance state.

Hypertension is one of the major risk factors for atherosclerotic coronary arterial and cerebrovascular disease [11–17]. However, only recently has hypertension been considered a major risk factor in the elderly (i.e., age 65 years or older). Hypertension in the elderly not only increases the risk of heart attack and stroke, but also increases the risk for congestive heart failure, occlusive peripheral vascular disease, aortic aneurysm, stroke, and renal failure [11–19].

This chapter reviews the definitions for the different types of hypertension commonly seen in the elderly, systolic, and diastolic. In addition, a brief discussion of the epidemiologic and pathophysiologic processes underlying each of these forms of hypertension is presented as well as a review of the pertinent literature supporting the various therapeutic interventions for each form, underscoring specific recommendations.

Definitions

For the purpose of this discussion, an elderly person is defined as an individual who is 65 years of age or older. It is this segment of our population that has been and continues to be identified as having the greatest growth in numbers in the coming decades [12,17,20].

Isolated systolic hypertension, according to the Joint National Committee's fourth report, is defined as a systolic pressure elevation in excess of 139 mmHg with a diastolic pressure of less than 90 mmHg [17]. Patients whose systolic pressure is between 140–159 mmHg are said to have isolated *borderline systolic hypertension*; but if the systolic pressure is 160 mmHg or greater (with diastolic pressure of less than 90 mmHg), the patient has had *isolated systolic hypertension* [17]. *Diastolic hypertension* exists if the diastolic pressure is 90 mmHg or greater [17].

A definitive diagnosis of mild to moderate hypertension should not be based on a single blood pressure measurement [17,18,20–22]. Initially, elevated readings should be confirmed on at least two subsequent office visits when the diastolic pressure was 90 mmHg or greater, or a systolic pressure was 140 mmHg or greater. This is because the arterial pressure is a variable that may be affected by multiple extraneous factors. Blood pressure should be measured in a standard fashion so that the values obtained are reliable. If the pressure reading is alarmingly elevated, the physician must use clinical judgment as to initiating therapy. Table 9.1 summarizes the classification of arterial hypertension by arterial pressure levels. If a question remains regarding the significance between office blood pressure readings and their relationship to target organ involvement, home pressures on a 24-hour blood pressure monitor may be helpful in resolving the question [20–22].

Epidemiology

Estimates of the prevalence of both isolated systolic and diastolic hypertension in the elderly depend upon the definition. The 1976–1980 National Health and Nutrition Examination survey defined hypertension as an average of three blood pressure measurements equal to or greater than 160/90 mmHg taken on a single occasion [17,23]. This survey documented the prevalence of hypertension in elderly white and black individuals (age 65–74 years)

Table 9.1 Classification of arterial hypertension by arterial pressure levels. (From The Joint National Committee on Detection, Evaluation and Treatment of High Blood Pressure [17])

Pressure range (mmHg)	Class
Systolic (when diastolic pressure is <90)	
<140	Normal blood pressure
140–159	Borderline ISH
≥160	ISH
Diastolic	
<85	Normal blood pressure
85–89	High normal blood pressure
90–104	Mild hypertension
105–114	Moderate hypertension
≥115	Severe hypertension

ISH, isolated systolic hypertension.

to be 44% and 60%, respectively. These prevalence estimates, however, are considerably higher if the blood pressure thresholds are lowered to ≥140/≥90. Using the latter definitions, prevalence of hypertension was 63% and 76% for elderly white and black populations, respectively (Table 9.2).

Because of this high prevalence of elevated arterial pressure in the elderly, many physicians and other professionals have made the invalid inference that the increase of arterial pressure (systolic or diastolic) that is so common during the aging process is normal and innocuous. This clearly is not the case; there is a continuous rise in systolic and diastolic pressures in the elderly population (with aging) in westernized populations. This pressure increase is neither a physiologic nor an inconsequential phenomenon as increased risk is clear [1,18]. However, it does not mean that all individuals subjected to this risk should receive treatment and this must be demonstrated. Furthermore, many prospective multicenter studies have reported that reduction of elevated arterial pressure, either by pharmacologic or nonpharmacologic means, is associated with improved overall (total) morbidity and mortality as well as cardiovascular morbidity and mortality [11–19,24,25].

Table 9.2 Prevalence of hypertension among noninstitutionalized men and women, black and white, aged 65–74 years, 1976–1980. (From The Working Group on Hypertension in the Elderly [3])

	Blood pressure ≥160/95 mmHg* (%)	Blood pressure ≥140/90 mmHg† (%)
Black women	72.8	82.9
Black men	42.9	67.1
White women	48.3	66.2
White men	37.5	59.2
Total blacks	59.9	76.1
Total whites	43.7	63.1
Total (all races)‡	45.1	64.3

* Defined as the average of three blood pressure measurements 160 mmHg or greater (systolic) and/or 94 mmHg or greater (diastolic) taken on a single occasion or the self-reported taking of antihypertensive medication.
† Defined as the average of three blood pressure measurements 140 mmHg or greater (systolic) and/or 90 mmHg or greater (diastolic) taken on a single occasion or the self-reported taking or antihypertensive medication.
‡ Includes races in addition to blacks and whites.

Isolated systolic hypertension

Epidemiology

By 1990, at least 29 million people in the United States will be 65 years or older [17]. Forty-five percent of these patients will have isolated systolic hypertension as defined as a blood pressure of ≥160/≥95 mmHg, and two-thirds of these 29 million people will have hypertension, if the disease is defined as a blood pressure ≥140/≥90 mmHg [17]. It is clear from these epidemiologic reports that control of arterial pressure is critical for prevention of major catastrophic illnesses and mortality in this aging population.

Epidemiologic studies also demonstrate that isolated systolic hypertension in the elderly imparts a two-fold greater risk of death when the involved individuals are compared to normotensive control subjects with respect to age, race, and sex [12,23,24]. In fact, the most common cause of mortality in this population is related to cardiovascular and cerebral events [13–19,25].

A number of epidemiologic studies have evaluated the risk of cardiovascular and cerebral events stemming from uncontrolled hypertension [11–19,23]. A 2-year follow-up of participants (age 55–74 years) with isolated systolic hypertension in the Framingham Heart Study demonstrated a two- to five-fold excess risk of cardiovascular death [12]. In the Chicago Stroke Study, the 3 year incidence of stroke was two-times and one-half-times greater in those patients with isolated systolic hypertension [11]. Lastly, the 1979 Build and Blood Pressure Study reported a 51% excess mortality rate among individuals with isolated systolic hypertension [19]. It is of particular importance to underscore that each of the foregoing studies demonstrated that systolic pressure elevation was a better predictor of cardiovascular complications than the usual clinical risk, diastolic pressure elevation.

Studies evaluating the risk of many catastrophic complications of hypertension such as stroke, coronary heart disease, and renal failure have been significantly reduced with the introduction of antihypertensive therapy [11–19,26]. These studies have been translated into a decreased occurrence of fatal strokes and myocardial infarction of almost 50% and 35%, respectively, in the United States over the past decade. This reduced complication of stroke as a result of effective antihypertensive therapy has been known for sometime [27]. Public health data have been extended recently with respect to myocardial infarction in the elderly. Results from the European Working Party Study on Hypertension in the Elderly demonstrated a 60% reduction in fatal myocardial infarction associated with antihypertensive therapy [14].

Pathophysiology

To gain insight into an appropriate therapeutic approach for this particular form of hypertension, one needs to understand its systemic, hemodynamic, and pathophysiologic changes. Etiologic evaluation of arterial hypertension in the elderly is similar to that which occurs in younger patients, although sudden onset in older patients should suggest occlusive renal arterial disease.

In studies by Adamopoulos et al. [28], a comparison of systemic hemodynamic changes in younger (<35 years) and older (>35 years) individuals with systolic arterial pressure elevation were compared hemodynamically with normotensive individuals of the same age, race, and sex. Even though systolic pressures were elevated (by design of the study), and patients with diastolic pressure elevation were excluded, the patients with isolated systolic hypertension had significantly higher diastolic pressures than their age- and sex-matched normotensive control subjects. Furthermore, the elevated systolic pressure in the younger individuals was associated with a hyperdynamic circulation, i.e., increased heart rate, elevated cardiac output, and a greater index of left ventricular contractility. The older patients had a significantly lower cardiac output and left ventricular ejection fraction that was associated with a greatly increased total peripheral resistance (Fig. 9.1). Finally, intravascular volume was normal in the younger patients but significantly contracted in the older subjects. Using a similar study design, Simon et al. [29] addressed the role of large arterial compliance as it related to systolic hypertension. This group of investigators demonstrated a significant reduction in large vessel compliance in patients greater than 51 years of age as estimated from the monoexponential blood pressure time curve during diastole.

Fig. 9.1 Hemodynamic indices in 27 younger (>35 years) and 19 older patients (>35 years) with systolic hypertension. The older patients have greater vascular resistance and a lower cardiac index than the younger group. (From Adamopoulos et al. [28].)

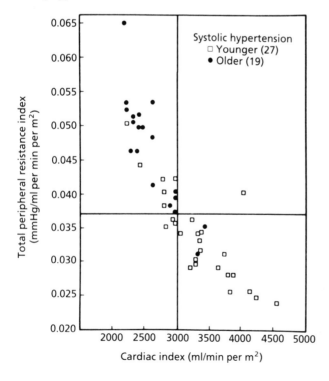

To initiate a rationale for hypertension therapy in the elderly patient, one must understand the role hypertension plays in contributing to the aging process as well as physiologic changes inherent with aging; both aging and hypertension result in similar cardiovascular and renal responses (Table 9.3). One of these responses is a decrease in baroreflex sensitivity which results in peripheral venous pooling, particularly in the splanchnic circulation after a meal. This results in reduced venous return and reduction of orthostatic fall of arterial pressure, which is not infrequently present in the elderly population and a cause of syncope [1,5−7,30].

Renal function also diminishes with aging. Specifically, renal blood flow (RBF) and glomerular filtration rate (GFR) decrease and renal excretory function may even become impaired [31−35]. These changes were evaluated in the Baltimore Longitudinal Study of Aging that demonstrated from age 30 years onward there was a progressive reduction of creatinine clearance from approximately $130-90$ ml/min per $1.73\,m^2$ [34]. Long-term evaluation of these subjects followed for 3 years, duplicating this trend and indicating that, with each decade, the slope of reduction of creatinine clearance is remarkably constant (and progressive) from ages $40-80$ years.

These decreases in cardiovascular and renal homeostatic function must be appreciated before determining an optimal therapeutic program for the individual elderly patient [35,36].

Table 9.3 The renal, cardiovascular, and endocrine alterations associated with the aging process (heart rate remains unchanged)

Increased
Peripheral vascular resistance
Arterial rigidity
Serum catecholamines

Decreased
Renal blood flow
Glomerular filtration rate
Plasma renin activity
Sodium conservation
Renal mass
Cardiac stroke index
Cardiac output
β-adrenoreceptor sensitivity
Baroreceptor sensitivity

Treatment

Two major questions arise from the foregoing consideration.

1 Will pharmacologic control of isolated systolic pressure elevation result in a reduced morbidity and mortality?
2 If so, what are the best agents for this control?

In general, initial management of all hypertension — (isolated systolic or diastolic) — merits consideration of dietary sodium restriction, weight control, moderation of alcohol consumption, and smoking cessation [17,37]. These nonpharmacologic modalities may not only reduce arterial pressure and overall cardiovascular risks, but may also reduce the need for drug therapy (or higher doses of that therapy) [17]. Therefore, drugs should be used only if the nonpharmacologic approaches are unsuccessful in achieving adequate blood pressure control (i.e., ≤139/≤89). In some patients, for example, sodium restriction (≤90 mmol/day) can reduce systolic pressure by as much as 15 mmHg [38].

Most of the major trials to date, concerned with the management of systolic hypertension, have involved thiazide diuretics [39−42]. A recent, small, multicenter feasibility trial conducted by the National Heart, Lung, and Blood Institute concluded that a large study using a thiazide diuretic was suitable [40]. This feasibility study showed excellent control of isolated systolic pressure elevation; however, reduced morbidity and mortality, albeit close to statistical significance, was not demonstrated in this small and short study. These findings justified the merits for initiating the Systolic Hypertension in the Elderly Program (SHEP) study. This is a prospective, double-blind, placebo-controlled trial to determine whether antihypertensive therapy in elderly patients with isolated systolic hypertension reduces cardiovascular as well as overall morbidity and mortality. Preliminary results from this study indicate that 80% of the 551 patients are still enrolled and being followed after 34 months. Side-effects from medication thus far have been infrequent and patient adherence has been excellent. Those receiving therapy have shown a greater fall in blood pressure than those assigned to the placebo group [41]. Furthermore, the recent conclusion of the study demonstrates a 36% reduction in cardiovascular events [43]. Diuretics, because of reasons mentioned earlier, may not always be ideal for this patient population. Although efficacious, these agents cause orthostatic hypotension, sexual dysfunction, dehydration, and

syncope. Furthermore, they may produce hyponatremia, hypokalemia, and other metabolic alterations. These biochemical alterations may predispose the patient to ventricular dysrhythmias and the risk of sudden death [44]. Carbohydrate intolerance and unfavorable changes in lipoprotein patterns have also been reported [44]. In spite of these reports, however, the Hypertension Detection Follow-Up Program reported a similar side-effect profile between young and older individuals receiving diuretics [45]. Therefore, although these agents clearly have been shown to be efficacious as single agents for management of systolic hypertension, their side-effect profile may result in greater catastrophic morbidity to this patient population. Hence, further studies evaluating these and other agents, for example, angiotensin-converting enzyme inhibitors and calcium antagonists, should be initiated to assess the efficacy of these drugs as single agents for the management of systolic hypertension in the elderly. Meanwhile, periodic biochemical checks of sodium, potassium, glucose, lipid levels, calcium, creatinine, and other factors should be carried out, and those patients receiving diuretics or other agents associated with these or other changes.

Calcium antagonists as single agents for management of hypertension in the elderly have received recent clinical attention [46]. They are appropriate for this group of patients since older patients with hypertension characteristically have enhanced peripheral vascular resistance, some reductions in cardiac output, and lower plasma renin activity (Table 9.3). Furthermore, some authors have reported that elderly individuals achieve better blood pressure control with calcium antagonists when compared to β-adrenergic receptor blockers or angiotensin-converting enzyme inhibitors — agents that control blood pressure adequately in younger hypertensives [47].

Many reports including the 1988 Joint National Committee on Detection, Evaluation, and Treatment of High Blood Pressure have suggested the use of calcium antagonists as single, first-line agents in treatment of elderly hypertension [17]. Among this class of agents, the report included diltiazem, nifedipine, nitrendipine, and verapamil. In addition, nicardipine, a more recently developed calcium antagonist, was used in 31 elderly patients, aged 57−95 years to assess tolerance and efficacy [48]. This study evaluated patients with systolic and mild diastolic hypertension and found that the effect to lower blood pressure was significantly greater than placebo and that the active agent was tolerated well. Orthostatic hypotension was not observed during the 4-week trial, nor were other significant side effects such as changes in plasma renin activity or electrolyte balance noted. Stressman et al. [49] evaluated a "slow-release" form of nifedipine as monotherapy in 21 elderly hypertensives over an 8-week period. The systolic blood pressure in this group decreased by 12−15%. Another recent study by Jansen et al. [50] comparing nitrendipine and hydrochlorothiazide as single agents for treatment of hypertensive patients over the age of 70, demonstrated that both agents effectively reduced blood pressure. Hydrochlorothiazide, on the other hand, produced elevated levels of plasma glucose, uric acid, and plasma renin activity, whereas plasma potassium levels decreased. The only side-effects noted with the calcium antagonist were edema and flushing and the response of blood pressure and heart rate to upright posture were not significantly different between treatment groups.

Angiotensin-converting enzyme inhibitors have also been evaluated in elderly patients [51,52]. They lower arterial pressure in patients with isolated systolic hypertension [51]. However, since plasma volume and plasma renin activity tend to be less in these individuals [53], some authors have suggested that their antihypertensive effects may be minimal [52,54].

Other agents such as β-blockers and direct-acting smooth-muscle relaxing vasodilators (e.g., hydralazine) have also been used in the elderly population for reduction of systolic pressure. However, some authors have suggested that the β-blockers may be associated with myocardial depression and cognitive disturbances, depression, and confusion in elderly populations [55]. However, these findings were not observed in elderly patients by the Hypertension Detection and Follow-Up Trials or other large multicenter studies [46,56]. Likewise, hydralazine may be associated with significant sympathetic nervous system stimulation, orthostatic hypotension, and sodium retention [57]. However, in the Veterans Administration Cooperative Study which utilized and included elderly hypertensive patients, the drug hydralazine was generally well tolerated without any significant untoward effects [58].

Other agents, such as the centrally active sympathetic drugs (e.g., methyldopa, clonidine, and guanfacine) are associated with side-effects such as sedation, lethargy, and dry mouth. These untoward effects may mitigate their use in this group of patients [57]. Prazosin, a peripheral α-receptor blocker also effectively reduces pressure in the elderly [57]. However, the orthostatic hypotension (whether with the initial dose or with increasing dosages) may be a very real side-effect in limiting its usefulness in older patients who may already have a higher incidence of postural hypotension prior to initiating any therapy [57].

One therapeutic approach
Since data from large clinical trials are still pending, and those that are available are limited, we suggest that therapy should be individualized, tailored to each patient, without making broad generalizations with regard to large patient populations. Studies have clearly shown that the diuretics and calcium entry blockers effectively reduce systolic pressure in patients with isolated systolic hypertension. The central and peripheral adrenergic inhibitors and β-blockers also are effective. Therefore, since most antihypertensive agents reduce systolic arterial pressure, it is worthwhile to consider using a single agent for coexistant diseases in addition to hypertension in the same patient (e.g., cerebrovascular disease, coronary arterial disease, peripheral arterial insufficiency, etc.). If possible, one drug or a combination of agents that may be given once daily approaches the ideal from a patient adherence consideration.

We generally use calcium antagonists as single agents to treat hypertension in patients with coexistent coronary, cerebral, or peripheral vascular disease. Once the dose of a single agent has been maximized and arterial pressure not well controlled, a second once daily agent (e.g., β-blocker, diuretic, angiotensin-converting enzyme inhibitor, or even a second calcium antagonist) may be prescribed. Low-dose hydrochlorothiazide (12.5 mg/day) minimizes biochemical side-effects seen with higher doses and may provide a reduction of 10−15 mmHg in systolic pressure [40,41]. In specific patient populations, (e.g., patients with angina pectoris or history of myocardial infarction) long-acting diltiazem is preferred, particularly in patients with coronary disease who have had a history of a non-Q-wave myocardial infarction [59]. We try to avoid diuretic agents (especially in higher doses) in patients receiving digitalis or with a history of dysrhythmias, because of possible electrolyte-induced disturbances that may exacerbate underlying rhythm disturbances, or precipate sudden death. We are, likewise, particularly careful with the use of diltiazem and other calcium antagonists in patients with a history of arteriovenous nodal disease or severe cardiac failure.

In patients with diabetes mellitus, we generally prefer an angiotensin-converting enzyme inhibitor or a calcium antagonist, both of which reduce glomerular hydrostatic pressure [60,61], if proteinuria is severe and/or edema present. However, if these agents do not control high blood pressure adequately or if renal functional impairment is present, a loop-acting diuretic may be added to augment the antihypertensive effects of the initially prescribed drug, as well as help control peripheral edema. If this combination fails to achieve adequate arterial pressure control, the combined use of an angiotensin-converting enzyme inhibitor with a calcium entry antagonist is a reasonable selection [59,60].

Lastly, some degree of atherosclerosis is present in most elderly patients with westernized societies. Calcium antagonists have attenuated this process in experimental animals [62,63], and they may provide long-term protection from premature calcinosis, especially in smokers and patients with diabetes [62,63]. In any event, these agents are effective for attenuating symptoms in patients with occlusive coronary arterial disease. Thus, this class of drugs may be particularly protective against cardiovascular and other end-organ vascular disease in elderly patients with atherosclerosis.

Diastolic hypertension

Epidemiology

The prevalence of diastolic hypertension (diastolic pressure equal to or greater than 90 mmHg) in patients older than age 65 years is approximately 50% [17]. In general, 90–95% of patients with hypertension have no identifiable cause for their elevated pressure; they have primary or essential hypertension [20]. The remaining patients have secondary hypertension produced by a specific abnormality, and occlusive (atherosclerotic) disease of the renal artery is always a consideration [20].

Reduction of cardiovascular morbidity and mortality has been shown to occur with effective pharmacologic treatment of essential hypertension in the elderly [3,4,11–19]. The European Working Party on High Blood Pressure in the Elderly, which consisted of 840 patients with essential hypertension, demonstrated that treatment

reduced cardiovascular mortality by 38%, and this resulted in a 60% reduction of fatal myocardial infarction [14]. Fatal and nonfatal stroke was reduced by 46% in the Hypertension Detection Follow-up Program [13], and the Australian trial demonstrated a 26% reduction in stroke associated with treatment [15]. Finally, the Japanese Trial of Mild Hypertension in the Aged showed a significant reduction in cardiovascular complications in a small group of patients ($n = 32$) followed for 2 years [64].

The use of 24-hour blood pressure monitoring for predicting cardiovascular complications from hypertension is under active investigation. One recent study utilizing continuous 24-hour blood pressure monitoring of elderly patients with essential hypertension, demonstrated significantly lower daytime ambulatory systolic pressures at home than those obtained in the office [22]. However, two different patterns of blood pressure response emerged during the evening. In one group of patients, both systolic and diastolic pressures fell further during sleep; conversely, in a smaller subgroup, systolic pressures were similar to those obtained in the office and the diastolic pressures did not fall [21]. It was of particular interest that the prevalence of clinical cardiovascular complications was 43% in those with the nocturnal fall in pressure, but 100% in those with the nocturnal increase in systolic pressure [21]. This study suggests the importance of considering the overall 24-hour blood pressure fluctuations. Furthermore, it may have certain therapeutic implications concerning the need for restoring normal pressure control to prevent events related to morbidity and mortality.

Pathophysiology

The causes of hypertension in the elderly are similar to those encountered in younger age groups [20]. However, given the nature of occlusive vascular disease in the aging individual, there may be a greater number of patients with secondary hypertension that results from occlusive atherosclerotic renal arterial disease as compared with younger patients [1]. Although renal arterial disease may be the most common form of secondary hypertension in the young (excluding drug-related causes), elderly patients who develop occlusive arterial disease may never have had hypertension earlier in life. Alternatively, occlusive renal arterial disease may develop in patients with pre-existing and well-controlled hypertension that suddenly becomes more difficult to manage [20]. Thus, it is important not to exclude this possibility of occlusive renal arterial disease in the elderly patient with new or exacerbating hypertension.

Other causes of hypertension in younger populations should also be considered in the elderly. These include thyroid disease, hypercalcemic disorders, release of humoral agents from malignant tumors, pheochromocytomas, and hyperaldosteronism [20]. Certain drugs may also elevate arterial pressure and these include steroidal and nonsteroidal anti-inflammatory agents, nosedrops (α-adrenergic agonists), β-adrenergic receptor agonists, cyclosporine, and others [57,65,66].

Essential hypertension is not attributable to a specific cause. However, in recent years we have learned much about the pathophysiologic mechanisms underlying the disease. Arterial pressure is maintained at normal levels by means of a homeostatic balance of a wide variety of pressor and depressor mechanisms. These mechanisms are summarized in Table 9.4. Abnormal participation in one or more of these factors results in an elevated blood pressure through changes in the contribution of the others in the mosaic [20]. As a result, most authorities consider essential hypertension as a multifactorial disease. Among the pressor mechanisms that participate in essential hypertension are the adrenergic nervous system or alterations in catecholamine synthesis, release or reuptake; the renopressor system; altered regulation of fluid and electrolyte metabolism possibly through subclinical renal parenchymal disease or by humoral factors that directly affect this balance by renal parenchymal function; and reduced distensibility of the great vessels by atherosclerosis. Recent studies also support the role for various depressor systems (e.g., the kallikrein−kinins system, prostaglandins, atrial natriuretic hormone, etc.) in controlling arterial pressure [20].

The two hemodynamic determinants critical for determining arterial pressure are cardiac output and total peripheral resistance. Cardiac output is a product of two variables, heart rate, and the stroke volume; the latter may be affected by the state of myocardial contractility and venous return to the heart. Vascular resistance may be increased through the active participation of a wide variety of mechanisms, such as, adrenergic factors, the renopressor system, or any other circulating hormonal or humoral factors (Table 9.4).

To determine the effect of aging in patients with essential hypertension, two separate studies compared the

Table 9.4 Mechanisms of altering vascular resistance. (From Frohlich [20])

CONSTRICTION

Active
Adrenergic stimulation
Catecholamines: norepinephrine, epinephrine
Renopressor: angiotensin II
Cations: Ca^{2+}, K^+ (high levels)
Humoral substances: vasopressin, serotonin

Passive
Edema: extravascular compression
Vessel wall waterlogging
Increased blood or plasma viscosity
Obstruction (proximal): thrombosis, embolus
Cold

DILATATION

Active
Prostaglandins
Catecholamines: epinephrine (low dose), dopamine
Kinins: bradykinin, kallidin
Histamines
Peptides: atrial natriuretic factor, insulin, secretin, intestinal polypeptide, parathormone
Cations: K^+ (low levels), Mg^{2+}
Metabolites: adenosine, Krebs intermediate metabolites, acetate

Passive
Reduced blood or plasma viscosity
Increased tonicity
Heat

hemodynamic indices of younger (<42 years) and older (≥65 years) aged patients who were matched with respect to mean arterial pressure, race, sex, and body surface area [67,68]. This analysis indicated that cardiac output, heart rate, stroke volume, intravascular volume, and RBF were lower in the older age group, whereas the total peripheral and renal vascular resistances and left ventricular mass were higher in the elderly patients. Cardiac mass and the degree of left ventricular hypertrophy were greater in the elderly patients with hypertension, but their RBF was significantly lower.

These studies also showed that increased total peripheral resistance was reflected in higher systolic and diastolic pressures, and resulted in a structural adaptation of the left ventricle to the progressively increasing afterload through a process of concentric hypertrophy [68−71].

However, the elderly person, even if normotensive, also develops some degree of cardiac enlargement which may be related to ventricular hypertrophy, collagen, or amyloid deposition or other factors [71]. Thus, cardiac enlargement may be related to the coexistence of ischemic heart disease, to altered responsiveness of the aging myocardium to adrenergic stimulation, or other factors [1,5,20,69–71].

One important hemodynamic consideration relating the heart in the elderly patient with hypertension concerns the Pascal relationship. Myocardial oxygen consumption is directly related to left ventricular wall tension, the physical factor that is the product of left ventricular diameter and the systolic pressure generated within this contractile chamber [72,73]. In hypertension, and even in the elderly normotensive individual, there is an increased chamber diameter, cardiac mass, and wall thickness of the left ventricle [74–76]. Thus, when both tension-dependent factors coexist, they serve to increase

further the oxygen demand of the left ventricle whether the hypertension is isolated systolic or is comprized of both systolic and diastolic hypertension (Fig. 9.2). These considerations provide a sound physiologic explanation for the development of coronary arterial insufficiency in the patient with hypertension and a rationale for the therapeutic reduction of arterial pressure in these patients, even if only mild diastolic hypertension is present. This is even further enhanced if occlusive coronary arterial disease coexists, thereby reducing the oxygen supply to the ventricle with increased demand.

Plasma volume is usually expanded in normotensive or hypertensive patients with exogenous obesity, but this does not occur in most patients with essential and certain secondary forms of hypertension [30,77–82]. These changes are also observed in elderly patients with essential hypertension. Furthermore, the role of the renopressor system seems to be attenuated in elderly individuals resulting in a less inverse relationship between plasma

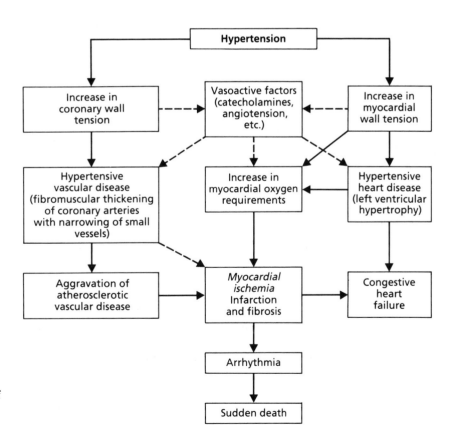

Fig. 9.2 The interrelationship between hypertension and the clinical sequelae of occlusive coronary artery disease. (From Dunn & Frohlich [72].)

volume and plasma renin activity in elderly patients with essential hypertension [83,84]. Thus, these findings might provide an explanation for the responsiveness of elderly individuals with hypertension, particularly those with isolated systolic hypertension to diuretics [84].

Treatment

The benefits of treating diastolic hypertension in the elderly are well established [11–19,45,85–88], and the goal of treatment in the elderly is similar to that of younger patients, i.e., reduction of diastolic pressures to levels below 90 mmHg. A Veteran Administration study involving patients over 59 years of age revealed that the incidence of morbid events observed over an average period of 3.3 years was extremely high. Antihypertensive therapy, however, significantly attenuated morbidity even in those patients whose diastolic pressures were in the range of 90 and 104 mmHg [89,90]. Furthermore, patients who had major complications secondary to hypertension, prior to the initiation of treatment, benefitted most from therapy.

The value of antihypertensive therapy in hypertensive survivors of stroke has been assessed in two separate studies [91,92]. The Hypertensive Stroke Cooperative Study demonstrated that the overall recurrence of strokes was not affected by antihypertensive therapy; however, data for patients age 70 years and older suggested a beneficial effect of therapy [91]. In a study by Carter [92] antihypertensive therapy produced a 50% reduction in the overall mortality of patients with diastolic hypertension, and those with good blood pressure control had the best outcome. Unfortunately, the number of elderly patients in this study was too small, so that a beneficial effect could not be demonstrated in those over 65 years of age.

Evidence for each group of antihypertensive drug used for therapy in elderly patients is reviewed below.

Diuretics

Many studies using diuretics have demonstrated their efficacy in hypertension for the elderly [12–15,40–42]. Low-dose thiazide diuretics alone or in combination with a potassium-sparing agent (e.g., triamterene, amiloride) have been effective for control of hypertension with minimal side-effects. However, most but not all, studies demonstrate a reduction in cardiovascular morbidity and mortality with the use of these agents. Although diuretics reduced arterial pressure in elderly hypertensive patients, they did not always prevent heart attack or stroke; in fact, in some studies the diuretics may have contributed to increased cardiovascular complications, possibly associated with hypokalemia [86].

Thiazide diuretics, which act primarily on the distal tubule, are preferred to the "high ceiling," loop diuretics because of their longer duration of action in patients with good renal function. The major side-effect of diuretics reported in these studies was hypokalemia, and this effect was dose-dependent. One study indicated that the thiazides (12.5 mg/day), provided excellent control of arterial pressure with minimal effect on potassium [40].

Another complication of the thiazide diuretics is carbohydrate intolerance. Deterioration of glucose tolerance, associated with thiazide diuretics, occurred to a varying extent in elderly patients after some years of therapy [44]. Clinical diabetes mellitus, however, was unlikely unless the patients had abnormal carbohydrate tolerance prior to initiation of therapy [44].

Lastly, the danger of volume depletion in elderly patients receiving diuretics remains an unresolved consideration. Volume status of elderly patients seems to be reduced, and agents that may aggravate this state may result in more profound and prolonged hypotension.

Beta-blockers

If particular care is taken to exclude patients in whom this group of drugs might be contraindicated, the β-adrenergic receptor blocking agents are well tolerated in elderly patients. The Metoprolol in Elderly Hypertension Patient Study (and other similar studies using β-adrenergic blocking agents) showed that when administered properly, and careful attention is given to side-effects, these agents were generally well tolerated and effective for control of blood pressure [93–95]. However, recent evidence suggests that the clinical response of the elderly to these agents may be different from that of younger patients. Thus, responsiveness to β-adrenergic blocking drugs may be reduced in the elderly [96]. Furthermore, there are important pharmacokinetic alterations related to the handling of propanolol in both acute and chronic situations in the elderly; plasma levels tend to be higher in older patients [97]. Elderly patients have different volumes of distribution and increased bioavailability secondary to alterations in "first-pass" metabolism of these compounds [97]. Kendall et al. [98] found a marked variation between elderly and younger patients; the older patients tended to have higher plasma levels of propranolol. Thus, higher plasma levels of β-blockers may be expected to occur in elderly patients. When initiating β-adrenergic blocker therapy in the elderly, lower initial and final doses should be the suggested rule.

Sympatholytic agents

Methyldopa, in short-term studies, minimally reduces cardiac output in elderly patients and is well maintained with few side-effects other than sedation [99]. The afterload reduction with these agents overrides any negative ionotropic effect. Methyldopa also reduces left ventricular mass, an effect that may reflect its antihypertensive as well as nonhemodynamic effects [100].

Clonidine, another central α2-agonist may have transient negative ionotropic effect on the left ventricle, and this should also be considered in elderly patients [101]. Once the patient is maintained on a low dose of clonidine, the drug tolerance is usually excellent. No significant renal or other hemodynamic parameters are altered in elderly patients receiving clonidine [102]. Rebound hypertension upon sudden withdrawal of the drug and sedation are two troublesome effects of this agent that should be kept in mind.

Prazosin reduces left ventricular afterload in patients with hypertension and possibly preload in patients with cardiac failure [57]. Based on these considerations, this postsynaptic α-blocker may be an alternative selection for an elderly hypertensive. However, prazosin is also associated with orthostatic hypotension especially in predisposed elderly patients, and tachyphlaxis may occur in patients with cardiac failure [57]. Thus, we do not generally select this agent as first-line therapy in elderly patients with hypertension.

Reserpine is an agent that is less used today primarily because of its side-effects that include depression, extrapyramidal tract symptoms, and nightmares [57]. However, the Veterans Administration reports indicated that it was well tolerated when used in low doses with diuretics [85].

Calcium antagonists

This class of agents includes verapamil, diltiazem, nifedipine, nitrendipine, and a number of other newer agents under study. They are well known to have antihypertensive as well as antianginal properties [46]. They reduce arterial pressure through a fall in total peripheral resistance, and their effect on heart rate and cardiac output is variable. Elderly patients with hypertension very often suffer concomitant coronary arterial disease as well as low-grade congestive heart failure [103–105]. Therefore, these agents may be an excellent choice for this age group. Verapamil, in particular, seems to be more effective in older and low renin patients than in comparable younger age groups. Nevertheless, its tolerance in the aged may be limited by its propensity to produce constipation [103–105]. In contrast to diuretics, the calcium antagonists, especially diltiazem, also offer the advantage of some cardioprotection by attenuating the influx of calcium ions into the cardiac myocyte [106]. They may also reduce left ventricular mass [100,103,107]. These agents also preserve renal filtration fraction and some (for example, diltiazem, nitrendipine) may reduce glomerular hydrostatic pressure [70].

An inhibiting effect on platelet aggregation that has been reported for verapamil and nifedipine together with certain preliminary experimental evidence suggests that these drugs may have the potential to prevent arteriosclerosis [62,63]. However, long-term clinical studies have not been done to examine this effect.

Angiotensin-converting enzyme inhibitors

These agents reduce arterial pressure through a fall in total peripheral resistance without affecting cardiac output [108]. Angiotensin-converting enzyme inhibitors decrease ventricular afterload, left ventricular mass, and are useful in cardiac failure. Therefore, they may become important in the management of hypertension in the elderly. Their effect, according to some investigators, may be dependent upon circulating plasma renin activity, which is usually lower in elderly hypertensive patients unless they also have congestive heart failure. Low-dose diuretic therapy may be necessary to potentiate the antihypertensive effects in these agents [108–110]. However, their usefulness in patients with low-plasma renin activity, expanded plasma volume, or in anephric subjects, may relate to their putative effects on local tissue renin angiotensin systems including vessel, heart, and brain [100].

Vascular smooth-muscle relaxants (hydralazine, minoxidil)

These agents are less useful in the elderly, particularly

because of their propensity to expand intravascular volume coincidental with their hypotensive action and a tendency towards palpitations and headaches [20,57]. Reflex tachycardia in the elderly may not be as great a problem in the elderly with less sensitive baroreceptor function as it is in younger people [57]. However, the pharmacokinetics of hydralazine require frequent dosing [57] and the edema and hirsutism associated with minoxidil preclude its use in this population [57].

One therapeutic approach

When an elderly patient with hypertension requires treatment, several factors require consideration, including the patient's renal functional status, age, race, and gender. In addition to these factors, other considerations such as single-agent therapy, the lowest clinical and biochemical side-effect profile, and cost of drug should also be taken into account. This section will focus on specific disease entities, i.e., coronary artery disease, diabetes mellitus, cardiac failure, and the effect of hypertension control in these groups. It will concentrate on specific agents for management of hypertension and how they may fit the criteria mentioned above to optimize not only patient compliance but cardiovascular and renal function.

Coronary artery disease

There is a fairly large prevalence of coronary artery disease as well as occlusive peripheral vascular disease in elderly patients with hypertension, particularly if they are also smokers [12,14,17,45]. Many studies have shown in nonelderly populations that control of blood pressure will lead to improved cardiac function and alleviation of symptomatic coronary artery disease as well as a decrease in coronary morbidity and mortality [12,14,17,111].

Our approach to an elderly patient with coronary artery disease or peripheral vascular disease with hypertension and a smoking history is to encourage cessation of smoking, and attempt blood pressure control with a calcium antagonist. Alternatives to this as first-line therapy would include an angiotensin-converting enzyme inhibitor or β-blocker, the latter particularly if there is a prior history of myocardial infarction. Many studies have shown that calcium antagonists significantly improve myocardial function secondary to its effects on myocardial oxygen demand and inhibition of calcium influx [112,113]. These effects are true in both white and black

Table 9.5 Antihypertensive therapies reported to decrease left ventricular hypertrophy

Drug class	Specific agents
Sympatholytic agents	Reserpine
Central α2-receptor agonists	Clonidine, α-methyldopa
β-adrenergic receptor blockers	Propranolol, atenolol, metoprolol, naldolol
Combined α- and β-receptor antagonists	Labetalol
Angiotensin-converting enzyme inhibitors	Captorpil, enalapril, lisinopril
Calcium channel antagonists	Diltiazem, nifedipine, verapamil

patients, and there does not seem to be a difference between genders with these agents [105,114,115].

New compounds are available such as long-acting verapamil, diltiazem, nicardipine, isradipine, nitrendipine, and on the horizon, long-acting nifedipine. These agents are usually administered once or twice daily (nicardipine, three times daily). Unlike other agents such as β-adrenoreceptor blockers, when peripheral vascular disease coexists it will not be exacerbated by these agents and may even be improved [113]. Studies from the European Working Party that examined elderly patients with coronary artery disease found them to do well on β-adrenoreceptor blockers [14].

Lastly, both aging and long-standing hypertension are associated with left ventricular hypertrophy [116–118]. The clinical significance of regression of left ventricular hypertrophy is not known. However, it is a well-known independent risk factor for cardiovascular morbidity and mortality [100]. Most agents, if used for a long enough period of time, will decrease cardiac mass except for minoxidil, hydralazine, and diuretics. Those known to decrease left ventricular hypertrophy within weeks are summarized in Table 9.5. These agents are more expensive than the once daily diuretics that could be used in these circumstances [119]. However, diuretics may be associated with metabolic side-effects.

Diabetes mellitus

Generally, elderly patients with Type II noninsulin-dependent diabetes mellitus with hypertension require aggressive blood pressure and blood sugar control. Many studies have shown in younger diabetic populations that aggressive blood pressure management will also improve glycemic control [120,121]. The major clinical problem in those patients is impaired renal function and significant proteinuria that may result in edema. Studies have shown that the angiotension-converting enzyme inhibitors may significantly attenuate proteinuria as well as control arterial pressure [122,123]. Certain calcium antagonists may also reduce hydrostatic pressure similar to the angiotensin-converting enzyme inhibitors and could decrease proteinuria in this setting [61]. There does not seem to be any difference in response of black and white patients to angiotensin-converting enzyme inhibitors or calcium antagonists with hypertension and diabetes [113,114]. Furthermore, the calcium antagonists have been shown in our studies and others to preserve, or actually improve, renal hemodynamics in the elderly hypertensives as well as serve as an excellent first-line drug [46–50,61,124–126]. Therefore, we generally select either a long-acting angiotensin-converting enzyme inhibitor or a long-acting calcium antagonist, such as diltiazem or verapamil, for our hypertensive patients with diabetes mellitus.

Agents, such as minoxidil or other direct-acting vascular smooth-muscle vasodilators, are usually avoided because of their volume expanding effects, potential exacerbation of edema, and eventually attenuation of their antihypertensive effects [20,56]. Prazosin may also be avoided because some diabetic patients frequently have orthostatic hypotension secondary to autonomic neuropathy [127].

Diuretics, in this group of patients, are useful because they also help with edema management. However, these patients should have close monitoring of renal function when started on these agents. If there is a significant renal impairment, serum creatinine concentrations of equal to or greater than 2 mg/dl in an elderly patient, a loop-acting diuretic may be used to achieve diuresis [44]. However, the high-ceiling (loop) diuretics usually are of short duration in action and then must given twice (or more) daily for appropriate management of edema and pressure control.

Congestive heart failure

Congestive heart failure is another "high renin" state, and patients with early congestive heart failure (New York Heart Classes I and II) and with associated mild degrees of hypertension will be markedly improved with treatment. The best agents, based on studies that have evaluated various antihypertensive agents in this clinical setting, are the angiotensin-converting enzyme inhibitors with or without adding diuretic agents [17]. Calcium antagonists may also be valid choices in patients with higher left ventricular ejection fractions (approximately 40%) [59]. Calcium antagonists improve afterload and myocardial contractile ability and have been shown to be beneficial in this age group. However, cases have been reported of calcium antagonists precipitating congestive heart failure in people with marginal myocardial function [128]. Therefore, we suggest calcium antagonists in people that have fairly good myocardial function and angiotensin-converting enzyme inhibitors as our first-base selection.

The diuretics of choice in this clinical situation may be the high-ceiling or loop diuretics since edema management and natriuresis are major concerns in the patient with cardiac failure, especially in the elderly population. Beta-adrenoreceptor antagonists are to be used with extreme caution for fear of aggravating the cardiac failure.

Recently, vasodilator therapy, along with nitrates, has been shown effective to reducing arterial pressure in patients with cardiac failure [129]. However, they generally require frequent dosing and the problem of tachyphylaxis associated with nitrate therapy must be considered.

In conclusion, we feel strongly that hypertension in the elderly patient should be treated, and in this way significantly reduce morbidity and mortality in this population. Furthermore, therapy should be tailored for each individual patient with emphasis on coexisting cardiovascular, renal, or other underlying diseases (e.g., diabetes mellitus, coronary, renal and peripheral arterial disease, chronic obstructive lung disease, etc). We should recognize that elderly patients normally have altered adrenoreceptor and baroreceptor function. In addition, they have altered cardiac and renal responses to various stimuli as well as drug metabolism when compared to a younger population. Therefore, careful consideration of the physiologic status of the patient, coexisting diseases, and the overall medical history of the patient will insure optimal and wise selection of therapy and consequent response to the treatment. Following these guidelines, hopefully elderly patients will achieve improved blood pressure control with decreased morbidity and mortality and a better quality of life.

References

1 Lipsitz LA. Abnormalities in blood pressure homeostasis associated with aging and hypertension. In Horan MJ, Steinberg GM, Dunbar JB, et al., eds. Blood Pressure Regulation and Aging, New York: Biomedical Info. Corp., 1986:201–212.

2 Curb JD, Borhani NO, Schnaper H, et al. Detection and treatment of hypertension in older individuals. Am J Epidermiol 1985;121:371–376.

3 The Working Group on Hypertension in the Elderly. Statement on hypertension in the elderly. J Am Med Assoc 1986;256:70–74.

4 Kannel WB. Blood pressure and the development of cardiovascular disease in the aged. In Chaird FI, Dall J, Kennedy RD, eds. Cardiology and Old Age. New York: Plenum Press, 1976:127–138.

5 Kawanamoto-A, Shimada K, Matsubayashi K, et al. Cardiovascular regulatory functions in elderly patients with hypertension. Hypertension 1989;13:401–407.

6 Lakatta EG. Age-related alterations in the cardiovascular response to adrenergic mediated stress. Fed Proc 1980; 39:3173–3177.

7 Rowe JW, Troen BR. Sympathetic nervous system and aging in man. Endocr Rev 1980;1:167–179.

8 Crane MG, Harris JJ. Effect of aging on renin activity and aldosterone excretion. J Lab Clin Med 1976;87:947–959.

9 Stern N, Beahm E, McGinty D, et al. Dissociation of 24 hour catecholamine levels from blood pressure in older men. Hypertension 1985;7:1023–1029.

10 National Center for Health Statistics. Blood Pressure Levels of Persons 65–74 Years. United States, 1971–1974, Series 11, No. 203. Rockville: National Center for Health Statistics, 1977.

11 Shekelle RB, Ostfeld AM, Klawans HL Jr. Hypertension and risk of stroke in an elderly population. Stroke 1974;5: 71–76.

12 Kannel WB. Implications of Framingham study data for treatment of hypertension: Impact of other risk factors. In Laragh JH, Buhler FR, Seldin DW, eds. Frontiers of Hypertension Research. New York: Springer-Verlag, 1981: 167–178.

13 Hypertension Detection and Follow-up Program Cooperative Group: Five year findings of the Hypertension Detection and Follow-up Program III. Reduction in stroke incidence among persons with high blood pressure. J Am Med Assoc 1982;247:633–638.

14 Amery A, Birkenhager W, Brixho P, et al. Mortality and morbidity results from the European Working Party on High Blood Pressure in The Elderly Trial. Lancet 1985;1: 1349–1356.

15 National Heart Foundation of Australia: Treatment of mild hypertension in the elderly. Report by the Management Committee. Med J Aust 1981;2:398–402.

16 Kannel WB, Dawber TR, Sorlie P, et al. Components of blood pressure and risk of atherothrombotic brain infarction: The Framingham Study. Stroke 1976;7:327–334.

17 Joint National Committee on Detection, Evaluation, and Treatment of High Blood Pressure. Hypertension in the elderly. Arch Intern Med 1988;148:1023–1038.

18 Ostfeld AM. Epidemiology of hypertension in the elderly. In Horan MJ, Steinberg GM, Dunbar JB, et al., eds. NIH Blood Pressure Regulation and Aging. New York: Biomedical Info. Corp., 1986:3–10.

19 Anon. Blood Pressure Study 1979. Chicago Society of Actuaries and Association of Life Insurance Medical Directors of America, 1980.

20 Frohlich ED. Hypertension in the Elderly. Curr Prob Cardiol 1988;13:315–367.

21 Kobrin I, Dunn FG, Oigman W, et al. Essential hypertension in the elderly: Circadian variation of arterial pressure. In Weber MA, Drayer JM, eds. Ambulatory Blood Pressure Monitoring. Steinkoff: Darmsstadt, 1984:181–185.

22 Tochikubo O, Miyazaki N, Yamada Y, et al. Mathematical evaluation of 24 hour blood pressure variability in young, middle-aged, and elderly hypertensive patients. Jpn Circ J 1987;51:1123–1130.

23 Drizd T, Dannenberg A, Engel A. Blood pressure levels in persons 18–74 years of age in 1976–1980 and trends in blood pressure from 1960–1980 in the United States. Vital Health Stat [11],1986.

24 Frohlich ED. Multicenter clinical trials: Potential influence of consumer education. Hypertension 1987;9(Suppl. III): 75–79.

25 Straessen J, Fagard R, Van Hoof R, et al. Mortality in various intervention trials in elderly hypertensive patients. A review. Eur Heart J 1988;9:215–222.

26 Intersociety Commission for Heart Disease Resources. Primary preparation of the atherosclerotic diseases. Circulation 1970;42:A55–A95.

27 Baumbach GL, Heistad DD. Cerebral circulation in chronic arterial hypertension. Hypertension 1988;12:89–95.

28 Adamopoulos PN, Chrysanthakopoulis SG, Frohlich ED. Systolic hypertension: Nonhomogeneous diseases. Am J Cardiol 1975;36:697–701.

29 Simon AC, Safar MA, Levenson JA, et al. Systolic hypertension: Hemodynamic mechanisms and choice of antihypertensive treatment. Am J Cardiol 1979;44:505–511.

30 Messerli FH, Sundgaard-Riise K, Ventura HO, et al. Essential hypertension in the elderly: Haemodynamics, intravascular volume, plasma renin activity, and circulating catecholamine levels. Lancet 1983;2:983–985.

31 Hollenberg NK, Adams DF, Solomon HS, et al. Senescence

and the renal vasculature in normal man. Circ Res 1974; 34:309–316.

32 Hollenberg NK, Adams DF. The renal circulation in hypertensive disease. Am J Med 1976;60:773–784.

33 Krakoff LR. Renal and adrenal mechanisms pertinent to hypertension in an aging population. In Horan MJ, Steinberg GM, Dunbar JB, et al., eds. *Blood Pressure Regulation and Aging*. New York: Biomedical Info. Corp., 1986:161–172.

34 Rowe JW, Andres R, Tobin JD, et al. The effect of age on creatinine clearance in men: a cross-sectional and longitudinal study. J Gerontol 1976;31:155–163.

35 Epstein M. Effects of aging on the kidney. Fed Proc 1979; 38:168–179.

36 Lindeman RD, Tobin JD, Shock NW. Association between blood pressure and the rate of decline in renal function with age. Kidney Int 1984;26:861–868.

37 Kaplan N. Nonpharmacologic therapy of hypertension. Med Clin North Am 1987;71:921–933.

38 Grabbe DE, Hofman A. Does sodium restriction lower blood pressure? Br Med J 1986;293:27–30.

39 O'Malley K, O'Brien E. Management of hypertension in the elderly. N Engl J Med 1980;302:1397–1400.

40 Hulley SP, Furberg CD, Gurland B, et al. Systolic hypertension in the elderly program: antihypertensive efficacy of chlorthalidone. Am J Cardiol 1985;56:913–920.

41 Perry HM Jr, McDonald HR, Hulley SB, et al. Systolic hypertension in the elderly program. Pilot study (SHEP-PS): Morbidity and mortality experience. J Hypertens 1986; 41(Suppl. 6):S21–S23.

42 Smith WM. Isolated systolic hypertension in the elderly. Curr Med Res Opin 1982;8(Suppl. 1):19–29.

43 SHEP Cooperative Research Group. Prevention of stroke by antihypertensive drug treatment in older persons with isolated systolic hypertension: Final results of the Systolic Hypertension in the Elderly Program. JAMA 1991;265: 3255–3264.

44 Friedman PA. Clinical use of diuretics. Semin Nephrol 1988;8:198–212.

45 Hypertension Detection and Follow-up Program Cooperative Group: Five year findings of the hypertension detection and follow-up program. J Am Med Assoc 1979;242: 2562–2577.

46 Pieplio RW, Sowers JR. Antihypertensive therapy in the geriatric patient: A review of the role of calcium channel blockers. J Clin Pharmacol 1989;29:193–199.

47 Buhler FR. Cardiovascular regulation as a function of age. Determinants of antihypertensive treatment based on beta blockers and calcium inhibitors. Arch Mal Coeur 1985;27: 83–90.

48 Forette F, Bellet M, Henry JF, et al. Effect of nicardipine in elderly hypertensive patients. Br J Clin Pharmacol 1985; 20:125S–129S.

49 Stressman J, Leibel B, Yagil Y, et al. Nifedipine in the treatment of hypertension in the elderly. J Clin Pharmacol 1985;25:193–196.

50 Jansen RWM, Van Lier HJJ, Hoelnagels WHL. Nitrendipine versus hydrochlorothiazide in hypertensive patients over 70 years of age. Clin Pharmacol Ther 1989;45:291–298.

51 Woo KS, Kim T, Vallance-Owen J. A single-blind randomized cross-over study of angiotension-converting enzyme inhibitors and triamterene and hydrochlorothiazide in the treatment of mild to moderate hypertension in the elderly. Arch Intern Med 1987;147:1386–1389.

52 Pool JL, Nelson EB, Taylor AA. Clinical Experience and rationale for angiotension-converting enzyme inhibition with lisinopril as the initial treatment for hypertension in older patients. Am J Med 1988;85(Suppl. 3B):19–24.

53 Vardan S, Dunsky MH, Hill NE, et al. Systemic systolic hypertension in the elderly: correlation of hemodynamics, plasma volume, renin, aldosterone, urinary metanephrine, and response to thiazide therapy. Am J Cardiol 1986;58: 1030–1034.

54 Corea L, Bentivoglio M, Verdecehia P, et al. Converting enzyme inhibitor vs. diuretic therapy as first therapeutic approach to the elderly hypertensive patient. Curr Ther Res 1984;36:347–351.

55 Greenblatt DJ, Shader RI. On the psychopharmacology of beta-adrenergic blockade. Curr Ther Res 1972;14:615–625.

56 Report by the Management Committee: The Australian therapeutic trial in mild hypertension. Lancet 1980;1: 1261–1267.

57 Blaschke TF, Melmon KL. Antihypertensive agents and the drug therapy of hypertension. In Goodman AG, Goodman LS, Gilman A, eds. *The Pharmacological Basis of Therapeutics*, 6th edn. New York: MacMillan Publishing Co., 1980:778–826.

58 Veterans Administration Cooperative Study: Effects of treatment on morbidity in hypertension. J Am Med Assoc 1967;121:1028–1034.

59 Gibson RS, Young PM, Boden WE, et al. Diltiazem Reinfarction Study Group. Prognostic significance and beneficial effect of diltiazem on the incidence of early recurrent ischemia after non-Q wave myocardial infarction: results from the multicenter diltiazem reinfarction study. Am J Cardiol 1987;60:203–209.

60 Hostetter TH, Rennke HG, Brenner BM. The case for intra-renal hypertension in the initiation and progression of diabetic and other glomerulopathies. Am J Med 1982;72: 345–380.

61 Isshiki T, Amodeo C, Messerli FH, et al. Diltiazem maintains renal vasodilation without hyperfiltration in hypertension: Studies in essential hypertensive man and the spontaneously hypertensive rat. Cardiovasc Drug Ther 1987;1: 350–366.

62 Weinstein DB, Heider JG. Antiatherogenic properties of calcium antagonist. Am J Cardiol 1987;59:B163–B172.

63 Weinstein DB, Heider JG. Protective action of calcium channel antagonists in atherogenesis and experimental

vascular injury. Am J Hypertens 1989;2:205−212.

64 Kuramoto K, Matsushita S, Kuwajiwa I, et al. Prospective study on the treatment of mild hypertension in the aged. Jpn Heart J 1981;22:75−85.

65 Bakris GL, Kern S. Renal hemodynamic effects of nonsteroidal antiinflammatory agents in man. Am Fam Physician 1989;40:199−204.

66 Myers BD. Cyclosporine nephrotoxicity. Kidney Int 1986; 30:964−974.

67 Messerli FH, Glade LB, Dreslinski GR, et al. Hypertension in the elderly: Hemodynamic, fluid volume, and endocrine findings. Clin Sci 1981;61:S393−S394.

68 Messerli FH, Sundgaard-Riise K, Ventura HO, et al. Essential hypertension in the elderly: Haemodynamics, intravascular volume, plasma renin activity, and circulating catecholamines. Lancet 1983;2:983−985.

69 Lakatta EG, Gerstenblith G, Angell CS, et al. Diminished ionotropic response of aged myocardiuim to catecholamines. Circ Res 1975;36:262−269.

70 Lakatta EG, Gerstenblith G, Angell CS, et al. Prolonged contraction duration in aged myocardium. J Clin Invest 1975;55:61−65.

71 Lakatta EG. Alterations in the cardiovascular system that occur in advanced age. Fed Proc 1979;38:163.

72 Dunn FG, Frohlich ED. Hypertension and angina pectoris. In Yu PN, Goodwin JF, eds. Progress in Cardiology. Philadelphia: Lea & Febiger, 1978:163−196.

73 Sarnoff SJ, Braunwald E, Welch GH Jr, et al. Hemodynamic determinants of oxygen consumption of the heart with special reference to the tension time index. Am J Physiol 1958;192:148−153.

74 Gerstenblith G, Weisfeldt ML, Lakatta EG. Age changes in myocardial function and exercise response. Prog Cardiovasc Dis 1976;19:1−21.

75 Sjogren AL. Left ventricular wall thickness determined by ultrasound in 100 subjects without heart disease. Chest 1971;60:341−346.

76 Gardin JM, Henry WL, Savage DP, et al. Echocardiographic evaluation of an older population without clinically apparent heart disease (abstr.). Am J Cardiol 1977;39:277.

77 Frohlich ED, Messerli FH, Reisin E, et al. The problem of obesity and hypertension. Hypertension 1983;5(Suppl. III):71−78.

78 Messerli FH, Christie B, de Carvalho JGF, et al. Obesity and essential hypertension: Hemodynamics, intravascular volume, sodium excretion, and plasma renin activity. Arch Intern Med 1981;141:81−84.

79 Messerli FH, Sundgaard-Riise K, Reisin E, et al. Disparate cardiovascular effects of obesity and arterial hypertension. Am J Med 1983;74:808−812.

80 Tarazi RD, Frohlich ED, Dustan HP. Plasma volume in men with essential hypertension. N Engl J Med 1968;278: 762−766.

81 Tarazi RC, Dustan HP, Frohlich ED. Relation of plasma to interstitial fluid volume in essential hypertension. Circulation 1969;40:357−361.

82 Tarazi RC, Dustan HP, Frohlich ED, et al. Plasma volume and chronic hypertension: Relationship to arterial pressure levels in different hypertensive diseases. Arch Intern Med 1970;125:835−842.

83 Schmieder RE, Frohlich ED, Messerli FH. Pathophysiology of hypertension in the elderly. In Abrams WB, Frohlich ED, eds. Cardiology Clinics, vol. 4. Philadelphia: WB Saunders Co., 1986:235−243.

84 Frohlich ED, Messerli FH. Systolic hypertension in the elderly. In Safar M, Simon A, Weiss YA, eds. Arterial and Venous Systems in Essential Hypertension. The Netherlands: Martinus Nijhoff, 1987:105−114.

85 Veterans Administration Cooperative Study Group on Antihypertensive Agents. Effects of treatment on morbidity in hypertension III. Influence of age, diastolic pressure, and prior cardiovascular disease. Circulation 1972;45: 991−1004.

86 Multiple Risk Factor Intervention Trial Research Group. Benfari RC, Sherwin R, eds. The Multiple Risk Factor Intervention Trial (MRFIT): the methods and impact of intervention over four years. Prev Med 1981;10:387−553.

87 Stamler J. Risk factor modification trials: Implications for the elderly. Heart J 1988;9(Suppl. D):9−53.

88 Applegate WB. Hypertension in elderly patients. Ann Intern Med 1989;12:901−905.

89 Veterans Administration Cooperative Study Group on Antihypertensive Agents: Effects of treatment on morbidity in hypertension. II: Results in patients with diastolic blood pressures averaging 90 through 114 mmHg. J Am Med Assoc 1970;213:1143−1152.

90 Veterans Administration Cooperative Study Group on Antihypertensive Agents: Effects of treatment on morbidity in hypertension. III: Influence of age, diastolic pressure, and prior cardiovascular disease; further analysis of side effects. Circulation 1972;45:991−1003.

91 Hypertension−Stroke Cooperative Study Group. Effect of antihypertensive treatment on stroke recurrence. J Am Med Assoc 1974;229:409−18.

92 Carter AB. Hypotensive therapy in stroke survivors. Lancet 1970;1:485−489.

93 Wikstrand J, Westergren G, Berglund G, et al. Antihypertensive treatment with metoprolol or hydrochlorothiazide in patients aged 60−75 years. Report from a double-blind international multicenter study. J Am Med Assoc 1986; 255:1304−1310.

94 Wikstrand J, Berglund G. Antihypertensive treatment with beta-blockers in patients aged over 65. Br Med J 1982;285: 850−851.

95 Hartford M, Wendelhag I, Berglund G, et al. Cardiovascular and renal effects of long-term antihypertensive treatment. J Am Med Assoc 1988;259:2553−2557.

96 Lakatta EG. Diminished beta-adrenergic modulation of

cardiovascular function in advanced age. In Abrams R, Frohlich ED, eds. *Cardiology Clinics.* Philadelphia: WB Saunders Co., 1986:49−57.

97 Castleden CM, George C. The effect of aging on hepatic clearance propranolol. Br J Clin Pharmacol 1979;7:49−54.

98 Kendall MJ, Brown D, Yates RA. Plasma metropolol concentrations in young, old, and hypertensive subject. Br J Clin Pharmacol 1977;4:497−499.

99 Messerli FH, Sundgaard-Riise K, Reisin E, *et al.* Dimorphic cardiac adaptation to obesity and arterial hypertension. Ann Intern Med 1983;99:757−761.

100 Frohlich ED. The first Irvine H Page Lecture: The mosaic of hypertension: past, present, and future. J Hypertens 1988; 6:2−11.

101 Mroczek WJ, Davidov M, Finnerty FA Jr. Intravenous clonidine in hypertensive patients. Clin Pharmacol Ther 1973;14:847−851.

102 Cohen IM, O'Connor DT, Preston RA, *et al.* Reduced renovascular resistance by clonidine. Clin Pharmacol Ther 1979;26:572−577.

103 Buhler FR. Age and cardiovascular response adaptation: Determinants of an antihypertensive treatment concept primarily based on beta-blockers and calcium entry blockers. Hypertension 1983;5:94−100.

104 Frohlich ED. Calcium channel blockers: A new dimension in antihypertensive therapy. Am J Med 1984;77:45−51.

105 Nicholson JP, Resnick LM, Laragh JH. The antihypertensive effect of verapamil at extremes of dietary sodium intake. Ann Intern Med 1987;107:329−334.

106 Owen NE, Feinberg H, LeBreton JN. Epinephrine induces Ca^{2+} uptake in human blood platelets. Am J Physiol 1980; 239:H483−H488.

107 Katz AM, Reuter H. Cellular calcium and cardiac cell death. Am J Cardiol 1979;44:188−190.

108 Frohlich ED. Angiotensin-converting enzyme inhibitors: Present and future. Hypertension 1989;13(Suppl. I): I125−I130.

109 Guillevin L, Lardoux MD, Corrol P. Effects of captopril on blood pressure, electrolytes, and certain hormones. Clin Pharmacol Ther 1981;29:699−704.

110 Frohlich ED, Cooper RA, Lewis EJ. Review of the overall experience of captopril in hypertension. Arch Intern Med 1984;144:1441−1444.

111 O'Kelly BF, Massie BM, Tabau JF, *et al.* Coronary morbidity and mortality, pre-existing silent coronary artery disease and mild hypertension. Ann Intern Med 1989;110: 1017−1026.

112 Frishman WH, Charlap S. Calcium channel blockers for combined systemic hypertension and myocardial ischemia. Circulation 1987;75(Suppl. V):V154−V162.

113 Cubeddu LX. Calcium channel blockers as monotherapy in hypertension. In Epstein SE, ed. *Current Status of Calcium Channel Blockers in Hypertension.* New York: Biomedical Info. Corp., 1986:65−83.

114 Cubeddu LX, Aranda J, Singh B, *et al.* A comparison of verapamil and propranolol for initial treatment of hypertension: Racial differences in response. J Am Med Assoc 1986;256:2214−2221.

115 Resnick LM, Nicholson JP, Laragh JH. Calcium metabolism and the renal−aldosterone system in essential hypertension. Fed Proc 1986;45:2739−2745.

116 Yin FCP. The aging vasculature and its effect on the heart. Age Aging 1980;12:137−214.

117 Gerstenblith G, Frederiksen J, Yin FCP. Echocardiographic assessment of a normal adult aging population. Circulation 1987;56:273−278.

118 Lakatta EG. Alterations in the cardiovascular system that occur in advanced age. Fed Proc 1979;38:163−167.

119 Stason WB. Cost and quality trade-offs in the treatment of hypertension. Hypertension 1989;13(Suppl. I):I145−I148.

120 Ferrannini E, Buzzigoli G, Bonadonna R, *et al.* Insulin resistance in essential hypertension. N Engl J Med 1987; 317:350−357.

121 Modan M, Halkin H, Almog S, *et al.* Hyperinsulinemia: a link between hypertension, obesity, and glucose intolerance. J Clin Invest 1985;75:809−817.

122 Tagama Y, Kitamolo Y, Futake G, *et al.* Effect of captopril on heavy proteinuria in azotemic diabetics. N Engl J Med 1985;313:1617−1620.

123 Anderson S, Rennke HG, Brenner BM. Therapeutic advantage of converting enzyme inhibitors in arresting progressive renal diseases associated with systemic hypertension in the rat. J Clin Invest 1986;77:1993−2000.

124 Giles TD, Massie BM. Role of calcium antagonists as initial pharmacologic monotherapy for systemic hypertension in patients over 60 years of age. Am J Cardiol 1988;61: H13−H17.

125 Bakris GL, Barnhill BW, Sadler R. Treatment of arterial hypertension in diabetic man: importance of therapeutic selection. Kidney Int 1992;41:346−352.

126 Demarie B, Bakris GL. Effects of different calcium antagonists on proteinumia associated with diabetes mellitus. Ann Intern Med 1990;113:987−988.

127 Leichter SB, Baumgardner B. Effects of chronic prazosin therapy on intermediate metabolism in diabetic patients. J Cardiovasc Pharmacol 1981;55:38−42.

128 Winniford MD, Hillis LD. Calcium antagonists in patients with cardiovascular disease. Medicine 1985;64:61−73.

129 Cohn JN, Archibald DG, Ziesche S, *et al.* Effect of vasodilator therapy on mortality in chronic congestive heart failure. Results of a Veterans Administration Cooperative Study. N Engl J Med 1986;314:1547−1552.

10

Clinical assessment and management of mild to severe hypertension in the elderly

C. Venkata S. Ram

Disability from cardiovascular disease is a major problem in the elderly. Systemic hypertension is the predominant risk factor predisposing to cardiovascular morbidity and mortality among the elderly population. Cardiovascular mortality in elderly hypertensives is approximately three times higher compared to normotensives in the same age group. Approximately 40–60% of all cardiovascular diseases in the elderly are attributable to systemic hypertension. The proportion of elderly people in our population is steadily increasing. At the present, it is estimated that between 10 and 15% of the population of most western countries are older than 60 years. It has been further estimated that a substantial part of a physician's professional life will be spent in taking care of elderly patients. The number of people in the elderly age group is increasing at a much faster rate than the overall population. The elderly also consume over one-third of the health expenditures in the United States even though they represent an approximate 12% of the population. Systemic hypertension is perhaps the most potent risk factor for congestive heart failure, coronary artery disease, and cerebral vascular disease, which are the major causes of cardiovascular morbidity and mortality in the population over age 65 [1]. Contrary to previous belief, cardiovascular disease is not an inevitable consequence of aging. Prevention of cardiovascular disease in the elderly would likely decrease chronic disability and premature mortality, and might also improve their quality of life. Because of these considerations, more attention should be devoted to the identification, management, and monitoring of cardiovascular disease in the elderly population.

In order to explore the pathophysiologic significance of elevated arterial blood pressure in the elderly, it is necessary to determine the levels of systolic and diastolic blood pressure that constitute "hypertension for this age group." Hypertension can be generally considered as that level of blood pressure beyond which the benefits of therapy exceed the risk. The Joint National Committee on Detection, Evaluation, and Treatment of High Blood Pressure has recommended that the diagnosis of hypertension in adults be made when the average of two or more diastolic blood pressures on at least two separate visits is 90 mmHg or higher, or when the average of multiple systolic blood pressures on two or more subsequent visits is consistently greater than 140 mmHg [2]. This definition may not be strictly applicable to the elderly population. According to the Working Group on

Table 10.1 Classification of hypertension in the elderly, based upon the level of systolic and diastolic blood pressure

	Blood pressure (mmHg)	
Classification	Systolic	Diastolic
Combined hypertension	>160	>90
Borderline hypertension	140–159	>90
Predominant systolic hypertension	>(DBP − 15) × 2	>90
Isolated systolic hypertension	>160	<90

DBP, diastolic blood pressure.

Hypertension in the Elderly, an average systolic blood pressure >160 mmHg and/or average diastolic blood pressure ≥90 mmHg on three consecutive visits constitutes the diagnosis of hypertension [3]. Table 10.1 (see also Chapter 5) provides a classification of hypertension in the elderly based upon the level of systolic and diastolic blood pressure. The importance of disproportionate systolic hypertension is still being debated, although there is convincing evidence to suggest that patients with systolic hypertension are predisposed to cardiovascular complications. Those with isolated systolic hypertension are at increased risk of cardiovascular morbidity and mortality, although the diastolic blood pressure may be completely normal. The problem of isolated systolic hypertension will be discussed subsequently. Prevalence estimates of either combined hypertension or isolated systolic hypertension obviously depend on the number of blood pressure measurements taken, the level of blood pressures used for definition, and the population studied [4–6]. Consequently, prevalence rates decrease as the number of patients and the number of times the blood pressure measurements are taken increases. As shown in Tables 10.2 and 10.3, prevalence estimates of hypertension are significant in the elderly but also can vary substantially. More elderly blacks and women are hypertensive than are whites and men.

Table 10.3 Prevalence of hypertension among noninstitutionalized men and women (black and white, aged 65–74 years, 1976–1980)*. (From The Working Group on Hypertension in the Elderly [3])

	Blood pressure over 160/95 mmHg (%)	Blood pressure over 140/90 mmHg (%)
Black women	72.8	82.9
Black men	42.9	67.1
White women	48.3	66.2
White men	37.5	59.2
Total blacks	59.9	76.1
Total whites	43.7	63.1
Total all races	45.1	64.3

* Defined as the average of three blood pressure measurements taken on a single occasion or those who reported taking antihypertensive medication.

Risks of hypertension in the elderly

A number of epidemiologic studies have clearly demonstrated the increased risk of cardiovascular events as-

Table 10.2 Prevalence of hypertension in people more than 65 years old

Study (Reference)	Type of hypertension	Race	Cut-off value	Number of measurement	Prevalence estimate (%)
HANES	DH	W	DBP > 95 mmHg	One	>40
		B			>50
HDFP	DH	W	DBP > 90 mmHg	Two	>11
		B			>26
SHEP	SH	W	SBP > 160 mmHg	Two	>10

HANES, Health and Nutrition Examination Survey; HDFP, Hypertension Detection and Follow-up Program; SHEP, Systolic Hypertension in the Elderly Program (pilot); DH, diastolic hypertension; SH, systolic hypertension; W, white; B, black; DBP, diastolic blood pressure; SBP, systolic blood pressure.

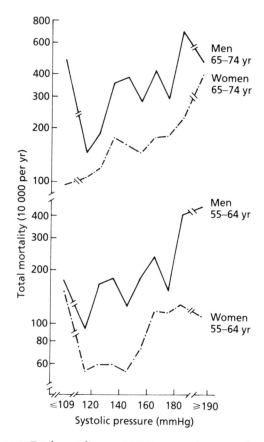

Fig. 10.1 Total mortality per 10 000 per year in men and women, aged 55–64 and 65–74 in the Framingham Study according to initial systolic pressure in mmHg. (From Kannel *et al.* [8].)

Table 10.4 Six-year mortality rates by blood pressure classification at screening of men aged 50–57 years

Age	All causes (per 1000)		Coronary artery disease (per 1000)	
	ISH	Diastolic hypertension	ISH	Diastolic hypertension
50–54	62.3	38.0	33.1	15.5
55–57	101.4	52.0	49.8	20.6

ISH, isolated systolic hypertension.

of isolated systolic hypertension in middle-aged men carried a greater risk of coronary artery disease than did the presence of purely diastolic hypertension [10] (Table 10.4). It has become evident that both systolic and diastolic blood pressures exert independent cardiovascular risks and thus neither isolated systolic hypertension nor diastolic hypertension can be ignored. Although with advancing age systolic blood pressure level increases (Fig. 10.2), both systolic and diastolic blood pressures are strong risk factors for future development of cerebrovascular events [11,12]. Taken together, epidemiologic observations implicate the level of systolic blood pressure as the single greatest risk factor for increased cardiovascular disease in the elderly. It should

sociated with untreated hypertension in the elderly, including those with isolated or predominantly systolic hypertension. These data have confirmed that not only the diastolic blood pressure but also the level of systolic blood pressure is an important determinant in the development of hypertension-related cardiovascular complications. Observations obtained from the Society of Actuaries and the Framingham Study clearly suggest that for people older than 65 years in age, systolic pressure elevations are more predictive of cardiovascular morbidity and mortality than are the elevations of diastolic blood pressure [7–9] (Fig. 10.1). These observations were also subsequently confirmed in the Multiple Risk Factor Intervention Trial which demonstrated that the presence

Fig. 10.2 Average age trends in systolic blood pressure for cross-sectional and longitudinal (cohort) data in the Framingham Study. (From Kannel *et al.* [9].)

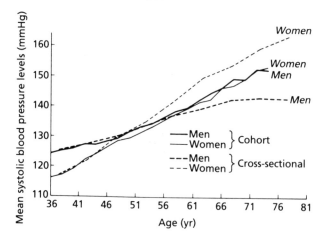

also be emphasized that the level of blood pressure clearly interacts with other concomitant known cardiovascular risk factors such as hyperlipidemia and cigarette smoking.

In addition, left ventricular hypertrophy is more prevalent in the elderly and correlates with increased systolic blood pressure. Left ventricular hypertrophy is associated with a number of cardiovascular complications. The presence of multiple risk factors in the elderly, therefore, substantially increase the risks of cardiovascular mortality. The occurrence of other risk factors makes the treatment of hypertension especially important. Since there is no controversy about the risk of systolic hypertension, at least two questions should be considered.

1 What is the ideal means of achieving control of systolic hypertension?

2 Will the control of elevated systolic blood pressure in the elderly result in reduced morbidity and mortality?

The presumption that medical treatment of isolated systolic hypertension may reduce cardiovascular morbidity and mortality in the elderly is currently being tested in at least three major clinical trials — the Systolic Hypertension in the Elderly Program (SHEP) being conducted in the United States, the trial conducted by the Medical Research Council in the United Kingdom, and the so-called Syst-Eur Trial being conducted in Europe [13]. The aim of these randomized trials is to determine whether antihypertensive drug therapy is associated with a reduction in cardiovascular complications. The preliminary results of the pilot SHEP study demonstrate that a significant difference in systolic pressure can be achieved when elderly hypertensives receive antihypertensive drug therapy. Initial analysis of the SHEP results indicate that morbidity and mortality can be significantly reduced as a result of therapy [14]. In a statewide survey of current clinical practices of family physicians and general internists, it was noted that a majority of physicians used drug therapy for patients with isolated systolic hypertension [15].

The risk of hypertension in the elderly has been the subject of a number of epidemiologic studies. There is a growing consensus that elevated arterial blood pressure in the elderly poses a major risk factor for the development of cardiovascular disease in this age group. Whereas the value of treating diastolic hypertension has been previously established [16], the ultimate benefit of treating systolic hypertension remains to be determined.

Pathophysiologic considerations

Systemic hypertension, by definition, is a hemodynamic disorder. The hemodynamic changes in elderly patients with hypertension are not uniform. From a physiologic angle, to some extent, hypertension-related and age-related cardiovascular changes appear to be similar. In both instances, there is an increase in left ventricular mass, a decrease in left ventricular diastolic filling, and a decrease in arterial compliance [17–20]. It may not always be possible to clearly distinguish the age-related cardiovascular changes from those observed in hypertension. The presence of arterial hypertension signifies an augmented risk in the elderly population. The pathophysiologic hallmark of established hypertension, in general, is increased systemic vascular resistance. In a longitudinal study conducted by Lund-Johansen [21], systemic hemodynamics were measured in a group of men with untreated essential hypertension. These subjects were followed for 17 years, and hemodynamic measurements were obtained during the period of observation. In this important longitudinal study, there was a progressive fall in cardiac output mainly due to a reduction in the stroke volume and a gradual increase in peripheral vascular resistance. This study provided an important landmark in the clinical hemodynamic status of patients with untreated hypertension. When the hemodynamic changes were compared between elderly hypertensive subjects and normotensive patients, it was evident that in the former, peripheral resistance was markedly increased, whereas the cardiac output, the stroke volume, and the blood volume declined [22].

In a carefully conducted study, Messerli et al. [23] studied hemodynamic characteristics of younger and older patients with hypertension. These authors noted that the heart rate, stroke volume, and cardiac output were significantly lower, and total peripheral vascular resistance significantly higher in the elderly than in younger subjects (Table 10.5). In the same study, elderly patients, even with mild hypertension, had remarkable left ventricular hypertrophy. In another study involving elderly patients with isolated systemic hypertension, Vardan et al. [24] noted that although the cardiac output and stroke volume in this population varied widely, peripheral vascular resistance was uniformly elevated. Although in these and other studies the number of patients was small, the hemodynamic changes point to

Table 10.5 Pathophysiologic differences in hypertensive patients (mean ± SD). (From Messerli *et al.* [23])

	Elderly	Young	*P* values
Age (yr)	73 ± 7	32 ± 7	By design
Systolic pressure (mmHg)	182 ± 32	153 ± 23	$<10^{-5}$
Mean arterial pressure (mmHg)	114 ± 17	113 ± 16	By design
Diastolic pressure (mmHg)	81 ± 11	93 ± 14	$<10^{-5}$
Cardiac output (l/min)	4.70 ± 1.04	6.22 ± 1.20	$<10^{-5}$
Total peripheral resistance (units)	26 ± 7	19 ± 4	$<10^{-5}$
Stroke volume (ml)	71 ± 18	88 ± 23	<0.001
Heart rate (beats per min)	67 ± 10	72 ± 8	<0.02
Total blood volume (l)	4.10 ± 0.8	4.64 ± 1.0	<0.05
Renal blood flow (ml/min)	674 ± 92	1110 ± 296	<0.001
Renal vascular resistance (units)	1691 ± 153	1012 ± 33	$<10^{-5}$
Norepinephrine (pg/ml)	418 ± 209	331 ± 182	NS
Epinephrine (pg/ml)	95 ± 89	98 ± 76	NS
Dopamine (pg/ml)	63 ± 78	62 ± 63	NS
Plasma renin activity (μg/ml per min)	0.454 ± 0.38	1.154 ± 0.87	<0.05

NS, not significant.

the importance of elevated peripheral vascular resistance as the determinant of hypertension in this age group. This pathophysiologic correlate obviously has important implications with regards to the choice of therapy. As the arterial pressure and the total peripheral vascular resistance rise in elderly patients with hypertension, there is a progressive contraction of plasma volume [25]. Although there is contraction of intravascular volume, the renin−angiotensin system responsiveness is impaired, which results in a distorted relationship between these counter-regulatory mechanisms. Whereas the elderly patients with hypertension might respond fairly well to administration of a diuretic, it should be remembered that any unwanted degree of further loss of body sodium and water might cause serious problems in some individuals.

As discussed elsewhere in this textbook, renal function progressively declines with aging (Fig. 10.3) [26]. Like cardiac output, the renal blood flow (RBF) also decreases with age [27,28]. Generally, the RBF decreases by approximately 10% per decade of life after adulthood. It appears that the diminution in RBF is more evident in the cortical area sparing the medulla, which might explain the increase in renal filtration fraction (FF) which occurs with advancing age. The most significant impairment of renal function with advancing age is a progressive

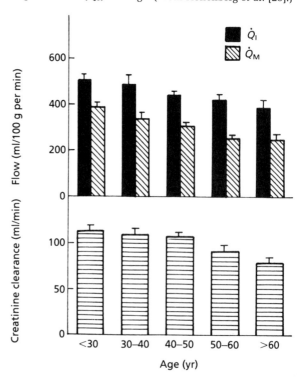

Fig. 10.3 Change in mean renal blood flow (Q_m) and rapid-component flow (Q_1) with age. (From Hollenberg *et al.* [26].)

decrease in the glomerular filtration rate (GFR) after the age of 40 years [29]. It is possible that these data might not be entirely accurate because the measurement of GFR is based on endogenous creatinine clearance, a factor that also decreases with the aging process.

In the elderly patients, not only the basal plasma renin levels are low but the responsiveness of renin to stimulatory maneuvers is also blunted [30–32]. Thus, the majority of the elderly hypertensives have either low or normal plasma renin activity. The percentage of elderly hypertensives with elevated plasma renin levels is probably low. These considerations might dictate the therapeutic options in the long-term management of hypertension in the elderly. Elderly people are also less able to excrete sodium, and the ability of the kidney to mount the release of antidiuretic hormone declines with age.

Why should we treat hypertension in the elderly?

Not long ago, most clinicians were reluctant to treat hypertension in the elderly on the presumption that elevated blood pressure in this group was a normal phenomenon associated with aging due to progressive atherosclerosis and loss of elasticity in blood vessels. Antihypertensive therapy was even thought to cause problems rather than provide therapeutic benefit. There is emerging consensus to suggest that active therapy should be considered for elderly patients with documented hypertension. The treatment initially could include nonpharmacologic means, and based upon clinical evaluation, drug therapy might be necessary. As a result of this revised therapeutic philosophy, most elderly hypertensives in the United States at present are receiving drug therapy [33].

The basis for this therapeutic change comes from several studies that have shown that treatment reduces cardiovascular morbidity and mortality in elderly patients with diastolic hypertension. The Veterans Administration Cooperative Study, Australian National Blood Pressure Study, Hypertension Detection and Follow-up Program, and the European Working Group on Hypertension in the Elderly studies have demonstrated the possible benefit of treating diastolic hypertension in the elderly [16,34–37] (Fig. 10.4). The European Working Party on Hypertension in the Elderly is particularly

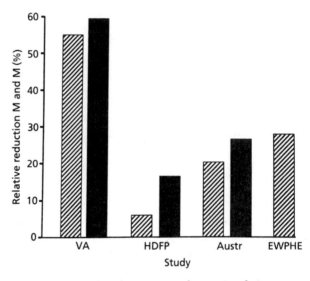

Fig. 10.4 Impact of antihypertensive therapy in relative reduction (intervention compared with control) of cardiovascular morbidity (VA), mortality (HDFP), and combined cardiovascular morbidity and mortality (M and M), (Austr and EWPHE) for participants younger than age 50 (cross-hatched bars) compared with older than age 60 (solid bars). VA, Veterans Administration Cooperative study; HDFP, Hypertension Detection and Follow-up Program; Austr, Australian Trial on Mild Hypertension; EWPHE, European Working Party on Hypertension in the Elderly. Cardiovascular morbidity in each study represents total nonfatal cardiovascular and cerebrovascular events reported. (From Applegate [37].)

relevant since it examines the benefit of antihypertensive therapy in patients over age 60 years with moderate hypertension. In this study, fewer cardiovascular deaths were reported in the treated group compared to those on placebo up until age 80. So far, the European Working Party on Hypertension in the elderly is the only placebo-controlled study that has shown decreased coronary mortality with antihypertensive therapy in the elderly hypertensive patients (Fig. 10.5). In this study, a total of 840 patients were randomized to receive either active drug treatment or placebo after a run-in period of 1 month. Patients with active drug were treated with one or two capsules of a combination of 25 mg of hydrochlorothiazide and 50 mg triamterene, and if the blood pressure was not controlled, e.g., systolic <160, diastolic <90 mmHg after 4 weeks, they were given α-methyldopa beginning with 250 mg titrated up to 2000 mg daily. Approximately 70% of the patients were female and the

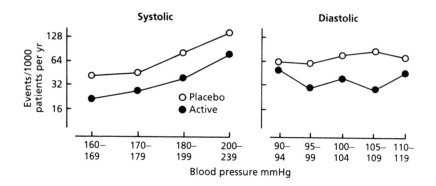

Fig. 10.5 Data from the European Working Party on Hypertension in the Elderly. Cardiovascular study terminating events in systolic blood pressure groups (obtained at randomization) show a steady increase both in placebo-treated and actively treated subjects. This trend is absent in diastolic blood pressure groups, indicating that systolic pressure overrides diastolic pressure as a risk factor in (these) patients aged 60 years and over. (From Amery *et al.* [16].)

mean age of the study population was 72 years. Whereas the overall mortality was not reduced as a result of antihypertensive therapy, the cardiovascular mortality was significantly lower in patients who received therapy. Careful avoidance of hyperkalemia may have been a factor in the ultimate benefit accrued in the study, but no firm evidence was presented.

So far, no interventional trial has been completed concerning the effects of treating isolated systolic hypertension. The Systolic Hypertension in the Elderly Program, examined the effect of drug therapy vs. placebo in over 8000 elderly patients with isolated systolic hypertension; the pilot study, however, has shown the efficacy of fairly lower doses of antihypertensive therapy in treating systolic hypertension with an excess of 80% of patients achieving a therapeutic goal. At least one clear-cut conclusion has already become available from this study — it should be possible to reduce the systolic blood pressure with relatively modest therapy in most patients. As discussed above, data indicate that systolic blood pressure tends to override diastolic blood pressure in exerting cardiovascular risk in the elderly. Since the aging process itself may predispose the patient to atherosclerotic disease, it is tempting to associate the increased risk with arterial rigidity rather than with systolic pressure *per se.* This view is not supported by the Framingham data which showed the deleterious consequences of systolic pressure are not directly connected with arterial rigidity, as estimated from pulse wave configuration. Completion of ongoing therapeutic trials concerning systolic hypertension will no doubt culminate in providing new guidelines for treating hypertension in relation to the level of blood pressure.

Clinical evaluation of elderly patients with hypertension

Although the general approach to the management of hypertension in the elderly is grossly similar to the guidelines described for other age groups, special attention should be paid to certain key points in the aging patient. Obviously, a thorough clinical examination should be performed to document the extent of target organ damage and to identify concomitant risk factors. It is also important to determine the patient's standing blood pressure as well, because of the greater incidence of postural hypertension in the elderly [38,39] which sometimes might be aggravated by therapy. Some elderly patients might also have reduced baroreceptor function which may influence the therapeutic approach. The counterregulatory sympathetic responses to hypotension may be attenuated which may result in serious consequences.

Elderly hypertensive patients, in contrast to normotensives, demonstrate an increased prevalence of severe internal carotid artery disease [40]. Whether such patients are predisposed to develop cerebral ischemia as a result of lowering the arterial blood pressure is speculated. Nevertheless, the problem of carotid artery occlusion in elderly patients should be taken into consideration in the management of hypertension.

Another clinical consideration of considerable importance is the phenomenon of spontaneous postprandial production in blood pressure that occurs in elderly people [41] (Fig. 10.6). It has been recognized that blood pressure homeostasis in elderly patients changes after the consumption of a meal. This so-called spontaneous postprandial hypotension may be responsible for the high

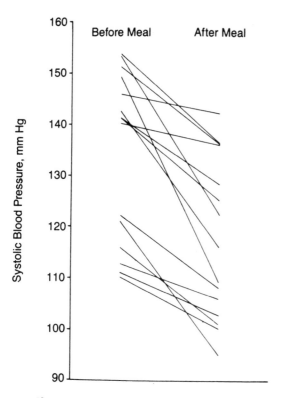

Fig. 10.6 Changes in systolic blood pressure from before to after meal ingestion for elderly subjects (omitted is one subject whose values went from 159 mmHg). Values are means of three before- and three after-ingestion measurements, as described in text. (From Peitzman & Berger [41].)

frequency of syncopal episodes that occur in some elderly patients. Due to baroreceptor dysfunction, the postprandial fall in blood pressure may not be compensated by an increase in the reflex heart rate. This problem can be alleviated to some extent by advising the patient to ingest smaller quantities of food at more frequent intervals. Whether drug therapy influences the degree and duration of postprandial hypotension has not been carefully studied. The estimation of arterial blood pressure by indirect means might be erroneous in some elderly patients with rigid, calcified arteries that do not collapse under the balloon cuff. Pseudohypotension should be suspected in someone with significant increases in arterial blood pressure levels and when there is no clinical evidence of target organ damage. One can also perform Osler's maneuver to document pseudohypotension. This maneuver is considered to be positive when the radial pulse remains palpable after the cuff is inflated well above the systolic level. The presence of left ventricular hypertrophy in elderly patients with hypertension certainly dictates aggressive therapeutic approach.

Generally, extensive work-up is not necessary to uncover secondary causes of hypertension in the elderly unless there are obvious clinical or laboratory signs. Sudden onset or worsening of hypertension after age 60 might signify renal arterial disease from atherosclerotic stenosis. If the patient's general health is stable, work-up to uncover renal vascular disease should be undertaken in selected individuals. Since some patients might have renal artery stenosis which may be amenable to angioplasty or aortorenal bypass, renovascular hypertension should be considered as a potential secondary cause based upon the clinical criteria.

Management

As in other age groups, the initial step in the therapy of hypertension in the elderly could be by nonpharmacologic means. These include maintenance of ideal body weight, moderate restriction of sodium to 2 g daily, reduction of alcohol intake, and regular aerobic isotonic exercise. Elderly patients appear to be sensitive to dietary sodium restriction or to the use of low doses of diuretic [42]. Since alcohol abuse is not uncommon in the elderly [43], a recommendation should be made to limit daily consumption of alcohol to no more than 30 ml or 1 ounce — preferably equal to two usual portions of beer, wine, or spirits. It is possible that with careful application of nonpharmacologic therapy the blood pressure might improve in many patients, and even in those who may not reach therapeutic goal, such as approach might compliment the effects of drug therapy.

Guidelines for drug therapy and management

If nondrug therapies do not reduce the blood pressure or if immediate treatment of hypertension is warranted, the following guidelines should be applied for drug therapy of elderly patients with hypertension.
1 Multiple (at least three) blood pressure readings should be obtained on different days before labelling the patient as having hypertension. At times the blood pressure in

the elderly can be labile and often decreases with repeated measurements. Ideally, the patient should have rested for at least 10 min prior to the blood pressure measurement being taken.

2 The blood pressure cuff should be inflated to 250 mm or higher to avoid the ausculatory gap. Initial and follow-up blood pressure readings should be obtained in the supine (or sitting) and standing positions at each visit to detect and prevent an unwanted degree of orthostatic hypotension. In most instances, monotherapy should be begun with small doses and the increments be made only after careful assessment of response to therapy.

3 The choice of therapy should be based on the clinical evaluation of the patient with particular reference to the hemodynamic and volume status of the patient.

4 Drugs which can be given once or twice daily should be chosen to sustain patients' compliance with the treatment program.

5 Excessive reduction in blood pressure should be avoided. For those patients who have isolated systolic hypertension, an attempt should be made to lower the blood pressure to systolic 160 mmHg if the patient can tolerate the treatment.

Since elderly patients represent a special category, pharmacologic treatment of hypertension can be especially challenging because of several age-related factors which influence drug metabolism and drug effects (Table 10.6). For example, absorption of medications and volume of distribution may change with increasing age. Altered drug metabolism may predispose the patients to develop adverse effects. Many elderly patients are also likely to be taking several drugs concurrently and drug interactions might occur causing considerable confusion in the management. With advancing age, lean body muscle mass decreases and fat as a percentage increases. These factors tend to reduce the total volume of fluid in which drug is distributed, consequently, causing an increase in drug concentration. Another issue concerning the drug distribution in the elderly is related to the level of circulating proteins, especially albumin which is significantly lower in the elderly than in younger people. This may result in greater concentration of non-bound drug which may cause therapeutic or adverse effects in the elderly. The status of liver function might also change the drug metabolism. Even though a patient may not have underlying liver disease, the actions of one medication on hepatic function may alter the metabolism

Table 10.6 Processes which might be expected to alter in the elderly and have resulting influences on pharmacokinetics. The well-known effects are described in the text but some have yet to be studied

Absorption	Gastric pH
	Gastric emptying
	Intestinal motility
	Intestinal surface area
	Intestinal blood flow
Distribution	Protein binding
	Regional blood flow
	Cardiac output
	Tissue and organ uptake and binding
Metabolism	Hepatic blood flow
	Extraction of drugs by the liver
	Amounts and activity of drug-metabolizing enzymes
	Transport of drugs and metabolites from the liver
Elimination	Renal blood flow
	Active tubular secretion
	Tubular reabsorption

of others, thereby increasing the propensity to develop adverse drug interactions. The kidneys are the main route of elimination of many cardiovascular drugs. In the elderly patients, as we discussed earlier, the renal function decreases. Since the GFR declines with age, the drug excretion might be delayed. All of these factors should be considered in prescribing cardiovascular drugs to the elderly. By providing optimal therapy with the understanding of pharmacokinetic actions of the drug, therapeutic objectives can be achieved with minimal discomfort to the patient.

In the past, considerable emphasis was placed on the age-dependency as a factor in the therapeutic effectiveness of certain antihypertensive drugs. However, a careful analysis of the published literature indicates that age *per se* may have only a small role in determining the therapeutic response to most antihypertensive drugs [44]. When larger numbers of patients are studied, both the old and the young demonstrate equal responses to antihypertensive drug therapy. Blacks, however, respond less favorably to β-blockers and angiotensin-converting enzyme inhibitors, but coadministration of a diuretic will often augment the efficacy of these drugs. There is no single universally acceptable drug which is effective in the treatment of hypertension in the elderly. The choice of therapy should be based upon the clinical and laboratory evaluation and after consideration of patients' concomitant medications and medical conditions.

Diuretics

Diuretics were previously widely recommended as first choice in treating elderly hypertensives. However, this recommendation is subject to considerable reassessment and revision because there is no conclusive evidence that diuretics are more effective in the elderly than in other population groups. Furthermore, the plasma volume in the elderly might already be low and indiscriminate use of diuretics might further worsen the hemodynamic status of the patient. Nevertheless, some clinical trials have confirmed the antihypertensive efficacy of diuretics in elderly patients with hypertension. The Systolic Hypertension in the Elderly Program and the European Working Party on Hypertension in the Elderly studies have noted that elderly patients tolerate diuretic therapy without experiencing significant adverse reactions. The major advantages of diuretics in the elderly are their usefulness in the presence of congestive heart failure and other edematous conditions, their low cost, and their ability to potentiate the antihypertensive actions of other drugs. However, these advantages should be balanced by potentially serious side-effects such as hypokalemia, hyponatremia, and azotemia. It would be advisable to use the lowest dose, for example, starting with 12.5 mg hydrochlorothiazide or its equivalent. Little therapeutic benefit, if any, is seen beyond 25–50 mg of hydrochlorothiazide [45]. Since GFR decreases with age, thiazide diuretics may have a decreased natriuretic effect, especially in the presence of renal insufficiency. Loop diuretics are generally more effective in inducing natriuresis when renal function is compromised.

Beta-adrenergic blocking agents

Because of their antihypertensive and antianginal effects, β-blockers enjoyed widespread application in the management of cardiovascular diseases. Initial studies in the elderly hypertensive patients suggested that β-blockers as a group are less effective in reducing the blood pressure [46,47]. Although the evidence is not entirely clear that β-blocking drugs lower the blood pressure solely by renin suppression, there is evidence that patients with normal or high renin levels respond much better than those with low levels. The activity of the renin–angiotensin system tends to decline with age, therefore, the response to β-adrenoreceptor blockade may be blunted. Many studies, however, have found significant falls of blood pressure in elderly subjects when β-adrenergic blocking drugs are administered. The Veterans Administration Cooperative Study and the International Multicenter Study of Metoprolol Vs. Hydrochlorothiazide have clearly shown the antihypertensive efficacy of β-blockers in elderly patients [48,49]. In a large study [50], 884 hypertensive patients older than 60 years of age were randomized to receive either atenolol, with or without a diuretic, or no treatment. Over a 10-year period of observation, atenolol, with or without a diuretic, reduced blood pressure significantly compared to the control group and was well-tolerated. Furthermore, the incidence of all strokes was significantly reduced by 58% of that in the control group. And there was no evidence that β-blockers aggravated or precipitated congestive heart failure in the treated group. The occurrence of myocardial infarction was not reduced by treatment, in general, although there were fewer cardiovascular events in the treated patients. Beta-blockers might have a therapeutic role in those patients who may have concomitant coronary artery disease [51]. The known potential adverse effects of β-blocking drugs should be carefully considered in choosing this class of drugs in the elderly. These include atrial ventricular conduction delay, negative inotropic and chronotropic effects, increased peripheral vascular resistance, and unfavorable alteration of the lipid profile. The elderly are also at higher risk for the known side-effects of β-blockers on the central nervous system. These agents may exacerbate depression in the elderly. In addition to depression, β-blockers might cause a number of other neurophysiologic side-effects [52]. Beta-blockers might also precipitate and/or worsen the symptoms of claudication in patients with peripheral vascular disease. Given the large spectrum of potential adverse side-effects, β-blocker use in the elderly should be monitored.

Alpha-adrenergic blockers

Alpha-adrenergic receptor antagonists have proven to be useful in the treatment of hypertension. The present generation of α-adrenergic blocking drugs selectively block the postsynaptic or α-adrenergic receptor which causes a reduction in the peripheral vascular resistance. At present, there are three α-adrenergic blocking drugs available for the treatment of hypertension—prazosin, terazosin, and doxazosin. This class of drugs produces desirable hemodynamic consequences in elderly hypertensive patients including a decrease in the peripheral vascular resistance without invoking reflex tachycardia. Additionally, the postsynaptic α-adrenergic blocking drugs have a favorable effect on lipid profile and are generally devoid of central side-effects. Few systematic studies of α-adrenergic blocking drugs in elderly hypertensive patients have been performed. From a pure hemodynamic point of view, α-adrenergic blockers would seem useful also in elderly hypertensive patients. As a rule, peripheral vascular resistance is elevated in elderly hypertensive patients, whereas, the absence of reflex tachycardia upon exposure to α-adrenergic blocking drugs is a suitable attribute of this class of compounds. It appears that α-adrenergic blocking drugs are at least as effective in the elderly as in the younger hypertensive adults. Further clinical experience is necessary to delineate the precise role of α-adrenergic blocking drugs in the long-term treatment of hypertension in the elderly. By the virtue of their mechanism of action, these drugs might cause some degree of postural hypotension if high doses are used initially or if rapid dosage increments are made. This problem can be easily avoided by initiating the treatment with a small dose, by titrating the dosage carefully, and by monitoring the patient's standing blood pressure. A major advantage of α-adrenergic blocking drugs which may be particularly relevant to the elderly is that they do not impair the cerebral blood flow [53], and they also cause significant regression of left ventricular hypertrophy [54].

Centrally acting agents

Central-acting α-agonists such as α-methyldopa, clonidine, quanabenz, and guanfacine, decrease the sympathetic outflow from the brain and thereby cause a reduction in systemic blood pressure. Although these drugs may be effective in the treatment of hypertension in the elderly, their clinical use has declined because of their propensity to cause central nervous system side-effects such as sedation and dry mouth. The availability of effective and safe alternate agents with a better clinical profile has caused the usage of centrally acting drugs to decline over the last few years.

Direct arterial vasodilators

Direct arterial dilators such as hydralazine and minoxidil are potent antihypertensive agents. Minoxidil is much more powerful than hydralazine in causing peripheral vasodilation and is, therefore, reserved for the treatment of refractory hypertension with or without renal impairment. These drugs are not useful as monotherapy because of their hemodynamic consequences, namely, reflex tachycardia, and fluid retention, which would require concomitant administration of an α-adrenergic drug and a diuretic, respectively. The role for direct vasodilators in the management of uncomplicated hypertension is rather limited. However, in selected patients, they exert profound antihypertensive effects when used in combination with a β-blocking drug and a diuretic.

Angiotensin-converting enzyme inhibitors

Because of their unique mechanism of action, angiotensin-converting enzyme (ACE) inhibitors have been gaining increasing use in the treatment of hypertension. At the present time, there are three ACE inhibitors available for clinical use in hypertension—captopril, enalapril, and lisinopril—which differ mainly in the duration of their action, and only lisinopril has a duration of action that permits once a day administration. Because plasma renin activity tends to fall with increasing age, it has been speculated that ACE inhibitors may not be effective in lowering the blood pressure of elderly hypertensive patients. However, it is also known that pretreatment plasma renin activity is not a reliable predictor of long-term therapeutic benefit of ACE inhibitors. Angiotensin-converting enzyme inhibitors may have some attractive effects on cardiac function in the elderly since these agents have been shown to be remarkably effective in the treatment of congestive heart failure, and they also cause reversal of left ventricular hypertrophy. Contrary to earlier claims about the ineffectiveness of ACE inhibitors in the treatment of hypertension in the elderly, many reports have confirmed their usefulness in this population [55–57]. Angiotensin-converting enzyme inhibitors provide a number of advantages which include lack of central nervous system side-effects, orthostasis, and peripheral vascular symptoms. Angiotensin-converting enzyme inhibitors cause reversal of left ventricular hypertrophy, and they are also useful in the treatment of hypertension complicated by congestive heart failure. When prescribing ACE inhibitors in the elderly, certain potential adverse effects should be considered and an effort made to avoid them by proper selection of patients. Since side-effects of ACE inhibitors can be dose-related, the dosage for the elderly must be selected cautiously. Angiotensin-converting enzyme inhibitors might worsen renal function in patients with significant renal artery stenosis (especially bilateral), congestive heart failure, and hyponatremia. Atherosclerotic renal artery stenosis is not unusual in elderly patients and clearly represents an enhanced risk of provoking renal failure when elderly patients are given ACE inhibitors. Therefore, it is a good clinical practice to monitor the renal function (serum creatinine) within 7–10 days after initiating ACE inhibitor therapy in elderly patients. These agents can also sometimes cause hyperkalemia. Nonproductive cough is being increasingly recognized as a common problem with ACE inhibitor therapy. The administration of a diuretic enhances the efficacy of ACE inhibitor therapy.

Calcium antagonists

Calcium antagonists, which were originally introduced as antianginal drugs, are rapidly becoming popular in the management of hypertension. From a theoretical point of view, these drugs are of great importance because of their beneficial hemodynamic, anti-ischemic, and antiatherogenic actions. A number of clinical studies have attested to the antihypertensive efficacy of calcium antagonists in the treatment of geriatric hypertension [58–62]. Since many elderly patients might have concomitant cardiovascular disease, calcium antagonists provide distinct therapeutic advantages. Plasma half-life of calcium blocking drugs is prolonged in elderly patients and this property can be useful in the selection of proper dosage requirements in older patients. Calcium antagonists possess a pharmacodynamic spectrum that blocks many of the pathophysiologic abnormalities found in old age. Despite some earlier assertions, there is no convincing evidence that age is an independent predictor of hypotensive efficacy of calcium antagonists. In fact, calcium antagonists as antihypertensive agents are effective in all age groups [62]. Not only are calcium blocking drugs useful in the chronic treatment of mild to moderate uncomplicated hypertension, but as in other age groups, acute administration of nifedipine has been shown to promptly reduce severe hypertension in elderly patients [64]. There are currently four calcium antagonists which are available for the treatment of hypertension: diltiazem,

verapamil, nifedipine, and nicardipine. The dihydropyridine derivatives (nifedipine and nicardipine) are more potent than other calcium blocking drugs for the treatment of hypertension and they do not exert negative chronotropic and inotropic effects. They may cause reflex tachycardia, flushing, headache, and peripheral edema. The gastrointestinal therapeutic system formulation of nifedipine is associated with fewer vasodilatory adverse effects. Since verapamil and diltiazem may reduce cardiac contractility and arteriovenous nodal conduction, they should be used with great caution in combination with a β-blocker, especially in those patients whose cardiac function is already compromised. These agents may also cause constipation. As a pharmacologic class, calcium antagonists offer important advantages in the treatment of hypertension in the elderly and have few contraindications. Importantly, these drugs do not alter electrolytes or lipids and do not cause postural hypotension or central nervous system side-effects. In patients with co-existing coronary artery disease, calcium blocking drugs might be especially useful. There is also evidence to suggest that calcium blocking drugs might have anti-atherosclerotic and vasculoprotective effects [65]. A recent study [66] showed that left ventricular mass was reduced in elderly patients with hypertension to a greater extent with verapamil than with atenolol therapy (Fig. 10.7). The reversal of left ventricular hypertrophy caused by verapamil was associated with improved cardiac function. In general, all calcium antagonists tend to cause regression of left ventricular hypertrophy in hypertension.

Complicated and severe hypertension

If an elderly patient has refractory hypertension, unresponsive to the administration of two or three antihypertensive drugs, such a patient should be carefully evaluated to identify the possible causes for resistance to therapy. Refractory hypertension is not unusual in patients with significant target organ damage and dysfunction—such as, congestive heart failure and renal impairment. If these complications are present, treatment should be tailored appropriately to reverse the target organ damage, if possible. In patients with congestive heart failure and/or renal insufficiency, administration of a potent dose of a diuretic is often necessary to obtain optimal response to other antihypertensive drugs. When

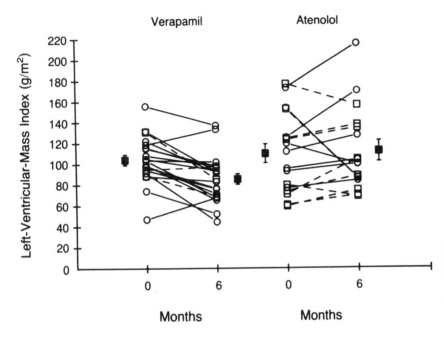

Fig. 10.7 Individual and mean changes in the left ventricular mass index from base line to the 6-month follow-up, as determined by two-dimensional echocardiography. (From Schulman *et al.* [66].)

the traditional use of antihypertensive drugs does not achieve blood pressure reduction, consideration should be given to the use of more potent drugs such as minoxidil in selective patients. Based upon the clinical course of the patient, work-up to exclude renal artery stenosis should be undertaken in elderly patients with severe, new onset, or refractory hypertension.

"Hypertensive emergencies" are relatively uncommon in the elderly population. However, it is important to recognize that critical elevations in blood pressure levels might cause serious damage to vital organs and, therefore, prompt treatment is necessary to prevent the serious consequences that may otherwise occur [67]. Any form of hypertension, if not properly treated, may cause a crisis, the main determinant being the blood pressure itself rather than the etiology of hypertension. In some clinical circumstances the abruptness of the increase in blood pressure is more important than its absolute level. The examples of conditions that constitute so-called hypertensive emergencies are shown in Table 10.7. Diagnosis of hypertensive crisis is made after careful evaluation of the patient to determine the status of target organ function. Upon the conclusion of clinical evaluation, appropriate treatment should be instituted promptly and the choice for drug therapy should be strictly individualized based

upon the condition at hand and the hemodynamic status of the patient. Antihypertensive drugs which are useful in the immediate management of hypertensive crisis are listed in Tables 10.8 and 10.9.

Table 10.7 Examples of hypertensive emergencies and urgencies

Hypertensive emergencies	Hypertensive urgencies
Hypertensive encephalopathy	Hypertension associated with coronary artery disease
Acute aortic dissection	Accelerated and malignant hypertension*
Pulmonary edema	Severe hypertension in kidney transplant patients
Pheochromocytoma crisis	Postoperative hypertension
Monoamine oxidase inhibitor + tyramine interaction	Uncontrolled hypertension in patients who require emergency surgery
Intracranial hemorrhage	

* Can be classified as either hypertensive emergency or hypertensive urgency.

Table 10.8 Acute oral therapy for the management of severe hypertension

Drug	Route and dose	Onset	Duration	Comments
Nifedipine	10–20 mg p.o. or sublingual	5–15 min	3–5 hours	Generally good response. Short duration of action, optimal dosage not standardized
Clonidine	0.2 mg p.o. initial then 0.1 mg/hour, up to 0.8 mg total	½–2 hours	6–8 hours	Prominent sedation
Captopril	6.5–25 mg p.o.	15 min	4–6 hours	Generally good, sometimes excessive response
Minoxidil	5–10 mg p.o.	30–60 min	12–16 hours	Tachycardia, fluid retention

Table 10.9 Parenteral drugs for hypertensive emergencies

Drug	Route and dose	Onset	Offset	Comments
Nicardipine	5–15 mg/hour i.v.	5–15 min	Continuous during infusion	May cause reflex tachycardia. Has a number of advantages over drugs because of its mechanism of action
Nitroprusside	i.v. infusion per 0.25 µg/kg per min to 8 µg/kg per min	s	Continuous duration infusion	Thiocyanate toxicity may occur with prolonged (>48 hours) or high dose infusion (>15 µg/kg per min) (particularly in renal insufficiency)
Labetalol	i.v. 20 mg q 10 min (can go to 80 mg doses); max cumulative dose 300 mg	5 min or less	3–6 hours	Prompt response. Can be followed with same drug taken orally
Hydralazine	10–20 mg i.m./i.v.	10–30 min	2–4 hours	May precipitate angina, myocardial infarction

Conclusion

The percentage of elderly patients in western societies is steadily increasing because of improved general health. However, cardiovascular diseases, especially those associated with hypertension, are responsible for significant morbidity and mortality in the elderly. The hypertension-related complications are especially prominent in the elderly because they might aggravate the pathophysiologic processes that are associated with the aging process. The biophysiology of the aging process is a complex phenomenon. Age-related physiologic changes *per se* may contribute to morbidity and mortality in elderly patients. The presence of hypertension might accentuate the age-related vascular disease.

In elderly patients, one can witness a wide spectrum of hypertensive diseases including mild to moderate hypertension, isolated systolic hypertension, refractory hypertension, and hypertensive emergencies. There is clear-cut evidence that diastolic hypertension in the elderly should be lowered. The issue of treating isolated systolic hypertension has been a subject of considerable debate during the last few years. There is growing consensus to suggest that, not only is systolic hypertension a powerful risk factor for cardiovascular disease, but its treatment might provide important benefits to the patient. More precise guidelines for the long-term treatment of isolated systolic hypertension are likely to be available from the Systolic Hypertension in the Elderly Program (SHEP) and other studies.

Recently concluded clinical trials have affirmed the benefits of treating both the diastolic as well as isolated systolic hypertension in the elderly. In SHEP, low dose antihypertensive drug therapy reduced the incidence of stroke by 36% [68]. In the Swedish Trial in Old Patients (STOP), antihypertensive therapy conferred highly significant reductions in cardiovascular morbidity and mortality in patients aged 70–84 [69]. More recently, the Medical Research Council (MRC) trial in elderly patients with hypertension concluded that effective therapy lowers the risk of stroke, coronary events, and all cardiovascular events [70]. These clinical trials clearly offer the proof of benefit that can be expected as a consequence of blood pressure reduction in the elderly with chronic hypertension.

Elderly hypertensives can be effectively treated with currently available antihypertensive drugs. While using cardiovascular drugs in the elderly, attention should be paid not only to the benefits but also to the potential adverse effects, which can be avoided in most instances. There is considerable enthusiasm for the utility of newer antihypertensive drugs such as calcium antagonists in the treatment of hypertension. Whether application of these newer agents protects against cardiovascular complications in the elderly remains to be seen by prospective experience. The absence of adverse hemodynamic and metabolic side-effects makes the use of newer antihypertensive drugs such as calcium antagonists and ACE inhibitors particularly attractive. With rational use of nondrug and drug therapies, elderly hypertensives can have their blood pressure reduced to safe levels. As in other age groups, the ultimate goal of treating elderly hypertensives is not only to lower elevated arterial blood pressure, but to prevent premature cardiovascular morbidity and mortality. Even a modest control of hypertension per decade of life may sharply decrease the number of elderly hypertensives and may possibly decrease the hypertension-associated morbidity and mortality in this important segment of our population.

References

1 Kannel WB, Gordon T. Evaluation of cardiovascular risk in the elderly: the Framingham Study. Bull NY Acad Med 1978;54:573–591.

2 Joint National Committee. The 1988 Report of the Joint National Committee on Detection, Evaluation, and Treatment of High Blood Pressure. Arch Intern Med 1988;148:1023–1038.

3 Working Group on Hypertension in the Elderly. Statement on hypertension in the elderly. J Am Med Assoc 1986;256:70–74.

4 Five-year findings of the Hypertension Detection Follow-up Program. Hypertension, Detection, Follow-up Cooperative Group. J Am Med Assoc 1979;242:2562–2577.

5 Vogt TM, Ireland CC, Black D, et al. Recruitment of elderly volunteers for multicenter clinical trial: the SHEP pilot study. Controlled Clin Trials 1986;7:118–133.

6 Drizd T, Dannenberg AL, Engel A. Blood Pressure Levels in Persons 18–74 Years of Age in 1976–1980, and Trends in Blood Pressure from 1960 to 1980 in the United States. Hyattsville, Maryland: United States Department of Health and Human Services, 1986:DHHS publication No. (PHS) 86–1684. (Vital Health Statistics Series, No. 11).

7 Build and Blood Pressure Study. Chicago: Society of Actuaries, 1959.

8 Kannel WB, Gordon T, Schwartz MJ. Systolic versus diastolic blood pressure and risk of coronary heart disease: The Framingham Study. Am J Cardiol 1971;27:335–346.

9 Kannel WB, Dawber TR, McGee DL. Perspective on systolic hypertension: The Framingham Study. Circulation 1980;71:1179–1182.

10 Rutan G, Kuller LH, Neaton JD, et al. Mortality associated with diastolic hypertension and isolated systolic hypertension among men screened for the Multiple Risk Factor Intervention Trial. Circulation 1988;77:504–514.

11 Shekelle RB, Ostfeld AM, Kiawans HL Jr. Hypertension and risk of stroke in an elderly population. Stroke 1974;5:71–75.

12 Kannel WB, Wolf PA, McGee DL, et al. Systolic blood pressure, arterial rigidity, and risks of stroke: The Framingham Study. J Am Med Assoc 1981;245:1225–1229.

13 Isolated systolic hypertension in the elderly (editorial review). J Hypertens 1990;8:393–405.

14 Perry HM Jr, Smith WM, McDonald RH, et al. Morbidity and mortality in the systolic hypertension in the elderly program (SHEP) pilot study. Stroke 1989;20:4–13.

15 Breckenridge MB, Kostis JB. Isolated systolic hypertension in the elderly: results of a statewide survey of clinical practice in New Jersey. Am J Med 1989;86:370–375.

16 Amery A, Birkenhager W, Brixko P, et al. Mortality and morbidity results from the European Working Party on High Blood Pressure in the Elderly trial. Lancet 1985;1:1349–1354.

17 Horan MJ, Steinberg GM, Dunbar JB, *et al.* Summary of NIH workshop on blood pressure regulation and aging. Hypertension 1986;8:178–180.

18 Gerstenblith G, Fleg JL, Becker LC, *et al.* Maximum left ventricular filling rate in healthy individuals measured by gated blood pool scans: effective age (abstr.). Circulation 1983;68(Suppl. III):110–111.

19 Gerstenblith G, Fredriksen J, Yin FCP, *et al.* Echocardiographic assessment of a normal adult aging population. Circulation 1977;56:273–278.

20 Lakette EG. Do hypertension and aging have a similar effect on the myocardium? Circulation 1987;75:169–177.

21 Lund-Johansen P. Heart pump function and total peripheral resistance in mild essential hypertension—a 17 year follow-up study. In Folkow B, Nordlander M, Straver B-E, *et al.* eds. *Hypertension: Pathophysiology and Clinical Implications of Early Structural Changes.* Sweden: Hassle, Molndal, 1985:392.

22 Terasawa F, Kuramoto K, Ying LH, *et al.* The study on the hemodynamics in old hypertensive subjects. Acta Gerontol Jpn 1972;56:47.

23 Messerli FH, Sundgaard-Riise K, Ventura HO, *et al.* Essential hypertension in the elderly: hemodynamics, intravascular volume, plasma renin activity, and circulating catecholamine levels. Lancet 1983;2:983–986.

24 Vardan S, Dunsky MH, Hill E, *et al.* Systemic systolic hypertension in the elderly: correlation of hemodynamics, plasma volume renin aldosterone, urinary metanephrines, and response to thiazide therapy. Am J Cardiol 1986;58:1030–1034.

25 Frohlich ED, Messerli FH. Systolic hypertension in the elderly. In Safar M, London G, Simon A, eds. *Arterial and Venous Systems in Essential Hypertension.* Paris: Martinus Nijhoff, 1987:105–114.

26 Hollenberg NK, Adams DF, Solomon HS, *et al.* Senescence and the renal vasculature in normal man. Circ Res 1974;34:309.

27 Goldring W, Chasis H, Ranges HA, *et al.* Relations of effective renal blood flow and glomerular filtration to tubular excretory mass in normal man. J Clin Invest 1940;19:739.

28 Davies DF, Shock NW. Age changes in glomerular filtration, effective renal plasma flow, and tubular excretory capacity in adult males. J Clin Invest 1950;29:496.

29 Rowe JW, Andres RA, Tobin FD, *et al.* The effect of age on creatinine clearance in man. A cross-sectional and longitudinal study. J Gerontol 1976;31:155.

30 Scott P, Giese J. Age and the renin–angiotensin system. Acta Med Scand 1983;676(Suppl.):45–51.

31 Luft FC, Grim CE, Fineberg N, *et al.* Effects of volume expansion and contraction in normotensive whites, blacks, and subjects of different ages. Circulation 1979;59:643–650.

32 Noth RH, Lassman MN, Tan SY, *et al.* Age and the renin–angiotensin system. Arch Intern Med 1977;137:1414–1417.

33 Havlik RJ, LaCroix AZ, Kleinman JC, *et al.* Antihypertensive drug therapy and survival by treatment status in a national survey. Hypertension 1989;13(Suppl. I):I28–I32.

34 Veterans Administration Cooperative Study Group on Antihypertensive Agents: effects of treatment on morbidity in hypertension. II. Results in patients with diastolic blood pressure averaging 90 through 114 mmHg. J Am Med Assoc 1970;213:1143–1152.

35 Management Committee. The Australian therapeutic trial in mild hypertension. Lancet 1980;1:1261–1267.

36 Hypertension Detection and Follow-up Program Cooperative Group: Five-year findings of the Hypertension Detection and Follow-up Program. J Am Med Assoc 1979;242:2562–2571.

37 Applegate WB. Hypertension in elderly patients. Ann Intern Med 1989;110:901–915.

38 Caird FI, Andrews GR, Kennedy RD. Effect of posture on blood pressure in the elderly. Br Heart J 1973;35:527–530.

39 Goldstein IB, Shapiro D. Cardiovascular response during postural changes in the elderly. J Gerontol 1990;45:M20–M25.

40 Lewis RR, Padayachee TS, Ariyanayagam RP, *et al.* Prevalence of severe internal carotid artery disease in hypertensive elderly patients. J Hypertens 1988;6(Suppl. 1):S33–S36.

41 Peitzman SJ, Berger SR. Postprandial blood pressure decrease in well elderly persons. Arch Intern Med 1989;149:286–288.

42 Niarchos AP, Laragh JH. Effects of diuretic therapy in low-, normal-, and high-renin isolated systolic systemic hypertension. Am J Cardiol 1984;53:797–801.

43 West LJ, Maxwell DS, Noble EP, *et al.* Alcoholism and aging. Ann Intern Med 1984;100:405–416.

44 Kaplan NM. Critical comments on recent literature: age and the response to antihypertensive drugs. Am J Hypertens 1989;2:213–215.

45 Materson BJ, Cushman WC, Goldstein G, *et al.* Treatment of hypertension in the elderly: I. Blood pressure and clinical changes. Results of a Department of Veterans Affairs Cooperative Study. Hypertension 1990;15:348–360.

46 Bühler FP, Burkart F, Lütold BE, *et al.* Antihypertensive beta blocking action as related to renin and age: a pharmacologic tool to identify pathogenetic mechanisms in essential hypertension. Am J Cardiol 1975;36:653.

47 Bühler FR, Bertel O, Lütold BE. Simplified and age-stratified antihypertensive therapy based on beta blockers. Cardiovasc Med 1978;3:135.

48 Freis ED. Age and antihypertensive drugs (hydrochlorothiazide, bendroflumethiazide, nadolol, and captopril). Am J Cardiol 1988;61:117–121.

49 Wikstrand J, Westergren G, Berglund G, *et al.* Antihypertensive treatment with metoprolol or hydrochlorothiazide in patients aged 60 to 75 years. J Am Med Assoc 1986;255:1304–1310.

50 Coope J, Warrender TS. Randomised trial of treatment of

hypertension in elderly patients with primary care. Br Med J 1986;293:1145.

51 Gonzalez DG, Ram CVS. Geriatric hypertension: antihypertensive therapy in coronary artery disease. Geriatrics 1987;42:45−48.

52 Dimsdale JE, Newton RP, Joist T. Neurophysiologic side effects of β-blockers. Arch Intern Med 1989;149:514−525.

53 Ram CVS, Meese R, Kaplan NM, et al. Antihypertensive therapy in the elderly. Effects on blood pressure and cerebral blood flow. Am J Med 1987;82(Suppl. 1A):53−57.

54 Ram CVS. Regression of left ventricular hypertrophy in hypertension with alpha-adrenergic blockade: physiologic basis and therapeutic implications. J Hypertens 1989; 7(Suppl. 6):S98−S99.

55 Jenkins AC, Knill JR, Dreslinski GR. Captopril in the treatment of the elderly hypertensive patient. Arch Intern Med 1985;145:2029−2031.

56 Tuck ML, Katz LA, Kirkendall WM, et al. Low dose captopril in mild to moderate geriatric hypertension. J Am Geriatr Soc 1986;34:693−696.

57 Woo J, Woo KS, Vallance-Owen J. The use of angiotensin-converting enzyme (ACE) inhibitor enalapril in treatment of mild to moderate hypertension in the elderly. Br J Clin Pract 1987;41:845−847.

58 Ben-Ishay D, Leibel B, Stessman J. Calcium channel blockers in the management of hypertension in the elderly. Am J Med 1986;81(Suppl. 6A):30−34.

59 Bohmer F, Barousch R, Reinfrank J. Treatment of isolated systolic hypertension in the elderly with verapamil slow-release 240 mg. J Cardiovasc Pharmacol 1989; 13(Suppl. 4):S45−S46.

60 Myburgh DP, Gordon NF. Comparison of diltiazem and atenolol in young, physically active men with essential hypertension. Am J Cardiol 1987;60:1092−1095.

61 Leehey DJ, Hartman E. Comparison of diltiazem and hydrochlorothiazide for treatment of patients 60 years of age or older with systemic hypertension. Am J Cardiol 1988;62:1218−1223.

62 Montamat SC, Abernethy DR. Calcium antagonists in geriatric patients: diltiazem in elderly persons with hypertension. Clin Pharmacol Ther 1989;45:682−691.

63 Ram CVS. Calcium antagonists as antihypertensive agents are effective in all age groups. J Hypertens 1987;5(Suppl. 4): S115−S118.

64 Adler AG, Leahy JJ, Cressman MD. Management of perioperative hypertension using sublingual nifedipine. Experience in elderly patients undergoing eye surgery. Arch Intern Med 1986;146:1927−1930.

65 Ram CVS. Antiatherosclerotic and vasculoprotective actions of calcium antagonists. Am J Cardiol 1990;66:I29−I32.

66 Schulman SP, Weiss JL, Becker LC, et al. The effects of antihypertensive therapy on left ventricular mass in elderly patients. N Engl J Med 1990;322:1350−1356.

67 Ram CVS. Management of hypertensive emergencies: changing therapeutic options. Am Heart J 1991;122:356−363.

68 SHEP Cooperative Research Group. Prevention of stroke by antihypertensive drug treatment in older persons with isolated systolic hypertension. Final results of the Systolic Hypertension in the Elderly Program (SHEP). JAMA 1991; 265:3255−3264.

69 Dahlöf B, Lindhold LH, Hansson L, et al. Morbidity and mortality in the Swedish Trial in Old Patients with Hypertension (STOP-Hypertension). Lancet 1991;338:1281−1285.

70 MRC Working Party. Medical Research Council trial of treatment of hypertension in older adults: principal results. Br Med J 1992;304:405−412.

11

Rationale for nonpharmacologic treatment of hypertension in the elderly

Priscilla Kincaid-Smith

Hypertension is so common in the elderly in western communities that it has been regarded by some not as a disease but as one end of a normal distribution curve.

At a conservative estimate and depending upon the definitions of "hypertension" and of "elderly" some 50% of elderly people are hypertensive. The percentage of people aged over 65 has increased dramatically in the past 100 years (Fig. 11.1) and this increase is continuing; hence the number of hypertensive people in the community is increasing [1].

Both systolic and diastolic blood pressure are elevated in many elderly people but isolated systolic hypertension which is present in 30% of the elderly [1] is also associated with an increase in morbidity and mortality.

As recently as 1981 a paper appeared entitled "Hypertension in the elderly—has the time come to treat?" [2] but in the interval since 1981, partly as a result of large controlled trials of treatment, the vast majority of publications now support active treatment of hypertension in the elderly.

Most publications on hypertension in the elderly are either epidemiologic studies documenting increased prevalence and the risks of raised blood pressure or they address the question of treatment of hypertension.

Clinical features of hypertension in the elderly

Elderly patients with mild hypertension are commonly asymptomatic but as the severity of the hypertension increases the symptoms which they develop are similar to those in younger patients. Patients with malignant hypertension commonly present with headache, visual symptoms, cerebrovascular episodes, or left ventricular failure. Dyspnea on exertion and headache are among the more common symptoms of those with severe nonmalignant hypertension; however, the first presentation may be with a stroke.

The aging process and other concurrent disease processes may obscure some of the physical findings in elderly patients. Retinal arterioles may show arteriosclerotic changes in normotensive patients over age 60. Heart failure may be due to a combination of ischemic heart disease and hypertension.

The hemodynamic, fluid volume, and endocrine changes seen in the elderly patient with hypertension are shown in Table 11.1 [3].

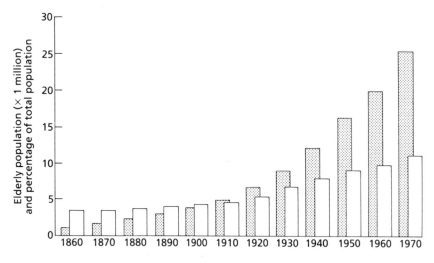

Fig. 11.1 Total population of the United States over 65 years of age (□) and their percentage of the total population (▨). (From Julius [1].)

Table 11.1 Physiologic characteristics of the elderly hypertensive

---

Reduced cardiac output and myocardial reserve
Reduced aortic elasticity and baroreceptor sensitivity
Increased peripheral resistance
Reduced intravascular volume
Increased susceptibility to orthostatic hypotension
Reduced regional blood flow
Reduced renal and hepatic function
Reduced plasma renin activity
Increased plasma catecholamine levels

These features are relevant because they made it difficult to treat hypertension with the ganglion blocking or sympathetic blocking drugs in the early years of antihypertensive therapy because elderly patients could not tolerate the postural hypotension induced by these agents.

Underlying cause of hypertension

In the elderly as in other age groups, if there is an underlying cause of hypertension it is usually renal.

The increased prevalence of renal disease in elderly people documented above and the fact that most chronic renal diseases are associated with hypertension, means that a relatively high proportion of patients have underlying renal disease, but no appropriate study could be found which documents what percentage of elderly patients with hypertension has underlying renal disease. Certain renal disease such as atheroma are very common indeed and renal artery stenosis should always be considered in any elderly patient who abruptly develops hypertension or has loin or abdominal bruits. Renal artery stenosis is also the most frequent cause of renal failure in the elderly. It should also be considered in any patient who has impaired renal function.

Investigations in elderly patients with hypertension

The very large numbers of elderly patients with hypertension mitigates against any extensive search for an underlying cause. Endocrine causes are rare and among these diseases such as Cushing's disease or pheochromocytoma declare themselves through symptoms or physical signs.

Conn's syndrome or primary hyperaldosteronism may not be clinically apparent and this is one reason why plasma urea and electrolyte estimations should be done at the commencement of treatment. The presence of hypokalemia warrants further consideration of this diagnosis.

The urea and creatinine levels indicate if renal function is impaired and if further investigations are required. The urine should be examined for glucose and protein and by microscopy. Urine microscopy provides by far the most sensitive index of the presence of underlying renal disease [4].

The presence of an increased count of urinary erythro-

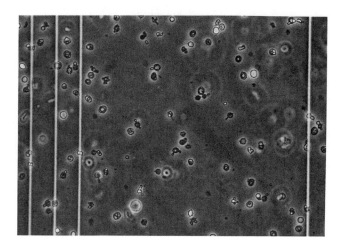

Fig. 11.2 One of glomerular erythrocytes.

cytes indicates glomerular disease (Fig. 11.2) and the presence of an excess of casts without an increase in erythrocytes indicates tubular interstitial or ischemic renal disease.

Clearly in the case of such a common disease as hypertension the number of patients subjected to further investigations after the simple blood and urine analysis referred to above must be carefully considered. If renal function is impaired and the urine deposit suggests a parenchymal disease, there may well be a case for further investigation.

If for example the urine contains 10^6 or more erythrocytes per ml the patient is very likely to have crescentic glomerular disease which is common in the elderly (Table 14.4) [4]. Because crescentic glomerulonephritis causes severe renal failure and responds well to treatment but can only be treated when the diagnosis based on a renal biopsy is known, appropriate investigation may include a renal biopsy.

If renal function is impaired and the urine deposit shows casts but no increase in cells the patient may have renal artery stenosis. Treatment of renal artery stenosis may not only improve the blood pressure but may reverse impaired renal function hence further investigations aimed at demonstrating renal artery stenosis may be justified.

Each case needs to be assessed on its own merits but in countries where dialysis is not freely available for elderly patients there may be an increased incentive to investigate for treatable renal disease if renal function is impaired.

Evidence from controlled trials that treatment for hypertension is of benefit in the elderly

Table 11.2 summarizes the results of earlier controlled trials of hypertension which were not designed specifically to examine the question of treatment in the elderly but from which information can be derived about this age group. Only one major trial was designed specifically to look at benefits of treatment of mild hypertension in patients over 60 years of age. The average age of patients in this study which was conducted by the European Working Party on high blood pressure in the elderly (EWPHE) was 72 years [5].

The results of this study are illustrated in Figure 11.3. In this study, 846 patients over the age of 60 were randomized to active treatment with triamterene and hydrochlorothiazide or placebo. If the blood pressure remained elevated, methyldopa was added to the treated group and matching placebo to the placebo group. On intention to treat analysis, there was a significant reduction in cardiovascular mortality ($P < 0.037$) due to a reduction in cardiac mortality ($P < 0.036$). In the double-blind part of the trial total mortality was not reduced but cardiovascular mortality was ($P < 0.023$) owing to a reduction in cardiac deaths ($P < 0.048$). Deaths from myocardial infarction were also reduced ($P < 0.043$). There was a highly significant reduction in cardiovascular terminating events 60% ($P < 0.0064$). In patients randomized to active treatment there were 29 fewer cardiovascular events and 14 fewer cardiovascular deaths per 1000 patient years.

This study is the only major placebo-controlled trial in which cardiac deaths and death from myocardial infarction have been reduced. One possible explanation for this may be the drugs used, namely, a potassium-sparing diuretic as first-line treatment and methyldopa as second-line treatment. Low potassium has been incriminated as a factor increasing cardiac deaths in some studies. In others the adverse effects of diuretics and β-blockers and plasma lipids have been blamed for an excess of cardiac deaths in the treated group. Methlydopa does not have this adverse effect [6].

Other smaller trials looking at the effects of treatment in the elderly or which included some elderly subjects provide some additional information about the benefit of treatment in this age group [7–9]. Systolic hyperten-

Table 11.2 Design and results of three trials which provide information on the value of antihypertensive drug therapy in subjects >60 years old with diastolic hypertension

Study	Age range	Composition of study groups	Statistical features	Range of diastolic blood pressure at entry	No. of patients (patient-years of follow-up)	Outcome per 1000 patient-years				Interpretation
						Active or stepped-care treatment		Placebo or referred-care treatment		
						Mortality	Morbidity* and mortality	Mortality	Morbidity* and mortality	
Veterans Administration Study (1970) [10]	60–75; 63% 60–79	"High-risk" complaint male veterans	Double-blind placebo-controlled	105–114 90–104	41(133) 40(130)	— —	49 131	— —	199 187	Suggests value of drug treatment in elderly, high-risk males. Difficult to generalize results to average elderly male hypertensives. Entry pressures probably underestimated the average level of diastolic blood pressure
Hypertension Detection and Follow-up Program (1979) [11]	60–69	Community-based random sample of "moderate risk" male and female participants	Open comparison of 2 methods of care (stepped-care and referred-care)	90–115+	2376(11 880)	25	—	30	—	Suggests value of special care system but difficult to evaluate effect of antihypertensive medications alone and difficult to generalize from special care system
Australian National Study (1980)	60–69; 69% 60–64	"Low-risk" male and female community volunteers	Single-blind placebo-controlled	95–109	582(2252)	6	32	8	44	Suggests benefit of drug treatment in low-risk elderly subjects, but mortality results based on only 16 deaths and most participants aged 60–64 years

* Since the criteria for assessable morbid events in each trial differed considerably, this information is best used for within-trial comparisons.

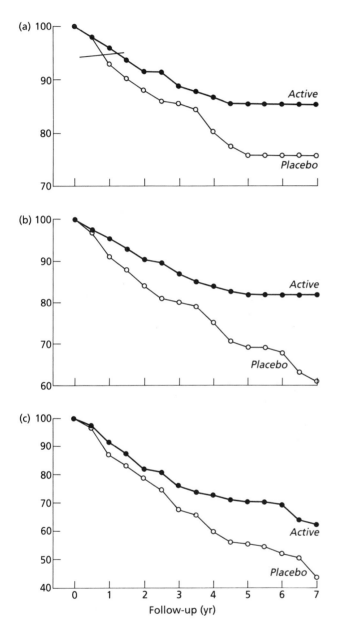

Fig. 11.3 Cumulative percentage of survivors without events calculated for the patients on randomized treatment by life-table method. (From Amery *et al.* [5].)

sion is more common in the elderly because the systolic blood pressure continues to rise after the age of 60, whereas diastolic does not [12]. Only a preliminary report of the study of systolic hypertension in the elderly has been published. This demonstrated that thiazide diuretics were effective and well tolerated [9]. The Australian Study also demonstrated that antihypertensive medication (chlorthiazide, methyldopa, pindolol, propranolol) was as well tolerated by older age patients as they were by those aged 30–60 years [7].

In the Medical Research Council trial of treatment in younger individuals it was necessary to treat over 800 patients for 1 year to prevent one stroke but far more clear-cut benefits were recorded in the EWPHE study where 14 fewer cardiovascular deaths occurred per 1000 patient years of treatment [5].

Attitudes on treating hypertension in elderly patients have always been more conservative than those concerning treatment in younger individuals but the results of the EWPHE study have convinced most investigators that hypertension should be treated in patients over 60 years of age.

Little information is available about the upper age limit which should be treated. The EWPHE trial included a subgroup over 80 years but this was small (155 patients). Most of these patients were women, many of whom run a more benign course in spite of significant blood pressure elevation. The trial did not demonstrate benefit in the subgroup over 80 but this may well have been due to a Type II error reflecting small numbers. There is some evidence from Scandinavia that hypertension in very old people is associated with reduced mortality.

In addition to the trial in systolic hypertension there are two other trials in progress which are looking at patients aged 65–84 years. These are a Medical Research Council Study in the United Kingdom and a Swedish trial in old patients.

Treatment of hypertension in the elderly

The major evidence of benefit of treatment of hypertension in elderly subjects derives from the EWPHE study [5]. It should be remembered that overall mortality was not reduced in this study but there was a reduction in both mortality due to cardiovascular causes and in cardiovascular events. Not only is this the only large placebo-controlled trial which demonstrates benefit in terms of reduction of cardiac mortality, but it is also the only trial which used a potassium-sparing diuretic.

Another much smaller study in which 84% of patients were over 50 years used a combination of methyclothia-

(a)

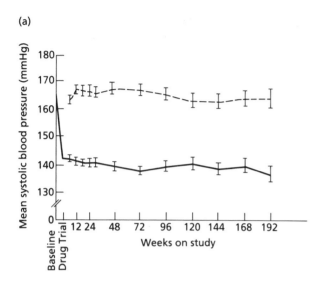

(b)

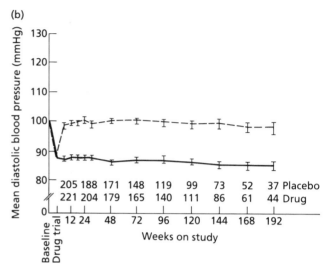

Fig. 11.4 Effect of treatment with methyclothiazide 5 mg plus deserpidine 0.5 mg (n = 233) [– – –] twice daily or placebo (n = 219) [———] on (a) mean systolic blood pressure and (b) mean diastolic blood pressure in elderly patients with mild hypertension. Numbers indicate the number of patients evaluated at each follow-up visit. (From Julius [1].)

zide (5 mg) and deserpidine (0.5 mg). A fixed dose was given twice daily. A highly significant reduction in systolic and diastolic blood pressure was achieved in this study (Fig. 11.4). There were 219 patients on placebo and 233 on treatment, and the study was continued over 3½ years; equal numbers of deaths occurred in the two groups, 26 in the treated group and 24 in the placebo group. Trial-end patients were also similar, 112 in the treated group and 123 in the placebo group. There was no reduction in the number of strokes but congestive heart failure was reduced, none occurring in treated patients [1]. The drugs were well tolerated.

In the Veterans Administration Study 1972 and the HDFP study in 1979 [11,13] there was some evidence that older patients seemed to benefit more than younger ones [14,15].

Attention to lipids and other risk factors

The morbidity and mortality of hypertension is due to coronary heart disease and strokes. In addition to hypertension the other two major risk factors for both these vascular lesions are an adverse serum lipid profile and smoking.

Elderly patients are much more likely to develop vascular complications than younger hypertensive patients.

The benefits of reduction in cholesterol levels in the elderly was addressed in the Los Angeles Veterans Administration Domiciliary Facility Study, a randomized controlled trial of 846 men (average age 65.5 years) who were free of signs of coronary heart disease at entry. Moderate serum cholesterol reduction was achieved by diet. Over 8½ years the incidence of severe atherosclerotic events (coronary cerebrovascular or peripheral vascular) was reduced by 31%. This study demonstrated benefit from reduction of serum cholesterol levels in this age group. The benefits in terms of reduced coronary and cerebrovascular disease derived from stopping smoking is very well documented in numerous studies [16].

Choice of method of treatment in hypertension in the elderly

Nonpharmacologic treatment

In all patients presenting with hypertension, which is judged to warrant treatment, consideration should be given to nonpharmacologic forms of therapy. As the number of elderly people with hypertension grows so does the size of the potential cost of treating these individuals with antihypertensive drugs. Not all nonpharmacologic forms of therapy are cheap but some which involve dietary modifications and other life style alterations are inexpensive.

Weight reduction

The evidence that weight reduction reduces the level of the blood pressure is overwhelming. The study of McMahon *et al.* [17] showed that weight loss achieved a larger blood pressure reduction than a β-blocking drug. Because of some of the difficulties involved in drug therapy in the elderly, considerable effort should be put into weight reduction in overweight elderly hypertensive patients before starting drug therapy. The effect of weight reduction is also seen in patients on treatment and those with severe hypertension [18,19].

Vegetarian diet

Vegetarians have lower blood pressures than meat eaters [20]. Although it has not been possible to document which component or components of a vegetarian diet reduce the blood pressure this reduction has been demonstrated in controlled cross-over studies [21]. Some elderly patients may prefer changing to a vegetarian diet to taking tablets and they should be advised of the potential benefits of a vegetarian diet before starting drug treatment, so that they can exercise this option.

Alcohol

The association between alcohol and hypertension has been recognized for some years [22]. Recently in a controlled cross-over study it has been clearly demonstrated that reduction in alcohol intake lowers blood pressure [23]. Elderly people before starting drug treatment for hypertension should be advised to reduce their alcohol intake.

Because many studies have shown that alcohol increases high-density lipoprotein cholesterol and that a low or moderate intake of alcohol may protect against ischemic heart disease [24], one to two standard drinks per day may be permitted. Although Shaper *et al.* [25] recently queried the benefits resulting from a low-alcohol intake, the balance of evidence suggests that it is beneficial as far as ischemic heart disease is concerned.

Sodium

The most controversial area in terms of nonpharmacologic therapy for treatment of hypertension, namely reduced salt intake, is also the one which is most widely recommended. Elderly patients are more susceptible than younger people to sodium depletion because they conserve sodium poorly and this postural hypertension is a moderately common side-effect of salt depletion in the elderly.

The intersalt study was designed to determine the relationship between blood pressure and sodium intake in 32 countries [26]. It showed that when adjustment is made for body mass index, alcohol intake, and potassium intake, a 100 mmol lower sodium intake is associated with an average systolic blood pressure which is lower by 2.2 mmHg. The potential reduction in blood pressure from reduced sodium intake at community level is therefore very small and in the elderly the potential side-effect of postural hypotension may cancel out any benefits in terms of blood pressure reduction achieved by sodium restriction. Not all hypertensive patients will reduce their blood pressure on a low-salt diet. In some studies as few as a third have shown a reduction in blood pressure, a third remained unchanged and in a third blood pressure showed a slight increase.

In an Australian-controlled cross-over study small reductions in systolic (3.5−5 mm) and diastolic (3−3.5 mm) blood pressure were achieved by reduction of sodium intake (average 67 mmol/day). Replacement of dietary sodium with sodium chloride capsules while subjects continued with the low-sodium diet did not restore the blood pressure to the previous level [27].

On the basis of these observations it may be reasonable to recommend that the effect of moderate reduction in dietary salt intake be monitored in elderly patients before starting antihypertensive drugs. Over 50% of patients are likely to show some slight reduction in systolic and diastolic blood pressure and if this reduction is not accompanied by side-effects such as postural hypotension it is worth continued sodium restriction.

Potassium

Epidemiologic studies have shown that the potassium intake in the diet varies inversely with the level of blood pressure [28].

Potassium supplements have achieved a fall in blood pressure in several controlled studies [29−31]. Tobian [32] has shown that a high-potassium intake reduces vascular lesions and strokes in stroke-prone rats.

There would seem to be sufficient reason to suggest

that an increase in potassium intake may be beneficial in elderly hypertensive subjects. An increase in potassium intake is usually more acceptable than reduction in sodium intake and hence compliance rates are better.

Calcium

As is the case of potassium there is an inverse relationship between blood pressure and dietary calcium intake.

Calcium supplements have achieved a modest reduction in blood pressure [33,34].

In advising elderly patients about increasing calcium intake care should be taken to avoid a high-cholesterol diet. In elderly women an increased calcium intake combined with oestrogen supplements has the additional benefit of reducing the risk of osteoporosis.

Relaxation therapy and biofeedback

Relaxation and biofeedback therapy are much more time consuming and labor intensive than dietary alterations which may reduce the blood pressure by nonpharmacologic techniques.

Relaxation therapy has been shown in a controlled trial to reduce the blood pressure over a 4-year period [35]. Biofeedback has also been shown to lower the blood pressure and may benefit the quality of life [36,37].

Overview of antihypertensive therapy in elderly hypertensive patients

Patients over the age of 60 respond to most groups of antihypertensive drugs.

Before drug therapy is commenced it is worth considering the use of nonpharmacologic methods of controlling the blood pressure.

References

1 Julius S. The therapeutic dilemma of hypertension in the elderly. Drugs 1988;36:7–17.

2 Radin AM, Black HR. Hypertension in the elderly: the time has come to treat. J Am Geriat Soc 1981;29:193–200.

3 Burris JF. Antihypertensive treatment in the elderly: Goals and options. Cardiovasc Rep Rev 1988;9:47–51.

4 Fairley KF. Urinalysis. In Schrier RW, Gottschalk CW, eds. *Diseases of the Kidney* New York: Little, Brown & Co., 1988:359.

5 Amery A, Birkenhager W, Brixko P, *et al.* Mortality and morbidity results from the European working party on high blood pressure in the elderly trial. Lancet 1985;1349–1354.

6 Onrot J, Wood AJJ. Hypertension in the elderly. The benefits of therapy. Hypertension 1984;76:46–57.

7 National Heart Foundation of Australia. Treatment of mild hypertension in the elderly. Med J Aust 1981;2:398–402.

8 Coope J, Warrender TS. Randomised trial of treatment of hypertension in elderly patients in primary care. Br J Med 1986;293:1145–1148.

9 Hulley SB, Furberg CD, Gurland B, *et al.* Systolic hypertension in the elderly program (SHEP): Antihypertensive efficacy of chlorthalidone. Am J Cardiol 1985;56:913–920.

10 Veterans Administration Cooperative Study on Antihypertensive Agents. Effects of treatment on morbidity in hypertension. II. Results in patients with diastolic blood pressure averaging 90 through 114 mmHg. J Am Med Assoc 1970;213:1143–1152.

11 Hypertension detection and follow-up program Cooperative group. Five-year Findings of the hypertension detection and follow-up program. II. Mortality by race-sex and age. J Am Med Assoc 1979;42:2572–2577.

12 Dyer AR, Stamler J, Shekelle RB, *et al.* Hypertension in the elderly. Med Clin North Am 1977;61:513–529.

13 Veterans Administration Cooperative Study Group on Antihypertensive Agents. Circulation 1972;45:991–1004.

14 Working group on hypertension in the elderly: Statement on hypertension in the elderly. J Am Med Assoc 1986;256:70–74.

15 Kannell WB. Treating hypertension in the elderly. Cardiovasc Med 1985:41.

16 Stamler J. Risk factor modification trials: Implications for the elderly. Eur Heart J 1988;9:9–53.

17 McMahon SW, Macdonald GJ, Bernstein L, *et al.* Comparison of weight reduction with metoprolol in treatment of hypertension in young overweight patients. Lancet 1985;1233–1236.

18 Reisen E, Abel R, Modan M, *et al.* Effect of weight loss without salt restriction on the reduction of blood pressure in overweight hypertensive patients. N Engl J Med 1978;298:1–6.

19 Ramsay LE, Ramsay MH, Hettiarachchi J, *et al.* Weight reduction in a blood pressure clinic. Br J Med 1978;2:244–245.

20 Rouse IL, Beilin LJ. Vegetarian diet and blood pressure. J Hypertens 1984;2:231–240.

21 Margretts BM, Beilin LJ, Vandongen R, *et al.* Vegetarian diet in mild hypertension: a randomised controlled trial. Br J Med 1986;293:1468–1471.

22 Beilin LJ, Vandongen DB. Alcohol-related hypertension in mild hypertension: From drug trials to practice. In Strasser T, Ganten D, eds. *Mild Hypertension* New York: Raven Press, 1987:147–157.

23 Puddey IB, Beilin LJ, Vandongen R. Regular alcohol use raises blood pressure in treated hypertensive subjects: A

randomised controlled trial. Lancet 1987;647–651.

24 Stampler ME, Colditz GA, Willett WC, *et al.* A prospective study of moderate alcohol consumption and the risk of coronary disease and stroke in women. N Engl J Med 1988; 319:267–273.

25 Shaper AC, Wannamethee G, Walker M. Alcohol and mortality in British men: explaining the U-shaped curve. Lancet 1988;1267–1273.

26 Intersalt Cooperative Research Group. Intersalt: an international study of electrolyte excretion and blood pressure. Results for 24 hour urinary sodium and potassium excretion. Br J Med 1988;297:319–328.

27 Australian National Health and Medical Research Committee management committee: Diet study in mild hypertension. In Strasser T, Ganten D, eds. *Mild Hypertension.* New York: Raven Press, 1987:165–180.

28 Langford HG. Potassium and its role in the aetiology and therapy of hypertension. In Blaufox MD, Langford HG, eds. *Bibliotheca Cardiologica 41 Nonpharmacologic Therapy of Hypertension.* Basel: S Karger, 1987:57–58.

29 Kaplan NM, Carnegie A, Raskin P, *et al.* Potassium supplementation in hypertensive patients with diuretic-induced hypokalemia. N Engl J Med 1985;312:746–749.

30 McGregor GA, Smith SJ, Markandu ND, *et al.* Moderate potassium supplementation in essential hypertension.

Lancet 1982:567–570.

31 Zoccali C, Cumming AMM, Hutcheson MJ, *et al.* Effects of potassium on sodium balance, renin, noradrenaline, and arterial pressure. J Hypertens 1985;3:67–72.

32 Tobian L. High potassium diets markedly protect against stroke deaths and kidney disease in hypertensive rats, a possible legacy from prehistoric times. Can J Physiol Pharmacol 1986;64:840–848.

33 Belizan JM, Villar J, Pineda O, *et al.* Reduction of blood pressure with calcium supplementation in young adults. J Am Med Assoc 1983;249:1161–1165.

34 McCarron DA, Morris CD. Blood pressure response to oral calcium in persons with mild to moderate hypertension: A randomized, double-blind, placebo-controlled, crossover trial. Ann Intern Med 1985;103:825–831.

35 Patel CH, Marmot MG, Terry DJ. Controlled trial of biofeedback-aided behavioural methods in reducing mild hypertension. Br J Med 1981;282:2005–2008.

36 Marmot MG. Psychosocial factors and blood pressure. In Bulpitt CJ, ed. *Handbook of Hypertension.* vol. 6. *Epidemiology of Hypertension*: Elsevier, 1985:89–103.

37 Kincaid-Smith P. Strategies to reduce cardiovascular risk in the hypertensive patient: lifestyle, hypertension and the risk of CHD. In press.

12

Pathophysiology and management of electrolyte disturbances in the elderly

John W. Rowe
Kenneth L. Minaker
Moshe Levi

Introduction

As discussed in detail elsewhere (see Chapter 2) in this volume, normal aging, in the absence of disease, is associated with substantial loss of renal function. This age-related impairment is most evident in glomerular filtration rate (GFR) and certain aspects of renal tubular function. Under normal circumstances, renal function in healthy older individuals is adequate to maintain fluid and electrolyte balance within normal range. However, this homeostatic capacity is impaired in the presence of physiologic stress or disease. This chapter will review the influence of aging on the adaptive reserve mechanisms responsible for maintaining the constancy of the volume and composition of the extracellular fluid and will discuss the management of fluid and electrolyte disturbances in elderly people.

Sodium balance

Sodium conserving ability

The ability of the aged kidney to conserve sodium in response to reduced salt intake is impaired. Clinical studies have shown that when placed on a very low-sodium diet (10 mmol/Na per day) healthy elderly individuals reduce urinary sodium excretion much less promptly than their younger counterparts, but are able, over time, to come into balance and reduce urinary sodium losses to 10 mmol/day [1] (Fig. 12.1). This sluggish response to abruptly impaired intake, such as often accompanies surgery or acute illness, can have major clinical consequences and result in substantial overall reduction in extracellular fluid volume and effective circulating blood flow. Clearance studies in young and elderly subjects have shown a decreased distal tubular capacity for sodium reabsorption in the elderly [2]. Contributors to this distal tubular dysfunction might include anatomic changes in the aging kidney such as interstitial fibrosis, as well as functional and hormonal changes including increased medullary blood flow, decreased renin−angiotensin−aldosterone activity, decreased Na−K−ATPase activity, or increases in atrial natriuretic peptide effects.

There are important age-related alterations in the renin−angiotensin−aldosterone system. Basal plasma renin concentration or activity is decreased by 30−50% in elderly subjects in spite of normal levels of renin

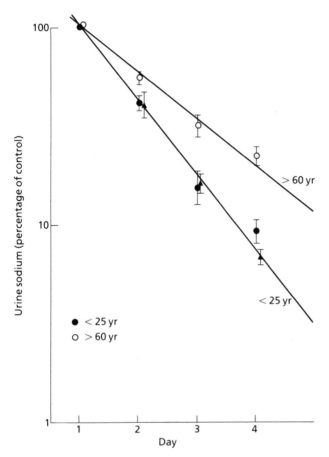

Fig. 12.1 Response of urinary sodium excretion to restriction of sodium intake in normal humans. The mean half-time for eight subjects of 60 years of age was 30.90 ± 2.8 hours, exceeding the mean half-time of 17.6 ± 0.7 hours for subjects under 25 years of age. ($P = 0.01$.) (From Epstein & Hollenberg [1].)

substrate [3,4]. In response to maneuvers designed to stimulate renin secretion (e.g., upright posture, 10 mmol/day sodium intake, and furosemide administration), the age difference in plasma renin activity are further amplified [3–8] (Fig. 12.2a). There is a similar 30–50% decrease in plasma aldosterone levels in elderly subjects during recumbency and normal sodium intake, which also becomes more pronounced during upright posture, sodium restriction, and furosemide administration [4,8–10] (Fig. 12.2b). Studies in young and elderly subjects have shown marked improvement in distal tubular sodium reabsorption in the elderly following

treatment with aldosterone [11]. The age-related aldosterone deficiency appears to be related to the renin–angiotensin deficiency and not to intrinsic adrenal gland defects, since both plasma aldosterone and cortisol responses to corticotropin (adrenocorticotropic hormone (ACTH)) infusion are normal in the elderly [10].

Thus, during sodium restriction, impaired angiotensin II and/or aldosterone response may reduce renal tubular reabsorption in the elderly.

Sodium excreting ability

Excessive sodium retention and volume overload are commonly encountered problems in elderly patients. Both the excretory capacity for sodium and the circadian variation in excretion are influenced by age. Short-term intravenous sodium loading reveals distinct age-related differences in sodium excretion. Individuals older than 40 years excrete slightly less sodium per 24 hours following a 2 liter normal saline load than do race-, sex-, and size-matched subjects below 40 years of age [12–14] (Fig. 12.3). In addition, the older subjects excrete a significantly greater portion of the sodium load at night than do their younger counterparts. The age-related decrease in GFR is probably the major factor limiting the aged kidney's capacity to excrete an acute sodium load. The potential roles of additional factors, including intrarenal hemodynamics, renal nerve activity, and activities of intrarenal α-adrenergic system, renin–angiotensin–aldosterone, dopamine, and prostaglandins have not been elucidated.

Studies in the aged rat confirm the clinical experience that the natriuretic efficiency is impaired in the aged following isotonic saline or blood expansion [15,16]. It is interesting to note that a recent study found a significant age-related decrease in number of renal dopamine D_1 receptors but not dopamine D_2 receptors [17]. The possible role of the alteration in renal dopamine receptor activity in the impaired natriuresis, however, remains unstudied.

Atrial natriuretic peptide (ANP)

Several very recent studies have suggested a possible role of alterations in ANP secretion in mediating the age-related alterations in sodium balance. In view of the striking changes in ANP with aging and implications for several aspects of fluid and electrolyte balance, this area will be reviewed in detail below. Additional discussion

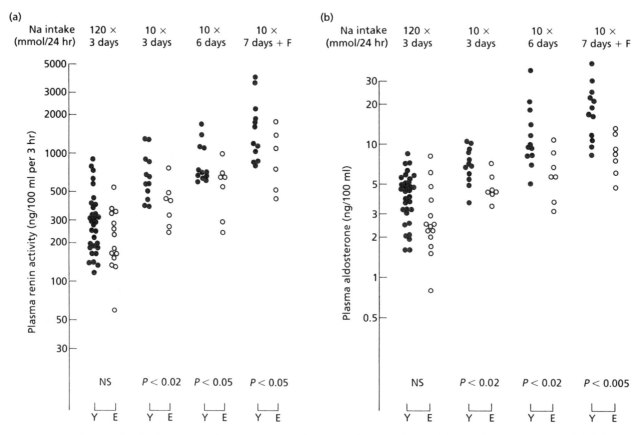

Fig. 12.2 Distribution of individual supine plasma renin (a) and aldosterone values (b) before and during progressive sodium depletion in young and elderly healthy subjects. Y, young subjects; E, elderly subjects. Values indicating statistical significance refers to difference between young and elderly subjects. Plasma renin activity values are those obtained in incubation pH 5.7. (From Crane & Harris [4].)

of ANP and aging is also found in Chapter 7 of this volume.

It was long suspected that in addition to aldosterone and vasopressin, a "third factor" was involved in the regulation of sodium balance and extracellular fluid volume. Numerous studies have now documented that peptides isolated from atria are modified in concentration by water and salt deprivation. These cause profound diuresis, natriuresis, and reduction in blood pressure. In humans, ANP exists as a 126 amino acid prohormone stored primarily in atrial myocytes with a 28 amino acid active circulating peptide form. Atrial natriuretic peptide is released in response to a variety of maneuvers that increased atrial pressure. The most striking effects of physiologic actions of ANP are sustained increases in

GFR, free water clearance and natriuresis without a corresponding increase in renal blood flow (RBF). These effects are believed to be secondary to alterations in intrarenal blood flow and are independent of changes in total RBF or tubular sodium transport [18,19]. Atrial natriuretic peptide decreases blood pressure by vasodilatation and possibly through direct modulation of baroreceptor reflexes [20]. Cardiac output is decreased by several mechanisms, primarily the vasodilatory effect of ANP resulting in lowered cardiac filling pressures. Plasma volume is decreased by the ANP-mediated renal effects of sodium and free water loss as well as a translocation of fluid from plasma to interstitial spaces secondary to an ANP-mediated increase in capillary permeability [18]. This latter effect, the "edemagenic effect" [20], may be

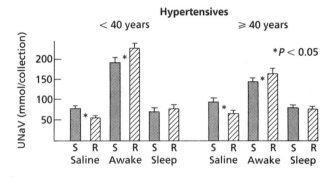

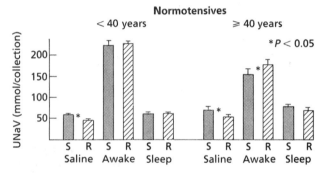

Fig. 12.3 Natriuretic responses following volume expansion. Sodium-sensitive individuals exhibited "exaggerated natriuresis" during the 4-hour saline load. By the following morning, balance was restored. S, sensitive; R, resistant; UNaV, urinary sodium excretion. (From Luft *et al.* [14].)

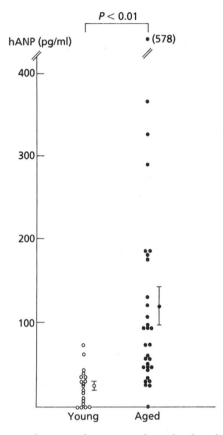

Fig. 12.4 Circulating atrial natriuretic factor levels in healthy young and aged individuals. (From Ohashi *et al.* [23].)

particularly important in the elderly. Atrial natriuretic peptide also directly antagonizes the components of the counterbalancing vasoconstrictive sodium-retentive hormonal systems, through inhibition of the secretion of aldosterone and vasopressin [20–22].

Altered ANP physiology in healthy and frail elderly people
Studies in carefully selected subjects have shown that the healthy elderly have basal circulating ANP levels three to five times those of the healthy young [22–24]. The variability within the elderly is very large in these studies and in all series some healthy elderly people have ANP levels similar to young adults (Fig. 12.4). In one study in a large long-term care facility, baseline ANP levels in clinically stable patients with evidence of cardiovascular disease were twice the levels seen in healthy elderly people. In this institutionalized population, sig-

nificant independent risk factors for elevated ANP included advancing age, atrial fibrillation, and administration of nitrates or diuretics [25].

Several possible mechanisms for the increased levels of ANP in the elderly deserve consideration. These include the following.

1 Aging is a state of increased effective extracellular fluid volume. This view is supported by the coexisting elevations of ANP and the suppression of renin levels in the elderly.

2 Elevated ANP is secondary to enhanced sensitivity of the atrial afferent system for ANP release.

3 End-organ resistance to ANP actions induce feedback stimulation of ANP release in the elderly.

This would help explain several age-related effects including the decrease in GFR and impaired ability to excrete a sodium load (secondary to resistance to the renal vascular effects of ANP), the increase in systolic blood pressure (due to resistance to the antagonization of angiotensin/norepinephrine mediated vasoconstriction of large arteries), and the age-related enhancement of vasopressin secretion with osmotic stimulation (to counterbalance the suppressive effect of ANP on vasopressin secretion [22]. In this regard, and also relevant to the preceding discussion on sodium balance, preliminary evidence from Clark *et al.* [26] suggest that renal sodium excretion in the healthy elderly is relatively resistant to physiologic elevations of ANP.

While the clinical implications of age-related increases in ANP have not yet been elucidated, several intriguing possibilities deserve careful study. Specifically, the role of ANP in enhancing edema development in elderly people, and, through its inhibition of arginine vasopressin (AVP), in facilitating nocturnal diuresis, have obvious implications for the management of very common clinical problems in this age group. It is important to note that neither edema formation nor AVP inhibition, are dependent upon the responsiveness of the renal vasculature in elderly people to ANP.

Another major issue currently under investigation relates to the possible value of ANP levels as predictors of future cardiovascular morbidity or mortality in the elderly. Davis *et al.* [27] recently reported the results of a prospective study relating ANP levels and clinical history to future clinical course in 339 elderly residents of a long-term care facility. In this very old, frail, but clinically stable study population, 15% of individuals developed at least one episode of congestive heart failure over the course of 1 year. Baseline ANP levels were over twice as high in those developing congestive failure than in those who did not. While a prior history of heart failure was a strong risk factor for future heart failure, within this previously affected high risk group, elevated ANP levels increased the prediction of heart failure. For the patients with prior heart failure, the risk of another episode was nearly 75% if ANP was high, whereas the risk fell to 20% if ANP was low [27]. These findings, which require verification and further study, suggest that clinically stable elderly people represent a physiologically heterogeneous group, and that measures of ANP may be helpful in identifying those individuals who are at greatest risk for clinical decompensation, especially during times of clinical stress.

Water balance

Renal concentrating ability

Renal concentrating ability is well known to decline with age in humans [28–31] (Fig. 12.5). In several studies the maximal urine osmolality, measured following 12–24 hours of dehydration, was inversely related to age [28,30]. In one study, the maximal urine osmolality was 1109 mosmol per kg in 31 subjects 20–39 years old, compared to 1051 mosmol per kg in 48 subjects 40–59 years old, and 882 mosmol per kg in 18 subjects 60–79 years old [31]. It is interesting to note that the age-related decline in concentrating ability did not correlate with

Fig. 12.5 Maximum urine osmolality in healthy young men, hospitalized controls, and patients with ulcer, showing a decrease with age. The solid line represents the regression slope for hospitalized patients. (From Lindeman *et al.* [30].)

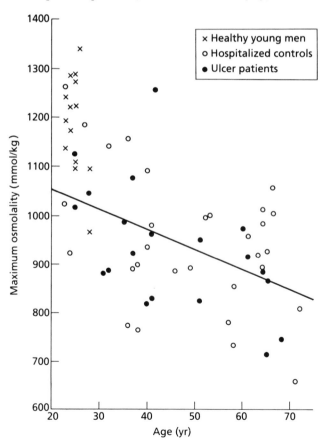

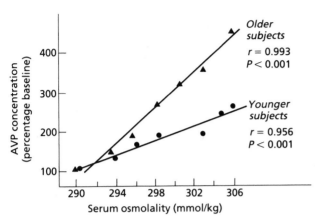

Fig. 12.6 Correlation between serum osmolality and AVP concentration in young and old subjects during a 2-hour intravenous infusion of 3% NaCl at the rate of 0.1 ml/kg per min. The points represent main values of osmolality and AVP at successive 20 min intervals in each age group. (From Helderman *et al.* [32].)

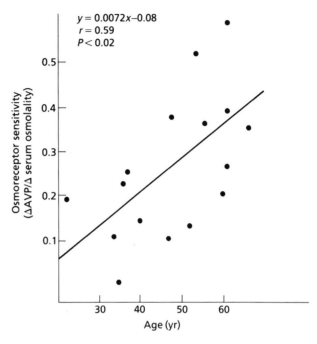

Fig. 12.7 The relationship between age and osmoreceptor sensitivity (AVP/serum osmolality). The slope of plasma AVP concentration in pg/ml on serum osmolality in mosmol/kg was computed and plotted for each subject. (From Helderman *et al.* [32].)

the age-related decline in the GFR [28,31]. While this age-related deficit in water conservation can easily be demonstrated in physiologic studies, it is likely to be of only minor clinical consequence since very old healthy individuals maintain substantial concentrating capacity.

Studies in humans suggest that the concentrating defect is due to an intrarenal defect rather than a failure in the osmotic-induced release of AVP [29,32,33]. Following intravenous infusion of hypertonic saline (3% NaCl) in nine young (21−49 years) and three old (54−92 years) subjects, plasma AVP levels rose 4.5 times the baseline in the older men compared to 2.5 times the baseline in the younger, despite similar free water clearances [32] (Fig. 12.6). The slope of the plasma AVP concentration (percentage baseline) vs. serum osmolality, an index of the sensitivity of the osmoreceptor, was significantly increased in the older subjects (Fig. 12.7). In addition, in the same study, intravenous infusion of ethanol resulted in a progressive decline in plasma AVP levels in the young subjects, but failed to have a similar effect in the older subjects. In contrast to osmotic stimulation, volume−pressure-mediated AVP release has been found to decrease with age and appears to be absent in many healthy elderly people [34]. An additional factor which may influence AVP levels and impair water conservation in the elderly is the previously discussed increase in

ANP levels with age, since ANP has been demonstrated to suppress AVP release in response to hyperosmolality in young and old individuals [22] (Fig. 12.8).

Studies in humans reveal an age-related increase in solute excretion and osmolar clearance during dehydration [31]. This phenomenon, which may be a reflection of an impaired solute transport by the ascending loop of Henle, may be responsible for the impairment in urine concentrating ability in elderly subjects. This possibility is supported by clearance studies during water-diuresis that demonstrate a decrease in the sodium chloride transport in the ascending loop of Henle in elderly subjects [2,11]. This defect in solute transport by the thick ascending limb of Henle's loop could diminish inner medullary hypertonicity and thereby impair urinary concentrating ability. A relative increase in medullary blood flow as suggested by the xenon wash-out studies [35] could also increase removal of solutes from the medullary interstitium and thereby contribute to the decreased maximal urinary osmolality.

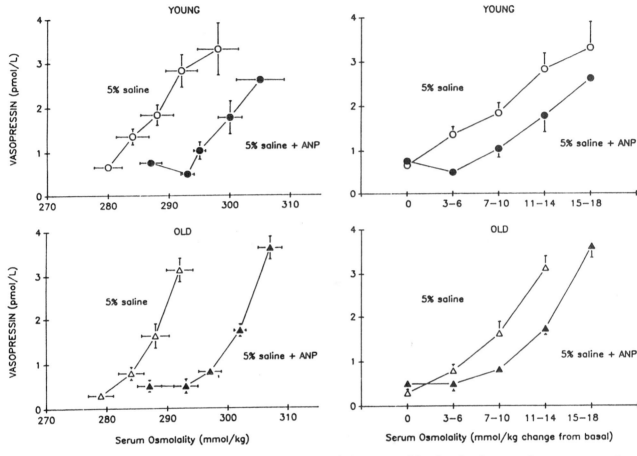

Fig. 12.8 Plasma vasopressin responses during infusion of 5% saline and 5% saline + ANP in young and old individuals. The left panels depict absolute osmolality and right panels depict change in osmolality from baseline. Atrial natriuretic peptide significantly suppressed osmostimulated vasopressin release. (From Clark *et al.* [22].)

Studies in the aging rat, however, suggest that impaired responsiveness of the collecting duct cells to AVP, rather than diminished inner medullary hypertonicity, is responsible for the concentrating defect [36]. The maximal urinary concentration following a 40-hour dehydration period and exogenous vasopressin administration was markedly impaired. Clearance studies revealed a normal solute-free water formation (C_{H_2O}/GFR as a function of V/GFR), but impaired solute-free water reabsorption of (T^c H_2O/GFR as a function of C_{osm}/GFR), implying normal solute transport by the ascending limb and decreased water transport by the collecting duct. In fact, inner medullary solute content in the old and young rats was identical.

Studies with inner medullary slices in rat and mice have revealed an age-related impairment in AVP-induced cAMP generation [37,38]. The threshold dose of AVP required to elicit a significant rise in cAMP was greater in older animals with a shift in the dose−response curve to the right in old mice [38]. In both rats and mice the maximum cAMP level in older animals was decreased compared with that in younger animals. Studies in the rat suggested that the chronically increased levels of circulating AVP may result in down-regulation of the renal AVP receptors and thus may be responsible for the age-related impairment in cAMP response to AVP [39,40]. A recent study in mice, however, found no age-related differences in the number of receptors or their affinity for

AVP, and suggested that the decreased cAMP response is probably due to postreceptor mechanisms [41].

Thirst in the elderly

The age-related impairments in renal-concentrating and sodium-conserving ability are associated with increased incidence of volume depletion and hypernatremia in the elderly [42]. Under normal physiologic conditions, increased thirst and fluid intake are natural defense mechanisms against volume depletion and hypernatremia. A deficit in thirst and regulation of fluid intake in the elderly, however, may further contribute to the increased incidence of dehydration and hypernatremia.

Recent studies confirm the long-held clinical observation that thirst and fluid intake is impaired in the elderly [43–46]. In a series of studies by Minaker et al. [45], the osmotic threshold for thirst during hypertonic saline infusion was much higher in healthy elderly subjects than their younger counterparts, with many apparently normal elders not reporting thirst despite elevations of plasma osmolality to levels over 300 mosmol/kg. In studies of water ingestion after intravenously induced hyperosmolality, elderly individuals demonstrated marked reductions, when compared to the young group in their water intake and rate of return of plasma osmolality to baseline [46]. Finally, the same investigators evaluated the influence of free access to water on prevention of osmolality during hypertonic saline infusion. Despite equivalent increases in plasma volume, the older group displayed significantly less water intake and greater increases in plasma osmolality than the younger group [47]. As discussed later in this chapter, thirst may also be severely impaired in patients with a prior history of stroke who do not have cognitive impairment or evidence of hypothalamic or pituitary dysfunction [48].

The complication of age-related decreases in thirst by systemic illnesses and dementia in many frail elderly patients clearly place them at risk for the development of severe water deficiency.

Renal diluting ability

Renal diluting ability is also impaired as a function of aging [27,29,49]. In water-diuresing subjects, minimal urine osmolality is significantly higher, 92 mosmol per kg in the elderly subjects (ages 77–88), when compared to 52 mosmol per kg in the young subjects (ages 17–40). Free water clearance (C_{H_2O}) is also decreased: 5.9 ml per min in elderly subjects compared to 16.2 ml per min in the young subjects. While the impairment in C_{H_2O} is largely due to the decrease in GFR, when C_{H_2O} is factored for GFR, C_{H_2O}/GFR is, however, still decreased in the older subjects [29,49]. Mechanisms of the impaired diluting ability in the elderly have not been well studied; in addition to the major role of impaired GFR, inadequate suppression of AVP release or impaired solute transport in the ascending loop of Henle may also play a role.

Potassium balance

Studies on the effects of aging on renal and extrarenal adaptation to high potassium loads or dietary potassium deprivation in the human are lacking. Two different studies, however, have found that both total body potassium and total exchangeable potassium [25] decreases with age in both sexes and that the decrease is more marked in women than in men. This decrease may relate to the decrease in muscle mass with advancing age.

Studies of the effects of aging on potassium adaptation in the rat show the efficiency of kaluretic response to intravenous infusion of potassium chloride and the rise in plasma potassium are not influenced by age [16]. In response to high dietary potassium intake, however, the efficiency of kaluretic response to intravenous potassium chloride was impaired in the rat, with a significantly greater plasma potassium. Following bilateral nephrectomy, the rise in plasma potassium concentration was also higher in the aged rats who were on a high potassium, but not normal potassium intake. The renal and extrarenal impairment in potassium adaptation was associated with significant decreases in renal and colon $Na-K-ATPase$ activity [16]. Whether these findings also apply to human aging remains to be determined.

Over the past several years there has been substantial attention paid to extrarenal potassium disposal. Rosa et al. [50] demonstrated in humans that β-adrenergic mechanisms were responsible for potassium disposal during potassium infusion. This study was conducted on healthy individuals across the adult age range (ages 23–85) and the authors found no effect of age on the extrarenal potassium disposal or the effect of β-adrenergic blockade. In another study, Minaker & Rowe [51] evaluated the effects of insulin level, β-adrenergic blockage, and age on potassium homeostasis during hyperinsulinemia. These investigators showed that increasing steady state levels of insulin are associated with dose-dependent declines in plasma potassium during the first hour of insulin infusion, but that during the second hour of insulin infusion plasma potassium continued to decline at the lowest insulin doses but began to rise at the highest insulin dose levels. This finding suggests the presence of a regulatory mechanism influencing insulin-mediated alterations in plasma potassium. The effect was not influenced by β-adrenergic blockade or aging [51]. Taken together, these studies suggest that hormonal regulation of extrarenal potassium homeostasis is generally intact in aging despite the marked impairment in renal potassium excretions in elderly people.

Fluid and electrolyte disorders in the elderly

General principles

Physicians skilled in the clinical care of the elderly are familiar with five general principles that guide diagnosis and management. Application of these principles to clinical disorders of volume and composition of extracellular fluid are essential for their successful management.

First, the symptoms of disordered regulation of volume and composition of extracellular fluid are often vague. Many diseases in the elderly present with nonspecific signs and symptoms not clearly attributable to a particular organ system. The clinical approach requires an awareness of the increased frequency of severe clinical disorders of this type in the elderly, and a low threshold to obtain measures of blood urea nitrogen, creatinine, and electrolytes in all sick patients. Clinical estimates of central peripheral volume remain important features of the clinical examination. However, assessment of volume contraction is notoriously imprecise in the elderly owing to laxity of skin and hypotension under basal conditions (up to 30% of all elderly people).

The second principle is that elderly patients delay seeking medical assistance because of altered cognition, decreased level of consciousness, impaired mobility, reclusiveness, and/or depression. This delay results in more advanced clinical deterioration in which subtle early findings will generally be lacking. When early signs of severe deterioration are present, initial management should be concurrently associated with aggressive pursuit of existing records, looking for prior similar episodes and response to previous treatment. These are the most helpful guides for ongoing care. Even when such records

are available, contacting family members is often of substantial additional value to clarify the time course of the development of symptoms and patterns of changes in function and behavior. This is particularly helpful if seizures or falls have been witnessed, fluid intake behaviour has changed, or patterns of medication intake are recorded.

The third principle is to consider any influence of medications in elderly patients. The most common drug group causing hospital admission in elderly patients is diuretics. Even low doses of these drugs can cause harm. Often secondary effects of other medications being taken concurrently worsen the clinical state (e.g., sedatives being taken when hyponatremia has produced mild confusion). Clinically, drugs that inhibit the thirst mechanism and the synthesis and release of AVP, including most of the sedatives and major tranquilizers, and drugs that inhibit the renal tubular action of AVP, especially lithium and demeclocycline, are therefore best avoided. The use of osmotic diuretics, enteral feeding containing high protein and glucose, and bowel cathartics should also be carefully monitored in the elderly. The evaluation of every older person must therefore include a careful review of all medications being taken, with appropriate adjustment of dosages made.

The fourth concern for elderly people with disorders of regulation of volume and composition of extracellular fluid is their often-narrowed homeostatic physiologic reserve. As previously discussed, this leads to "medical fragility." It is almost unique to the elderly that therapy for dehydration without careful monitoring can lead to significant volume overload. Similarly, administration of fluid or osmotic loads, such as during intravenous pyelography, may result in the rapid development of fluid overload and cardiovascular decompensation in previously apparently stable elderly people. Because there is great variation in reserve function among patients, therapy must include frequent careful monitoring for the development of adverse side-effects. If possible, full characterization of organ reserve is often warranted. This is accomplished by determining baseline creatinine clearance and renal sodium conservation in an elderly patient with modest elevation of creatinine, once stabilized during a hospital admission. Until appropriate biomarkers of reserve capacity become available, this type of testing is justified.

The final principle is to be aware of the ever-present

potential for a previously subclinical cascade of multiple pathologies to declare themselves during therapy. The development of focal neurologic signs or delirium subsequent to an episode of dehydration is more likely in the elderly because of a greater vulnerability due to compromised baseline cerebral blood flow or cognitive function. Similar concerns apply for the appearance of seizures during hypernatremia (and its correction), or ischemic limbs during volume depletion.

Hypernatremia

The incidence of severe hypernatremia among the elderly exceeds one case per hospital per month [52]. The variety of contributing causes (Tables 12.1–12.3), high mortality rate and incidence of neurologic sequelae associated with hypernatremia are striking [53]. Clinical experience suggests that institutionalized, cognitively impaired elderly individuals are very susceptible to hypernatremia. The previously discussed breakdown in thirst defense mechanisms, both in terms of sensation of thirst and access to fluids, may contribute to the water deficit (Table 12.3). The diagnostic difficulty of separating psychiatric disease from electrolyte disorders is illustrated by a report of four elderly patients admitted to a psychiatric service with symptoms of psychomotor agitation and confusion. All were found to have profound hypernatremia (mean Na^+, 162 mmol/liter) in the absence of excessive thirst, acute illness, or focal neurologic findings. Symptoms improved with correction of the free water deficit [54]. Physical restraints and excessive use of

Table 12.1 Factors associated with hypernatremia. (From Synder *et al.* [42])

Factor	Percentage of patients
Febrile illness	70
Infertility	40
Surgery	21
Nutritional supplementation	20
Intravenous solutes	18
Diabetes mellitus	15
Diarrhea	11
Gastrointestinal bleeding	9
Diuretics	9
Diabetes insipidus	7
Dialysis-related	3

Table 12.2 Causes of increased fluid loss in the elderly. (From Davis & Minaker [53])

Chronic or acute infections

Excessive urinary losses
   Diuretic misuse
   Glycosuria
   Hypercalciuria
   Mannitol
   Radiographic contrast agents
   Elevated blood urea nitrogen
   Diabetes insipidus
      Central (pituitary)
      Nephrogenic
   Hypoaldosteronism
      Addison's disease
      Hyporeninemic hypoaldosteronism
   Suppressed vasopressin
      Phenytoin
      Ethanol
      Postatrial tachyarrhythmia

Postobstructive diuresis

Gastrointestinal losses
   Upper gastrointestinal tract
      Vomiting
      Nasogastric damage
      Enteral alimentation with hypertonic fluids
   Lower gastrointestinal tract
      Laxative abuse/bowel preps
      Infectious/secretory
      Surgical bypass/fistulas
      Ischemic bowel
      Colectomy

Excessive blood loss

Environment-related fluid loss
   Heat wave
   Hypothermia

Compartmental fluid shifts
   Hypoalbuminemia
   Pancreatitis
   Ascites
   Anaphylaxis
   Burns
   Hypertonic peritoneal dialysate

sedatives and major tranquilizers probably contribute to hypodipsia among the institutionalized elderly.

Hypodipsia is commonly associated with pathology of the hypothalamus or pituitary gland [55], but exceptions

Table 12.3 Causes of decreased fluid intake in the elderly. (From Davis & Minaker [53])

Limited access to fluids
    Physical restraints
    Mobility restriction
    Poor visual acuity

Fluid restriction
    Preprocedure
    Prevention on incontinence/nocturia/aspiration
    Therapy for edema or hyponatremia

Altered sensorium
    Decreased consciousness level
        Sedatives, neuroleptics, narcotics
        Structural and metabolic central nervous system insults
        Febrile illness
    Decreased level of awareness
        Dementia, delirium
        Mania, psychosis, depression

Gastrointestinal disorders
    Swallowing disorders
    Bowel obstruction
        Mechanical
        Metabolic
        Ischemic
    Anticholinergic medication

Alteration in thirst mechanism
    Primary adipsia
    Medication-related
        Cardiac glycosides
        Amphetamines
    Associated with focal central nervous system pathology

occur [48]. Six cases of hypodipsia-induced hypernatremia have been reported in otherwise alert elderly individuals with a history of previous stroke, but no hypothalamic or pituitary pathology. The subjects, aged 68–91, were admitted with a mean plasma osmolality of 363 mosmol/liter and evidence of volume depletion. Despite such potent stimuli, none was thirsty. Mental status examinations were normal and there was no evidence of aphasia or physical inability to obtain water [48]. This intriguing report prompts consideration of alterations in thirst mechanisms of elderly patients with a variety of central nervous system diseases.

Many renal diseases impair urine-concentrating ability. Renovascular and glomerular disease accelerate the age-related decline in GFR. When GFR decreases to below 60 ml/min, urinary concentrating ability is significantly limited. Obstructive uropathy secondary to prostatic hyperthophy, chronic pyelonephritis, renal amyloidosis, and tubulointerstitial disease associated with the excretion of Bence–Jones protein in multiple myeloma are conditions frequently seen in advanced age that further reduce renal concentrating ability. Chronically ill elderly patients are also at risk for protein–calorie malnutrition and sodium depletion, both of which further reduce medullary tonicity [55]. Decreased protein intake limits the availability of urea, which constitutes 50% of medullary hypertonicity. Sodium depletion prompts enhanced proximal sodium reabsorption and limits sodium delivery to the ascending limb, where active chloride and passive sodium movement constitute the initial step in the countercurrent mechanism. Hyperosmolar hyperglycemic nonketotic coma is a consequence of uncontrolled diabetes seen almost exlusively among elderly individuals and is associated with an osmotic diuresis, hypotonic renal water losses, and frequently, hypernatremia [56].

Hypertonicity results in brain shrinkage, capillary hemorrhages, and permanent neurologic injury if deficits are severe and prolonged [53]. Failure to recognize concomitant volume deficits or overly cautious estimates of cardiovascular reserve may delay therapy. Since water distributes itself across all membranes, only 8% of infused free water remains in the intravascular space. Data on the rapidity with which hypernatremia can safely be corrected are lacking for elderly patients. Rapid correction of hypertonicity to serum osmolality of approximately 300 mosmol/kg, which can then be followed by a more gradual repletion of free water deficits over 36–48 hours, is accepted practice. If not promptly diagnosed and treated, hypernatremia leads to coma, seizures, and death [53]. In fact, in adults, acute elevation of serum sodium above 160 mmol per liter is associated with a 75% mortality. Even in the absence of death, the neurologic sequelae can be severe in the elderly. It is also important to keep in mind that mental status may recover very slowly after hyperosmolality in the elderly, even when fluid and electrolyte balance is promptly normalized. Recognition of this delay will inhibit unnecessary additional clinical testing, such as computerized axial tomography scans and the like.

Hyponatremia

Age-related alterations in the maximum diluting capacity

of the senescent kidney are less than decreases in concentrating capacity, yet hyponatremia is the most commonly encountered electrolyte disturbance among elderly individuals.

The age-related impairment in maximal diluting ability and the enhanced osmotic release of AVP are associated with a high incidence of hyponatremia in the elderly. A random sampling of 160 patients in a chronic disease facility showed that 36 patients had hyponatremia, with a mean serum sodium of 120 mmol/liter, and 27 of these patients were symptomatic [57]. Another survey of hospitalized patients in a 683-bed geriatric unit during a 10-month period revealed that 77 patients or 11% of elderly individuals were found to have serum sodium concentration of less than 130 mmol/liter. Sixty-one percent of those individuals were symptomatic or had plasma sodium concentration below 130 mmol/liter [58]. Diuretics, especially the combination of hydrochlorothiazide and amiloride, and hypotonic intravenous fluid administration caused the hyponatremia in 56 of these patients. Forty-seven of these patients were symptomatic and the mortality rate for the hyponatremic patients was twice the overall rate for the geriatric unit.

The symptoms of hyponatremia are vague and nonspecific, consisting of lethargy, confusion, agitation, weakness, and anorexia with resultant delays in diagnosis and treatment. Arieff et al. [59] have determined that symptoms are related to both the magnitude and rate of development of hyponatremia. Subclinical brain edema (which occurs after a 7% increase in brain water) can be demonstrated at sodium concentrations below 125 mmol/liter. This can result in seizures or permanent neurologic injury. Hyponatremia may be associated with symptoms outside the central nervous system. Kunze & Brown [60] reported that decrements in serum sodium concentration of 5−12% were associated with diminished carotid sinus baroreflex sensitivity in animals. As a possible clinical manifestation of this phenomenon, Caird et al. [61] have implicated hyponatremia as an etiologic factor in the postural hypotension observed among elderly individuals.

Diseases and drugs contribute significantly to the striking prevalence of hyponatremia among the elderly. Older individuals carry a disproportionate burden of illnesses associated with hypovolemic and hypervolemic hyponatremias [62]. Age has been implicated as a factor in the syndrome of idiopathic excess vasopressin secretion where volume status is generally euvolemic to slightly expanded [63]. In this syndrome, the resultant hyponatremia is attributable to "vasopressin leak" and is seen in the absence of conditions or medications commonly associated with the syndrome of inappropriate vasopressin secretion. Both anesthesia and surgery predispose older individuals to hyponatremic states. One report describes 11 elderly patients with postoperative hyponatremia caused by sustained vasopressin secretion plus the administration of hypotonic fluids [64]. In a study of chlorpropamide-induced hyponatremia in a general clinic population, advanced age was a dominant risk factor for emergence of severe hyponatremia associated with this drug [65]. In the study by Sunderam & Mankikar [58], 14% of hyponatremia cases were caused by excessive administration of intravenous hypotonic fluids.

Other conditions with protean manifestations in the elderly, such as tuberculosis and hypothyrodism, are often overlooked and are commonly associated with hyponatremia caused by excessive vasopressin secretion.

The well-known effect of thiazide diuretics to impair the renal diluting ability under normal physiologic conditions seems to be compounded in the elderly with a pre-existing renal diluting defect [34]. In addition, thiazide diuretics when used in combination with the sulfonylurea chlorpropamide, which is known to potentiate the peripheral action of vasopressin, have synergistic effects in impairing the renal diluting ability. In practice, drugs or agents that stimulate the nonosmotic release of AVP, or drugs that potentiate the renal tubular action of AVP must be therefore used with extreme caution in the elderly.

The role of diuretics, especially thiazides, in the impairment of free water excretion has been well described [66]. In one series, 64% of hyponatremic elderly patients admitted with hyponatremia had diuretics identified as the causative agent [58]. In another large series, diuretic therapy was implicated in the development of severe hyponatremia in 44% of patients older than 65 years of age [67]. Clinical observations indicate that the development of hyponatremia may be surprisingly rapid (less than 72 hours) in some apparently otherwise well elderly people after initiation of diuretics.

The associated morbidity and mortality of hyponatremia is very significant. Ashraf et al. [68] reported on seven elderly patients in good health who were placed on thiazide-like diuretics for hypertension. Within 16 days of initiating therapy, all developed profound symptomatic hyponatremia (Na^+, 105 ± 9 mmol/liter). Death (two cases) and permanent neurologic injury (two cases) resulted. Although such severe sequelae are unusual, the elderly experience them at a disproportionately high rate.

The signs and symptoms of hyponatremia are most likely related to cellular swelling and cerebral edema caused by the water movement as a result of the lowering of extracellular fluid osmolality. Patients may present with symptoms of lethargy, apathy, disorientation, muscle cramps, anorexia, nausea, or agitation, and signs ranging from depressed deep tendon reflexes to pseudo-bulbar palsy and seizures [9]. Differentiation of these symptoms from primary neurologic or psychiatric disease in the elderly is important so that one can promptly institute appropriate therapy and avoid severe neurologic sequelae, including central pontine myelinolysis.

The above evidence suggests that the first step in treating elderly patients with hyponatremia is the discontinuation of medications or intravenous fluids that are frequent accompaniments of this condition. Proper therapeutic measures, such as fluid restriction or low-dose demeclocycline (300 mg once or twice daily), can then be used. The impressive morbidity and mortality that accompany severe hyponatremia (Na < 120 mmol/liter), particularly among the elderly, warrant an aggressive initial approach using hypertonic saline to increase serum sodium above 125 mmol/liter.

Altered potassium balance

Hypokalemia and hyperkalemia are frequent accompaniments of acute or chronic illness in the elderly, and are often precipitated by or aggravated by administration of medications. The presence of a renal acidification defect, and a decreased activity of the renin–angiotensin–aldosterone system may be the cause of the increased incidence of Type 4 renal tubule acidosis, or the syndrome of hyporeninemic hypoaldosteronism in the elderly. In addition, largely because of the age-related reduction in GFR, the elderly are also at increased risk for developing hyperkalemia with potassium-sparing diuretics, including triamterene, aldactone, and amiloride, as well as drugs that inhibit the renin–angiotensin system, especially nonsteroidal anti-inflammatory agents, β-blockers, converting enzyme inhibitors, heparin, and cyclosporine

[69–71]. One often overlooked but important cause of hyperkalemia in the elderly is modest gastrointestinal bleeding. The high potassium content of erythrocytes can lead to substantial intestinal potassium absorption which overwhelms the impaired capacity of the aging kidney to execute potassium especially when RBF is further impaired subsequent to the blood loss. While management of potassium imbalance in the elderly is similar to that in younger adults, special attention must be paid to elimination of any offending medications, careful testing for gastrointestinal bleeding, and awareness of the tendency of the elderly to "overshoot" during potassium repletion for hypokalemia with resultant hyperkalemia.

References

1 Epstein M, Hollenberg NK. Age as a determinant of renal sodium conservation in normal man. J Lab Clin Med 1976; 11–417.

2 Macias-Nuñez JF, Garcia-Iglesias C, Bonda-Roman A, et al. Renal handling of sodium in old people: A functional study. Age Ageing 1978;7:178–181.

3 Anderson GH, Springer J, Randall P, et al. Effect of age on diagnostic usefulness of stimulated plasma renin activity and saralasin test in detection of renovascular hypertension. Lancet 1980;II:821–824.

4 Crane MG, Harris JJ. Effect of aging on renin activity and aldosterone excretion. J Lab Clin Med 1976;87:947.

5 Cugini P, Murano G, Lucia P, et al. The gerontologic decline of the renin–aldosterone system: A chronobiological approach extended to essential hypertension. J Gerontol 1987; 42:461–465.

6 Hall JE, Coleman TG, Guyton AC. The renin–angiotensin system normal physiology and changes in older hypertensives. JAGS 1989;37:801–813.

7 Tsunoda K, Abe K, Goto T, et al. Effect of age on the renin–angiotensin–aldosterone system in normal subjects: Simultaneous measurement of active and inactive renin, renin substrate, and aldosterone in plasma. J Clin Endocrinol Metab 1986;62:384–389.

8 Weidmann P, De Myttenaere-Bursztein S, Maxwell MH, et al. Effect of aging on plasma renin and aldosterone in normal man. Kidney Int 1975;8:325–333.

9 Flood C, Gherondache C, Pincus G, et al. The metabolism and secretion of aldosterone in elderly subjects. J Clin Invest 1967;46:960–966.

10 Weidmann P, de Chatel R, Schiffmann A, et al. Interrelations between age and plasma renin, aldosterone and cortisol, urinary catecholamines, and the body sodium/volume state in normal man. Klin Wochenschr 1977;55:725–733.

11 Macias-Nuñez JF, Garcia-Iglesias C, Tabernero-Romo JM,

et al. Renal management of sodium under indomethacin and aldosterone in the elderly. Age Ageing 1980;9:165−172.

12 Luft FC, Fineberg NS, Miller JZ, *et al.* The effects of age, race, and heredity on glomerular filtration rate following volume expansion and contraction in normal man. Am J Med Sci 1980;279:15−24.

13 Luft FC, Weinberger MH, Grim CE. Sodium sensitivity and resistance in normotensive humans. Am J Med 1982;72: 726−736.

14 Luft FC, Weinberger MH, Fineberg MS, *et al.* Effects of age on renal sodium homeostasis and its relevance to sodium sensitivity. Am J Med 1987;82(Suppl. 1B):9−15.

15 Bengele HH, Mathias RS, Alexander EA. Impaired natriuresis after volume expansion in the aged rat. Renal Physiol Biochem 1981;4:22−29.

16 Friedman SA, Friedman CL. Salt and water balance in aging rats. Gerontologia 1957;1:107−121.

17 Galbusera M, Garattini S, Remuzzi G, *et al.* Catecholamine receptor binding in rat kidney: Effect of aging. Kidney Int 1988;33:1073−1077.

18 Brenner BM, Ballersmann BJ, Gunning ME, *et al.* Diverse biological actions of atrial natriuretic peptide. Physiol Rev 1990;70:665−599.

19 Weidmann P, Hasler L, Gnadinger MP, *et al.* Blood levels and renal effects of atrial natriuretic peptide in normal man. J Clin Invest 1986;77:734−742.

20 Volpe M, Odell G, Kleinert HD, *et al.* Antihypertensive and aldosterone lowering effects of synthetic atrial natriuretic factor in renin-dependent renovascular hypertension. J Hypertens 1984;2:313−315.

21 Goodfriend TL, Elliot ME, Atlas SA. Actions of synthetic atrial natriuretic factor on bovine adrenal glomerulosa. Life Sci 1984;35:1675−1682.

22 Clark BA, Elahi D, Fish L, *et al.* Atrial natriuretic peptide suppresses osmostimulated vasopressin release in young and elderly man. Am J Physiol 1991;261:E252−E256.

23 Ohashi M, Gujio N, Nawata H, *et al.* High plasma concentration of human atrial natriuretic peptide in aged man. J Clin Endocrinol Metab 1987;64:81−86.

24 McKnight JA, Roberts G, Sheridan B, *et al.* Aging and atrial natriuretic factor. J Hum Hypertens 1990;4:53−56.

25 Davis KM, Fish LC, Ten Cate AJ, *et al.* Determinants of basal atrial natriuretic peptide (ANP) in the institutionalized elderly. Gerontologist 1989;29:A6.

26 Clark BA, Fish LC, Davis KM, *et al.* Resistance to atrial natriuretic peptide (ANP) induced sodium excretion (NaXR) in the elderly. Gerontologist 1988;28:A141.

27 Davis KM, Fish LC, Clark BA, *et al.* Atrial natriuretic peptide (ANP) levels predict risk for congestive heart failure (CHF) in frail elderly. Gerontologist 1990;30:A44.

28 Dontas AS, Marketos S, Papanayioutou P. Mechanisms of renal tubular defects in old age. Postgrad Med J 1972;48: 295−303.

29 Lindeman RD, Lee TD, Jiengst MJ, *et al.* Influence of age, renal disease, hypertension, diuretics, and calcium on the antidiuretic responses to suboptimal infusions of vasopressin. J Lab Clin Med 1966;68:206−223.

30 Lindeman RD, VanBuren HC, Raisz LG. Osmolar renal concentrating ability in healthy young men and hospitalized patients without renal disease. N Engl J Med 1960;262: 1306−1309.

31 Rowe JW, Shock NW, DeFronzo RA. The influence of age on the renal response to water deprivation in man. Nephron 1976;17:270−278.

32 Helderman JH, Vestal RE, Rowe JW, *et al.* The response of arginine vasopressin to intravenous ethanol and hypertonic saline in man: The impact of aging. J Gerontol 1978;33:39−47.

33 Miller JH, Shock NW. Age differences in the renal tubular response to antidiuretic hormone. J Gerontol 1953;8: 446−450.

34 Rowe JW, Minaker KL, Sparrow D, *et al.* Age-related failure of volume-pressure-mediated vasopressin release. J Clin Endocrinol Metab 1982;661−664.

35 Hollenberg NK, Adams DF, Solomon HS, *et al.* Senescence and the renal vasculature in normal man. Circ Res 1974;34: 309−316.

36 Bengele HH, Mathias RS, Perkins JH, *et al.* Urinary concentrating defect in the aged rat. Am J Physiol 1981:F147−F150.

37 Beck N, Yu BP. Effect of aging on urinary concentrating mechanism and vasopressin-dependent cAMP in rats. Am J Physiol 1982;243:F121−F125.

38 Goddard C, Davidson YS, Moser BB, *et al.* Effect of aging on cyclic AMP output by renal medullary cells in response to arginine vasopressin *in vitro* in C57 BL/Icrfa mice. J Endocrinol 1984;103:133−139.

39 Handelmann GE, Sayson SC. Neonatal exposure to vasopressin decreases binding sites in the adult kidney. Peptides 1984;5:1217−1224.

40 Miller M. Increased vasopressin secretion: An early manifestation of aging in the rat. J Gerontol 1987;42:3−12.

41 Davidson YS, Davies I, Goddard C. Renal vasopressin receptors in aging C57 BL/Icrfa mice. J Endocrinol 1987;115: 379−385.

42 Snyder NA, Feigal DW, Arieff AI. Hypernatremia in elderly patients. Ann Intern Med 1987;107:309−319.

43 Miller PD, Krebs RA, Neal BJH, *et al.* Hypodipsia in geriatric patients. Am J Med 1982;73:354−356.

44 Phillips PA, Phil D, Rolls BJ, *et al.* Reduced thirst after water deprivation in healthy elderly men. N Engl J Med 1984; 311:753−759.

45 Minaker KL, Fish LC, Rowe JW. Altered thirst threshold during hypertonic stress in aging man. Gerontologist 1985; 25:A118.

46 Murphy DJ, Minaker KL, Fish LC, *et al.* Impaired osmostimulation of water ingestion delays recovery from hyperosmolarity in normal elderly. Gerontologist 1988;28:A141.

47 McAloon-Dyke M, David KM, Ckark BA, *et al*. Age-related failure to defend against hypertonicity. Gerontologist 1990; 30:A183.

48 Miller PD, Krebs RA, Neal BS, *et al*. Hypodipsia in geriatric patients. Am J Med 1982;73:354−356.

49 Crowe MJ, Forsling ML, Rolls BJ, *et al*. Altered water excretion in healthy elderly man. Age Aging 1987;16:285−293.

50 Rosa RM, Silva P, Young JB, *et al*. Adrenergic modulation of extrarenal potassium disposal. N Engl J Med 1980;302:431−433.

51 Minaker KL, Rowe JW. Potassium homeostasis during hyperinsulinemia: effect of insulin level, β-blockade, and age. Am Physiol Soc 1982;E373−E377.

52 Zierler KL. Hyperosmolders of water metabolism. Kidney Int 1976;10:117−132.

53 Davis KM, Minaker KL. Disorders of fluid and electrolyte balance. Princ Geriatr Med Gerontol 1990;110:1079−1083.

54 Jana DK, Romano-Jana L. Hypernatremic psychosis in the elderly: Case reports. J Am Geriatr Soc 1973;21:473−477.

55 Berl T, Anderson RJ, McDonald K, *et al*. Clinical disorders of water metabolism. Kidney Int 1976;10:117−132.

56 Arieff AI, Carroll HJ. Nonketotic hyperosmolar coma with hyperglycemia. Medicine (Baltimore) 1972;51:73−94.

57 Kleinfeld M, Casimur M, Borra A. Hyponatremia as observed in a chronic disease facility. J Am Geriatr Soc 1979;27:156−161.

58 Sunderam SG, Mankikar GD. Hyponatremia in the elderly. Age Ageing 1983;12:77−80.

59 Arieff AI, Llach F, Massry S. Neurologic manifestations and morbidity of hyponatremia: Correlation with brain waical of age on the renal response to water deprivation in man. Nephron 1976;17:270−278.

60 Kunze DL, Brown AM. Sodium sensitivity of baroreceptors. Circ Res 1978;42:714−720.

61 Caird FI, Andrews GR, Kennedy RD. Effect of posture on blood pressure in the elderly. Br Heart J 1973;35:527−530.

62 Narins RG, Jones ER, Stom MC, *et al*. Diagnostic strategies in disorders of fluid, electrolyte, and acid base homeostasis. Am J Med 1982;72:496−520.

63 Goldstein CS, Braunstein S, Goldfarb S. Idiopathic syndrome of inappropriate antidiuretic hormone secretion possibly related to advanced age. Ann Intern Med 1983;99:185−188.

64 Deutsch S, Goldberg M, Dripps RD. Postoperative hyponatremia with inappropriate release of antidiuretic hormone. Anesthesiology 1966;27:250−256.

65 Weissman P, Shenkman L, Gregerman R. Chlorpropramide hyponatremia. N Engl J Med 1971;284:65−71.

66 Zanuszewicz W, Heinemann H, Demartini F. A clinical study of effects of hydrochlorothiazide on renal excretion of electrolytes and free water. N Engl J Med 1959;261:264−269.

67 Fichman M, Vorherr H, Kleeman G. Diuretic-induced hyponatremia. Ann Intern Med 1971;75:853−863.

68 Ashraf N, Locksley R, Arieff A. Thiazide-induced hyponatremia associated with death or neurologic damage in outpatients. Am J Med 1981;70:1163−1168.

69 Meier DE, Myers WM, Swenson R, *et al*. Indomethacin-associated hyperkalemia in the elderly. J Am Geriatr Soc 1983;31:371−373.

70 Mor R, Pitilk S, Rosenfeld JB. Indomethacin- and moduretic-induced hyperkalemia. Isr J Med Sci 1983;19:535−537.

71 Walmsley RN, White GH, Cain M, *et al*. Hyperkalemia in the elderly. Clin Chem 1984;30:1409−1412.

13

Renal acidification and metabolic acidosis in the elderly

Stephen H. Norris
Neil A. Kurtzman

This article summarizes our current understanding of normal renal acidification, clinical tests of renal acidification, the evidence for an age-related renal acidification defect, and the pathophysiology, diagnosis, and treatment of the metabolic acidoses most prevalent in the geriatric population, with clinical examples of each.

In addition to renal acidification, aging affects all aspects of renal function [1–9]. It is associated with progressive reduction of renal blood flow (RBF) and glomerular filtration rate (GFR) [10–12], impaired urinary concentration and dilution [13–16], and reduced sodium conservation [17]. Similarly, tubular transport of glucose [18], amylase [19], and diodrast are decreased [10]. The clinical sequelae of acidosis are listed in Table 13.1.

Mechanisms of normal renal acidification

Proximal acidification and bicarbonate reclamation
(Fig. 13.1)
Proximal sodium reabsorption drives a Na-H exchanger on the apical (luminal) brush border membrane. About 80% of proximal acidification is therefore sodium-dependent [20]. Filtered bicarbonate meeting secreted hydrogen ions forms carbonic acid (H_2CO_3). H_2CO_3 is rapidly dehydrated to carbon dioxide (CO_2) by carbonic anhydrase on the apical membrane [21]. Inside the cell, CO_2 is again hydrated to H_2CO_3, H, and bicarbonate. Intracellular H is resecreted via the apical Na–H exchanger and bicarbonate enters the blood via a basolateral $Na–HCO_3$ cotransporter [22]. Under basal conditions virtually all filtered bicarbonate (~4000 mmol/day) is reclaimed by urinary acidification before reaching the distal nephron — 90% in the proximal tubule and 10% in the distal nephron. Bicarbonate reclamation and proximal acidification are stimulated by volume contraction, potassium and chloride depletion, decreased filtrate flow, metabolic acidosis, hypoparathyroidism, hypercalcemia (independent of parathyroid hormone (PTH) or vitamin D), increased circulating 1,25-$(OH)_2$-cholecalciferol (independent of PTH or plasma calcium), hypercapnea, hyperphosphatemia, and possibly hyperthyroidism. Because bicarbonate reclamation varies directly with fractional sodium reabsorption, there is no absolute tubular maximum (Tm) for bicarbonate. Under basal conditions (i.e., normal plasma bicarbonate, P_{aCO_2}, potassium, and volume) the Tm bicarbonate range is 24–28 mmol/liter in adults and 20–24 mmol/liter in children.

Table 13.1 Clinical sequelae of acidosis

Acute	Chronic
Hyperkalemia (mineral acidoses)	Impaired erythrocyte glycolysis and decreased 2,3-diphosphoglycerate
Hypercalcemia	
Protein wasting from antianabolic glucocorticoids increased muscle branched-chain ketoacid dehydrogenase increased decarboxylation of valine and leucine	Bony demineralization
	Malaise
	Fatigue
Inhibition of organic acid synthesis	
Increased catecholamine secretion	
Increased glucocorticoid secretion	
Hyperaldosteronism	
Hyperreninism	
Hypovolemia	
Increased pulmonary vascular resistance	
Diminished O_2–hemoglobin affinity	
Hyperventilation (Kussmaul breathing)	
Increased proximal Na^+ reabsorption	
Hyperuricemia (organic acidoses)	
Depressed myocardial contractility (pH < 7.20)	
Arteriolar dilatation	
Venular constriction	
Decreased myocardial response to catecholamines	
Tachycardia (mild acidosis)	
Bradycardia (pH < 7.10)	

Renal ammoniagenesis

Fifty to a hundred millimoles of "new" bicarbonate must be generated daily by the kidneys to replace buffer consumed by the fixed metabolic acids (sulfate and hydrochloric) produced by hepatic protein metabolism (Fig. 13.2). Because nearly all proximal acidification is expended in reclaiming filtered bicarbonate, most of this "new" bicarbonate must be generated in the proximal nephron by ammoniagenesis (NH_4^+, 40–200 mmol/day) [23] or in the distal nephron by titration of divalent phosphate (HPO_4^{-2}, 10 mmol/day) [24]. In the proximal tubule, glutamine delivery, mitochondrial glutamine entry, and α-ketoglutarate dehydrogenose, the rate-limiting step in renal ammonia-genesis, are pH-dependent (Fig. 13.3). Systemic acidosis and hypokalemia both produce intracellular acidosis that stimulates glutamine transport. In the mitochondria of the proximal tubular epithelium a mole of glutamine is metabolized to two moles of ammonia and bicarbonate. Removal of H from the body in the form of urinary NH_4^+ allows the bicarbonate generated by renal ammoniagenesis to replace the body's buffer deficit (Fig. 13.2). Any ammonia that escapes trapping and excretion in the urine is reabsorbed, returns to the liver, produces acid in the urea cycle, and may generate or perpetuate metabolic acidosis.

Distal acidification

Urinary ammonia trapping and excretion are dependent on distal acidification. About two-thirds of proximately secreted NH_4^+ is reabsorbed in the thick ascending limb (Fig. 13.4) and NH_4^+ dissociates to $NH_3 + H^+$. The H^+ is resecreted into the thick ascending limb and forms H_2CO_3 with the remaining 400 mmol of filtered bicarbonate, which is then reclaimed in the cortex. Medullary interstitial NH_3 is anionically resecreted into the descending limb (the countercurrent multiplier) and collecting tubules (the medullary ammonia shunt), where it buffers distally secreted protons, is trapped in the urine, and excreted as NH_4^+. Ammonia can therefore be excreted only if distal acidification, principally in the collecting tubule, is intact. Increasing or slowing the rate of distal proton secretion thereby causes the plasma bicarbonate (and pH) to rise or fall proportionally. Distal acidification (Fig. 13.5) is stimulated by increased urinary buffer (e.g., renal ammoniagenesis), distal delivery (e.g., sodium loading, volume expansion, or diuretic administration), metabolic acidosis, poorly reabsorbable anions (e.g., sulfate or phosphate), decreased potassium secretion, the electrical gradient or potential difference across the epithelium (increased by distal sodium reabsorption), mineralocorticoid activity, apical membrane proton ATPase activity, bicarbonate secretion, potassium depletion, and chloride depletion [25].

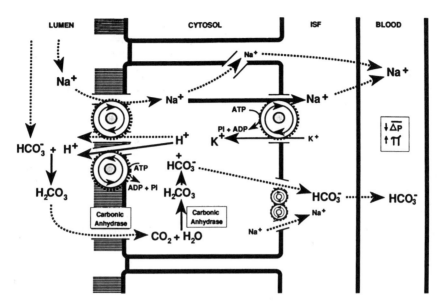

Fig. 13.1 Proximal acidification and reclamation of filtered HCO_3. Eighty percent of filtered Na^+ entering the proximal tubular cell does so via a brush border $Na^+ - H^+$ exchanger. One-third of intracellular Na^+ exits the cell passively, driven by high oncotic pressure (π) and low hydraulic pressure (ΔP) in the peritubular capillaries. These changes in the transtubular starling forces are brought about by diminished renal perfusion that stimulates angiotenisin II-mediated efferent arteriolar vasoconstriction. Two-thirds of intracellular Na^+ is actively transported by basolateral $Na^+ - K^+ - ATPase$ regardless of transtubular starling forces. Filtered HCO_3^- and secreted H^+ form luminal H_2CO_3, which is rapidly dehydrated to CO_2 by brush border carbonic anhydrase. Intracellular CO_2 is rehydrated to H^+ and HCO_3^-. Protons are secreted in exchange for Na^+ while reclaimed bicarbonate exits the cell via a basolateral Na^+-HCO_3^- cotransporter.

Conditions associated with antinatriuresis stimulate proximal acidification and HCO_3 reclamation and may thus produce or perpetuate metabolic alkalosis: e.g., severe volume contraction, congestive heart failure, hypoalbuminemia, hepatic cirrhosis, shock states, renal ischemia, urinary tract obstruction, acute glomerulonephritis, cellular dehydration, hypercalcemia, or severe depletion of potassium or chloride. Conditions that reduce proximal sodium reabsorption (e.g., Fanconi's syndrome) or reduce proximal acidification (e.g., acetazolamide) may lower the T_mHCO_3 below 22 mmol/liter, and induce bicarbonate wasting and hypokalemic, hyperchloremic metabolic acidosis (proximal renal tubular acidosis).

Clinical tests of distal acidification

Partial pressure of urinary CO_2 (U-P_{CO_2}) during bicarbonate loading

The distal tubular epithelium does not have carbonic anhydrase on its apical membrane. When distal bicarbonate delivery is increased by $NaHCO_3$ infusion (3 ml/min of a 1 M solution) to increase bicarbonaturia to <80 mmol/liter and urine pH > 7.8, a large proportion of H secreted in the collecting tubules is buffered by bicarbonate. Carbonic acid formed in the collecting tubule slowly dehydrates to CO_2 nonenzymatically in the terminal portions of the collecting system where the surface/volume relationship does not favor CO_2 reabsorption. The urine P_{CO_2} rises to 70 mmHg or greater and exceeds the blood P_{CO_2} by more than 30 mmHg during bicarbonaturia, as long as urinary acidification is intact [26].

U-P_{CO_2} during phosphate infusion

In highly alkaline urine (pH > 7.8), almost all phosphate is in its alkaline monohydric form (HPO_4^{-2}) and incapable of donating protons to bicarbonate. Inorganic phosphate (Pi, $HPO_4^{-2}/H_2PO_4^-$) both consumes and donates protons when the urine pH is near its pK, 6.8. When an infusion of $NaHCO_3$ raises the urine pH to only 6.8, the urine contains sufficient bicarbonate to generate CO_2, provided acidification is stimulated, but the urinary bicarbonate *per se* does not raise the U-P_{CO_2} as it does when the urine

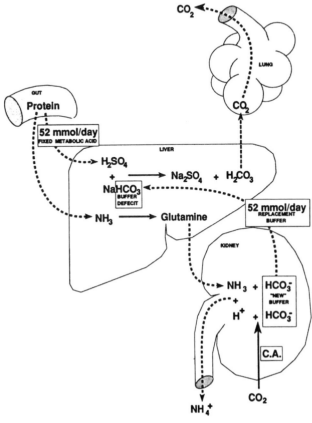

Fig. 13.2 Proton homeostasis via the hepatic−pulmonary−renal axis. The average acid−ash diet consumed in North America contains approximately 1 mol of amino acid residues that generate a net excess of about 52 mmol/day (range 0−100 mmol/day) of fixed metabolic (i.e., sulfuric and hydrochloric) acid. Unlike weak organic acids, "fixed" mineral acids are unable to regenerate bicarbonate *in situ* and thus create an equimolar buffer defect that must be replaced by "new" bicarbonate generated in the kidneys. Ammonia (NH_3) not utilized in the hepatic urea cycle is converted to glutamine. In the renal proximal tubule glutamine is reconverted to NH_3 and bicarbonate. Renally generated NH_3 is trapped in the urine as poorly reabsorbable ammonium ion (NH_4^+) by distal acidification. Excretion of renally generated ammonium allows the bicarbonate generated by renal glutamine metabolism to replace the buffer defect created by protein metabolism and thus maintains acid−base balance.

pH is >7.8 (see above). At a pH of 6.8, half of the urinary phosphate is in its acid dihydric form ($H_2PO_4^-$), capable of donating H to bicarbonate and forming CO_2. Neutral phosphate (1 mmol/liter total body water dissolved in

180 ml of 0.9% NaCl) is infused at a rate of 1 ml/min for 3 hours while 1 M $NaHCO_3$ is infused at a rate sufficient to raise the urine pH to 6.8 ± 0.5. This usually results in a two- to three-fold rise in plasma phosphate, raises urine phosphate to at least 20 mmol/liter, and increases U-P_{CO_2} to >70 mmHg, as long as distal acidification is intact [26].

Urine pH during sulfate infusion

As long as distal delivery is adequate and sodium reabsorption is avid (insured by administering 0.1 mg 9-α-fludrocortisone 12 hours prior to the test), infusion of 500 ml of 4% Na_2SO_4 over an hour induces a marked increase in the lumen-negative cortical collecting tubule transepithelial electrical gradient by delivering sodium accompanied by poorly reabsorbable anion. During sulfate loading voltage-enhanced distal acidification and potassium secretion cause the urinary ammonium and potassium to rise and the urinary pH to fall to <5.5 (usually <5.0) in subjects with intact distal acidification [25].

Urinary pH and U-P_{CO_2} after oral furosemide

The furosemide test has largely replaced the classical tests of urinary acidification (i.e., ammonium or calcium chloride loading or sodium bicarbonate, phosphate, or sulfate infusion) in most clinical situations because of its convenience, safety, and reliability. It avoids the side-effects and time required for acid loading, multiple-timed urine collections, and prolonged intravenous infusions. Furosemide primarily blocks chloride reabsorption through an apical Na−K−2Cl symporter in the thick ascending limb. Furosemide increases distal urine flow and sodium delivery and may also block chloride channels in the distal nephron. Increased distal sodium reabsorption increases the cortical collecting tubule transepithelial potential difference that facilitates distal acidification and potassium secretion [27]. In subjects with intact distal acidification the pH of urine collected under mineral oil 1−2 hours after a single 40 mg oral dose of furosemide falls to less than 5.5, the U−P_{CO_2} is <30 mmHg, and the urine/blood P_{CO_2} gradient (U−BP_{CO_2}) is negative [28].

Urinary anion gap

The amount of free H^+ (titratable acid) in the urine is small (~10 mmol/day) and collecting duct epithelia are incapable of maintaining a urine pH below 4.3. The total

Fig. 13.3 Renal ammoniagenesis. In the proximal tubule hepatically generated glutamine crosses the basolateral membrane via a pH-dependent transporter. Glutamine entry, the rate-limiting step in renal ammoniagenesis, is stimulated by hypokalemia and systemic acidosis, both of which induce intracellular acidosis. Renal ammoniagenesis is conversely inhibited by both hyperkalemia and systemic alkalosis. In the mitochondria glutamine is deaminated to glutamate and thence to α-ketoglutarate (α-KG). Through the Krebs cycle α-KG is metabolized to CO_2 and malate, which enters the cytososol to be incorporated into glucose via its three-carbon precursor, phosphoenolpyruvate. The CO_2 thus generated is hydrated to HCO_3^- and H^+. Ammonia and H^+ form ammonium ion (NH_4^+), which is secreted via a brush border Na–H exchanger, while the HCO_3 enters the blood via basolateral Na–HCO_3 cotransporter.

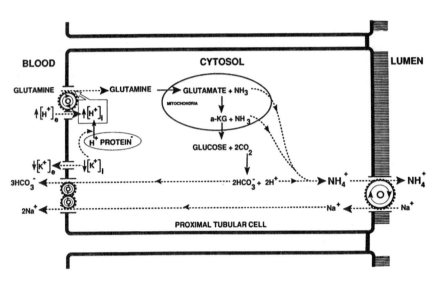

Fig. 13.4 Renal ammonium excretion. Most of the 40–200 mmol/day of NH_4^+ generated and secreted proximally is reabsorbed in the thick ascending limb through the potassium channels of the Na–K–2Cl cotransporter and by nonionic diffusion as NH_3. From the medullary interstitium NH_3 is resecreted into the thin descending loop (the countercurrent multiplier) and into the collecting tubule, where it becomes the major urinary buffer. Trapped in the collecting tubule as poorly reabsorbable NH_4^+, renally generated ammonia is excreted in the urine as long as distal acidification is intact. Whenever distal acidification is impaired, however, a portionate amount of ammonia is reabsorbed and returned to the liver, where it generates acid in the urea cycle.

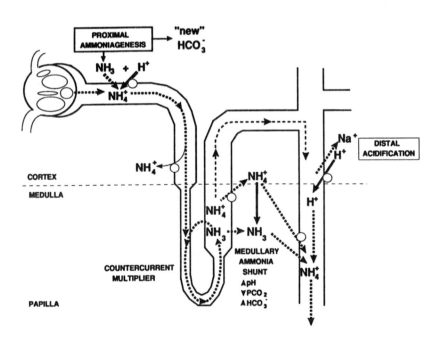

amount of acid excreted in the urine is the sum of urinary ammonium (40–200 mmol/day) plus titratable acid (mostly phosphoric), less any urinary bicarbonate (derived by the Henderson–Hasslebalch equation from urinary pH and P_{CO_2}). The H^+ contained in nonphosphate buffer (e.g., uric acid or creatinine) is inconsequential. Measuring the urine pH (i.e., titratable acid) alone may thus give a false impression of distal acidification (see

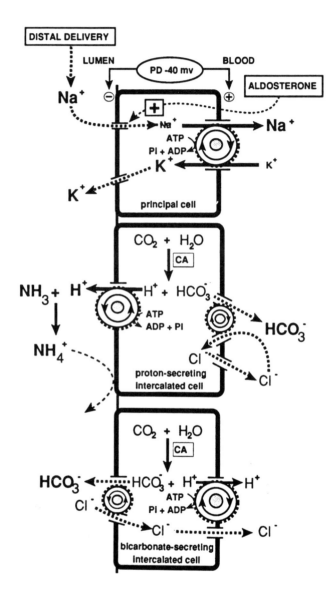

Fig. 13.5 Distal urinary acidification and tubular acidosis (dRTA). Reabsorption of Na$^+$ delivered to principal cells in the cortical collecting tubules is facilitated by an aldosterone-stimulated increase in apical, amiloride-sensitive Na$^+$ ion channels. Sodium flux, driven by basolateral Na$-$K$-$ATPase, generates a lumen-negative transepithelial potential difference (TPD) of about 40 mV under basal conditions. K$^+$ is passively secreted down its electrochemical gradient and H$^+$ is actively secreted from intercalated cells by luminal proton ATPase (the H$^+$ pump). Distal secretion of both K$^+$ and H$^+$ (i.e., hypokalemic alkalosis) may be facilitated by increasing distal solute delivery (e.g., diuretics), hyperaldosteronism, poorly reabsorbable anion (e.g., carbenicillin), and by severe potassium and chloride depletion.

Hypokalemic, pump-dependent dRTA with urine pH > 5.5 (i.e., diminished electromotive force of the H$^+$ pump) may be associated with familial Type I dRTA, chronic renal allograft rejection, collagen-vascular diseases, or toluene poisoning. Hypokalemic, gradient-dependent dRTA with urine pH > 5.5 (i.e., H$^+$ backleak) is only associated with amphotericin B nephrotoxicity.

Hyperkalemic, voltage-dependent dRTA (urine pH > 5.5) may be induced by decreased Na$-$K$-$ATPase activity (e.g., urinary tract obstruction or sickle cell anemia), or toxic doses of amiloride or lithium.

In states of decreased mineralocorticoid activity reduced Na$^+$ flux and TPD cause a mild form of hyperkalemic dRTA. Hypomineralocorticism and hyperkalemia diminish ammoniagenesis, reduce urinary buffer capacity, and further impair distal acidification while the urinary pH is appropriately low (<5.5). Type IV dRTA may be caused by hyporeninism (e.g., diabetes mellitus or cyclooxygenase inhibition), acetazolamide, selective hypoaldosteronism (e.g., ACE inhibitors, β-adrenergic receptor blockade, hypoinsulinism, or heparin administration), adrenal insufficiency (e.g., Addisonian crisis), or aldosterone resistance due to tubulointerstitial nephropathies.

discussion of diarrhea, below). In the absence of other unmeasured cation (e.g., lithium), the urine anion gap is a fair estimate of the urinary buffer capacity (i.e., ammonium).

In subjects with hyperchloremic metabolic acidosis, a negative urinary anion gap ([Na$^+$] + [K$^+$] − [Cl$^-$] <0) indicates normal ammonia generation and excretion, urinary buffer capacity, and distal acidification. In these subjects acidosis may be caused by gastrointestinal buffer losses (e.g., diarrhea), renal buffer losses (e.g., proximal tubular acidosis or administration of a carbonic anhydrase inhibitor), or exogenous mineral acid (e.g., administration of HCl, argenine HCl, or ammonium HCl). On the other hand, a positive urinary anion gap ([Na$^+$] + [K$^+$] − [Cl$^-$] >0) in an acidotic subject indicates deficient urinary ammonium but cannot distinguish a primary defect in buffer production/excretion from a primary defect in distal acidification that secondarily prevents trapping and excretion of urinary ammonia. Both urinary anion gap and pH are required to distinguish between the various defects of distal acidification [29].

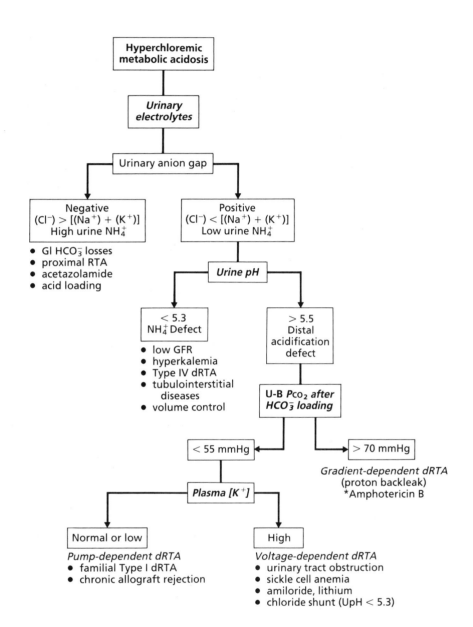

Fig. 13.6 Diagnostic algorithm for hyperchloremic metabolic acidosis.

Diagnostic algorithm for hyperchloremic metabolic acidosis (Fig. 13.6)

To determine whether hyperchloremia and hypobicarbonatemia are caused by normal anion gap metabolic acidosis, rather than dehydration and/or chronic respiratory alkalosis, obtain an arterial or arterialized capillary blood gas and correct the plasma chloride for hypernatremia, if any, by multiplying by (140/plasma [Na] >145 mmol/liter). In subjects with hyperchloremic metabolic acidosis a negative urinary anion gap ($[Na^+] + [K^+] - [Cl^-] < 0$) indicates normal ammonia generation and excretion, urinary buffer capacity, and distal acidification. In these subjects acidosis may be caused by gastrointestinal buffer losses (e.g., diarrhea), renal buffer losses (e.g., proximal tubular acidosis or administration of acetazolamide), or exogenous mineral acid (e.g., administration of HCl, argenine HCl, or ammonium HCl). On the other hand, a positive urinary anion gap ($[Na^+] +

$[K^+] - [Cl^-] > 0$) in an acidotic subject indicates deficient urinary ammonium but does not distinguish a primary defect in buffer production/excretion from a primary defect in distal acidification that secondarily prevents trapping and excretion of urinary ammonia. Both the urinary anion gap and pH are required to distinguish between the various defects of distal acidification [29]. When the urinary anion gap is positive in a subject with hyperchloremic metabolic acidosis a urinary pH < 5.3 is indicative of inadequate buffer production/excretion with intact acidification (e.g., renal failure, primary hyperkalemia, tubulointerstitial nephropathy, adrenal failure, selective aldosterone deficiency, or aldosterone resistance). A urinary pH > 5.5 suggests that inadequate buffer excretion may be caused by defective distal acidification. With a urinary pH > 5.5 and $U-P_{CO_2}$ > 70 mmHg after bicarbonate loading, H^+ backleak (e.g., amphoterecin B toxicity) is likely. When the $U-P_{CO_2}$ after bicarbonate loading is < 55 mmHg and the serum potassium is normal or low, pump-dependent distal renal tubular acidosis (dRTA) is likely (e.g., familial Type I dRTA, autoimmune diseases, toluene poisoning, or chronic renal allograft rejection). When the $U-P_{CO_2}$ is < 55 mmHg and the serum potassium is elevated, voltage-dependent dRTA is likely (e.g., sickle cell anemia, urinary tract obstruction, or amiloride or lithium toxicity).

Aging and renal acidification

Elderly individuals maintain normal acid−base balance under resting conditions [30]. With acid loading, however, an age-dependent renal acidification defect has been revealed [31−34]. Nephron loss was implicated in this phenomenon by one study because the GFR of elderly subjects was half that of young controls [33], although a decrease in GFR *per se* does not affect acidification. In another study of six healthy elderly male subjects (mean age 73, range 63−86 years) creatinine clearance (76 ± 14 ml/min per 1.73 m^2) and base-line acid−base balance and urinary acid excretion did not differ significantly from 29- to 35-year-old controls [34]. After acid loading with ammonium chloride the lowest urine pH achieved by the elderly group was 4.93 ± 0.07 (4.5 ± 0.14 in controls, $P < 0.02$), net acid excretion was 47.3 ± 7.26 μmol/min (78.6 ± 3.5 μmol/min in controls, $P < 0.01$), and net ammonia excretion was 26.0 ± 5.6 (47.8 ± 2.6 in controls, $P < 0.01$). Correcting ammonia excretion

for GFR, the difference was still significant (33.7 ± 2.4 μmol/min vs. 51.2 ± 8.7 μmol/min, $P < 0.05$), although titratable acid excretion corrected for GFR did not differ significantly between elderly and youthful groups. A group of five subjects aged 35−60 showed intermediate values. Other studies [35,36] have shown that aldosterone production declines with age. Mild hypoaldosteronism better explains the progressive, age-dependent hypoammoniagenesis disclosed by acid loading. Although not clinically relevant under basal conditions, diminished capacity to buffer and excrete an acid load might predispose elderly people to metabolic acidosis, should they be subjected to conditions that increase the acid load or further impair urinary acidification. Conditions most likely to produce overt metabolic acidosis in elderly patients include diarrhea, urinary tract obstruction, additional aldosterone deficiency or resistance, and renal failure.

Diarrhea

Of all the causes of hyperchloremic metabolic acidosis, diarrhea is the one most prevalent at any age. Each day 500−4000 ml of acidic gastric chyme, containing 25−520 mmol H^+, 40 mmol sodium, 4−70 mmol potassium, and 7−630 mmol chloride, is extensively modified during its passage through the small intestine [37]. Enterocytes absorb sodium and secrete H^+ via a brush border cation exchanger (Fig. 13.7). Chloride and bicarbonate traverse the brush border via an anion exchanger. The direction of specific anion flux in the various bowel segments depends on the interplay of basolateral Na−K−ATPase and Na−K−2Cl cotransport with selective permeability of the apical membrane to intracellular chloride. Chloride is secreted in the duodenum and jejunum and absorbed in the ileum and colon, whereas bicarbonate is absorbed in the duodenum and jejunum and secreted in the ileum and colon. The 600 ml of ileal fluid that reach the cecum daily contain approximately 75 mmol sodium, 6 mmol potassium, 45 mmol bicarbonate, and 36 mmol chloride. Stool water (100 ml/day) contains 4 mmol sodium, 9 mmol potassium, 3 mmol bicarbonate, 1.5 mmol chloride, and 8.5 mmol unmeasured anion (organic acid anions). Fermentation of unabsorbed carbohydrate by colonic bacteria generates organic acids (propionic, butyric, acetic, and lactic) that titrate secreted bicarbonate and create the stool anion gap. These organic anions are

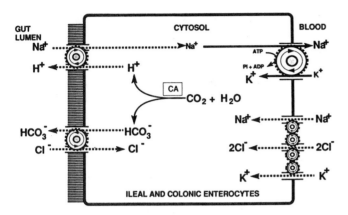

Fig. 13.7 Enteric electrolyte transport. Aldosterone-dependent Na$^+$ reabsorption through a luminal Na$-$H exchanger is driven by basolateral Na$-$K$-$ATPase. Depending upon luminal Cl$^-$ permeability and basolateral Na$-$K$-$2Cl cotransporter activity, Cl$^-$ may be either secreted (duodenum and jejunum) or absorbed (ileum and colon), while HCO$_3^-$ is transported in the opposite direction via a luminal HCO$_3$$-$Cl exchanger.

normally absorbed in the colon, metabolized to bicarbonate in the liver, and thus replace enterically secreted bicarbonate. The 3 mmol bicarbonate and 8.5 mmol organic anions (potential bicarbonate) in stool produce a basal net gastrointestinal alkali loss of only 11.5 mmol/day in the absence of diarrhea [38].

Diarrhea greatly increases sodium, potassium, bicarbonate, organic acid anion, and free water losses. Evacuation of this chloride-free solution results in volume contraction, hypernatremia, hypokalemia, and hyperchloremic metabolic acidosis. Volume contraction and hypobicarbonatemia stimulate renal NaCl reabsorption and shift chloride from intracellular to extracellular fluid, further augmenting hyperchloremia. Although diarrheal stool may be quite acidic, its loss nonetheless generates systemic acidosis because acid generated by colonic fermentation remains extracorporeal.

In addition to diagnosing and treating the cause of diarrhea, extracellular volume must be restored with isotonic NaCl, hyperosmolality is corrected with free water, and potassium is replaced with KCl. Replacement of diarrheal losses with tap water may result in profound hyponatremia. Each liter of diarrheal stool may be replaced with a liter of 5% dextrose in 0.225% (1/4 normal) NaCl, to which is added 40 mmol KCl and 45 mmol NaHCO$_3$ (one 50 ml ampule of 0.9 M). To avoid serious

hypokalemia from transcellular shifts, the plasma potassium should be raised to at least 3.0 mmol/liter before vigorously administering alkali. Alkali therapy becomes increasingly important as the arterial pH falls below 7.25 and the plasma bicarbonate falls below 10 mmol/liter, and is mandatory in patients with renal failure.

Case example

An 83-year-old woman was transferred to hospital from a nursing home after 12 days of a febrile illness, during which she had been passing up to six watery diarrheal stools per day. She was breathing deeply 34/min, blood pressure supine 90/50 mmHg, pulse 94/min, blood pressure sitting 84/60 mmHg, pulse 120/min, weight 43 kg, temperature 38.2°C. She was obtunded and confused, her buccal mucosa was desiccated, and forehead skin turgor was poor. Serum sodium 154 mmol/liter, potassium 3.4 mmol/liter, chloride 132 mmol/liter, tco$_2$ 10.0 mmol/liter, urea nitrogen 20 mg/dl, creatinine 1.5 mg/dl, and glucose 94 mg/dl. Arterial blood (breathing room air): pH 7.04, Pco$_2$ 26 mmHg, and Po$_2$ 63 mmHg. Urine pH 6.15, sodium 2 mmol/liter, potassium 14 mmol/liter, chloride 164 mmol/liter, creatinine 37.5 mg/dl, and osmolality 616 mosmol/kg.

Analysis

With orthostatic hypotension her estimated isotonic fluid loss is at least 15% total body water ($43 \times 0.55 \times 0.15 = 3.5$ liters 0.9% NaCl). She has additionally lost sufficient free water in excess of isotonic losses to raise the serum sodium from 140 to 154 mmol/liter (43×0.55 [154 $-$ 140]/140 = 2.365 liters 5% dextrose in water). Because the arterial blood pH should be raised to the 7.10$-$7.20 range to prevent cardiovascular instability, she should receive an ampule of bicarbonate (45 mmol) in the first liter of replacement fluid (5% dextrose in 0.45% NaCl). Because body potassium stores are depleted, she should also receive 20 mmol KCl per liter of replacement fluid. Half of her replacement fluid (3 liters) may be given during the first 12 hours. With maintenance fluid and replacement of ongoing losses (~2 liters 0.45% NaCl per day), her infusion rate should be 333 ml/hour. She should be monitored closely for signs of pulmonary congestion and the rate of infusion slowed, should it prove excessive. Low urinary sodium and high urinary creatinine and osmolality indicate that renal function is intrinsically intact, but that hypoperfusion has resulted in prerenal azotemia. The ratio of plasma urea nitrogen/creatinine is only 13 because of poor protein intake. Note that the urine pH was 6.15, despite severe systemic acidosis. A urine pH > 5.5 does not, in this case, indicate defective distal acidification because the urinary anion gap is −148 mmol/liter (2 + 14 − 164). After a few days of extra-renal metabolic acidosis (e.g., diarrhea) renal ammonia-genesis increases to >10 mmol/hour. As long as distal sodium delivery is adequate, a negative urinary anion gap (in the absence of other unmeasured cation, e.g., lithium) means that urinary ammonium production has increased sufficiently to raise the pH to 6.0, even though distal acidification in this acidotic subject is unimpaired. When a patient with chronic diarrhea becomes so volume-contracted that distal sodium delivery is extremely low and the urine essentially sodium-free, however, distal acidification may be impaired regardless of buffer production and distal nephron integrity.

Urinary tract obstruction

Voltage-dependent distal renal tubular acidosis caused by obstructive uropathy is the overt acidification defect most commonly encountered in elderly men [39]. Conditions that reduce sodium reabsorption in the cortical collecting tubule include obstructive uropathy, sickle cell anemia, and treatment with amiloride or lithium (although neither drug, administered in therapeutic doses, produces overt acidosis). Specifically, urinary tract obstruction decreases RBF and GFR, reduces the activity of Na−K−ATPase throughout the nephron, and decreases sodium reabsorption [40]. Inhibition of sodium reabsorption in the cortical collecting tubule lowers the trans-epithelial potential difference. Diminished luminal electronegativity slows secretion of cation (i.e., H⁺ and K⁺, Fig. 13.4). In urinary tract obstruction hyperchloremic metabolic acidosis is associated with an inappropriately high urine pH (>5.5), even after sulfate loading or furosemide administration, and the plasma potassium is elevated. The $U-P_{CO_2}$ does not exceed 70 mmHg ($U-BP_{CO_2}$ <30 mmHg) with either bicarbonate or phosphate loading. Voltage-dependent dRTA is treated by correction of underlying or associated factors (e.g., prostatic resection) and administration of 50−100 mmol of alkali per day (Table 13.2).

Case example

A 73-year-old man complained of increasing urinary frequency, nocturia, difficulty initiating micturation, and decreased force of the urinary stream over the past 6 months. During the 3 weeks prior to admission he experienced progressively severe fatigue, malaise, and

Table 13.2 Alkali preparations used to treat metabolic acidoses

Preparation	Anion	Alkali equivalent	Cation equivalent	
			Na⁺	K⁺
Hyperkalemic acidoses (incl. uremic acidosis)				
Sodium Bicarbonate (600 mg tab)	HCO₃	7 mmol/tab	7 mmol	
Baking Soda (6 tbsp/liter H₂O)	HCO₃	11 mmol/15 ml	11 mmol	
Bicitra	Citrate	15 mmol/15 ml	15 mmol	
Shohl's solution	Citrate	7 mmol/15 ml	7 mmol	
Hypokalemic acidoses				
Polycitra	Citrate	30 mmol/15 ml	15 mmol	15 mmol
Polycitra-K syrup	Citrate	30 mmol/15 ml		30 mmol
Kaon elixir	Gluconate	20 mmol/15 ml		20 mmol
K-Lyte effervescent tabs	Glu/HCO₃	25 mmol/tab		25 mmol
Kolyum liquid	Gluconate	17 mmol/15 ml		17 mmol
Potassium triplex	Glu/cit/HCO₃	45 mmol/15 ml		45 mmol

anorexia. He weighed 70 kg and his physical examination was within normal limits, but for dullness to percussion over the suprapubic area, a sense of urinary urgency when the bladder was palpated, and a smoothly enlarged prostate. Serum sodium 143 mmol/liter, potassium 6.2 mmol/liter, chloride 116 mmol/liter, tco_2 17 mmol/liter, urea nitrogen 54 mg/dl, creatinine 3.4 mg/dl, and glucose 124 mg/dl. Arterial blood (breathing room air) pH 7.32, Pco_2 34 mmHg, Po_2 73 mmHg. Urine pH 5.81, sodium 47 mmol/liter, potassium 23 mmol/liter, chloride 47 mmol/liter, creatinine 27 mg/dl, and osmolality 371 mosmol/kg. His electrocardiogram was within normal limits.

Analysis

This patient manifests all of the clinical and biochemical derangements characteristic of chronic obstructive uropathy i.e., renal insufficiency (GFR = $[140 - 73] \times 70/3.4 \times 72 = 19$ ml/min), hyperchloremic metabolic acidosis (plasma anion gap 16 mmol/liter), and hyperkalemia. A urine pH that is inappropriately high for his systemic pH (urine pH should be <5.5 when the arterial pH is <7.35) and decreased urinary ammonia (urine anion gap +23 mosmol/liter) are diagnostic of defective urinary acidification. The normal electrocardiogram indicates that the hyperkalemia is chronic and need not be treated emergently. After 500 ml of noninfected residual urine was evacuated through an indwelling urinary catheter the patient underwent uncomplicated transurethral prostatic resection. The acidosis and hyperkalemia resolved and the serum creatinine decreased to 1.3 mg/dl (GFR = $[140 - 73] \times 70/1.3 \times 72 = 50$ ml/min) over the ensuing weeks.

Mineralocorticoid deficiency/resistance (Type IV dRTA)

Because Type IV dRTA includes a heterogeneous group of distal acidification disorders, this imprecise and nondescriptive term should be abandoned. The adrenal gland may fail to secrete aldosterone in response to its usual agonists (angiotensin II or III, hyperkalemia, hyponatremia, adrenocorticotrophic hormone, neurotransmitters, melanocyte-stimulating hormone, β-endorphins, or vasopressin) with Addison's disease, heparin administration, insulinopenia, dopamine or somatostatin excess, volume expansion (atrial natriuretic factor), or β-

adrenergic blockade. The juxtaglomerular apparatus may fail to secrete renin in response to α- or β-adrenergic agonists, prostaglandins, etc., and renal prostaglandins may not be produced in response to angiotensin II, etc. if cyclo-oxygenase is inhibited by nonsteroidal anti-inflammatory agents or bradykinin production is reduced by diabetes mellitus or interstitial nephritis. Agiotensin-converting enzyme may be inhibited by captopril, enalopril, or lisinopril. All may result in relative hypoaldosteronism, hyperkalemia, and a mild hyperchloremic metabolic acidosis. Alternatively, the distal nephron may become refractory to normal or increased amounts of aldosterone. Aldosterone resistance may be inherited (e.g., pseudohypoaldosteronism with or without salt wasting) or acquired (e.g., spironolactone administration, cyclosporine nephrotoxicity, or tubulointerstitial nephropathies). Hypoaldosteronism and aldosterone resistance are clinically indistinguishable from each other and may be differentiated only by the level of plasma aldosterone. The normal ranges of plasma aldosterone in adults are 3–10 ng/dl supine and 6–22 ng/dl upright when the plasma potassium is normal. As a rule of thumb, the plasma aldosterone (ng/dl) divided by the plasma potassium (mmol/liter) normally exceeds 3.0.

After cytosolic receptor binding, aldosterone activates the gene that encodes for an apical membrane sodium transport protein or ion channel. By increasing sodium entry in states of diminished distal delivery, aldosterone enhances both H^+ and potassium secretion by increasing the transepithelial potential difference [41]. Because aldosterone deficiency also inhibits proton secretion in the inner medullary collecting duct where sodium reabsorption is passive and potential difference is lumen-positive, mineralocorticoid must be activating proton ATPase directly in this segment by a mechanism independent of its effect on sodium flux, potassium flux, and potential difference [42]. Aldosterone may directly enhance active proton secretion by changing membrane lipid composition to increase its fluidity. Aldosterone may increase the activity of $Na^+-K^+-ATPase$ directly or indirectly, by providing the enzyme with increased amounts of its intracellular substrate, sodium. Because aldosterone-independent sodium transport and the electromotive force of proton ATPase are unaffected, hypoaldosteronism induces hyperkalemia and mild hyperchloremic metabolic acidosis primarily by voltage effects whenever distal delivery is reduced [43].

Hyperkalemia inhibits passive transcellular potassium flux, increases cytosolic potassium, displaces cytosolic H^+, and raises the intracellular pH. Intracellular alkalosis, whether caused by hyperkalemia or alkalemia, reduces glutamine entry into proximal tubular cells and inhibits ammoniagenesis [44]. When associated with an acidification defect (e.g., the voltage effects of hypoaldosteronism), reduction of urinary buffer capacity contributes to the acidosis without further affecting potassium excretion. Because urinary buffer production is less than distal acidification in hypoaldosteronism, the urine pH is usually less than 5.5, despite voltage effects that diminish cortical collecting tubule proton conductance. Patients with hypoaldosteronism lower the urine pH normally (to <5.5) in response to acidemia, sulfate loading, or furosemide) and the urine P_{CO_2} rises appropriately to >70 mmHg with both bicarbonate and phosphate loading [45]. These metabolic derangements are exacerbated by diminished distal delivery (e.g., heart failure or salt depletion) and are ameliorated by increasing distal delivery (e.g., salt loading and/or diuretic administration) or administration of exogenous mineralocorticoid (e.g., 9-α-fludrocortisone acetate (Florinef^{TM}) 0.05-0.1 mg/day).

Case example

A 68-year-old woman had nonketotic diabetes controlled by diet, mild hypertension, and degenerative joint disease treated with ibuprofen 600 mg b.i.d and hydrochlothiazide 25 mg daily. When she was found to have a blood pressure of 178/105 on a routine office visit, 10 mg lisinopril was added to her regimen. Serum sodium was 133 mmol/liter, potassium 4.4 mmol/liter, chloride 100 mmol/liter, t_{CO_2} 23 mmol/liter, urea nitrogen 16 mg/dl, creatinine 0.9 mg/dl, and fasting glucose 134 mg/dl. Two weeks later serum sodium was 143 mmol/liter, potassium 6.2 mmol/liter, chloride 116 mmol/liter, t_{CO_2} 16 mmol/liter, urea nitrogen 34 mg/dl, creatinine 1.9 mg/dl, and fasting glucose 126 mg/dl. Her urine pH was 5.3.

Analysis

This patient likely has underlying mild, age-related hypoaldosteronism. In addition, diabetes commonly reduces renal bradykinin and produces hyporeninemic hypoaldosteronism. Thiazide diuretics cause volume contraction and stimulate prostaglandins. In diabetes and volume contraction, filtration pressure is largely dependent on uninhibited prostaglandin production. Cyclo-oxygenase antagonists inhibit renin-angiotensin II-aldosterone production by reducing prostaglandin synthesis in the juxtaglomerular apparatus. Despite these risk factors, she was able to maintain normal acid-base and potassium balance until stressed by yet a fourth risk factor, angiotensin-converting enzyme (ACE) inhibition. Diabetic afferent arterioles are unable to dilate normally in response to low perfusion pressure or reduction of efferent resistance. Functionally the response of diabetic kidneys to ACE inhibition is similar to that of kidneys whose blood supply is compromised by bilateral renal artery stenosis. Reduction of angiotensin II dilates the efferent arterioles, lowers filtration pressure, reduces GFR, slows distal delivery, and reduces sodium reabsorption in cortical collecting tubules. Without sufficient angiotensin II, response of the adrenal zona glomerulosa to hyperkalemia is blunted (especially in the presence of insulinopenia, β-adrenergic blockade, or heparin sodium), aldosterone production falls, and distal sodium reabsorption is further compromised. In the cortical collecting tubule both proton and potassium secretion are inhibited by voltage effects, the serum potassium rises, renal ammoniagenesis is reduced, and the patient develops hyperkalemic, hyperchloremic metabolic acidosis with an appropriately low urine pH.

Treatment in this case was gratifyingly simple. Stopping lysinopril and controlling blood pressure with clonidine restored GFR, acid-base balance, and plasma potassium to baseline. Incidentally, had she not been taking a diuretic, the consequences of ACE inhibition might have been worse, possibly fatal. Angiotensin-converting enzyme inhibition may be hazardous in elderly diabetics and requires careful monitoring of plasma urea nitrogen, creatinine, and potassium levels.

Renal failure

In chronic renal failure urinary acidification and ammoniagenesis increase up to four-fold in surviving nephrons as solute load per nephron is increased [46]. Proton homeostasis is maintained until more than half of the functioning nephrons are lost. Net ammonia excretion peaks at about 200 mmol/day, then begins to fall as GFR falls below 50%, although single-nephron ammoniagenesis may be maximal [47]. When the GFR falls to about 25%, the remaining intact nephrons are insufficient to maintain proton homeostasis and the patient becomes acidotic, unless dietary protein is restricted. Diminished clearance of organic acid salts (e.g., hippurate, guanidino-succinate, glucuronate, oxalate, etc.), cellular uptake of chloride, and increased proximal reclamation of filtered bicarbonate prevent the plasma chloride from rising. Uremic acidosis is usually associated with only a moderate rise in the plasma anion gap to 18−25 mmol/liter (ΔAG 2−9 mmol/liter) because single-nephron hyperfiltration and putative uremic natriuretic factors diminish proximal sodium reabsorption and lead to wasting of the poorly reabsorbable organic acid anions that otherwise would have been metabolized to bicarbonate. This is tantamount to losing bicarbonate or gaining protons. Titratable acidity may also fall in hypophosphatemic patients whose phosphate intake has been severely curtailed or who have taken in large amounts of phosphate binders ($Al[OH]_3$ gel, $CaCO_3$, or calcium citrate).

Extrarenal buffering, principally in bone, prevents the plasma bicarbonate from falling below 12−20 mmol/liter as the patient approaches end-stage renal failure. Increased extrarenal buffering, a manifestation of secondary hyperparathyroidism, is accomplished at the cost of bony demineralization and aggravation of renal osteodystrophy—an advantageous trade-off in terms of short-term survival, but a major source of morbidity in the chronic dialysis population [48]. Treatment of uremic acidosis should therefore never be neglected.

More severe acidoses are usually related to intercurrent obstructive uropathy, volume depletion, heart failure, tubulointerstitial nephropathies, diarrhea, diabetic keto-acidosis, toxins, hypoaldosteronism, or aldosterone resistance. Valuable clues that absolute or effective circulating volume may be contracted in a patient with renal failure are: worsening acidosis; $\Delta[HCO_3] > \Delta$ anion gap; hyperchloremia; and hyperkalemia. Although dissection and diagnosis of the mixed acid−base disorders encountered in patients with chronic renal failure may be challenging, treatment of uncomplicated uremic acidosis is usually straightforward and easily accomplished. Because the amount of buffer regenerated by the distal nephron is modest (1−1.5 mmol/kg per day), uremic acidosis is prevented or corrected with only 1.0−1.5 mmol/kg alkali (Table 13.2). Raising the plasma bicarbonate to normal prevents the anorexia, fatigue, malaise, protein wasting, and osteopenia caused by uremic acidosis.

Case example

A 72-year-old Afro-american man who had long-standing essential hypertension, congestive heart failure, and renal insufficiency was brought to the emergency room severely short of breath 3 weeks after running out of all medications, including digoxin 0.125 mg q.i.d., furosemide 20 mg b.i.d., and hydralazine 50 mg q.i.d. Two months previously his plasma sodium had been 143 mmol/liter, potassium 4.4 mmol/liter, chloride 108 mmol/liter, t_{CO_2} 25 mmol/liter, urea nitrogen 42 mg/dl, creatinine 2.5 mg/dl, and glucose 104 mg/dl. On admission he weighed 75 kg (last clinic weight 67 kg), blood pressure 185/125 mmHg, pulse 136/min and irregularly irregular, respirations 34/min and labored, temperature 37°C. Funduscopy revealed flat discs, hard exudates, and arteriolar narrowing. Neck veins were distended to the jaw line, fine inspiratory crepitant rales were auscultated over the lower half of both lung fields, and there was dullness to percussion with diminished breath sounds in the bases. An apical grade 3/6 holo-systolic murmur and an S3 gallop were auscultated at the cardiac apex, S1 intensity was variable, liver was enlarged and tender, and there was 3+ pitting, dependent leg edema. Plasma sodium was 132 mmol/liter, potassium 5.4 mmol/liter, chloride 111 mmol/liter, t_{CO_2} 8 mmol/liter, urea nitrogen 126 mg/dl, creatinine 5.6 mg/dl, glucose 127 mg/dl. Arterial blood (breathing O_2 by nasal prongs at 2 l/min) pH 7.28, P_{CO_2} 20 mmHg, PO_2 56 mmHg. Chest X-ray showed pulmonary congestion, bilateral pleural effusions, and cardiomegaly. Electrocardiogram showed narrow qrs complexes and atrial fibrillation with a rapid ventricular response. Urine pH 5.32, sodium 15 mmol/liter, potassium 14 mmol/liter, chloride 19 mmol/liter, creatinine 22 mg/dl, osmolality 315 mosmol/kg.

Analysis

This elderly hypertensive with underlying heart disease and renal insufficiency (GFR = $[140 − 72] \times 67/2.7 \times 72$) = 23 ml/min) presented with atrial fibrillation, severe hypertension, and pulmonary edema after running out of his medications 3 weeks previously. The plasma urea nitrogen had quadrupled and the plasma creatinine had doubled (prerenal azotemia). He was hyperkalemic with combined hyperchloremic metabolic acidosis and respiratory alkalosis (hypoxemia). Fractional excretion of sodium was 2.8% ($15 \times 5.6 \times 100/132 \times 22$), compatible with renal underperfusion in a patient with chronic renal insufficiency. The usual acid–base disturbance associated with renal failure is a high-anion gap metabolic acidosis, yet his anion gap was normal ($132 + 5.4 - 111 - 8 = 18.4$ mmol/liter). All may be explained by heart failure.

Under baseline conditions his surviving nephrons were hyperfiltering and producing a maximum amount of ammonia. A high rate of distal delivery and maximal urinary buffer capacity stimulated distal acidification and potassium secretion sufficiently to maintain acid–base and potassium balance. When effective circulating volume was contracted by heart failure, renal perfusion diminished, GFR and distal delivery fell, and distal acidification and potassium secretion were reduced. In addition, hyperkalemia reduced renal ammoniagenesis and urinary buffer capacity.

When the heart failure was treated by digitalization, diuresis, and afterload reduction with hydralazine, renal function, plasma potassium, and acid–base balance returned to baseline.

References

1 Kaysen GA, Myers BD. The aging kidney (review). Clin Geriatr Med 1985;1:207–222.

2 Epstein M. Aging and the kidney: clinical implications. Am Fam Physician 1985;31:123–137.

3 Bonomini V, Vangelista A. Structural and functional renal changes in the elderly (review). Contrib Nephrol 1988; 61:73–81.

4 Euans DW. Renal function in the elderly (review). Am Fam Physician 1988;38:147–150.

5 Beck LH. Renal function and disease in the elderly. Del Med J 1988;60:363–364, 367–368.

6 Sarkar S, Kushal M, Manshramani GG, et al. Renal function in the geriatric age group. J Assoc Physicians India 1986;34:345–347.

7 Brown WW, Davis BB, Spry LA, et al. Aging and the kidney (review). Arch Intern Med 1986;15:211–213.

8 Meyer BR, Bellucci A. Renal function in the elderly (review). Cardiol Clin 1986;4:227–234.

9 Lindeman RD. The aging kidney. Compr Ther 1986; 12:43–49.

10 Davies DF, Shock NW. Age changes in glomerular filtration rate, effective renal plasma flow, and tubular excretory capacity in adult males. J Clin Invest 1950;29:496–507.

11 Kafetz K. Renal impairment in the elderly: a review. J R Soc Med 1983;76:398–401.

12 Larsson M, Jagenburg R, Landahl S. Renal function in an elderly population. A study of S-creatinine, ^{51}Cr-EDTA clearance, endogenous creatinine clearance and maximal tubular water reabsorption. Scand J Clin Lab Invest 1986; 46:593–598.

13 Deutsch S, Goldberg M, Dripps RD. Post-operative hyponatremia with the inappropriate release of antidiuretic hormone. Anesthesia 1966;27:250–256.

14 Rowe JW, Shock NW, DeFronzo RA. The influence of age on the renal response to water deprivation in man. Nephron 1976;17:270–278.

15 Davis PJ, Davis FB. Water excretion in the elderly (review). Endocrinol Metab Clin North Am 1987;16:867–875.

16 Thirst and osmoregulation in the elderly (editorial). Lancet 1984;2:1017–1018.

17 Epstein M, Hollenberg NK. Age as a determinant of renal sodium conservation in normal men. J Lab Clin Med 1976; 87:411–417.

18 Miller JH, McDonald RK, Shock NW. Age changes in the maximal rate of renal tubular reabsorption of glucose. J Gerontol 1952;7:196–200.

19 Brohee D, Rondelez L, Bain H, et al. Kidney aging and renal excretion of amylase. Gerontology 1982;28:386–391.

20 Aronson PS. Mechanisms of active H^+ secretion in the proximal tubule. Am J Physiol 1983;245:F647–F659.

21 Maren TH. Current status of membrane-bound carbonic anhydrase. Ann NY Acad Sci 1980;341:246–258.

22 Sasaki S, Berry CA. Mechanism of bicarbonate exit across the basolateral membrane of the rabbit proximal convoluted tubules. Kidney Int 1983;23:A238.

23 Halperin ML. How much "new" bicarbonate is formed in the distal nephron in the process of net acid excretion? (editorial review). Kidney Int 1989;35:1277–1281.

24 Halperin ML. Metabolism and acid–base physiology. J Artif Organs 1982;6:357–362.

25 Kurtzman NA. Acquired distal renal tubular acidosis. (Nephrology Forum). Kidney Int 1983;24:807–819.

26 Halperin ML, Goldstein MB, Haig A, et al. Studies on the pathogenesis of Type 1 (distal) renal tubular acidosis as revealed by the urinary PCO_2 tensions. J Clin Invest 1974;53:669–677.

27 Hropot M, Fowler N, Karlmark B, et al. Tubular action of diuretics: distal effects on electrolyte transport and acidification. Kidney Int 1985;28:477–489.

28 Batlle DC, Sehy JT, Roseman MK, et al. Clinical and pathophysiologic spectrum of acquired distal renal tubular acidosis. Kidney Int 1981;20:389–396.

29 Goldstein MB, Bear R, Richardson RMA, et al. The urine anion gap: a clinically useful index of ammonia excretion. Am J Med Sci 1986;292:198–201.

30 Shock NW, Yiengst MJ. Age changes in the acid–base equilibrium of the blood of males. J Gerontol 1950;5:1–5.

31 Hilton JG, Goodbody MF, Kruesi OR. The effect of prolonged administration of ammonium chloride on the blood acid–base equilibrium of geriatric subjects. J Am Geriat Soc 1955; 3:697–703.

32 Adler S, Lindeman RD, Yiengst MJ, *et al*. Effect of acute acid loading on urinary acid excretion by the aging human kidney. J Lab Clin Med 1968;72:278−289.

33 Agarwal BN, Cabebe FG. Renal acidification in elderly subjects. Nephron 1980;26:291−295.

34 Crane MG, Harris JJ. Effect of aging on renin activity and aldosterone excretion. J Lab Clin Med 1976;57:947−959.

35 Weidmann P, DeMythenau-Bursztein S, Maxwell MH, *et al*. Effect of aging on plasma renin and aldosterone in normal man. Kidney Int 1975;8:325−333.

36 Binder HJ. Absorption and secretion of water and electrolytes by small and large intestine. In Sleisenger MH, Fordtran JS, eds. *Gastrointestinal Disease. Pathophysiology Diagnosis Management*, 4th edn. Philadelphia: WB Saunders Co., 1989:1022−1045.

37 Makhlouf GM. Electrolyte composition of gastric secretion. In Johnson LR, ed. *Physiology of the Gastrointestinal Tract*. New York: Raven Press, 1981:551−566.

38 Wrong O, Metcalf-Gibson A. The electrolyte content of feces. Proc R Soc Med 1965;58:1007−1009.

39 Batlle DC, Arruda JAL, Kurtzman NA. Hyperkalemic distal renal tubular acidosis associated with obstructive uropathy. N Engl J Med 1981;304:373−380.

40 Sabatini S, Kurtzman NA. Enzyme activity in obstructive uropathy: Basis for salt wastage and the acidification defect. Kidney Int 1990;37:79−84.

41 Wingo CS, Kokko JP, Jacobson HR. Effects of *in vitro* aldosterone on the rabbit cortical collecting tubule. Kidney Int 1985; 28:51−57.

42 Dubose TD Jr, Cflisch CR. Effect of selective aldosterone deficiency on acidification in nephron segments of the rat inner medulla. J Clin Invest 1988;82:1624−1632.

43 DiTella PJ, Sodhe B, McCreary J, *et al*. Mechanism of the metabolic acidosis of selective mineralocorticoid deficiency. Kidney Int 1978;14:466−477.

44 Kuwahara M, Sasaki Sei, Shiigai T, *et al*. Glutamine transport in the rabbit proximal straight tubule: effect of acute acid pH. Kidney Int 1986;30:340−347.

45 Batlle DC. Hyperkalemic hyperchloremic metabolic acidosis associated with selective aldosterone deficiency and distal renal tubular acidosis. Sem Nephr 1981;1:260−274.

46 Bricker NS, Klahr S, Lubowitz H, *et al*. Renal function in chronic renal disease. Medicine 1965;44:263−288.

47 Maclean AJ, Hayslett JP. Adaptive change in ammonia excretion in renal insufficiency. Kidney Int 1980;17:595−606.

48 Arruda JAL, Alla V, Rubinstein H, *et al*. Parathyroid hormone and extrarenal acid buffering. Am J Physiol 1980;239: F533−F535.

Renal disease in the elderly

Priscilla Kincaid-Smith

Aging and the kidney

The kidneys reduce considerably in weight with age from around 250 g each in a young adult to less then 200 g in an 80-year-old [1]. With this reduction in size there is an increase in the number of sclerosed glomeruli [2−4]. Within remaining glomeruli the mesangial matrix is increased although there is no increase in cells [5]. Capillary wall basement membrane thickness also increases with age in rats but not in humans [6,7]. Progressive glomerular sclerosis occurs in aging Sprague−Dawley rats but this has not been convincingly demonstrated in humans [8]. Renal tubules diminish in size with age so that there is relative crowding of glomeruli resembling the change seen in ischemia [9].

Arteries and arterioles show increased fibroelastic and hyaline intimal thickening with age but these are very variable and do not necessarily reduce the size of the lumen [9]. Radiographic studies, however, show an increasing prevalence of reduction in calibre as well as tortuosity of arteries [10,11]. Both glomerular filtration rate (GFR) and renal blood flow (RBF) decreases progressively from the age of 30 [12]. At age 80 the creatinine clearance is below 100 ml/min per 1.73 m^2.

Ability to conserve sodium falls in elderly subjects. This makes such individuals susceptible to sodium depletion on sodium-restricted diets (13). Renal-concentrating abilities also decline with age [14]. Elderly subjects are less efficient in excreting an acid load than young subjects [15]

A major implication of the above changes in renal function with aging relates to the dose of drugs administered to the elderly when excretion of a drug is mainly renal. The susceptibility of aged people to toxic effects of drugs cannot, however, be totally explained by the changes in renal function. Elderly people seem particularly susceptible to toxic effects of certain groups of drugs such as sulphonamides, aminoglycosides, radiocontrast media, and nonsteroidal anti-inflammatory drugs.

Specific renal diseases which effect the elderly

Neoplasms

Renal cell carcinoma

This is the commonest renal neoplasm accounting for 85% of all renal tumors and accounting for 2.3% of male and 1.6% of female cancer deaths in the United States. The most important predisposing factor is cigarette smoking.

The classic clinical triad of presenting features, namely a mass in the flank, loin pain, and hematuria, occur late and many patients have secondary spread at the time of diagnosis.

Perineoplastic symptoms are commonly associated with renal carcinoma. These include fever, anemia, erythrocytosis, and hypercalcemia.

Diagnosis is based on the finding of nonglomerular erythrocytes in the urine and on imaging techniques. Computed tomography scanning with contrast has replaced other imaging techniques as the definitive method of diagnosis of renal cell carcinoma [16].

Surgical removal is the treatment of choice. Although many trials of chemotherapy are in progress there is no standard accepted therapy for advanced renal cell carcinoma. Interferon has been used but although a 25% response rate has been claimed, side-effects are common as they are with chemotherapeutic regimes [17].

Uroepithelial tumors of the renal pelvis, ureter, and bladder

Most urothelial tumors occur in the bladder where they may affect the kidney by obstructing one or both ureters.

Tumors of the urothelium in the pelvis and ureter account for 10–15% of tumors of the kidney. Classically, they occur predominantly in males with a 2 : 1 male to female ratio; however, in those secondary to analgesic nephropathy and Balkan nephropathy the sex incidence is reversed with a 2 : 1 ratio of females to males.

Various chemicals including aniline dyes have been implicated as causing urothelial tumors which are also more frequent in smokers.

Most patients present with nonglomerular hematuria which is usually macroscopic and may be accompanied by clot colic. Urinary tract infection and obstruction may complicate the course.

Urine cytology may reveal malignant cells. Imaging techniques used to locate the tumor included intravenous and intravenous pyelography. Treatment is surgical removal. The response to chemotherapy is poor.

Other renal tumors such as sarcomas are rare.

Prostatic carcinoma

The effect of these tumors on the kidney is through obstruction to the urethra or the ureters.

Prostatic carcinoma is the second commonest tumor in males and prevalence is age-related; so-called latent carcinoma of the prostate at autopsy is found in 45% of 80-year-old men.

Symptoms are similar to those seen with benign prostatic hypertophy and the diagnosis is made on rectal examination.

Treatment depends upon the stage of the disease and includes surgical excision, hormonal chemotherapeutic, and radiation therapy.

Other renal lesions due to malignancies

Glomerular disease and neoplasms. Lee *et al.* [18] first described the association between cancer and the nephrotic syndrome. They found that 10.9% of 101 patients with the nephrotic syndrome had an associated malignancy. Most patients had membranous glomerulonephritis and in a subsequent study from the same group, Hopper [19] found a 6% prevalence of cancer among 82 patients with membranous glomerulonephritis. Row *et al.* [20] reported cancer in 10.6% of patients with membranous glomerulonephritis. Because cancer selects patients in older age groups, most of these patients have been over the age of 60. Many different carcinomas have been associated with the nephrotic syndrome: colon, breast, stomach, and ovaries being the most frequent.

Tumor cell antigens have been detected in glomeruli from patients with membranous glomerulonephritis [21]. Carcinoembryonic antigen has also been demonstrated in membranous glomerulonephritis [22].

These observations suggest a causal relationship between the cancer and the glomerulonephritis.

Hodgkin's disease has frequently been reported in association with the nephrotic syndrome, usually minimal lesion nephrotic syndrome, but these patients are not necessarily elderly.

Nonglomerular complications of malignancies. Tumors may invade the kidney and produce renal manifestations, even renal failure occasionally, through replacement of renal parenchyma.

The hypercalcemia associated with malignancy may cause impaired renal function in association with calcium oxalate deposits in the parenchyma.

Myeloma and other diseases associated with paraproteins may cause renal failure in which tubular obstruction by casts is present. The casts have a particular "fractured" appearance.

Following treatment of malignancy, acute renal failure may ensue due to either uric acid crystal deposition in the renal tubules or to nephrotoxic effects of antineoplastic drugs.

Renal vascular disease

The prevalence of atheroma of the renal arterial system increases with age and causes narrowing of the main renal arteries and their branches as well as atheromatous emboli in smaller arterial branches and arterioles. As with all atheromatous disease this is more commonly seen in men than in women.

Renal artery stenosis

Atheromatous renal artery stenosis is relatively less frequent in women but is seen as a frequent complication in patients with analgesic nephropathy [23].

Not only is atheromatous renal artery stenosis a lesion frequently associated with hypertension in the elderly but it is the commonest cause of end-stage renal failure in patients over 65 [24].

A high prevalence of renal artery stenosis has been recorded in men undergoing coronary angiography for coronary artery disease [25].

Smoking is strongly associated with atheromatous renal artery stenosis [26].

The clinical sign with the greatest significance in patients with renal artery stenosis is a bruit in the loin or abdomen. Renal artery stenosis is much more likely to be present if the patient has severe hypertension with retinal hemorrhages exudates and papilledema [27].

Investigation may reveal a low serum potassium, a high plasma renin activity, and imaging may reveal a smaller kidney on the side of the stenosed renal artery. Renal blood flow is usually reduced on the ischemic side but the definitive method of diagnosis of renal artery stenosis is a renal angiogram.

Treatment may involve nephrectomy where there is little function in the kidney distal to renal artery stenosis, but because atheroma is widespread in such patients and the disease may be bilateral, preservation of renal function is important. This can be achieved by operative vascular surgical correction of the lesion or by percutaneous balloon dilatation. Although successful dilatation may be achieved in 89% of cases (Table 14.1) cure of hypertension is only reported in 28% with almost 60% showing some improvement [28–33].

Percutaneous angioplasty has also been performed for preservation of renal function. In one large series all of whom had serum creatinine levels above 2 mg%, the serum creatinine fell in 63% of the 75% successfully dilated, 20% of cases showed an increase in serum creatinine level which may well have been due to atheromatous embolization occurring in distal vessels during the procedure [34]. Serious complications of cholesterol embolization are commonly reported following angioplasty [30].

Hypertension associated with atheromatous renal artery stenosis can be adequately treated by antihypertensive drugs. Converting enzyme inhibitors are very effective in such patients because of the high plasma renin activity. Patients may be very sensitive to converting enzyme inhibitors which must therefore be given cautiously. A more serious complication is the permanent total occlusion of the renal artery which occurred in 40% of patients in one series [35]. The same permanent loss of function in the ischemic kidney has been reported in experimental renal artery stenosis treated with converting enzyme and inhibitors.

Atheromatous emboli

Atheromatous emboli are increasingly being recognized as a cause of renal failure—a diagnosis often missed in the past.

The patients who develop renal failure from atheromatous emboli are elderly and mainly males.

We have recently reported a group of eight elderly males who developed renal failure due to atheromatous emboli. As in other series the long-term outlook for renal function in these patients was very poor. Renal choles-

Table 14.1 Clinical results with renal angioplasty. The percentages for cured, improved, and failed are expressed relative to the number of patients who were successfully dilated

Author [reference]	Number of patients	Successfully dilated (%)	Cured (%)	Improved (%)	Failed (%)
Fibromuscular dysplasia					
Sos *et al.* [28]	31	27(87)	16(59)	9(33)	2(7)
Tegtmeyer *et al.* [29]	21	21(100)	13(62)	8(38)	0(0)
Geyskes *et al.* [30]	21	21(100)	10(48)	10(48)	1(5)
Martin *et al.* [31]	11	8(73)	5(63)	1(13)	2(25)
Grim *et al.* [32]	10	9(90)	5(56)	4(44)	0(0)
Mean		90	58	35	7
Atheroma (unilateral nonostial)					
Schwarten *et al.* [33]	54	49(91)	23(47)	25(51)	1(2)
Geyskes* *et al.* [30]	44	44(100)	21(48)	19(43)	4(9)
Sos *et al.* [28]	20	15(75)	4(27)	9(60)	2(13)
Martin *et al.* [31]	15	13(87)	2(15)	4(31)	7(54)
Grim *et al.* [32]	15	15(100)	1(7)	7(47)	7(47)
Tegtmeyer *et al.* [29]	13	11(84)	3(27)	8(73)	0(0)
Mean		89.5	28.5	57	21

* Includes some patients with bilateral disease.

terol emboli may occur after trauma, angiographic, and other procedures involving catheterization of the aorta and after surgical procedures involving the abdominal aorta [36].

There may be manifestations of involvement of other organs by emboli including peripheral gangrene, gastrointestinal bleeding, retinal ischemia, and cerebral emboli. Fever, a raised erythrocyte sedimentation rate, and eosinophilia may be present.

The renal failure which follows atheromatous embolization usually happens a week or more after the precipitating cause. The most common precipitating event in our experience has been abdominal angiography, and whereas renal failure from contrast media happens immediately after angiography, renal failure due to atheromatous emboli may be delayed for up to 3 weeks.

Analgesic nephropathy and the effects of nonsteroidal anti-inflammatory drugs (NSAIDs)

Analgesic nephropathy is essentially a disease of middle-aged and elderly women (Fig. 14.1) [37]. The incidence of this condition as a cause of end-stage renal failure has declined following control of the sales of over-the-counter

analgesic mixtures and compounds; the age of new patients presenting with end-stage renal failure has increased over this period. Over the period during which the number of cases due to over-the-counter analgesics has declined, there has been an increase in the number of elderly patients presenting with acute and chronic renal failure due to nonsteroidal anti-inflammatory drugs.

The clinical features of analgesic nephropathy include the renal manifestations of renal papillary necrosis (hematuria, loin pain, renal colic, ureteric obstruction, and acute and chronic renal failure) which are commonly complicated by infection. Other associated clinical features are hypertension, peptic ulceration, anemia, and psychotic disturbances [38–41].

A diagnosis is based on a history of prolonged excessive analgesic intake and the demonstration of renal papillary necrosis either by finding necrotic material in the urine or more commonly by demonstration of characteristic radiologic features of renal papillary necrosis. The treatment is to cease analgesic abuse which leads to reversal of all clinical features, and to recovery or stabilization of renal function in a high percentage of cases [42].

An important concept in the diagnosis of renal papillary

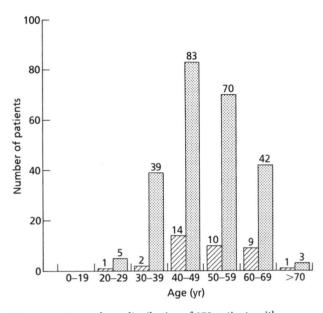

Fig. 14.1 Age- and sex-distribution of 279 patients with analgesic nephropathy. The female to male ratio is 6.5/1. Analgesic nephropathy is rare under the age of 30 years, the peak occurrence being in the fourth and fifth decades of life. Stippled bars denote female patients; hatched bars denote male patients. (From Nanra *et al.* [37].)

necrosis is the fact that if the papillae do not separate and remain *in situ* there are no characteristic radiologic changes seen [43].

This is particularly important in the type of renal papillary necrosis which is being seen with increasing frequency in older patients taking NSAIDs. Papillary necrosis is well recorded as a toxic effect of NSAIDs [44,45]. Renal papillary necrosis is also produced experimentally by NSAIDs.

We [46] have seen an increasing number of elderly patients presenting with impairment of renal function which develops during treatment with NSAIDs. Some of those patients have acute renal failure and recover and these are discussed below; others progress to end-stage renal failure.

Those who develop permanent deterioration in renal function and in whom an autopsy is done have renal papillary necrosis [47]. This can sometimes be demonstrated on a renal biopsy or by characteristic calcification in papillae, seen on computed tomography scanning. Only occasionally in patients on NSAIDs do the papillae

separate, enabling a diagnosis to be made on the basis of finding necrotic tissue in the urine or on characteristic radiologic changes of renal papillary necrosis.

Renal papillary necrosis is found at autopsy in a high percentage of patients with rheumatoid arthritis who are taking NSAIDs [47,48], and many of these patients are elderly, as are most other patients who present with chronic renal failure while taking NSAIDs. Treatment is, if possible, to withdraw the NSAID, but as most of these patients are taking such medications for chronic painful osteoarthritis or rheumatoid arthritis, it is difficult to find alternative anti-inflammatory or pain-relieving treatment for long-term use.

Acute renal failure, and acute interstitial nephritis and the nephrotic syndrome resulting from NSAIDs
There are two distinct syndromes of acute renal failure resulting from NSAIDs which are particularly liable to occur in elderly people.

The first of these for which elderly patients are a higher risk group is often associated with other predisposed factors, such as salt depletion, diuretics, cardiac failure, and other high renin states. Renal failure may be prerenal and recover quickly or may progress to acute tubular necrosis which recovers in 10–14 days. This syndrome can be looked upon as related to hemodynamic factors leading to renal ischemia and through that mechanism to acute renal failure. Any NSAID may cause this syndrome and reported cases tend to reflect the drug which is most commonly prescribed in a particular area at the time.

The second syndrome is more complex and involves an idiosyncratic reaction to a NSAID. Particular drugs have been incriminated in most reported cases, fenoprofen has caused two-thirds of reported cases and most other cases have been attributed to zomepirac or tolmetin. One or two cases have been attributed to most other NSAIDs [45]. This syndrome may occur 2–10 months after the patient starts taking the NSAID in question and renal failure is usually accompanied by the nephrotic syndrome. Renal biopsy shows interstitial nephritis often with few or no eosinophils in the infiltrate. This syndrome may respond promptly to steroids [46] but without treatment renal failure may be prolonged and even permanent.

Obstructive lesions
Obstructive lesions in elderly patients may be due to any obstructive causes, however, the commonest seen in

males is benign prostatic hypertrophy, whereas in females ureteric obstruction due to pelvic tumor — particularly invasive cervical carcinoma — is a frequent cause.

Benign prostatic hypertrophy

Benign prostatic hypertrophy is such a common disorder in males that it could be regarded as more normal than the gradual atrophy of the prostate, which commences at the age of 40 in the small percentage of men who do not develop prostatic hypertrophy. Benign prostatic hypertrophy has special relevance for the elderly because its prevalence rises to 95% in the eighth decade [49]. The probability of a 40-year-old man requiring an operation by the time he is 80, is about 10% [50,51].

The major disorder in benign prostatic hypertrophy is increasing bladder outlet resistance to urine flow. The symptoms associated with obstruction are reduction in the calibre and force of the stream, hesistancy in initiating urine flow, postvoiding, dribbling, incomplete emptying of the bladder, and eventually, urine retention.

Impaired renal function develops with an increasing obstruction.

The definitive diagnosis depends on rectal examination which reveals a firm elastic enlargement of the prostate. The size of the prostate on the rectal examination does not help in assessing the degree of bladder neck obstruction. Urinalysis is necessary to exclude infection and renal function tests and an intravenous pyelogram are performed to document the degree of impairment of renal function and the degree of upper urinary tract obstruction. A postvoiding film demonstrates the amount of residual urine as well as the size of the prostatic filling defect.

Treatment is primarily surgical, however, α-blocking drugs like prazosin can reduce the degree of bladder neck obstruction and improve symptoms in patients awaiting surgery or in those in whom surgical treatment is contraindicated.

Other obstructive lesions

Any obstructive lesion can affect the elderly. Those related to neoplasms such as retroperitoneal tumor, infiltrative bladder, or pelvic neoplasms are particularly likely to cause obstruction in the elderly. There has been a suggestion that retroperitoneal fibrosis is due to leakage from atheromatous lesions in the aorta and this occurs mainly in older age groups.

Other renal diseases in the elderly

Glomerular disease in the elderly

The prevalence of proteinuria increases with age and proteinuria is significantly associated with a higher mortality [51].

In people aged 65–84 years proteinuria is present in a very high percentage of cases, 37% of men and 31% of women. This contrasts with 3% for men and 6% for women aged 22–41 [52]. Some of this proteinuria in the elderly may be due to bacteriuria which also increases in elderly people. The subjects with proteinuria are more frequently hypertensive.

The nephrotic syndrome in the elderly

Bolton [53] compared biopsies in patients 60 years and older examined on their service, with those under 60 over a 10-year period.

When 63 biopsies in patients over 60 with the nephrotic syndrome were compared with 180 biopsies from those under 60, there were surprisingly few differences in histologic categories. Only amyloid disease was significantly more frequent in those over 60 (Table 14.2).

It is perhaps surprising that the diagnosis of renal vein thrombosis does not appear in the above series. In a group of 76 patients with renal vein thrombosis whom we studied, all but two were over 50 and six were over 60 years of age [9].

The indications for treatment of the nephrotic syndrome in elderly people does not differ from that in other adults. The susceptibility to thrombosis and other complications of the nephrotic syndrome together with the hypoalbuminemia, hypercholesteremia, and oedema associated with the nephrotic syndrome usually warrant treatment in our view.

The minimal lesion nephrotic syndrome can be reversed by steroids or cyclophosphamide and because of the relative lack of complications which disturb the patient taking cyclophosphamide compared with those seen with steroids in the elderly, we prefer cyclophosphamide treatment. The steroid dose is 50–60 mg/day for 10–14 days when the nephrotic state usually reverses abruptly. Dosage is then reduced to zero over 6 weeks. Cyclophosphamide is used in a dose of 1 mg/kg per day and continued for 8–12 weeks. Response is more gradual.

Membranous glomerulonephritis has been shown in a controlled trial to respond to high-dose alternate-day

Table 14.2 Incidence of histologic lesions associated with nephrotic syndrome in patients <60 and >60 years of age

Histologic diagnosis	Age (years)		Total
	60	≥60	
Membranous glomerulopathy	55(30%)	21(33%)	76
Minimal-change disease	49(27%)	13(21%)	62
Focal glomerular sclerosis	32(18%)	10(16%)	42
MPGN/GN	18(10%)	6(10%)	24
Amyloidosis	13(7%)	9(14%)	22
Diabetic nephropathy	13(7%)	4(7%)	17
Total	180	63	243

Ratio of <60/≥60 = 2.86.
MPGN, membranoproliferative glomerulonephritis; GN, glomerulonephritis.

Table 14.3 Comparative incidence of the different renal diseases in 115 elderly patients (older than 60 years) and 455 patients younger than 60 years

Diagnosis	Elderly adults (60 years and older) (%)	Other patients (<60 years) (%)
Idiopathic crescentic glomerulonephritis	16.5	4.0
Membranous glomerulonephritis	13.0	4.5
Minimal change nephrotic syndrome	7.8	7.0
Focal proliferative/mesangiopathic glomerulonephritis	6.0	10.5
Diffuse proliferative glomerulonephritis	4.0	2.2
Chronic glomerulonephritis	4.0	7.0
Membranoproliferative glomerulonephritis	1.7	9.2
Glomerulosclerosis	13.0	10.5
Vasculitis	5.0	3.0
Amyloidosis	4.0	1.0
Wegener's granulomatosis	3.0	0.2
Systemic lupus erythematosus	1.7	13.8
Other systemic diseases	8.6	12.0
Miscellaneous	8.6	15.0

steroids [54]. In an Australian collaborative controlled trial, cyclophosphamide combined with dipyridamole and warfarin was shown to reverse the nephrotic syndrome and improve renal function [55].

Ponticelli *et al.* [56] showed similar reversal of the nephrotic syndrome and improvement in function to that reported with cyclophosphamide, using methylprednisolone therapy, alternating with chlorambucil.

Of these three treatments we prefer the one used in the Australian Study which is remarkably free from side-effects in elderly patients, with the nephrotic syndrome if the dose of cyclophosphamide of 1 mg/kg per day is adjusted to keep the total blood leukocyte count above 3500 ml. In our experience high-dose steroids are associated with unacceptable side-effects in the elderly. Chlorambucil is probably far more likely to induce malignancies than cyclophosphamide. Both cyclophosphamide and chlorambucil cause azoospermia in males and interfere with ovarian function in females but these side-effects are clearly of no consequence in this age group.

Mesangiocapillary glomerulonephritis was relatively infrequent in Bolton's series [53] and has almost disappeared as a disease entity in several western countries including Australia.

Controlled trials have demonstrated benefit in mesangiocapillary glomerulonephritis using aspirin, warfarin, and dipyridamole [57,58].

Amyloidosis has been shown in a controlled trial to respond to alternative methylprednisolone and melphalan and as this is the only proven treatment for amyloid it is the one which we would recommend.

Diabetic nephropathy is an increasing cause of the nephrotic syndrome and renal failure in the elderly and is discussed below.

In focal glomerulosclerosis which has so far proved resistant to treatment, we have recently conducted a controlled trial of treatment and demonstrated benefit in terms of a reduction in proteinuria and increase in the serum albumin level using cyclosporine A. However, these changes are cyclosporine A-dependent and reverse when the drug is withdrawn.

Glomerulonephritis in the elderly

All forms of glomerulonephritis have been recorded in the elderly and in a study comparing the percentage of 115 patients over age 60 with 455 patients under age 60, Moorthy & Zimmerman [59] documented some interesting differences (Table 14.4). Idiopathic crescentic glomerulonephritis was the diagnosis in 16.5% of those over age 60 and only 4% under age 60. Membranous glomerulonephritis was more frequent in older patients but membranoproliferative glomerulonephritis much less frequent. Wegener's granulomatosis was 10 times more frequent in patients over 60 than those under 60. In spite of the fact that autoantibodies increase with age, the diagnosis of systemic lupus erythematosus was rare in those over 60 compared to younger patients.

The treatment of some of these conditions is discussed in the section on nephrotic syndrome. Several forms of glomerulonephritis which are the most responsive to treatment, feature significantly in Table 14.4. These are diffuse crescentic glomerulonephritis, Wegener's granulomatosis, and vasculitis. The latter two conditions respond well to both cyclophosphamide and prednisolone treatment. If diffuse crescents are present in these or in idiopathic glomerulonephritis, plasma exchange in addition to cyclophosphamide and prednisolone is very effective treatment [60–63].

Diabetic glomerulosclerosis

Although this disease does not appear in Table 14.3 as a lesion documented on renal biopsy, this is because of the selection of patients included in these biopsy series.

Diabetic glomerulosclerosis is a distressingly common disease. About 50% of insulin-dependent diabetes mellitus is accompanied by continuous proteinuria after 20 years [64]. Only 28% of diabetics lived for 10 years after the onset of proteinuria prior to the availability of dialysis [65].

The frequency of diabetic glomerulosclerosis in noninsulin-dependent diabetes mellitus is more relevant to the discussion of renal disease in the elderly and its frequency is much less clearly documented than that in insulin-dependent diabetes mellitus. Every year since registries commenced, the percentage of patients on dialysis in the United States with Type II diabetes and diabetic glomerulosclerosis has increased. In 1990 it is predicted that no less than 50% of all end-stage renal failure in the United States requiring dialysis will be due to diabetes and the majority of these are elderly Type II diabetes. Similar trends have been observed elsewhere.

No problem more urgently requires attention in the field of prevention of renal failure than that of diabetic glomerulosclerosis.

It has been well documented that control of hypertension slows progression in diabetics [66]. There is some preliminary evidence which is mainly experimental that converting enzyme inhibitors are particularly beneficial in slowing progression of diabetic glomerulosclerosis.

Urinary tract infection and reflux nephropathy

The prevalence of bacteriuria has increased in the elderly.

In males, bacteriuria is rare under the age of 50, but is present in 3.6% of men over 70 [67]. The prostate is the usual source of infection in males and in recurrent, persistant urinary tract infection, even in elderly males prostatic infection is usually present [68].

The increased prevalence of urinary tract infection with age is less well documented in women; however, in both sexes some 25–30% of elderly subjects in nursing homes have bacteriuria [69].

In elderly subjects as in younger age groups bacteriuria is a marker for impaired renal function [70]. But the reason for this association is no more clear-cut in this age group than in others.

More importantly, bacteriuria in the elderly is associated with reduced survival [70]; however, treatment of bacteriuria is associated with a high relapse rate and is not generally recommended unless there is an associated urinary tract abnormality.

Among associated abnormalities obstructive lesions are the most important because of the risk of septicemia in a patient with an infected obstructed kidney.

Among other common forms of renal parenchymal scarring renal papillary necrosis is discussed above, and in this condition, if the ureter is obstructed, the risks of a septicemic death are high.

Reflux nephropathy—an important diagnosis in children and young women—is rarely diagnosed in patients over 50 [71].

Increased susceptibility to nephrotoxic agents

The susceptibility of elderly patients to nephrotoxicity of NSAIDs is discussed above. It has also been well documented that elderly subjects have an increased susceptibility to amminoglycosides toxicity [72]. It has also been reported that the elderly are more likely to develop nephrotoxicity following radiocontrast media [73].

An increased susceptibility to nephrotoxic side-effects of antibacterial drugs has been implied but not well documented.

References

1 Tanchi H, Tsusboi K, Okutomi J. Age changes in the human kidney of different races. Gerontolgia 1971;17:87.

2 Kaplan C, Pasternack B, Shah H, et al. Age-related incidence of sclerotic glomeruli in human kidneys. Am J Pathol 1975;80:227–234.

3 McLachlan MSF, Gutherie JC, Anderson CK, et al. Vascular and glomerular changes in the aging kidney. J Pathol 1977;121:65–78.

4 Sworn MJ, Fox M. Donor kidney selection for transplantation: relationships between glomerular structure, vascular supply, and age. Br J Urol 1972;44:377–383.

5 Sorensen FH. Quantitative studies of the renal corpuscles. IV. Acta Path Microbiol Immunol Scand 1977;85:356–366.

6 Bolton WK, Sturgill BC. Spontaneous glomerular sclerosis in aging Sprague–Dawley rats. II. Ultrastructural studies. Am J Pathol 1980;98:339–350.

7 Shock NW. Homeostatic disturbances and adaptations in aging. Bull Schweiz Akad Med Wiss 1969;24:284–298.

8 Bolton WK, Benton FR, Maclay JG, et al. Spontaneous glomerular sclerosis in aging Sprague–Dawley rats. I. Lesions associated with mesangial IgM deposits. Am J Pathol 1976;85:277–302.

9 Kincaid-Smith P, ed. The Kidney—a Clinicopathological Study. Oxford: Blackwell Scientific Publications, 1975:13.

10 Davidson AJ, Talner LB, Downs WB. A study of the angiography appearance of the kidney in an aging normotensive population. Radiology 1969;92:975–983.

11 Griffiths GJ, Cartwright GO, McLachlan MSF. Estimation of renal size from radiographs: Is the effort worth while? Clin Radiol 1975;26:249–256.

12 Hollenberg NK, Adams DF, Solomon HS, et al. Senescence and the renal vasculature in normal man. Circ Res 1974;34:309–316.

13 Epstein M, Hollenberg NK. Age as a determinant of renal sodium conservation in normal man. J Lab Clin Med 1976;87:411–417.

14 Lewis WH Jr, Alving AS. Changes with age in the renal function in adult men. Am J Physiol 1938;123:500–515.

15 Adler S, Lindeman RD, Yiengst MJ, et al. The effect of acute acid loading on the urinary excretion of acid by the aging human kidney. J Lab Clin Med 1968;72:278–289.

16 Richie JP, Garnick MB, Seltzer S, et al. Computerized tomography scan for diagnosis and staging of renal cell carcinoma. J Urol 1983;129:1114–1116.

17 Quesada JR, Swanson DA, Trindade A, et al. Renal cell carcinoma: antitumour effects of leucocyte interferon. Cancer Res 1983;43:940–947.

18 Lee JC, Yamauci H, Hooper C. The association of cancer and the nephrotic syndrome. Ann Intern Med 1966;64:41–51.

19 Hopper J. Tumor-related renal lesions. Ann Intern Med 1974;81:550–551.

20 Row PG, Cameron JS, Turner DR, et al. Membranous nephropathy: Long-term follow-up and association with neoplasia. Q J Med 1975;44:207–239.

21 Couser WG, Wagonfield JB, Spargo BH, et al. Glomerular deposition of tumour antigen in membranous nephropathy

associated with colonic carcinoma. Am J Med 1974;57: 962–970.

22 Borochovitz D, Kam WK, Nolte M, *et al.* Adenocarcinoma of the palate associated with nephrotic syndrome and epimembranous carcinoembryonic antigen deposition. Cancer 1982;49:2097–2102.

23 Kincaid-Smith P. Analgesic nephropathy in Australia. In Kuhn K, Brod J, eds. *Contributions to Nephrology: Interstitial Nephropathies*, 6th Symposium on Nephrology. vol. 16. Basel: Hanover Karger, 1978:57–64.

24 Canadian Dialysis Registry, 1985.

25 Vetrovec GW, Cowley MJ, Landwehr DM, *et al.* High prevalence of renal artery stenosis in hypertensive patients with coronary artery disease. J Am Coll Cardiol 1984;3:518.

26 Maxwell MH, Bleifer KH, Franklin SS, *et al.* Cooperative study of renovascular hypertension: Demographic analysis of the study. J Am Med Assoc 1972;220:1195–1204.

27 Davis BA, Crook JE, Vestal RE, *et al.* Prevalence of renovascular hypertension in patients with grade III or IV hypertensive retinopathy. N Engl J Med 1979;301: 1273–1276.

28 Sos TA, Pickering TG, Sniderman K, *et al.* Percutaneous renal angioplasty in renovascular hypertension due to atheroma or fibromuscular dysplasia. N Engl J Med 1983;309:274–279.

29 Tegtmeyer CJ, Elson J, Glass TA. Percutaneous transluminal angioplasty: The treatment of choice of renovascular hypertension due to fibromuscular dysplasia. Radiology 1982; 143:631–637.

30 Geyskes GG, Puylaert CBAJ, Oei HY, *et al.* Follow-up study of 70 patients with renal artery stenosis treated by percutaneous transluminal dilation. Br Med J 1983;287: 333–336.

31 Martin EC, Mattern RF, Baer L. Renal angioplasty for hypertension: Predictive factors for long-term success. Am J Radiol 1981;137:921–924.

32 Grim CE, Luft FC, Yune HY, *et al.* Percutaneous transluminal dilation in the treatment of renal vascular hypertension. Ann Intern Med 1981;95:439–442.

33 Schwarten DE, Yune HY, Klatte EC, *et al.* Clinical experience with percutaneous transluminal angioplasty (PTA) of sclerosed renal arteries. Radiology 1980;135:601–604.

34 Pickering TG, Laragh JH, Sos TA. Renovascular hypertension. In Strauss MB, Welt LG, eds. *Diseases of the Kidney*, 2nd edn. New York: Little, Brown, & Co., 1971.

35 Atkinson JB, Brown JJ, Cumming AM. Captopril in the management of hypertension with renal artery stenosis: The long term effect as a prediction of surgical outcome. Am J Cardiol 1982;49:1460–1466.

36 Fraser I, Ihle B, Kincaid-Smith P. Renal failure due to cholesterol emboli. Aust NZ J Med 1991;21:418–421.

37 Nanra RS, Stuart-Taylor J, de Leon AH, *et al.* Kidney Int 1978;13:79–92.

38 Dawborn JK, Fairley KF, Kincaid-Smith P, *et al.* The association of peptic ulceration, chronic renal disease and analgesic abuse. Q J Med 1966;35:69–83.

39 Kincaid-Smith P. Pathogeneses of the renal lesion associated with the abuse of analgesics. Lancet 1967;1:850–862.

40 Kincaid-Smith P. Analgesic nephropathy. Ann Intern Med 1968;68:949–953.

41 Kincaid-Smith P. Analgesic nephropathy: a common form of renal disease in Australia. Med J Aust 1969;2:1131–1135.

42 Kincaid-Smith P, Nanra RS, Fairley KF. Analgesic nephropathy: a recoverable form of chronic renal failure. In Kincaid-Smith P, Fairley KF, eds. *Renal Infection and Renal Scarring.* Melbourne: Mercedes Publishing Services, 1971:385–400.

43 Fairley KF, Kincaid-Smith P. Renal papillary necrosis with a normal pyelogram. Br Med J 1968;1:156–157.

44 Prescott LF. Analgesic nephropathy: A reassessment of the role of phenacetin and other analgesics. Drugs 1982;23: 75–149.

45 Kincaid-Smith P. Effects of nonnarcotic analgesics on the kidney. Drugs 1986;32:109–128.

46 Champion De Crespigny PJ, Becker GJ, Ihle BU, *et al.* Renal failure and nephrotic syndrome associated with sulindac. Clin Nephrol 1988;30:52–55.

47 Nenra RS, Kincaid-Smith P. Renal papillary necrosis in rheumatoid arthritis. Med J Aust 1975;1:194–197.

48 Nanra RA, Kincaid-Smith P. Experimental renal papillary necrosis (RPN) with nonsteroid anti-inflammatory analgesics. In Haschek H, ed. *Phenacetin Abuse 1973*. International Symposium on problems of phenacetin abuse. Vienna: Facta Publications, 1973:67–88.

49 Harbitz TB. Histology of the prostate in elderly men. Acta Pathol Microbiol Scand 1972;80:756–768.

50 Lytton B, Emery JM, Harvard BM. The incidence of benign prostatic obstruction. J Urol 1968;99:639–645.

51 Hodkinson HM, Exton-Smith AN. Factors predicting mortality in the elderly in the community. Age Aging 1976;5:110–115.

52 Mimica M, Durakovic Prica L, Bule LJ. Proteinuria in samples of younger and older persons in the population. Acta Med Yugosl 1981;35:165–172.

53 Bolton WK, Westervelt FB Jr, Sturgill BC. Nephrotic syndrome and focal glomerular sclerosis in aging man. Nephron 1978;20:307–315.

54 Collaborative Study of the Adult Idiopathic Nephrotic Syndrome. N Engl J Med 1979;301:1301–1306.

55 Mathew TH. The treatment of idiopathic glomerulonephritis. In Becker GJ, Atkins RC, Kincaid-Smith PS, eds. *Preceedings of the Second Asian Pacific Congress of Nephrology*. Melbourne: Dominion Press, 1983:164–172.

56 Ponticelli C, Zucchelli P, Imbasciati E, *et al.* Controlled trial of methylprednisolone and chlorambucil in idiopathic membranous nephropathy. N Engl J Med 1984;310:946–950.

57 Donadio JV, Anderson CF, Michell JC, *et al.* Membranoproliferative glomerulonephritis: A prospective clinical trial of platelet-inhibitor therapy. N Engl J Med 1984;310:1421–1426.

58 Zimmerman SW, Moorthy AV, Dreher WH, *et al.* Prospective trial of warfarin and dipyridamole in patients with membranoproliferative glomerulonephritis. Am J Med 1983; 75:920–927.

59 Moorthy AV, Zimmerman SW. Renal disease in the elderly: clinicopathologic analysis of renal disease in 115 elderly patients. Clin Nephrol 1980;14:223–229.

60 Walker RG, Becker GJ, d'Apice AJF, *et al.* Plasma exchange in the treatment of glomerulonephritis and other renal diseases. Aust N Z J Med 1986;16:828–838.

61 Becker GJ, d'Apice AJF, Walker RG, *et al.* Plasmapheresis in the treatment of glomerulonephritis. Med J Aust 1977;2: 693–696.

62 Walker RG, d'Apice AJF, Kincaid-Smith P, *et al.* Plasmapheresis in Goodpasture's syndrome with renal failure. Med J Aust 1977;1:875–879.

63 Walker RG, Scheinkestel C, Becker GJ, *et al.* Clinical and morphological aspects of the management of crescentic antiglomerular basement membrane antibody (anti-GBM) nephritis/Goodpasture's syndrome. Q J Med New Series 1985;34:75–89.

64 Knowles HC. Discussion: Vascular and visual complications. Kidney Int 1974:6:41–46.

65 Caird FI. Survival of diabetics with proteinuria. Diabetes 1961;10:178–181.

66 Mogensen C. Long-term antihypertensive treatment inhibiting progression of diabetic nephropathy. Br Med J 1982;285–685–688.

67 Kunin CM, ed. *Detection, Prevention and Management of Urinary Tract Infections*, 3rd edn. Philadelphia: Lea & Febiger, 1979:47.

68 Stamey TA, ed. *Pathogeneses and Treatment of Urinary Tract Infections.* Boston: Williams & Wilkins, 1980:342–429.

69 Sherman FT, Tucci V, Libow LS, *et al.* Nosocomial urinary-tract infections in a skilled nursing facility. J Am Geriatr Soc 1980;28:456–461.

70 Dontas AS, Kasviki-Charvati P, Papanayiotou PC, *et al.* Bacteriuria and survival in old age. N Engl J Med 1981; 304:939–943.

71 El-Khatib M, Becker GJ, Kincaid-Smith P. Reflux nephropathy and primary vasicoureteral reflux in adults. Q J Med 1990;284:1241–1253.

72 Moore RD, Smith CR, Kipsky JJ, *et al.* Risk factors for nephrotoxicity in patients treated with aminoglycosides. Ann Intern Med 1984;100:352–357.

73 Byrd L, Sherman RL. Radiocontrast-induced acute renal failure: A clinical and pathophysiologic review. Medicine 1979;58:270–279.

15

Glomerular disease in the elderly

Richard J. Glassock

Introduction

The elderly patient may be afflicted by many of the same glomerular disorders as one encounters in more youthful patients [1]. Nonetheless, certain disorders seem to have a rising prevalence with age or present in as unusually severe or atypical disease in the older individual. A review of the entire spectrum of glomerular disease is beyond the scope of this chapter; therefore, the focus will be on the clinical and pathologic features of the more common glomerular diseases seen in elderly patients.

Broadly speaking, glomerular disease can be divided into two categories, namely those which primarily involve the glomerular capillaries, and those in which glomerular involvement is secondary to a multisystem disease process [2]. Primary glomerular diseases which more commonly occur in the elderly than in younger patients include membranous glomerulonephritis and certain forms of glomerulosclerosis. Secondary diseases which commonly occur in the elderly include diabetic glomerulosclerosis (most often secondary to noninsulin-dependent diabetes mellitus), vasculitis, and amyloidosis. Table 15.1 provides a summary of the findings of Ramirez & Saba [3] who reported a series of renal biopsies performed in patients over the age of 60 years at the Tampa Veterans Administration Hospital between 1974 and 1982. Among 277 renal biopsies performed in such patients, 137 (49%) revealed primary glomerular disease, 59 (21%) revealed secondary glomerular disease, and the remainder revealed a variety of tubulointerstitial and/or noninflammatory vascular diseases or were unclassifiable. Table 15.2 shows the distribution of glomerular lesions found among patients presenting with the nephrotic syndrome over the age of 60 years and who underwent renal biopsy [1,3–5]. The relative paucity of diabetic glomerulosclerosis in this (and other) analyses is undoubtedly due to the fact that renal biopsy is a seldom used tool to establish this diagnosis. Most patients with diabetic glomerulosclerosis are diagnosed on clinical grounds alone.

For ease of presentation these disorders will now be reviewed in the context of the clinical syndromes with which they are most commonly associated; specifically, nephrotic syndrome, acute and/or rapidly progressive glomerulonephritis, and symptomless hematuria and/or proteinuria.

Table 15.1 Prevalence of various renal diseases as demonstrated by renal biopsy in patients over 60 years of age. (From Ramirez & Saba [3])

		n	Percentage of total
	Primary glomerular disease		
	Minimal change disease	16	6
	Membranous glomerulonephritis	57	21
	Focal glomerulosclerosis	12	4
	Membranoproliferative glomerulonephritis	13	5
	Mesangial proliferative glomerulonephritis	5	2
	Rapidly progressive (crescentic) glomerulonephritis	15	5
	Acute glomerulonephritis	5	2
	IgA nephropathy	14	5
	Total primary glomerular disease	137	49%
	Secondary glomerular disease		
	Amyloidosis	22	8
	Diabetic glomerulosclerosis	14	5
	Lupus nephritis	12	4
	Vasculitis (including Wegener's granulomatosis and Schöenlein−Henoch purpura)	7	3
	Scleroderma	2	1
	Goodpastures Syndrome	2	1
	Total secondary glomerular disease	59	21%
	Nonglomerular disease and unclassifiable	81	29%

Table 15.2 Prevalence of various glomerular lesions as demonstrated by renal biopsy in patients with nephrotic syndrome over 60 years of age. (From Moorthy & Zimmerman [1], Ramirez & Saba [3], Abrass [4], and Murray & Raij [5])

Lesion	n	Percentage of total
Membranous glomerulonephritis	65	38
Minimal change disease	41	24
Proliferative glomerulonephritis	18	10
Focal glomerular sclerosis	15	9
Amyloidosis	22	13
Others (including diabetic glomerulosclerosis)	11	6
Total	172	100

Nephrotic syndrome

The development of heavy proteinuria with consequent lowering of plasma albumin concentration and accompanying edema and hyperlipidemia is one of the most common clinical syndromes arising secondary to glomerular disease in the elderly [6]. Such patients most frequently present in a symptomatic form with weight-gain and edema, but occasionally they are discovered in the course of an investigation for another illness. Based upon renal biopsy data, the glomerular lesions which evoke the nephrotic syndrome in the elderly are varied (see also Table 15.2) but three lesions account for over 75% of all cases [7]. These are, in descending order of prevalence, membranous glomerulonephritis, minimal-change disease, and primary amyloidosis. Other lesions, including various proliferative glomerulonephritides and focal and segmental glomerulosclerosis account for 25% of cases or less.

Diabetic glomerulosclerosis

It should be emphasized that this analysis is biased by the indications for performance of renal biopsy in patients with nephrotic syndrome. As mentioned above, this bias undoubtedly accounts for the relative infrequency of diabetic glomerulosclerosis and other multisystem diseases (e.g., lupus nephritis) since renal biopsies are performed much less frequently, if at all, in patients presenting with nephrotic syndrome when the cause of the disorder is self-evident (e.g., diabetes mellitus). However, it is important to emphasize that one cannot always safely conclude that diabetes is the cause of glomerular disease in an elderly patient with noninsulin-dependent diabetes mellitus since several nondiabetic glomerular diseases (such as IgA nephropathy, membranous glomerulonephritis, and postinfectious glomerulonephritis) can coexist with diabetes mellitus in the elderly [8]. This subject is dealt with in greater detail in the chapter by Hostetter & Daniels (Chapter 17). Suffice to say that the development of nephrotic syndrome in an elderly patient with noninsulin-dependent diabetes should be definitively ascribed to a diabetes-related process *only* when the diabetes has been of known long duration (in excess of 5−10 years) and when extrarenal vascular complications are concomitantly present (such as proliferative diabetic retinopathy) in *absence* of features suggesting glomerulonephritis. Most patients with diabetic glomerulosclerosis as a cause of nephrotic syndrome will also have hypertension and some degree of impaired renal function. The severity of glucose intolerance, the urinary sediment, and biochemical tests of the serum are of little help in differentiating diabetic glomerulosclerosis from nondiabetic lesions in patients with nephrotic syndrome [9]. However, a very active "nephritic sediment" with dysmorphic hematuria *may* support the diagnosis of glomerulonephritis and highly selective proteinuria in a diabetic patient with nephrotic syndrome would support the diagnosis of minimal-change disease. However, one must be cautious in overinterpreting the urinary sediment, since several reports have emphasized the development of hematuria in patients who have biopsy-proven diabetic glomerulosclerosis [9]. While background retinopathy (microaneurysms and soft exudates) develop in the vast majority of elderly patients with long-standing diabetes mellitus, irrespective of whether clinically relevant diabetic glomerulosclerosis is present or not, proliferative retinopathy is strongly associated with the development of clinically overt diabetic glomerulosclerosis [10]. It remains to be established whether measurement of specific substances in the urine, such as the C5b-9 neoantigen, C3dg, interleukin 6, or platelet-derived antigens, will improve on the precision of pre-biopsy identification of nondiabetic glomerular lesions in the elderly patient presenting with nephrotic syndrome concomitantly with diabetes mellitus [11−13]. At the present time renal biopsy is the only certain way to make this differentiation.

Membranous glomerulonephritis

Among the common lesions underlying nephrotic syndrome in the elderly, membranous glomerulonephritis stands out as a most frequently encountered lesion with an overall prevalence ranging from 30−50%, averaging about 40% [1,3−5]. Among patients with idiopathic membranous glomerulonephritis, approximately 15−20% are over the age of 60 at the time of discovery of disease [2,6]. The reason for this high prevalence of membranous glomerulonephritis in the elderly is unknown. The gradual decline of immunocompetence with aging conceivably could be important. Most of the patients with membranous glomerulonephritis in the elderly have idiopathic disease, i.e., no cause is ever found. However, secondary forms of membranous glomerulonephritis (e.g., neoplasia, drug-induced, chronic viral infections) do seem to be more frequent in the elderly than in young patients [2,5]. Underlying malignancies, especially solid tumors, may account in part for the rising prevalence of secondary membranous glomerulonephritis in the elderly (see below) [14].

Idiopathic membranous glomerulonephritis in the elderly produces clinical manifestations which parallel those found in younger patients. Approximately 80–85% of patients demonstrate heavy proteinuria and nephrotic syndrome with milder degrees of proteinuria in the remainder [2]. The glomerular filtration rate (GFR) is often mildly impaired, perhaps due to complicating arterionephrosclerosis. Edema may be quite severe, particularly in the presence of concomitant cardiac failure or poor nutrition. Biochemical changes in the serum reflect the loss of plasma proteins in the urine and have little diagnostic significance. Complement levels are normal. Fluorescent antinuclear antibody may be non-specifically slightly elevated especially in patients over the age of 65. Urinary C5b-9 neoantigen excretion may be increased [11]. Hepatitis B surface antigen may be found in the serum, especially in patients from endemic areas (such as the Far East), in patients who have received blood transfusions, or who are chronic intravenous drug abusers [2].

Renal biopsies reveal the typical features of membranous glomerulonephritis with capillary walls thickened by epimembranous electron dense deposits containing immunoglobulins [2]. These electron dense deposits may be small in early disease (Stage I) but with the progression that they coalesce and are associated with a basement membrane reaction (Stage II) disease. More advanced forms of membranous glomerulonephritis may present with glomerulosclerosis and significant capillary wall thickening on light microscopy. The extraglomerular vessels demonstrate varying degrees of arterionephrosclerosis. Focal interstitial fibrosis and tubular atrophy is commonly found, particularly in those patients with advanced-stage disease or in those presenting with significant impairment of renal function. With long-standing disease the capillary wall may become greatly thickened and distorted giving rise to difficulties with diagnosis based on light microscopy alone. When a secondary form of membranous glomerulonephritis is present (e.g., lupus nephritis, chronic viral infection, or malignancies) electron dense deposits may also be found in the mesangial zones. C3 complement proteins may be found irregularly

in the glomerulus. C1q complement component deposition in the capillary loops is very often found in membranous glomerulonephritis secondary to systemic lupus erythematosis.

Although it is relatively easy to establish a diagnosis of membranous glomerulonephritis in an elderly patient with nephrotic syndrome through the use of renal biopsy, differentiation of primary and secondary forms may be difficult. Mild elevation of fluorescent antinuclear antibody, commonly found in elderly patients, may confuse the picture. Antidouble-stranded (native) DNA antibodies may often, but not invariably, be present when membranous glomerulonephritis is due to systemic lupus erythematosus. Other renal pathologic features, such as mesangial deposits, C1q deposits or tubuloreticular inclusions may be the only clue to underlying disease in certain patients [2]. Drugs (such as captopril, probencid, gold, and mercury) may occasionally be incriminated in the disease when a careful history is taken [2]. Such history must include questions concerning use of topical preparations of mercurial compounds and environmental exposure. Underlying malignancy is the most difficult diagnostic challenge. It is well known that 3–11% of patients with nephrotic syndrome due to membranous glomerulonephritis have an underlying malignancy, a prevalence much higher than expected [14,15]. Furthermore, removal of the tumor may induce a remission and relapses may develop with a recurrence of neoplasia. Approximately 70% of patients with malignancies associated with nephrotic syndrome have membranous glomerulonephritis. Therefore, the association of malignancy with nephrotic syndrome is not a chance event. Most would agree that the malignancies are causally related to the nephrotic syndrome but in a few instances the nephrotic syndrome, or its treatment, may have contributed to the development of a neoplasia rather than the reverse. Most often, the neoplastic process is evident prior to or at the onset of nephrotic syndrome; however, in about a third of the patients with membranous glomerulonephritis and neoplasia the tumor is not discovered until well after the diagnosis of membranous glomerulonephritis is established [15]. Such patients will be inadvertently and erroneously labeled as idiopathic disease and may receive therapy which in itself may augment the development of neoplasia. Therefore, a careful search for underlying cancer is indicated in all elderly patients with a diagnosis of nephrotic syndrome due to membranous glomerulonephritis. At a minimum this should consist of chest X-ray, a stool for occult blood, an abdominal computed tomography scan, and a careful search for adenopathy, skin lesions, abdominal and rectal masses. Females should have a careful breast and pelvic examination. Mammography should also be performed. More invasive tests such as flexible sigmoidscopy, upper gastrointestinal series, intravenous pyelograms are only indicated on a case by case basis. Serologic screening with carcinoembryonic antigens or α-fetoprotein has little value.

Renal vein thrombosis may complicate membranous glomerulonephritis in 5–50% of instances. The reason for this variability is unknown. When it occurs renal vein thrombosis usually develops in patients with serum albumin concentrations less than 2.0 g/dl. Most often no signs or symptoms referable to the kidney are present. Pulmonary emboli may occur but appear to be uncommon. Treatment consists of long-term anticoagulants.

The prognosis for membranous glomerulonephritis in the elderly is generally favorable. About 15–20% of patients will undergo a spontaneous remission of proteinuria and will maintain stable renal function. Approximately 20–40% will have persistent heavy proteinuria and will ultimately develop progressive renal impairment usually 3 years or more following discovery of disease. The remaining patients will either enter a partial remission of proteinuria or will have persisting nephrotic range proteinuria but with stable renal function. Because of the general benign course of membranous glomerulonephritis, elderly patients should only receive specific therapy if poor prognostic indicators are present at the time of discovery. These include urinary protein excretion in excess of 10 g/dl, elevated serum creatinine concentration, Stage II or Stage III disease on renal biopsy, and definite chronic tubulointerstitial lesions with fibrosis on renal biopsy.

Elderly patients with membranous glomerulonephritis may have a somewhat worse prognosis compared to younger patients. Patients with advanced irreversible renal failure at discovery should be treated with dialysis. Currently, glucocorticoids alone are not believed to exert any lasting beneficial effect on the course of membranous glomerulonephritis, except that pulse intravenous methylprednisolone may temporarily improve renal function in those with rapidly declining glomerular filtration. Combinations of alkylating cytotoxic agents (chlorambucil or cyclophosphamide) and oral or intravenous glucocorticoids have been associated with increased frequency of complete and partial remissions and stabilization or improved renal function [16]. Unfortunately, these studies included relatively few elderly patients so one cannot be sure that these findings are also applicable to the older age group. However, complications of these regimens in the elderly patient may be increased, especially the development of herpes zoster. Therefore, they should be used with caution and only when severe symptoms of the nephrotic syndrome or progressive renal failure require aggressive management.

Minimal-change disease

Minimal-change disease is the most common cause of nephrotic syndrome in infants and children but it is by no means rare in the elderly [1,3–5]. Most series have noted that 15–25% of cases of nephrotic syndrome due to primary glomerular disease in the elderly is consequent to minimal-change disease [6]. Clinically, minimal-change disease is characterized by heavy, highly selective proteinuria which often may have an abrupt onset. Typically, the GFR is normal or only slightly decreased. On rare occasions acute renal failure may supervene. Blood pressure is normal, although systolic hypertension may be seen in the elderly. The urinary sediment reveals hematuria in 10–20% of patients. Serum complement levels are normal. Renal biopsies may be difficult to interpret because of the superimposition of age-related vascular and chronic tubulointerstitial lesions. One should not attach too much significance to the finding of focal or global sclerosis in an elderly patient with nephrotic syndrome when other light microscopic, immunofluorescence, and electron microscopic findings are compatible with minimal-change disease.

As with children, minimal-change disease is a steroid responsive lesion in older adults and it has a relatively benign prognosis in most patients [2,6]. However, unlike children, longer periods of glucocorticoid therapy and perhaps higher doses are required in order to induce complete remissions [17]. An appropriate regimen might consist of prednisone 1 mg/kg per day or 80 mg/day (whichever is larger) given as a single morning dose for approximately 8 weeks, following which the patient is converted to an every other day dosage of approximately 0.5 mg/kg per day for an additional 8 weeks, unless a complete remission occurs during initial daily dosage. If a remission occurs during the initial daily prednisone period the patient can be converted to an every other day regimen approximately 1 week after the urine is completely free of protein on qualitative testing. Overall, 80–90% of older adult patients with minimal-change disease will enter a complete remission within 16–20 weeks of beginning therapy utilizing this protocol. However, 20–50% of patients will have subsequent relapses. Remissions of these first relapses will occur with retreatment but sometimes the requirement of multiple courses of therapy will eventually cause unacceptable degrees of steroid toxicity. In such patients who have frequent relapses and who have developed side-effects of repeated courses of glucocorticoids, cyclophosphamide therapy can be considered. Oral cyclophosphamide, 1.5–2.0 mg/kg per day, for 10–12 weeks can be administered following or in conjunction with a glucocorticoid-induced remission [16]. This therapeutic approach should be reserved for those patients who have displayed a frequently relapsing course. A 12-week regimen of oral cyclophosphamide is preferred for those patients with steroid dependence and relapses during steroid tapering [2]. Elderly patients with few symptoms whose edema can be readily controlled with small doses of diuretics alone should probably *not be given* steroids or cyclophosphamide because of the overall benign course of minimal-change disease and the fact that 20–30% of patients will likely enter a spontaneous remission within the first year following initial diagnosis. Both glucocorticoids and cytotoxic regimens should be reserved for symptomatic patients. While the risks of glucocorticoids and/or cytotoxic drug therapy in patients with minimal-change disease are relatively small, it is likely that the elderly patient will be more prone to the development of side-effects, such as reactivation of latent viral infections, aggravation of noninsulin-dependent diabetes mellitus, worsening of hypertension, depression, and osteoporosis.

Other primary glomerular lesions, such as focal and segmental glomerulosclerosis, membranoproliferative glomerulonephritis, and "pure" mesangial proliferative glomerulonephritis are encountered in only 10–20% of elderly patients with nephrotic syndrome [1,3–5].

Focal and segmental glomerulosclerosisis

Focal and segmental glomerulosclerosisis is a particular problem in diagnosis since the renal lesions which accompany aging are similar to the lesions of primary focal and segmental glomerulosclerosis [2,6]. Thus, a renal biopsy in an elderly patient must be interpreted with great caution. The glomerular changes of aging are often accompanied by arterionephrosclerosis and are more often global than segmental. Otherwise, the clinical findings, course, and response to therapy is not different in elderly patients. In comparison to younger patients only 20–30% of patients will experience a remission with glucocorticoid therapy. The long-term prognosis is poor, especially with very heavy proteinuria (>10 g/dl).

IgA nephropathy (Berger's disease)

IgA nephropathy is a rare occurrence in the elderly population; in most series less than 2–5% of patients with IgA nephropathy are over the age of 60 at initial presentation [2,18]. The most common clinical presentation of IgA nephropathy in the elderly is recurrent bouts of macroscopic hematuria sometimes accompanied by low-grade proteinuria. Nephrotic syndrome is a very unusual presentation. This entity will be discussed in further detail below.

Fibrillary and immunotactoid glomerulonephritis

Fibrillary glomerulonephritis and the related condition of immunotactoid glomerulonephritis are very uncommon glomerular lesions sometimes first diagnosed in the elderly population [2,19,20]. These patients may present with hematuria, heavy proteinuria, including the nephrotic syndrome, and reduced renal function. The distinctive feature in renal biopsy is the presence of fibrillar or microtubular structures, diameter 10–40 nm, in the subendothelial zones of the glomerular capilliaries [19,20]. By light microscopy there is often a lobular appearance to the glomeruli. These fibrillar or microtubular structures have no affinity for congo red and contain both immunoglobulins and complement [20]. At times the immunoglobulin deposits are monoclonal [19] and contain predominantly IgG4. The etiology and pathogenesis of these rare forms of glomerulonephritis is unknown. In some respects they resemble amyloidosis but the mechanisms responsible are believed to be quite different than those responsible for amyloidosis. The prognosis is overall unfavorable, however, some patients may exhibit stable renal function over long periods of time, particularly when urinary protein excretion is less than 3 g/day. There is no known effective treatment for these conditions [2].

Amyloidosis

Amyloidosis, both of the primary and secondary varieties, tends to be a disease of older individuals [2]. With control of many of the chronic infectious diseases such as tuberculosis and osteomyelitis, secondary amyloid is nowadays confined to rheumatoid arthritis and malignancies, most commonly multiple myeloma [21]. Primary amyloidosis is largely a disease of older adults, being very rare in individuals less than the age of 40. Nephrotic syndrome, often without any extra renal features, may be the presenting finding in primary amyloidosis. In fact, among several large series of patients presenting with an apparently idiopathic nephrotic syndrome over the age of 60, amyloidosis was found in renal biopsy in approximately 13% [1,3−5] of patients. The finding of carpal tunnel syndrome, unexplained cardiomegaly with heart failure or atrioventricular conduction defects, peripheral or autonomic neuropathy, hepatosplenomegaly, diarrhea with malabsorption, postural hypotension, or unexplained easy bruisability should increase one's suspicion of primary amyloidosis as a cause of nephrotic syndrome in an older patient. Laboratory tests may be unrevealing as many patients do not have detectable serum paraproteins. Urinary monoclonal light chain evaluation may be obscured by heavy albuminuria. Bone marrow aspirates generally are normal or show slight increase in plasma cells. Radioisotopic imaging with labeled amyloid P component may detect amyloid deposits in tissues [22]. Tissue biopsies must be preserved in absolute alcohol and fixed sections stained with congo red and examined under polarized light microscopy in order to make the diagnosis of amyloidosis. Electron microscopy is the preferred morphologic approach to diagnosis. The characteristic randomly oriented narrow microfibrils are found in the mesangium at the subendothelial spaces. Other tissues, such as the carpal ligaments, rectal mucosa, and abdominal subcutaneous fat may also be biopsied for diagnosis.

Patients with primary amyloidosis and glomerular involvement typically have heavy proteinuria with the usual biochemical features of nephrotic syndrome, however, lesser degrees of proteinuria may be encountered (see below). Progression to renal failure and complicating renal vein thrombosis is common [2]. Median survival from the onset of nephrotic syndrome is usually only 2−3 years. Therapy is generally unsatisfactory, but in the absence of contraindications the use of cyclical melphalan and prednisone perhaps combined with daily colchicine is probably warranted [23]. Some patients treated in this fashion may experience a reduction in proteinuria and stabilization of renal function but complete remissions are very rare. Massive proteinuria may be treated with combinations of angiotensin-converting enzyme inhibitors and nonsteroidal anti-inflammatory agents. Transplantation is feasible in some patients; however, recurrence of disease in the transplanted kidney may develop.

Systemic necrotizing vasculitis occurs with somewhat increased frequency in the elderly [24]. This lesion more commonly presents with rapidly progressive glomerulonephritis rather than nephrotic syndrome and will be discussed below.

Systemic lupus erythematosis (SLE)

Systemic lupus erythematosis with renal involvement is relatively uncommon in older populations and is more often a benign disorder with cutaneous hematologic or arthritic manifestations [2]. Fluorescent antinuclear antibody, as commented upon below, may appear as a nonspecific phenomenon of aging and one should be cautious about labeling renal disease in the elderly as due to SLE solely on the basis of seriologic findings. Other clinical and serologic manifestations of SLE should be present, including antibodies to double-stranded (native) DNA and/or antibodies to the Smith (Sm) antigen before making the diagnosis. The clinical, serologic, and histologic findings in the elderly patient with SLE resemble those of younger patients and the treatment is similar. Nephrotic syndrome is found most often in patients with the diffuse prolifesrative and membranous forms of lupus nephritis [2]. The prognosis for patients having onset of SLE with renal involvement over the age of 60 may be somewhat worse than the average with a higher prevalence of diffuse proliferative glomerulonephritis and progressive renal failure.

Rheumatoid arthritis

Rheumatoid arthritis may produce a specific glomerulopathy although most frequently nephrotic syndrome developing in a patient with rheumatoid arthritis can be ascribed to membranous glomerulonephritis, amyloidosis, or a complication of therapy, especially gold salts or nonsteroidal anti-inflammatory agents [2,25].

Mixed IgG/IgM essential cryoglobulinemia

Mixed IgG/IgM essential cryoglobulinemia with nephritis may develop in an elderly patient [2,26]. The formation of a monoclonal IgM antibody to a component of polyclonal IgG results in the development of large amounts of cryoprecipitable immune complexes in the serum. This disease, also known as essential mixed cryoglobulinemia (EMC) or Type II cryoglobulinemia, the polyclonal IgG, is presumably an antibody to an endogenous or exogenous antigen. In 10−30% of patients hepatitis B can be implicated as an environmental antigen inducing the disease. Rarely other environmental antigens may be implicated. However, most patients present with idiopathic disease. Older women are often affected. Approximately 25% of all patients are women over the age of 60 years. Fever, vasculitic skin rash, splenomegaly, polyarthralgias, abdominal pain, adenopathy, and strongly positive rheumatoid factor assays are common clinical features. Approximately 60−70% of patients will have overt renal involvement which includes hematuria, nephrotic syndrome, and progressive renal failure. Serum specimens obtained in warm test-tubes and spun in a warm centrifuge reveal large amounts of cryoimmunoglobulins (usually greater than 5 mg/ml). C4 levels are frequently low, C3 levels are often normal. Renal biopsies reveal proliferative glomerulonephritis, often of the lobular type, with extensive subendothelial deposits and monocytic infiltrates. The deposits contain the same proteins as the circulating cryoglobulins and may at times acquire a distinct fine structure on electron microscopy.

Currently, the preferred therapy is high-dose, pulse intravenous methylprednisolone at repeated intervals and maintenance low-dose alternate-day prednisone [27]. Adjunctive use of chlorambucil or cyclophosamide may be helpful in severe cases. Plasma exchange is of value for the acutely ill patient, especially with a very high circulating cryoimmunoglobulin level. Interferon therapy may be of value when underlying chronic hepatitis B infection can be diagnosed [28]. Overall, the prognosis is guarded, but complete remissions do occur and enthusiasm for aggressive therapy should be tempered especially in mild disease when seriologic findings, for example, normalization of C4 or disappearance of circulating cryoimmunoglobulins indicate the development of a re-

mission. Combined pulse methylprednisolone and cytotoxic drug therapy is primarily indicated for patients with severe nephrotic syndrome and progressive renal failure, especially when renal biopsies show the added feature of crescentic glomerulonephritis (see below).

Some patients with plasma cell dyscrasias elaborate only light chains, especially of the κ type [2,29]. These light chains may deposit in the kidney and in other tissues (especially heart, skin, and nerves) and provoke disease. Nephrotic syndrome with renal failure is a common manifestation of light chain disease. The serum protein electrophoresis fails to reveal a "M" protein spike, but urine will reveal monoclonal light chains, typically of the κ type. Renal biopsies demonstrate lesions resembling nodular diabetic glomerulosclerosis but the deposits contain the monoclonal light chain [2]. Overall the prognosis is poor, but some patients respond to steroid and cytotoxic agents given in protocols similar to that used for the treatment of multiple myeloma.

Benign and malignant neoplasms

A wide variety of benign and malignant neoplasms have been associated with nephrotic syndrome, especially in elderly patients [2,14,15]. The renal lesions underlying nephrotic syndrome vary widely but are most commonly membranous glomerulonephritis, focal and segmental glomerulosclerosis, proliferative glomerulonephritis, IgA nephropathy, vasculitis, crescentic glomerulonephritis, membranoproliferative glomerulonephritis, or minimal-change disease. Solid tumors such as carcinoma of the lung, breast, colon, kidney, prostate, bladder, skin, thyroid, and ovary seem most common [2]. Leukemia and lymphoma may also be associated with nephrotic syndrome. Hodgkin's disease renal cell carcinoma and mesothelioma are particularly associated with minimal-change disease [2]. In about two-thirds of cases the tumor will have been discovered *before* the onset of nephrotic syndrome or will be evident at the time of presentation. Any elderly patient presenting with the new onset of nephrotic syndrome should be carefully scrutinized for evidence of a neoplasia. A chest X-ray, stool for occult blood, abdominal computed tomography scan are indicated in most cases. On occasion surgical removal or chemotheraphy of the malignancy has been associated with remission. Relapses can occur on recurrence of the tumor.

Poststreptococcal glomerulonephritis

While acute poststreptococcal glomerulonephritis is an uncommon disorder provoking the nephrotic syndrome in the elderly patient, this diagnosis always needs to be kept in mind in elderly patients presenting with edema, pulmonary congestion proteinuria, and an abnormal urinary sediment [2,30−34]. This constellation of findings should especially raise a suspicion of acute glomerulonephritis in an older patient with no prior history of cardiac disease. Geriatric patients with acute poststreptococcal glomerulonephritis often have atypical presentations and may have severe or progressive renal failure. Presence of a nephritic sediment in a patient with obvious fluid load is a valuable clue. Serologic studies, such as sequential measurement of serum complement values (C3 and C4) antistreptolysin O titers, anti-DNAase or an antihyalinurondase antibody may be of help in establishing diagnosis. An elevated antistreptococcal enzyme antibody and a low C3 level is virtually diagnostic. Throat or skin cultures may reveal Group A β-hemolytic streptococci, but are not helpful in establishing the diagnosis in 20−30% of patients.

Infective endocarditis

Infective endocarditis may occur in older patients especially associated with colonic disease but is an uncommon cause of nephrotic syndrome [2]. Enterococci are common organisms in this situation. Renal failure, heavy proteinuria, nephritic urinary sediment, hypocomplementmia, positive rheumatoid factor, low level cryoglobulinemia, and low titers of fluorescent antinuclear antibody are commonly observed. When blood cultures are negative this disorder may be difficult to separate from vasculitis, systemic lupus erythematosis, and cryoglobulinemia.

Nonsteroidal anti-inflammatory agents

Nonsteroidal anti-inflammatory agents are increasingly being incriminated as a case of nephrotic syndrome in older patients. The lesion underlying this complication is typically minimal-change disease with interstitial nephritis [35]. Acute renal failure may also occur.

Rapidly progressive glomerulonephritis

This clinical syndrome consists of progressive renal failure often leading to end-stage renal disease in a few months, accompanied by urinary findings indicative of glomerulonephritis [2]. As with nephrotic syndrome, it may arise consequent to primary glomerular disease or develop secondarily to a multisystem disorder such as systemic necrotizing vasculitis.

This syndrome is a common cause of renal failure due to glomerulonephritis in the elderly. In the biopsy survey of Ramirez & Saba [3] approximately 15% of renal biopsies in patients over the age of 60 which revealed glomerulonephritis were obtained from patients with this clinical syndrome. The syndrome of rapidly progressive glomerulonephritis (RPGN) is frequently, but not necessarily, associated with extensive cellular proliferation in Bowman's space (crescents). Primary forms of RPGN may be further categorized on the basis of immunopathologic findings on renal biopsy [2]. Type I RPGN reveals linear deposits of IgG which represent binding of antiglomerular basement membrane (GBM) antibodies. Circulating anti-GBM antibodies are present in 80−90% of such patients. Type II RPGN reveals extensive granular deposits of IgG representing localization of immune complexes in the glomerular capillary bed. Such patients may reveal circulating immune complexes and depressed serum complement levels. Type III (RPGN) reveals very few immune deposits and for this reason is often called "pauci-immune" glomerulonephritis. This subcategory may be a *forme-fruste* of vasculitis since it very frequently (over 75%) is associated with circulating autoantibodies to neutrophil cytoplasmic antigens (see below). In three series of renal biopsies in patients over age of 60 who presented with RPGN 22% had Type I, 35% Type II, and 43% Type III disease [1,36,37].

Strictly speaking patients should only be categorized as primary RPGN when extrarenal findings can readily be attributed to the renal disease itself, e.g., edema, pulmonary congestion, nausea, etc. When multisystem involvement occurs, e.g., purpura or lung hemorrhage, then patients are more properly categorized as having secondary forms of RPGN. This categorization may be quite difficult as extrarenal organ involvement in secondary RPGN may be quite covert or not appear contemporaneously with renal involvement. Furthermore, renal biopsies may fail to reveal the extraglomerular vascular involvement (e.g., granulomatous vasculitis) which typifies a multisystem disease. In the elderly patient common forms of secondary RPGN include microscopic polyarteritis (MPA) (or hypersensitivity angitis), Wegener's granulomatosis, cryoglobulinemia systemic lupus erythematosis, infective endocarditis, and system necrotizing vasculitis secondary to neoplasia or drugs. Less common forms include the Churg–Strauss syndrome, Schönlein–Henoch purpura, and vasculitis secondary to chronic viral, bacterial, or fungal diseases. Mixed essential IgG/IgM cryglobulinemia may present as rapidly progressive glomerulonephritis with vasculitis. Antiglomerular basement membrane antibody disease commonly presents with associated pulmonary hemorrhage (Goodpasture's Syndrome), although many other forms of glomerulonephritis, including systemic lupus erythematosus, Schönlein–Henoch purpura, cryoimmunoglobulinemia, and vasculitis can also present with pulmonary hemorrhage. Those entities which occur more commonly on the elderly will now be discussed.

Vasculitis

Vasculitis is a very heterogenous group of disorders having in common inflammatory and destructive lesions of the arteries, arterioles, capillaries, venules, and/or veins [2,24]. In most series, patients over the age of 60 years comprise 30% or more of cases [23]. When the glomerular capillaries are involved both necrotizing, proliferative, and crescentic forms of glomerulonephritis may ensue. The most common renal lesion is a segmental necrotizing glomerular nephritis. Most commonly vasculitis involves several organ systems either simultaneously or sequentially. Extravascular granuloma formation is found in Wegener's granulomatosis. In addition to the kidney, the skin, lung, nervous system, joints, heart (coronary arteries), and abdominal viscera are involved. Palpable purpura (leukocytoclastic vasculitis) is a characteristic skin lesion. Abdominal findings, such as peritonitis, may develop as a result of ischemic necrosis and perforation of hollow viscera. Mononeuritis multiplex is a sign of peripheral nervous system involvement. When large to medium size vessels (arteries, arterioles) are involved (periarteritis nodosa) ischemia and aneurysms may develop. Small vessel (capillaries and venules) involvement produces urticaria, palpable purpura, and lung hemorrhage. Fever, malaise, and weight loss are common. The erythrocyte sedimentation rate may be greatly elevated (greater than 100 mmol/hour by the Westergren method). The white blood cell count is usually elevated. The eosinophilia is present in association with small vessel vasculitis but is usually absent in Schönlein–Henoch purpura and in Wegener's granu-

lomatosis. Low levels of rheumatoid factor, weakly positive fluorescent antinuclear antibody, and low levels of cryoglobulinemia are common. Serum complement levels are more often increased than decreased [24].

A very high percentage of patients with RPGN secondary to vasculitis 70–80%, will have circulating autoantibodies to antigens contained within the granules of neutrophil cytoplasm (antineutrophil cytoplasmic antibody (ANCA)) [38,39]. Two subtypes of these autoantibodies are recognized; one reacting with myeloperoxidase and the other reacting with an elastinolytic neutral proteinase. The former autoantibodies are strongly associated with crescentic glomerulonephritis due to microscopic polyarteritis and the Type III primary ("pauci-immune") crescentic glomerulonephritis [38]. The latter are strongly associated with Wegener's granulomatosis [39]. Periarteritis nodosa, systemic lupus erythematosis, Schönlein–Henoch purpura, and Churg–Strauss Syndrome are usually negative. Occasional patients with coexistent antiglomerular basement membrane and antineutrophil cytoplasmic antibodies have been described [40]. Pulmonary hemorrhage is particularly common when ANCA are of the IgM class [40]. Renal biopsies reveal segmental or diffuse necrotizing glomerulonephritis with crescents. Immunofluorescent studies for immunoglobulin deposits are usually negative. Granulomatous vasculitis is seen in the kidney and elsewhere, particularly in the lung, in Wegener's granulomatosis. IgA deposits in the skin and glomerular mesangium are found in Schönlein–Henoch purpura [2].

In the past, the prognosis for patients with vasculitis was very poor with death from renal failure or complications of vasculitic organ involvement occurring within several years from the time of diagnosis. With better serologic tools for diagnosis and with more aggressive management, long-term survival is now the rule. Many patients can be "cured" or be induced into long-term remissions. However, if therapy is delayed, irreversible scarring and fibrosis may limit recoverability. Relapses may occur if therapy is interrupted before remission is induced.

Currently, the therapy of vasculitis (including Wegener's granulomatosis) includes glucocorticoids and alkylating agents usually given in combination [41–45]. Oral glucocorticoids, prednisone, or prednisolone (1 mg/ kg per day or 60–80 mg/day) should be instituted promptly. Initiating therapy with pulses of intravenous methylprednisolone (0.5–1.0 g intravenously for 3–4 doses) may be appropriate for patients with very rapid progression or life-threatening extra renal disease, such as pulmonary hemorrhage. As soon as possible, cyclophosphamide 1.5−2.5 mg/kg per day should be begun. Lower dosage is used with severe renal failure and subsequent dosage is adjusted according to the white blood cell count in order to keep total leukocyte count greater than 3000−3500 cells per cm³. Initial intravenous boluses of cyclophosphamide, 750−1000 mg/m² surface area may be used for patients with severe disease, but care should be taken to reduce the dose by 50% if severe renal failure is present. Oral prednisone should be continued in gradually decreasing dosage for 3−6 months, and oral cyclophosphamide should be continued for approximately 1 year or more depending on the clinical and seriologic response. Long-term *oral* cyclophosphamide is the preferred therapy for Wegener's granulomatosis [41]. Patients should be followed very carefully with serial erythrocyte sedimentation rates, C-reactive protein, ANCA, urinalysis, and renal function tests. Severe proteinuria may persist despite serologic and clinical remission. If patients rapidly develop clinical remission and if serologic studies are repeatedly negative (including ANCA) it *may* be safe to gradually convert the patient from cyclophosphamide to azathioprine maintenance (2 mg/kg per day) at 3−6 months, but any relapses should be initially treated with oral cyclophosphamide. Pulse intravenous cyclophosphamide is associated with a greater frequency of relapses. The role of cyclosporine is uncertain, but this agent might be used in patients intolerant of cyclophosphamide who relapse on azathioprine and who are intolerant of cyclophosphamide. Plasmapheresis and/or high-dose immunoglobulins may be of value in patients presenting with dialysis-dependent renal failure [44]. The role of broad spectrum antibiotics, including trimethoprim sulfamethazole, in the management of patients with Wegener's granulomatosis remains uncertain; however, such drugs might be considered as a part of the maintenance program for patients who have entered into a remission with steroid−cytotoxic drug therapy. Complications of therapy with alkylating agents include hemorrhagic cystitis, bladder cancer, bone marrow suppression, herpes zoster, alopecia, and hepatitis. With prolonged therapy, it is likely that the patients are at increased future risk for the development of acute non-lymphocytic leukemia and/or lymphoma.

With prompt institution of aggressive therapy 85% or more of patients improve and the majority (70−75%) of these will enter a complete remission, often of a long-term nature [24]. Some patients later will slowly progress to end-stage renal disease accompanied by heavy proteinuria, hypertension, and little or no clinical evidence of active vasculitis. Such patients should be treated with low-protein diets and angiotensin-converting enzyme inhibitors. Patients who have received prolonged cytotoxic drug therapy should be carefully followed for signs of emerging malignancy, particularly nonlymphocytic acute leukemia, carcinoma of the cervix and/or vulva, and/or bladder carcinoma.

Anti-GBM-mediated disease

Anti-GBM-mediated disease is relatively uncommon in elderly patients. However, there is a rising prevalence of anti-GBM antibody mediated glomerulonephritis without pulmonary hemorrhage in women over the age of 60 [2,45]. Such patients may present with rapidly progressive glomerulonephritis and an active "nephritic" sediment. Renal biopsies reveal typical linear IgG deposits with extensive crescent formation. Circulating anti-GBM antibody (radioimmunoassay) is present in 80−90% of cases. The prognosis is poor if patients are dialysis-dependent, since therapy is nearly always ineffective when administered late in the course of disease. For patients with lesser degree of renal involvement therapy should consist of intensive plasma exchange combined with cyclophosphamide 2−2.5 mg/kg per day and prednisone 1.0 mg/kg per day [2]. Plasma exchange, approximately 3−4 liters, should be repeated daily for 1−2 weeks, and then slowly decreased in frequency depending upon the level of circulating anti-GBM antibody. Cyclophosphamide can usually be decreased and discontinued 30−60 days after initiation of therapy. Prednisone can often be discontinued after 3 months, if the patient has had a satisfactory response. If the serum creatinine is over 3.0 mg/dl at the time therapy is instituted only about 50−60% of patients will recover useful renal function.

"Asymptomatic" proteinuria and/or hematuria

The incidental finding of proteinuria and/or hematuria in an older patient is a relatively common event. Most often it occurs in connection with a "routine" physical examination or in connection with an evaluation for surgery or an intercurrent illness.

The approach to the patient differs according to the findings in urinalysis. Three general categories can be described.

Type 1. Hematuria only (isolated hematuria). No abnormal proteinuria is found despite quantitation.

Type 2. Proteinuria only (isolated proteinuria). No abnormal excretion of erythocytes is found on repeated quantitative urinalysis.

Type 3. Combined proteinuria and hematuria. Both abnormal quantitative proteinuria and erythrocyturia is present.

Isolated hematuria

The differential diagnosis of isolated hematuria is long and complex, but can be greatly simplified by classification into *glomerular* and *nonglomerular subtypes* based on morphology of erythrocytes in the urinary sediment [2,46]. Small, hemoglobin-poor, dysmorphic erythrocytes are characteristic of "glomerular" hematuria; whereas, normal-sized, hemoglobin-rich, biconcave discs are characteristic of nonglomerular hematuria. These changes are best evaluated by phase contrast microscopy of the urinary sediment. Alternative methods include automated cell-sorting and Wright's stain. The presence of nonglomerular hematuria in an elderly patient should prompt a thorough urologic evaluation for genitourinary tumors (particularly carcinoma of the bladder, kidney, or prostate) stones, infections, vascular malformations, or papillary necrosis. Such evaluation should *always* be preceded by abdominal ultrasound and/or computed tomography to exclude polycystic kidney disease. Dysmorphic hematuria is indicative of a renal origin, most often glomerulonephritis. The differential diagnosis includes IgA nephropathy, thin basement membrane disease, mesangial proliferative glomerulonephritis, resolving postinfectious glomerulonephritis, membranoproliferative glomerulonephritis, vasculitis, crescentic glomerulonephritis, or interstitial nephritis of the hypersensitivity variant.

IgA nephropathy (Berger's disease)

IgA nephropathy or Berger's disease is characterized by excessive glomerular mesangial deposition of IgA and IgG [2]. This lesion is distinctly uncommon in the elderly. It accounted for about 10% of the renal biopsy diagnoses in patients with primary glomerulonephritis in the series of Ramirez & Saba [3]. In most series less than 5% of patients with proven IgA nephropathy are over 65 at the time of diagnosis [2,47]. This rarity of IgA nephropathy in the older patient may be due to the reluctance to perform renal biopsies in elderly patients with isolated hematuria. Patients with IgA nephropathy frequently present with bouts of recurring macroscopic hematuria sometimes following upper respiratory infection including tonsilitis. The course of IgA nephropathy in the elderly probably is the same as that in younger patients, but little information is available to evaluate this question. No definitive therapy is available and about 15−20% of patients will ultimately develop progressive disease eventuating in end-stage renal disease.

Thin basement membrane nephropathy

Thin basement membrane nephropathy is characterized by excessive thinning of the peripheral glomerular basement membrane (<250 nm in thickness) [2,48]. It is characterized by persisting microscopic glomerular hematuria and a strong tendency for preservation of renal function. This disorder may be transmitted as an autosomal dominant trait. It is seldom found in patients over the age of 60.

Isolated proteinuria

Although there may be a tendency for protein excretion to increase with age, total 24-hour urinary excretion of greater than 150 mg/day can be regarded as abnormal proteinuria in the elderly patient [49]. Excretion of over 30 µg/min of albumin can also be considered an abnormal finding in an older patient. Asymptomatic patients who excrete between 30 and 200 µg/min of albumin in the urine often have underlying diabetes mellitus or nephrosclerosis secondary to hypertension.

Any elderly patient who is discovered to have isolated abnormal proteinuria on qualitative testing should be first investigated for a paraproteinemic state such as might occur with multiple myeloma or primary amyloidosis. This can best be accomplished by urinary protein electrophoresis and quantitative measurement of the lambda and κ chains of immunoglobulins by immunofixation. If the urine reveals predominantly albumin it is likely that a glomerular source is responsible; however, tubular proteinuria can be evaluated by determination of an albumin/β2-microglobulin excretion ratio. High values are indicative of glomerular disease. Asymptomatic patients having values for total protein excretion between

0.2 and 1.0 g/day predominantly albumin, probably do not require additional investigation if the urinary sediment, renal function, blood pressure, and plasma glucose are normal. If protein excretion is consistently above 1.0 g/day and no cause is found after careful study one could follow the patient with observation only. If renal function or urinary sediment is abnormal a renal biopsy may be indicated to further evaluate the patient and to aid in the determination of prognosis. Patients with greater than 3.5 g/day of protein in the urine become definite candidates for renal biopsy if a renal cause (e.g., diabetes, amyloidosis) is not found following a careful evaluation or if the urinary sediment is abnormal.

Proteinuria and hematuria

This combination of findings nearly always is indicative of renal parenchymal disease, especially if proteinuria exceeds 1.0 g/day and/or dysmorphic glomerular hematuria is recognized. Such patients ordinarily do not require a urologic evaluation and the investigation should be directed to identifying a primary or secondary glomerular disease, such as systemic lupus erythematosus, or membranous glomerulonephritis. These disorders are discussed in greater detail in preceding sections.

References

1 Moorthy AV, Zimmerman SW. Renal disease in the elderly: Clinicopathologic analysis of renal disease in 115 elderly patients. Clin Nephrol 1980;14:223–229.

2 Glassock RJ, Adler S, Ward H, et al. Primary glomerular disease; Secondary glomerular disease. In Brenner B, Rector F, eds. The Kidney, 4th edn. Philadelphia: WB Saunders Co., 1990:1182–1368.

3 Ramirez G, Saba SR. Primary glomerulonephritis in the elderly. In Zawado ET Jr, Sica D, eds. Geriatric Nephrology and Urology. Littleton: PSG Publishing Co., 1985:49–66.

4 Abrass CK. Glomerulonephritis in the elderly. Am J Nephrol 1985;5:409–418.

5 Murray BM, Raij L. Glomerular disease in the aged. In Nuñez JFM, Cameron JS, eds. Renal Function and Disease in the Elderly. London: Butterworths, 1987:298–320.

6 Cameron JS, Glassock RJ. The Nephrotic Syndrome. New York: M Dekker, 1988.

7 Zech P, Colon S, Pointet P, et al. The nephrotic syndrome in adults aged over 60: etiology, evolution and treatment of 76 cases. Clin Nephrol 1982;17:232–236.

8 Cavallo T, Pinto G, Rajaraman S. Immune complex disease complicating diabetic glomerulosclerosis. Am J Nephrol 1984;4:347–351.

9 O'Neill WM, Wallin JD, Walker PP. Hematuria and red cell casts in typical diabetic nephropathy. Am J Med 1983;74:329–392.

10 Klein R, Klein B, Moss S, et al. Wisconsin epidemologic study of diabestic retinopathy. V. Proteinuria and retinopathy in a population of diabetic persons diagnosed prior to age 30. In Friedman EA, L'Esperance EA, eds. Diabetic Renal–Retinal–Syndrome: Therapy. New York: Grune & Stratton, 1986:245–264.

11 Coupes BM, Short C, Ballardie F, et al. Measurement of urinary complement C5b-9 and C3 dg in human membranous nephropathy—a useful prediction of clinical course. J Amer Soc Nephrol 1990:559.

12 Richards NT, Gordon C, Richardson K, et al. Urinary I1–6: marker for mesangial proliferation? J Amer Soc Nephrol 1990:566.

13 Taira K, Hevitson T, Kincaid-Smith P. Urinary platelet factor 4 levels are raised in mesangial IgA glomerulonephritis but not in thin basement membrane nephropathy. J Amer Soc Nephrol 1990:343.

14 Eagen JW, Lewis EJ. Glomerulopathies of neoplasia. Kidney Int 1977;11:297–306.

15 Brueggemayer CD, Ramirez G. Membranous nephropathy, a concern for malignancy. Am J Kid Dis 1987;9:23–27.

16 Glassock RJ. The treatment of membranous glomerulonephritis. Semin Nephrol 1990;11:138–147.

17 Korbet S, Schwartz M, Lewis EJ. Minimal change glomerulopathy of adulthood. Am J Nephrol 1988;8:29–35.

18 Colasanti G, Banfi G, Barbiano di Belgiojosa G. Idiopathic IgA mesangial nephropathy: Clinical features. Contemp Nephrol 1984;40:147–158.

19 Korbet SM, Schwartz MM, Rosenberg B. Immunotactoid glomerulopathy. Medicine 1985;64:228.

20 Alpers CF, Rennke HH, Hopper J, et al. Fibrillary glomerulonephritis: an entity with unusual immunofluorescence features. Kidney Int 1987;31:786–787.

21 Kyle R, Bayrd E. Amyloidosis. Review of 236 cases. Medicine 1975;54:271.

22 Hawkins P, Myers M, Lavender J, et al. Diagnostic radionuclide imaging of amyloid: biological targeting by circulating human serum amyloid P compound. Lancet 1983; 1:1413–1416.

23 Kyle R, Wagoner RD, Holley D. Primary systemic amyloidosis: resolution of nephrotic syndrome with mephalan and prednisone. Arch Int Med 1982;142:1445–1449.

24 Serra-Cardus A, Cameron JS. Renal vasculitis in the aged. In Nuñez JFM, Cameron JS, eds. Renal Function and Disease in the Elderly. London: Butterworths, 1987:321–347.

25 Samuels B, Lee JC, Engleman EP, et al. Membranous nephropathy in patients with rheumatoid arthritis. Medicine 1978;57:319–327.

26 Tarantino A, de Vecchi A, Montaguino G, et al. Renal disease in essential mixed Cryoglobulinemia. Long-term follow-up of 44 patients. Q J Med 1987;50:1–19.

27 Ponticelli C, Minetti G, D'Amico G, eds. *Antiglobulins, Cryoglobulins and Glomerulonephritis*. Dordrecht: Martinus Nijhoff, 1986.

28 Davis G, Hoofnagle JH. Interferon in viral hepatitis: role in pathogenesis and treatment. Hepatology 1986;6:1038–1041.

29 Tubbs RR, Gephardt GN, MacMahon JT, *et al*. Light-chain nephropathy. Am J Med 1981;71:263–269.

30 Arieff AI, Anderson RJ, Massry SG. Acute glomerulonephritis in the elderly. Geriatrics 1971;26:74–84.

31 Lee HA, Stirling G, Sharpstone P. Acute glomerulonephritis in the middle-aged and elderly patient. Br Med J 1966;2: 1361–1363.

32 Boswell D, Eknoyan G. Acute glomerulonephritis in the aged. Geriatrics 1968;23:73–80.

33 Samiy AH, Fields RA, Merrill JP. Acute glomerulonephritis in elderly patients. Ann Intern Med 1961;54:603–609.

34 Sapir DG, Yardley JH, Walker WG. Acute glomerulonephritis in older patients. Johns Hopkins Med J 1968;32:145–152.

35 Garella S, Matarese R. Renal effects of prostaglandins and clinical adverse effects of nonsteroidal anti-inflammatory agents. Medicine 1984;63:165–181.

36 Beirne GJ, Wagnild JP, Zimmerman SW. Idiopathic crescentic glomerulonephritis. Medicine 1977;56:369–381.

37 Morrin P, Hinglais N, Nabarra B, *et al*. Rapidly progressive glomerulonephritis. A clinical and pathological study. Am J Med 1978;65:446–460.

38 Falk RJ, Jennette JC. Anti-neutrophil cytoplasmic autoantibodies with specificity for myeloperoxidase in patients with systemic vasculitis and idiopathic necrotizing and crescentic glomerulonephritis. N Engl J Med 1988;318:1651–1657.

39 Van der Woude FJ, Rasmussen N, Lobatto S. Autoantibodies against neutrophils and monocytes. A tool for diagnosis and marker of disease activity in Wegener's granulomatosis. Lancet 1985;1:425–527.

40 Savage COS, Lockwood CM. Antineutrophil antibodies in vasculitis. Adv Nephrol 1990;19:225–236.

41 Fauci AS, Haynes BF, Kat P, *et al*. Wegener's granulomatosis; prospective clinical and therapeutic experience with 85 patients for 21 years. Ann Intern Med 1983:76–98.

42 Serra A, Cameron JS. Clinical and pathologic aspects of vasculitis. Semin Nephrol 1985;5:55–62.

43 Hoffman GS, Leavitt R, Fleisher T, *et al*. Treatment of Wegener's granulomatosis with intermittent high-dose intravenous cyclophosphamide. Am J Med 1990;89: 403–410.

44 D'Apice AJF. Plasmapheresis for management of renal disease. In Massry S, Glassock R, eds. *Textbook of Nephrology*, 2nd edn. Baltimore: Williams & Wilkins, 1989:1521–1524.

45 Wilson C. The renal response to immunologic injury. In Brenner B, Rector F, eds. *The Kidney*, 4th edn. Philadelphia: WB Saunders Co., 1990:1095–1098.

46 Fairley KF, Birch DF. Hematuria. A simple method for indentifying glomerular bleeding. Kidney Int 1982;21: 105–109.

47 Clarkson AR. IgA nephropathy. In Andreucci VE, ed. *Topics in Renal Medicine*. Boston: Martins-Nyhoff, 1987.

48 Tiebosch ATMG, Frederik P, Van-Breda Vreisman P, *et al*. Thin basement membrane nephropathy in adults with persistent hematuria. N Engl J Med 1989;320:14–23.

49 Anderson S, Brenner BM. The aging kidney: Structure, function mechanisms and therapeutic implications. J Am Geriatr Soc 1987;35:590–593.

16

Tubulointerstitial nephropathies in the aged

Garabed Eknoyan

Derangements of renal structure and function primarily affect the vasculature, the glomerular tuft, or the rest of the kidney parenchyma which consists of the interstitium and tubules. Over the past four decades, diseases in which the primary renal lesions involve the interstitium and tubules, while sparing the vasculature and the glomeruli, have come to be identified as a distinct clinicopathologic entity which accounts for over one-third of the cases of chronic renal failure [1–3] and an increasing number of cases of acute renal failure [4–6]. Originally termed "interstitial nephritis" because of the prominence of interstitial edema, fibrosis, and cellular infiltrate noted on microscopic examination [7], they have since come to be known as "tubulointerstitial nephropathies" or "tubulointerstitial nephritis," which are more descriptive of the coexistent structural changes affecting the tubules and the accompanying tubular dysfunction, which accounts for much of their initial clinical and functional manifestations [3,6,8]. This is not to imply that glomerular function is spared in such cases. On the contrary, a reduction in glomerular filtration rate (GFR) is a presenting feature which occurs early in the acute forms and develops ultimately in the chronic forms of tubulointerstitial nephropathies. Conversely, tubulointerstitial lesions may be present in cases of primary vascular and glomerular diseases of the kidney. In fact, when present in such cases, the severity of tubulointerstitial changes shows a better correlation to the reduction of GFR, renal blood flow (RBF), and overall progression to renal failure [9–11].

Functional and structural correlates

As a rule, the lesions of tubulointerstitial nephritis (TIN) are confined to the cortex or medulla of the kidney and are focal in distribution. Consequently, the functional changes which develop depend upon the principal site of tubular injury and the segmental nature of tubular function. Essentially, lesions localized in the cortex will affect either the proximal or distal tubules and lesions localized in the medulla will affect the loops of Henle and collecting ducts. The aberration from normal function of the affected segment will then determine the tubular dysfunction encountered clinically (Table 16.1). Since the proximal tubules reabsorb the bulk of the filtered glucose, uric acid, bicarbonate, phosphate, amino acids, and low-molecular weight proteins, lesions that affect

Table 16.1 Functional and clinical manifestations of tubulointerstitial nephropathies

Primary injury site	Tubular dysfunction	Clinical manifestations	Clinical conditions	
			Acute	Chronic
Cortex				
Proximal tubule	↓ Reabsorption of: Na^+, HCO_3^-, PO_4, urate, glucose, amino acids	Proximal tubular acidosis Fanconi syndrome Hypophosphatemia Hypouricemia Renal glucosuria Aminoaciduria β2-microglobulinuria	Antibiotics Multiple myeloma Lymphomas Phenacetin	Multiple myeloma Heavy metals Transplant rejection
Distal tubule	↓ Secretion of: H^+, K^+ ↓ Reabsorption of: Na^+	Distal tubular acidosis Hyperkalemia Hypokalemia Salt wasting	Antibiotics Analgesics NSAIDs	Obstructive nephropathy Sickle hemoglobinopathy Amyloidosis Transplant rejection Sarcoidosis
Medulla	↓ Concentrating ability ↓ Reabsorption of: Na^+	Polyuria Nocturia Papillary necrosis Salt wasting	Analgesics Hypercalcemia Hyperuricemia Sulfonamides Infection	Analgesics Obstructive nephropathy Sickle hemoglobinopathy Amyloidosis Polycystic kidney disease Infection Transplant rejection

the proximal tubule will result in glucosuria (renal glucosuria), uricosuria, bicarbonaturia (proximal renal tubular acidosis), phosphaturia, amino aciduria, and β2-microglobulinuria. To the extent that sodium is the principal cation with which most of these anions are reabsorbed in the proximal tubules, there will also be a reduction in the amount of sodium that can be reabsorbed at this site. Since the cortical segments of the distal tubule secrete hydrogen and potassium and regulate the amount of sodium excreted, lesions that affect the distal tubule will result in reduction in the ability to acidify the urine (distal renal tubular acidosis) and to maintain the homeostasis of potassium (hyperkalemia) and sodium (salt wasting). Finally, since the loops of Henle and collecting ducts maintain the medullary tonicity and regulate the final concentration of the urine lesions that are localized to the medulla and papilla, they will reduce the ability to concentrate the urine (nephrogenic diabetes insipidus) and to regulate distal sodium reabsorption (salt wasting) [8,10,12].

Although this type of functional analysis can be useful in the localization of the principal sites of tubular injury, varying degrees of overlap in the site and severity of tubular lesions may be present in the same kidney, in which case different degrees of proximal, distal, and medullary dysfunction may be encountered clinically in any one patient. Furthermore, depending upon the severity and extent of the tubular lesions, derangements of tubular function may not be immediately apparent, and will go undetected unless they are specifically sought by careful scrutiny of laboratory results or probed by specific tests of tubular function. Independent of the tubular segment involved, a common feature of the tubular dysfunctions that result is the reduction in sodium reabsorption regardless of the principal site of injury. Hence the absence of sodium retention, a hallmark of glomerular diseases which are characterized by early edema and hypertension, both of which are usually absent in TIN except in the final stages of progressive renal failure, when the serum creatinine exceeds 5 mg/dl [8,12–14].

While disorders of tubular function and their clinical manifestations are useful in the diagnosis of TIN, in the final analysis the diagnosis of this clinicopathologic syndrome can be confirmed only by examination of renal tissue. The principal morphologic features of TIN are an increase in interstitial volume and varying degrees of infiltration by inflammatory cells (Table 16.2). In *acute* TIN the increase in interstitial volume is due to edema although fibrogenesis may begin by the seventh to the 10th day of persisting insult [15]. The degree of reduction in GFR correlates with the extent of cellular infiltrate [16]. If the injury is severe, tubular damage and dilatation are also present and azotemia is an early feature [6]. In the *chronic* form of TIN, interstitial fibrosis accounts for the increased interstitial volume and tubular atrophy is evident. The degree of reduction in GFR correlates with the severity and extent of the interstitial fibrosis rather than that of the cellular infiltrates [11,14,17]. As a rule, progression to renal failure is slow to develop and is

chracterized by the development of sclerotic glomeruli and periglomerular fibrosis [3].

Tubulointerstitial changes in the aging kidney

Age-dependent changes in the structure and function of the human kidney begin to develop by the middle of the fourth decade and evolve at an accelerated rate after the end of the seventh decade of life [18–23]. The significant reduction in functional renal mass reflected in the declining GFR, that occurs during this interval, is accompanied by minimal changes in total renal size, measured radiographically, indicating an increase in the interstitial volume. In fact, studies in humans and experimental animals have shown a marked increase in interstitial volume, fibrosis, and cellular infiltration in the aging kidney [22–27]. In a morphometric study of kidneys from healthy humans ranging in age from neonates to 90 years, it was found that the mean value for the percentage of cortical interstitial tissue was $12.8 \pm 5.1\%$ [28]. In those who were below the age of 36 years, the volume of interstitial tissue ($11.7 \pm 5.5\%$) was lower than in those who were over 36 years of age ($15.7 \pm 3.0\%$), but this

Table 16.2 Structural features of tubulointerstitial nephropathies

	Acute	Chronic
Interstitium		
Cellular infiltrates	$+ \rightarrow ++++$	$+ \rightarrow ++$
Edema	$++ \rightarrow ++++$	$\pm \rightarrow ++$
Fibrosis	$0 \rightarrow \pm$	$++ \rightarrow ++++$
Tubules		
Epithelium	Injury → necrosis	Atrophy
Basement membrane	Injury → disruption	Thickened
Shape	Preserved	Atrophy/dilatation
Casts	Rare/cellular	Common/hyalin
Glomerulus	Normal or foot process effacement	Sclerosis and periglomerular fibrosis
Vasculature	Minimal and reversible	Variable sclerosis irreversible
Kidney size	Normal or enlarged	Normal or shrunken

Number of + indicates severity of changes ranging from 0 for absent; +, minimal; ++, mild; +++, moderate; ++++, severe.

difference was not statistically significant. In another study, the relative amount of interstitial cortical tissue, measured by the point count method, was studied in two sets of kidney tissue from humans without renal disease [26]. The first set of 54 samples consisted of kidneys intended for transplantation and removed immediately after sudden death. The second set of 69 samples were obtained at autopsy. In both, the percentage of interstitial tissue was dependent on age ($P<0.001$) and followed the regression equations of $y = 12.4 + 0.11 \ x$ for donor kidneys, and $23.8 + 10 \ x$ for the kidneys obtained at autopsy. There was no difference due to sex. While morphometric studies of the medulla and papilla have not been done, the amount of collagen fibrils and fibrous tissue in these areas have been noted to be increased making microdissection of human kidneys difficult, particularly after the seventh decade [24,29]. Interstitial changes characterized by edema and fibrosis with a slight to moderate lymphocytic infiltrate have been noted as early as 8 months of age in the Lewis rat [30]. In another study of the same strain of rats, there was a significant correlation between the age of the animals and the amount of interstitial fibrosis ($r = 0.46$) and of infiltrates ($r = 0.36$) present in the kidneys [31].

A decrease in the number of tubules, a reduction in the volume and length of the proximal tubules, and an increase in the number of diverticuli of the distal convoluted tubules have been noted to occur in aging human kidneys [24]. Semiquantitative analysis of multiple histologic sections of rat kidneys have revealed a close correlation ($r = 0.63$) between age and tubular atrophy and damage [25]. Hyperplasia of the residual tubules, assayed by radioactive thymidine autoradiography, was increased in rats aged $24-30$ months as compared to age $12-18$ months, and there was a significant correlation between interstitial infiltrates and degree of thymidine uptake [25].

Experimental studies in the aging rat have revealed impairment in concentrating ability due to intrinsic renal tubular defect [32], reduced capacity to transport p-aminohippurate [33], compromised reabsorption of phosphate, glucose, and amino acids [34,35], and a decrease in $Na^+-K^+-ATPase$ [36]. A progressive loss of tubular function with increasing age, which is out of proportion to the decline in GFR, has also been noted in humans [37–41]. A decrease in the ability to maximally concentrate the urine [37], generate free water [37], con-serve sodium [38], reabsorb glucose [41], and excrete an acid load [39] have been described in the aging human kidney.

Thus, the functional changes observed in the aging kidney cannot be reduced to a mere loss of functional nephrons but appear to be the result of several differential and specific changes which preferentially affect tubular function. Taken together with the structural changes which affect the interstitium it is evident that the renal lesions of aging are in fact those of a tubulointerstitial nephropathy. Stated otherwise the very clinical and pathologic features that characterize TIN are subtly tinted by the aging process itself. Thus, even in the absence of any specific renal disease the older patient may manifest the rudiments of a classic tubulointerstitial nephropathy. On a more practical level it is fair to state that given their reduced reserves of tubular function, the elderly could be more prone to succumb to the ravages of TIN.

While no exact data is available on the incidence or prevalence of TIN in the elderly, given the slowly progressive nature of the chronic forms of TIN it is not unexpected to encounter a larger number of such cases in the older population. So far as the acute forms of TIN are concerned, the majority of which are due to drugs, it should not be unexpected to encounter them more frequently in the elderly who have a higher exposure to the therapeutic agents incriminated as a cause of acute TIN.

Acute tubulointerstitial nephropathies

The acute form of TIN was first reported in 1860 as a complication of β-hemolytic streptococcal infection in a case of scarlet fever in which examination of the kidney at autopsy revealed diffuse lymphocytic cell infiltration in the absence of bacterial invasion of the tissue [42]. Subsequent reports of similar findings in cases of diphtheria, scarlet fever, and other septic states were reviewed and summarized in 1896 by Councilman [7]. The principal focus of the article was on the origin and type of mononuclear cellular infiltrates of the lesions. Ironically, it is the antibiotic drugs introduced to treat streptococcal infection that have now emerged as a principal cause of acute TIN. In addition to its occurrence in association with infections and drugs, acute TIN may occur in a variety of systemic diseases and in some 10% of cases is idiopathic in nature (Table 16.3).

Table 16.3 Conditions associated with acute tubulointerstitial nephritis

Drugs

Antibiotics
  Penicillin, methicillin, ampicillin, cephalothin, rifampin, others

Sulfonamides

Nonsteroidal anti-inflammatory drugs
  Fenoprofen, ibuprofen, naproxen, others

Miscellaneous
  Phenytoin, furosemide, thiazides, cyclosporine, cimetidine, captorpil, allopurinol, triamterene

Infections

Direct, invasion of parenchyma

Indirect, systemic infection

Systemic disturbances

Metabolic: hyperuricemia, hypercalcemia

Lymphoproliferative disorders

Plasma cell dyscrasias

Collagen–vascular diseases

Idiopathic

Pathologic features

The succinct description of the lesions Councilman observed in the infection-associated acute TIN is as inclusive and accurate today as it was when he described it in 1869 as "an accute inflammation of the kidney characterized by cellular and fluid exudation in the interstitial tissue, accompanied by, but not dependent on, degeneration of the epithelium; the exudation is not purulent in character, and the lesions may be both diffuse and focal" [7].

The hallmark of acute TIN is an increase in interstitial volume mainly because of interstitial edema. Experimentally, fibrosis has been shown to set during the end of 1 week and may be detected clinically in cases that go undetected or untreated [15]. The interstitial cellular infiltrates which may be diffuse or focal, are invariably patchy in distribution even when the infiltrate is diffuse

in nature. The extent of interstitial infiltration has been shown to have a direct correlation to the serum creatinine level at the time of biopsy, and to the maximal serum creatinine attained during the course of the disease [16]. The infiltrates are most evident in the proximity of the tubular basement membrane. Foci of erosion and discontinuity of the basement membrane and infiltration into the subepithelial cells may show focal tubular swelling and degeneration. In severe cases there may be focally denuded areas of tubular basement membrane with sloughed necrotic epithelial cells in the lumen. Thus, in contrast to cases of acute tubular necrosis, in acute TIN the tubular injury principally affects the basilar surface of the epithelial cells. As a rule, immunofluorescent examination reveals no staining for any immunoglobulins or complement along the tubular basement membrane except in a minority of cases [16,43–46]. The majority (up to 70%) of the infiltrating cells are lymphocytes, some 10–12% are macrophages, and the remainder are fibroblasts, plasma cells, and polymorphonuclear leukocytes, including eosinophils [43]. The lymphocytes consist of both helper/inducer and cytoxic/suppressor cells, generally with a slight preponderance of the former subset of T cells. Immunohistologic studies indicate that up to 80% of the infiltrating lymphocyte cells are activated T cells and less than 20% of them are B cells [47–49]. The majority of the remainder of the mononuclear cells consists of plasma cells and macrophages [43–50]. It is the latter which when assembled in a concentric pattern form the noncaseating granulomatous lesions, with or without multinucleated giant cells, surrounded by fibroblasts that have been described in some cases of acute TIN [51]. Their presence is a reflection on the chronicity of the lesion and is generally associated with the more severe forms of renal failure [6,52]. Polymorphonuclear leukocytes are a rare constituent of the cellular infiltrate. When the polymorphonuclear leukocytes constitute greater than 5% of the infiltrating cells the prognosis is generally poor [16]. The presence of eosinophils can be diagnostic of drug-induced hypersensitivity nephritis, but bears no relationship to the severity or course of the disease.

As a rule, there are no glomerular changes although mesangial hyperplasia and sclerosis has been noted. Obviously, in the elderly these may reflect the age-related glomerular changes and may have no bearing on the acute TIN. In cases of acute TIN associated with massive proteinuria effacement of the foot processes will be present [6,15,50,52].

Drugs

Acute renal failure may be the consequence of two types of drug-induced tubulointerstitial lesions: dose-dependent tubular injury and drug-induced hypersensitivity nephritis. The former are due to a direct toxic effect of the drugs and will not be discussed here. The latter are due to a hypersensitivity reaction as evidenced by a number of characteristic features [6,15,50]. Specifically:

1 They occur in an unrelated group of agents.

2 They are not dose related.

3 They affect only a small number of those exposed.

4 The reaction recurs upon re-exposure to the same agent or one of its congeners.

5 The renal lesions are generally associated with clinical or laboratory evidence of a systemic hypersensitivity reaction.

6 There is increasing evidence for the activation of humoral and cellular immune response in well-studied cases.

The nature of the sensitizing antigen is not clear. It may be the drug itself, one of its metabolites, or a consequence of local tissue changes induced by the drug [15]. It is this type of hypersensitivity reaction to drugs that accounts for the majority of cases in acute TIN now encountered clinically.

First noted to occur in conjunction with the use of sulfonamides in the 1940s, the lesions of acute TIN were next observed with the penicillins which became available in the 1950s [6,15,50,53]. Since then antibiotics have emerged as the most commonly incriminated group of drugs as a cause of acute TIN. The most commonly incriminated agents are the *penicillin* cogeners, specially *methicillin*, and the other β-*lacatam derivatives*. In the majority of cases of methicillin-induced TIN the lesions occur after exposure to relatively large doses over an average period of 15 days, with a reported range of $10-45$ days [54]. It has been estimated that in patients who are exposed to the drug for more than 2 weeks the incidence of acute TIN is approximately 15% [54,55]. However, following subsequent exposure to methicillin or one of its congeners, acute TIN may develop within a much shorter period and pursue a more fulminant course of renal failure [56]. The initial observation by immuno-fluorescence of dimethoxyphenyl-penicilloyl (DPO), a

metabolic product of methicillin, and linear deposits of IgG and complement along the tubular basement membrane, and the detection of circulating antibodies to DPO led to the proposal that an antibody-mediated reaction was the cause of acute TIN [53,57]. However, DPO can also be demonstrated by immunofluorescence in the kidney of patients given penicillin ante-mortem who have no clinical or laboratory evidence of TIN [58]. The detection of circulating antitubular basement antibodies in some cases of methicillin-induced acute TIN has led to the suggestion that during their secretion in the proximal tubule either methicillin or one of its metabolites render the tubular basement immunogenic and thereby induce the formation of antibodies to the tubular basement membrane or interstititum [15,57]. However, the paucity of demonstrable immune complexes or antibody−tubular basement membrane in the vast majority of reported cases, in contrast to the overwhelming evidence for the presence of activated lymphocytes, clearly indicates a cell-mediated response as the principal mechanism of injury in acute TIN [15,59].

The idiosyncratic hypersensitivity reaction with multiple organ involvement (heart, lung, liver, and kidney) that occurs with *sulfonamides* [59,60] first observed in the 1940s had declined until its resurgence with the introduction of *trimethoprim-sulfamethoxazole* [6]. Its occurrence appears to be more common in the setting of reduced renal function. Hence, the predisposition of the elderly given their age-related decline in GFR and the high incidence of urinary tract infection for which trimethoprim-sulfamethoxazole is frequently prescribed. The predisposition to a hypersensitivity reaction to sulfonamides has been attributed to individual differences in metabolism, the reaction being more common in slow acetylators which results in the accumulation of drug metabolites that have been incriminated to elicit the immunologic response [61]. The propensity of patients with reduced renal function, as a variable independent of acetylating capacity, has also been attributed to the accumulation of the toxic metabolite [62].

Most cases of *rifampin*-induced acute TIN have occurred during intermittent therapy or following reinstitution of rifampin after a hiatus in its uncomplicated use [63], but can occur during continuous daily therapy [64]. Circulating antibodies to rifampin detected in most but not all cases of acute TIN probably represent an epiphenomenon since they have also been demonstrated in the sera of patients who do not develop an adverse reaction to the drug [65].

Although the exact incidence of drug-induced acute TIN is unclear, next to antimicrobials, *nonsteroidal anti-inflammatory drugs* (NSAIDs) are probably the most commonly incriminated agents [6,66]. This is of special relevance to the elderly since degenerative joint disease and arthralgias, for which they are treated with NSAIDs, is a fairly common problem in those over 65 years of age [67]. Over-the-counter availability of some NSAIDs only increases the risk of exposure in the population in general, and the elderly in particular. In fact, most cases of NSAID-induced acute TIN have been in patients who were older than 60 years [67]. Although their principal detrimental effect on renal function is hemodynamically mediated, as a result of inhibition of prostaglandin synthesis [68], they also induce a distinct form of acute TIN, which, unlike other forms of drug-induced TIN, is frequently associated with massive proteinuria [66,69–71]. In fact, most patients present with nephrotic syndrome, which precedes the renal failure, although renal failure without nephrotic syndrome occurs in about 15% of the cases. Following discontinuation of the causative NSAID, the renal failure improves well before the subsidence of the proteinuria, which may persist for months. Actually, slow recovery from NSAID-induced TIN is another feature that sets these agents apart from other forms of drug-induced acute TIN. Another distinguishing feature is the rarity of associated symptoms of hypersensitivity reaction, which occurs in only 20% of cases compared to an incidence of over 85% in other forms of drug-induced TIN. However, this may be a reflection on the salutary effect of NSAIDs on hypersensitivity reactions in general, rather than a feature unique to these groups of drugs. The duration of exposure is quite long, averaging 5–6 months, with a range of 2 weeks to 18 months. The propionic acid derivatives (fenoprofen, ibuprofen, naproxen) account for 75% of the cases reported in the literature [66–72].

A final group of drugs that should be singled out with regard to the elderly are *diuretics* because of their frequent use in cardiovascular diseases such as hypertension and congestive heart failure, which commonly afflict the older population. Diuretic-induced TIN is a rare occurrence, but it is more commonly associated with the use of thiazides and furosemide, both of which are structurally related to sulfonamides [73–75]. Although the renal insufficiency that occurs with the use of diuretics gener-

ally is prerenal in origin and consequent to diuretic-induced extracellular fluid volume depletion, the possibility of diuretic-induced acute TIN must be kept in mind in the differential diagnosis of azotemia that develops during the course of diuretic therapy.

Relatively few cases of TIN have been reported with *cimetidine*, *phenytoin*, *captopril*, and *phenobarbital*, none of which present a problem unique to the elderly (Table 16.3). The association noted with most of these agents is rare, based on isolated or single case reports, and the evidence for a causative role less than convincing in the absence of kidney biopsy particularly in the presence of the concurrent administration of several drugs.

Infection

Acute TIN may develop as a reaction to the invasion of the renal parenchyma by an infective organism or as a complication of a systemic infection in the absence of bacteremia or of direct renal parenchymal invasion by the infective organism [6]. The former is the more classic and at least morphologically the more common form encountered in the elderly in whom the incidence of urinary tract infection is increased [76]. The renal lesions are focal, sharply demarcated, confined to the affected lobules, and characteristically wedge-shaped with a radial distribution of the inflammatory infiltrate. The clinical features (sudden onset of fever, shaking chills, costovertebral tenderness, dysuria) and laboratory findings (leukocytosis, pyuria, bacteriuria, polymorphonuclear casts) are quite characteristic. The urine culture is almost always positive and in some the infective organism can be cultured from the blood. Enterobacteriaceae are by far the most common organism isolated from the urine, staphylococci are common in immunosuppressed individuals and diabetics, less common are fungal, parasitic, and viral infections [6,76]. In urinary tract obstruction renal function is well preserved except in the presence of infection. A defect in urine concentration and acidification may be present which will subside when the infection is controlled [77,78]. When the infection is bilateral and the kidneys are diffusely involved, an acute deterioration of renal function may occur [79,80].

The incidence of acute TIN due to systemic infections is unknown. Prior to the advent of antimicrobials, acute TIN was commonly observed at post-mortem in fatal cases of β-hemolytic streptococcal infections [7]. In the absence of septic shock, the fall in renal function that occurs in the presence of a systemic infection may be due to postinfectious glomerulonephritis or acute TIN [81,82]. The latter generally occurs early during the course of the disease, usually within the first 10–12 days, whereas glomerular lesions develop at least 2 weeks following the onset of the infection. In contrast to the radial distribution of the lesion of direct bacterial invasion, the infiltrative cells of acute TIN form circular bands around the vasculature and are more prominent at the corticomedullary junction [83].

Systemic diseases

Although less common than drugs and infection as a cause of acute TIN, systemic diseases may be complicated by acute renal failure due to TIN. The renal lesions may be the consequence of coexistent metabolic disturbances, the infiltrative nature of the primary disease, or the immunologic basis of the systemic disease (Table 16.3).

Metabolic disturbances

The two metabolic disturbances which are specially pertinent to the elderly are those of urate and calcium because of their frequent occurrence in association with malignancies that are common in older individuals.

The hypercatabolic state associated with lymphoproliferative or myeloproliferative disorders, particularly with rapid cell lysis during chemotherapy, invariably results in the sudden and massive overproduction of *uric acid*. The determinants of uric acid solubility are its concentration and pH of the medium. Supersaturation of the tubular fluid, specially in dehydrated individuals, as the increased load of uric acid becomes concentrated in the renal medulla, and the fact that the tubular fluid is acidified in the distal tubule are both conducive to the precipitation of uric acid crystals in the distal tubule [84]. The resultant inflammatory reaction of peritubular edema and infiltration are characteristic of acute TIN [85]. Concomitantly, uric acid sludge may precipitate in the renal plevis and ureters. The net effect is an acute deterioration of renal function and oliguria. The serum urate level in such cases is usually, but not invariably, higher than 20 mg/dl and the urine uric acid/creatinine ratio is greater than one [86]. Hyperphosphatemia, hypocalcemia, and hyperkalemia will also result from the cellular lytic process and should be corrected. This deleterious sequence of events is preventable by:

1 hydration to maintain a high flow rate of urine;
2 alkalinization of urine; and
3 reduction of uric acid load by inhibition of xanthine oxidase with allopurinol, instituted prior to chemotherapy [84].

The acute reduction in renal function that occurs in acute *hypercalcemia* is hemodynamic in nature, due to a direct effect of calcium on the renal vasculature and cardiovascular hemodynamics [87,88]. The structural changes, noted in experimental animals, consist of focal tubular injury with edema and inflammatory infiltration of the adjacent interstitium [89]. Whether similar lesions develop acutely in humans is not known.

Neoplastic infiltrative lesions

Lymphoproliferative disorders and plasma cell dyscrasias are the two malignancies in which acute TIN is a relatively common complication. The kidney is one of the most common extranodal sites of metastatic lymphomas. Swelling and infiltration of the kidney with mitotic cells is more common in non-Hodgkin's lymphomas and acute lymphoblastic lymphomas. The renal complications of plasma cell dyscrasias, a disease of the elderly, are a major cause of the morbidity and mortality of these patients [90–92]. The classic lesions of "myeloma cast nephropathy" results from excessive production of light chains and their precipitation as dimers in the distal tubule. The consequent injury, necrosis, and regeneration of tubular epithelial cells around the "myeloma casts," with interstitial edema, inflammatory infiltrate, and multinucleated giant cells around the affected tubules present the classic morphologic features of acute TIN (93,94).

Idiopathic tubulointerstitial nephropathies

In some 10–20% of cases presenting with reversible renal failure, with the finding on kidney biopsy of acute TIN, no evidence of drug exposure, infection, or systemic disease can be substantiated [95–96]. The outcome has been favorable in most cases with recovery occurring spontaneously or following steroid therapy. Uveitis has been described as a coexistent feature of some cases, but this has been in adolescent girls of pubertal age, and therefore, not pertinent to the elderly [97].

Chronic tubulointerstitial nephropathies

The differentiation of the renal lesions of chronic TIN, which had been indiscriminately attributed to chronic pyelonephritis, began in the early 1950s when the lesions of the kidney in cases of analgesic abuse were first characterized as being those of a chronic TIN and occurred in the absence of any evidence of infection [98–100]. The subsequent clarification of the criteria for the diagnosis of pyelonephritis and the demonstration that in the absence of obstruction renal parenchymal infection rarely results in renal insufficiency dispelled the untenable notion that pyelonephritis is the main cause of chronic TIN [80,101]. In fact, a diverse group of unrelated diseases have now come to be implicated as a cause of chronic TIN (Table 16.4).

Pathophysiologic features

The distinctive morphologic features of chronic TIN are an increase in the interstitial volume due to interstitial fibrosis and mononuclear cell infiltration accompanied by varying degrees of tubular degeneration, atrophy, and dilatation (Table 16.2). The lesions may be focal or diffuse, but as a rule are patchy in distribution and localized predominantly in the cortical interstitium. Glomerular changes which are usually absent or minimal in the early phases of the disease will ultimately develop and consist of sclerosis, obsolence, and periglomerular fibrosis [3,11,101]. The rate of deterioration of renal function depends to a great extent on the extent of interstitial fibrosis and on the primary disease, but is generally slow to develop and the early manifestations of renal involvement are those of tubular dysfunction [3,11,12,14]. The altered pattern of tubular function which is present will depend on the principal site of tubular injury caused by the underlying disease (Table 16.1). Because of the insiduous onset of renal failure, the lesions of TIN may go undetected until significant renal damage has occurred. Early in the course of the disease the classic features of glomerular dysfunction (edema, hypertension, and proteinuria) usually considered the hallmarks of kidney disease are absent, and careful scrutiny for the presence of any tubular dysfunction is essential for early diagnosis [3,8,12]. This is particularly important since most of these disorders result from potentially preventable or treatable causes, whose timely recognition can preclude the otherwise relentless progression to irreversible renal

Table 16.4 Conditions associated with chronic tubulointerstitial nephritis

Drugs
Analgesics, cyclosporine, lithium, *cis*-platinum

Urinary tract obstruction
Partial or complete

Hematopoietic disorders
Sickle cell hemoglobinopathy, lymphoproliferative disorders, plasma cell dyscrasias

Metabolic disorders
Diabetes mellitus, hypercalcemia, hyperuricemia, hyperoxaluria

Vascular disorders
Arteriosclerosis, atheroembolic disease

Infection
Bacterial, viral, fungal, mycobacterial

Immunologic disorders
Transplant rejection, systemic lupus erythematosus, Sjögren's syndrome, amyloidosis, cryoglobulinemia, Wegener's granulomatosis

Heavy metal exposure
Lead, cadmium, mercury

Heriditary disorders
Hereditary nephritis, polycystic kidney disease

Miscellaneous
Sarcoidosis, Balkan nephropathy, radiation nephritis

Idiopathic

damage. At the late stages of the disease when glomerular sclerotic lesions develop and the clinical hallmarks of glomerular dysfunction—hypertension, edema, and proteinuria—are present, progressive renal failure is the rule even when the causative factor of TIN is identified and removed [1,3,102].

Regardless of the inciting event the development and progression of TIN is immune-mediated [15]. While the exact immunologic mechanisms involved are less clearly defined than they are for the glomerulonephritides the available experimental and clinical evidence suggest a central role for altered cellular immunity. The inflammatory cell infiltrates are a mixture of lymphocytes, macrophages, and plasma cells [47]. Most of the lymphocytes are T cells. Sensitized T cells capable of damaging renal tubular epithelial cells and mediate fibrinogenesis have been demonstrated in experimental models of TIN [103,104]. The cellular infiltrates also release lymphokines which modulate the biogenesis of new cellular matrix [15]. In addition, exposure of native structural antigens, selective to the tubular basement or shared by the tubular and glomerular basement membrane, has been implicated in activating the humoral limb of the immune system [105,106]. Antibodies reactive with antigens present in the tubulointerstitial tissue and with Tamm—Horsfall protein have been demonstrated [105–107]. The local generation of antibodies by infiltrating cells has been suggested from transfer studies. However, evidence for circulating antibodies or immune complexes and their deposition in the kidney has been scarce and lacking.

Conceivably, the expected decline of most cell-mediated and humoral responsiveness of the immune system with advancing age could retard the progression of the immune-mediated diseases in older patients [108]. However, most cases of chronic TIN are encountered in the elderly, reflecting primarily the slowly progressive nature of a lesion initiated earlier in life, well before the involutionary stage of the immune system sets in.

The frequency with which each of the diseases listed in Table 16.4 accounts for the cases of chronic TIN encountered clinically remains to be established. The available data suggests that drugs and obstructive nephropathy account for most of the cases of chronic TIN that progress to renal failure and that the majority of these occur in older patients [1,14,109]. Nephrosclerosis is another principal cause of TIN in the elderly, but will not be discussed in this chapter since it is covered elsewhere in the book. Other causes of chronic TIN in the elderly that should be singled out are those associated with hematopoietic and metabolic diseases.

Drugs

Although prolonged exposure to a number of drugs such as cisplatinum, lithium, cyclosporine, and nitrosurea lead to TIN, by far the most common cause of drug-induced TIN is analgesic abuse. In fact, in some countries—such as Australia and New Zealand—analgesic abuse nephropathy is the most common cause of end-stage kidney disease [100,110].

First described in the 1950s in individuals who used analgesic compounds, the incriminating agent was initially considered to be phenacetin, the principal ingredient of the analgesic mixtures then in use [99,110–112]. Subsequent experimental studies, however, showed that phenacetin, acetominophen, and aspirin alone were only moderately nephrotoxic even when given in large doses, but that their nephrotoxicity was increased when they were given in combination, particularly if accompanied by water deprivation [100,110–112]. Of therapeutic relevance is the experimental observation that water diuresis protects renal injury from analgesics, whether administered singly or in combination [113,114]. This may well account for the epidemiologic studies which show that only a small percentage of analgesic abusers develop nephropathy, and for the clinical observation that the use of diuretics and laxatives predisposes abusers to analgesic nephropathy [115–117]. The therapeutic implication for analgesic abusers who refuse to discontinue analgesics is that increasing fluid intake may provide protection to the kidney [100]. The protective effect of forced diuresis derives from the fact that both aspirin and phenacetin, as well as its metabolites, attain high concentrations in the renal medulla and that water diuresis abolishes this medullary gradient [113,114,118,119]. This corresponds to the primary site of injury of analgesic abuse which begins at the papillary tip and classically presents with renal papillary necrosis [100]. The toxic effect of paracetamol and its conjugated metabolites derives from their oxidation in the kidney to reactive intermediates, which in the presence of a deficiency of reducing substances, such as glutathione, induce oxidative cell injury [100,118–121]. The propensity to renal injury of paracetamol is increased in the coexistence of salicylates, which uncouple oxidative phosphorylation and decrease the cellular generation of reducing substances at the very time that the reactive oxidative by-products of paracetamol are increased [100,120,122].

Analgesic abuse is more common in women, with a female/male ratio of 5:1. Dependence on other agents such as alcohol or psychotropic drugs is common, and a major personality disorder is present in one-third. The reason for analgesic abuse is headache, musculoskeletal complaints, or nondescript minor aches and pains [100,110,113].

As a rule, the degree of renal injury that occurs with analgesic abuse is directly related to the duration and quantity of analgesic mixtures consumed. With continued exposure to analgesic mixtures, the patchy lesions of TIN which begin in the papilla extend to the outer medulla and become more diffuse. Ultimately, the entire papilla becomes necrotic, is sequestered, and either sloughs or calcifies *in situ*. Cortical scarring, interstitial fibrosis, and atrophy then develop in the lobule of the necrotic medullary segments. The adjoining medullary rays hypertrophy and thereby impart the characteristic cortical nodularity of the ultimately shrunken end-stage kidney. This is a slowly progressive process that develops over several years after large quantities of analgesic mixtures have been consumed. The average dose consumed has been estimated to be about 10 kg over the course of 13 years. A cumulative dose of 3 kg, or a daily ingestion of 1 g/day, for more than 3 years has been considered as the minimum required to induce clinically evident renal failure due to analgesic nephropathy [100,110−113].

The decline in renal function is insidious in nature and slow to evolve. Inability to concentrate the urine is the earliest abnormality to develop. The consequent nocturia, polyuria, and low urinary specific gravity may go undetected, particularly in the elderly. Inability to acidify the urine is common. Bacteriuria is present in one-third of cases, but pyuria which is present in most is sterile. Hematuria is present in one-third, may be gross in the presence of renal papillary necrosis (RPN), but is generally microscopic. Proteinuria is modest and less than 1−2 g/day. The presence of massive proteinuria denotes the development of focal glomerulosclerosis and heralds a rapid deterioration of renal function. Anemia, which is disproportionate to the degree of renal insufficiency, should always increase the index of suspicion for analgesic abuse. Although an element of hemolysis may contribute to the anemia it is primarily due to gastrointestinal bleeding. Actually, gastrointestinal complaints of dyspepsia, with or without demonstrable peptic ulcers, may be a presenting complaint in one-third to one-half of cases [100,110−113].

Cessation of analgesic-use generally stops the progression of renal involvement and usually will lead to improvement of renal function. In some the disease may progress even after discontinuation of analgesic abuse. However, even after initiation of maintenance dialysis therapy, sufficient recovery of renal function may occur to warrant the discontinuation of dialysis. All patients with a history of analgesic use should be monitored for transitional cell carcinoma of the uroepithelium which afflicts 10% of them, even after discontinuation of analgesic use [123]. The development of unexplained and persistent hematuria in these individuals should always prompt careful scrutiny for uroepithelial malignancies [100].

Urinary tract obstruction

Tubulointerstitial changes invariably develop in the presence of urinary tract obstruction. Prostatic hypertrophy, neurogenic bladder, intra-abdominal tumors encasing the ureters, and retroperitoneal fibrosis are all diseases of the elderly that will obstruct the urinary tract. The classic symptoms and signs of complete obstruction need not be present. Partial obstruction or persistent residual incomplete obstruction after surgical repair of complete obstruction will result in renal dysfunction, the structural basis of which is TIN [124−126].

The initial tubular dilatation that results following obstruction is accompanied by an increase in the interstitial matrix and by interstitial cellular infiltration and proliferation. The monocytic infiltration enhances fibrogenesis and accounts for the exaggerated prostaglandin and thromboxane synthesis noted in experimental models of urinary tract obstruction [127]. Following acute obstruction, the initial and transient increase in RBF in the face of declining glomerular filtration is soon followed by a decline in total RBF with a disproportionate decrease in cortical blood flow. These changes in blood flow relate to that of the local production of prostanoids with the early increase due to prostaglandin E_2 and the subsequent decline to thromboxane A_2. The gradual increase in fibrosis with persistent obstruction eventually results in contraction and scarring of the kidneys [124−127]. The duration, severity, location, and coexistence of infection are the principal determinants of the magnitude of renal injury that will result. The more complete the degree of obstruction and the closer it is to the renal pelvis the greater is the injury to the renal parenchyma and the lower is the likelihood to reverse the changes in renal function after relief of the obstruction [128−133].

Distal tubular dysfunction is at the root of the functional abnormalities that develop. Inability to concentrate the urine and hyposthenuric polyuria due to nephrogenic diabetes insipidus is a common and early manifestation of obstruction. Enuresis may ultimately be superimposed as part of the complex of symptoms that develop with partial obstruction of the lower urinary tract, that is characteristic of prostatic hypertrophy in the elderly [124−126,128]. Hyperkalemic hyperchloremic acidosis is the other abnormality of distal tubular dysfunction that occurs. Its unexplained presence in elderly patients with mild degrees of renal insufficiency should always lead to the search for underlying obstructive nephropathy. It is multifactoral in origin and can be due to distal renal tubular acidosis with or without a selective deficiency of aldosterone or a relative decrease in ammonium excretion [134]. Recurrent urinary tract infection is common in the presence of obstruction and is another clue to the presence of occult obstruction of urine outflow. Microscopic pyuria and hematuria in the absence of casts and moderate proteinuria are the characteristic findings noted on urinalysis. Massive proteinuria is an ominous finding which indicates the development of focal glomerulosclerosis as a complication of long-standing obstruction [135].

Given the potential reversibility or arrest of the renal injury caused by obstruction, its early diagnosis and treatment is essential. Renal ultrasonography is a simple, noninvasive, and reasonably sensitive method of diagnosis which has proven quite useful in detecting obstruction. In some 10% of cases, the ultrasound may fail to detect obstruction [136]. Hence, the necessity of pursuing the diagnosis by more invasive retrograde studies in the presence of unexplained renal insufficiency [126].

Hematopoietic disorders

Sickle cell hemoglobinopathies
Sickle cell hemoglobinopathies are commonly associated with TIN and RPN [137]. However, the renal sequelae and general ravages of these inherited abnormalities manifest themselves at a relatively young age, and, except for those with the trait, would be unusual in elderly individuals. The initiating event is a vascular occlusive lesion that affects the medullary vasculature [138]. The subsequent injury is ischemic in origin and to the extent that these lesions are more severe in the renal medulla will result in RPN [111]. The initial functional changes are those of concentrating defect and distal tubular dysfunction [139,140]. As the lesions progress, renal insufficiency ultimately supervenes [137,138].

Lymphoproliferative disorders
The kidneys are commonly infiltrated by abnormal cells in lymphoproliferative disorders [90]. Renal involvement is common with acute lymphoblastic leukemia and non-Hodgkin's lymphomas but rare in Hodgkin's disease [91]. The infiltrates are localized to the interstitium and result in various forms of tubular dysfunction. When the infiltrates are extensive, diffuse renal failure will result and may be the presenting symptom [92]. Certainly, the presence of renal failure in enlarged kidneys should lead to the consideration of this possibility.

Plasma cell dyscrasias
The excessive production of light chain proteins in plasma cell dyscrasias, a disease of the elderly, will result in TIN [93,141]. The excretion of light chain proteins in the urine results in their precipitation as dimers in the acid environment of the distal tubule [142]. The classic appearance of the myeloma-cast nephropathy is peritubular infiltrates of inflammatory cells, multinucleated giant cells, and interstitial fibrosis [141].

Reabsorption of the light chains in the proximal tubule and consequent cellular toxicity accounts for the proximal tubular dysfunction that may be noted in some cases [92]. Interstitial and perivascular deposition of paraproteins either as amyloid fibrils or fragments of light chains also contribute to the tubulointerstitial nephritis of these patients [143]. The renal injury is directly related to the load of light chains presented to the kidneys, hence, the importance of early treatment before progression to severe renal failure. Plasmapheresis has been shown to be particularly effective in such cases [144]. In addition to the deleterious effect of increased excretion of light chains, hypercalcemia, hyperuricemia, and plasma cell infiltration can contribute to the decline in renal function of these patients [93,145].

Metabolic disorders

The kidney, as the major organ for the excretion of calcium, oxalate, and uric acid becomes the target organ affected in disorders in the metabolism of these substances [145]. It is their precipitation in the kidney that initiates the sequence of events which begins as focal injury, but depending on the load presented and its chronicity ultimately results in the classic structural changes of chronic TIN: interstitial fibrosis, mononuclear cell infiltration, and tubular atrophy. In all three, nephrolithiasis is another complication, which, by inducing partial obstruction and predisposing to infection, can contribute to the development of TIN discussed in the preceding section on urinary tract obstruction.

Miscellaneous

Tubulointerstitial nephritis is a prominent feature of a variety of other disorders (Table 16.4). These are relatively uncommon and the renal involvement is principally a partial component of a more generalized systemic disease. An exception to this is the transplanted kidney whose rejection, be it acute or chronic, results in TIN. This is one instance where both the humoral and cellular limbs of the immune system come to bear on the kidney. The humoral reaction is directed toward the renal vasculature while the cellular limb is reflected in the interstitial infiltration by activated lymphocytes. As a result tubulointerstitial lesions are almost a universal finding in the transplanted kidney [106]. The use of cyclosporine in treatment of rejection can initiate TIN indepedent of the rejection process [3,115].

Finally, it should be noted that in some 10–15% of patients who present with renal insufficiency with biopsy-proven TIN, the disease remains idiopathic in nature despite the most thorough work-up [1,14,109].

References

1 Murray TG, Goldberg M. Chronic interstitial nephritis: Etiologic factors. Ann Intern Med 1975;82:453–459.

2 Rostand SG, Kirk KA, Rutsky EA, *et al.* Racial differences in the incidence of treatment for end-stage renal disease. N Engl J Med 1982;306:1276–1279.

3 Eknoyan G. Chronic tubulointerstitial nephropathies. In Schrier RW, Gottschalk CW, eds. *Diseases of the Kidney*, 4th edn. Boston: Little, Brown & Co., 1988:2191–2221.

4 Wilson DM, Turner DR, Cameron JS, *et al.* Value of renal biopsy in acute intrinsic renal failure. Br Med J 1976;2: 459–461.

5 Mustonen J, Pasternack A, Helin H, *et al.* Renal biopsy in acute renal failure. Am J Nephrol 1984;4:27–31.

6 Eknoyan G. Acute renal failure associated with tubulointerstitial nephropathies. In Brenner BM, Lazarus JM, eds. *Acute Renal Failure*, 2nd edn. New York: Churchill Livingstone, 1988:491–534.

7 Councilman WT. Acute interstitial nephritis. J Exp Med 1898;3:303–420.

8 Cogan MG. Tubulointerstitial nephropathies: A pathophysiologic approach. West J Med 1980;132:134–140.

9 Schainuck LI, Stricker GE, Cutler RE, *et al.* Structural–functional correlations in renal disease. II. The correlations. Hum Pathol 1970;1:631–641.

10 Bohle A, Mackensen-Haen S, Gise H. Significance of tubulo-interstitial changes in the renal cortex for the excretory function and concentration ability of the kidney: A morphometric contribution. Am J Nephrol 1987;7:421–433.

11 Mackensen S, Grund KE, Sindjic M, *et al.* Influence of the renal cortical interstitium on the serum creatinine concentration and creatinine clearance of different chronic sclerosing interstitial nephritis. Nephron 1979;24:30–34.

12 Cogan MG. Classification and patterns of renal dysfunction. Contemp Issues Nephrol 1983;10:35–48.

13 Blythe WB. Natural history of hypertension in renal parenchymal disease. Am J Kidney Dis 1985;5:A50–A56.

14 Eknoyan G, McDonald MA, Appel D, *et al.* Chronic tubulo-interstitial nephritis: Correlation between structural and functional findings. Kidney Int 1990;38:736–743.

15 Neilson EG. Pathogenesis and therapy of interstitial nephritis. Kidney Int 1989;35:1257–1270.

16 Laberke HG, Bohle A. Acute interstitial nephritis. Correlation between clinical and morphological findings. Clin Nephrol 1980;14:263–271.

17 Magil AB, Tyler M. Tubulo-interstitial disease in lupus nephritis. A morphometric study. Histopathology 1984;8: 81–87.

18 Pelz KS, Gottfried SP, Paz E. Kidney function studies in old men and women. Geriatrics 1965;20:145–149.

19 McLachlam MSF. The aging kidney. Lancet 1978;2: 143–146.

20 Epstein M. Effects of aging on the kidney. Fed Proc 1979; 38:168–172.

21 Brown W, Davis BB, Apry LA, *et al.* Aging and the kidney. Arch Intern Med 1986;146:1790–1796.

22 Anderson S, Brenner BM. The aging kidney: Structure, function, mechanisms and therapeutic implications. J Am Geriatr Soc 1987;35:590–593.

23 Beck LE. Kidney function and disease in the elderly. Hosp Pract 1988;15:75–90.

24 Darmady EM, Offer J, Woodhouse MA. The parameters of the aging kidney. J Pathol 1973;109:195–207.

25 Sworn MJ, Fox M. Renal age change in the rat compared with human renal senescence. An autoradiography study. Invest Urol 1974;12:140–145.

26 Kappel B, Olsen S. Cortical interstitial tissue and sclerosed glomeruli in the normal kidney, related to age and sex. Virchows Arch (Pathol Anat) 1980;387:271–277.

27 Haley DP, Bulger RE. The aging male rat: Structure and function of the kidney. Am J Anat 1983;167:1–13.

28 Dunnill MS, Halley W. Some observations on the quantitative anatomy of the kidney. J Pathol 1973;110:113–121.

29 Tauchi H, Tsuboi K, Okutomi J. Age changes in the human kidney of different races. Gerontologia 1971;17:87–97.

30 Goldstein RS, Tarloff JB, Hook JB. Age-related nephropathy

in laboratory rats. FASEB J 1988;2:2241—2251.

31 Bell RH, Borjesson BA, Wolf PL, *et al.* Quantitative morphological studies of aging changes in the kidney of the Lewis rat. Renal Physiol Biochem 1984;7:176—184.

32 Bengele HH, Mathias RS, Perkins JH, *et al.* Urinary concentrating defect in the aged rat. Am J Physiol 1981;240:F147—F150.

33 Adams JR, Barrows CH. Effect of age on PAH accumulation by kidney slices of female rats. J Gerontol 1963;18:37—40.

34 Cerman B, Pratz J, Poujeol P. Changes in anatomy, glomerular filtration, and solute excretion in aging rat kidney. Am J Physiol 1985;248:R282—R287.

35 Kiebzak GM, Sacktor B. Effect of age on renal conservation of phosphate in the rat. Am J Physiol 1986;251:F399—F407.

36 Proverbio F, Proverbio T, Marin R. Ion transport and oxygen consumption in kidney cortex slices from young and old rats. Gerontology 1985;31:166—173.

37 Lindeman RD, Lee TD, Yiengst MJ, *et al.* Influence of age, renal disease, hypertension, diuretics, and calcium on the antidiuretic responses to suboptimal infusions of vasopressin. J Lab Clin Med 1966;68:206—222.

38 Epstein M, Hollenberg NM. Age as a determinant of oral sodium conservation in normal man. J Lab Clin Med 1976;87:411—417.

39 Adler S, Lindeman RD, Yiengst MJ, *et al.* Effect of acute acid loading on urinary acid excretion by the aging human kidney. J Lab Clin Med 1968;72:278—289.

40 Davies DF, Shock NW. Age changes in glomerular filtration, effective renal plasma flow, and tubular excretory capacity in adult males. J Clin Invest 1950;29:496—507.

41 Miller JH, McDonald RK, Shock NW. Age changes in the maximal rate of renal tubular reabsorption of glucose. J Gerontol 1952;7:196—200.

42 Bieriner A. Ein ungervohnlicker Fall von Scharlach. Virchows Arch (Pathol Anat) 1860;19:537—549.

43 Olsen TS, Wasseff NF, Olsen HS, *et al.* Ultrastructure of the kidney in acute interstitial nephritis. Ultrastruct Pathol 1986;10:1—16.

44 Klassen J, Andres GA, Brennan JC, *et al.* An immunologic renal tubular lesion in man. Clin Immunopathol 1972;1:69—89.

45 Appel GB, Woda BA, Neu HC, *et al.* Acute interstitial nephritis associated with carbenicillin therapy. Arch Intern Med 1978;138:1265—1267.

46 Kleinknecht D, Kanfer A, Morel-Maroger L, *et al.* Immunologically mediated drug-induced acute renal failure. Controlled Nephrol 1978;10:42—52.

47 Mampaso FM, Wilson CB. Characterization of inflammatory cells in autoimmune tubulointerstitial nephritis in rats. Kidney Int 1983;23:448—457.

48 Boucher A, Droz D, Adafer I, *et al.* Characterization of mononuclear cell subsets in renal cellular interstitial infiltrates. Kidney Int 1986;29:1043—1049.

49 Gimenez A, Mampaso F. Characterization of inflammatory cells in drug-induced tubulointerstitial nephritis. Nephron 1986;43:239—240.

50 van Ypersele de Strihou C. Acute oliguric interstitial nephritis. Kidney Int 1979;16:751—765.

51 Mignon F, Mery J, Mougenot B, *et al.* Granulomatous interstitial nephritis. Adv Nephrol 1984;13:219—245.

52 Kleinknecht D, Vahille PH, Morel-Maroger L, *et al.* Acute interstitial nephritis due to hypersensitivity. An up-to-date review with report of 19 cases. Adv Nephrol 1983;12:277—308.

53 Baldwin DS, Levine BB, McCluskey RT, *et al.* Renal failure and interstitial nephritis due to penicillin and methicillin. N Engl J Med 1968;279:1245—1252.

54 Ditlove J, Weidmann P, Bernstein M, *et al.* Methicillin nephritis. Medicine 1977;56:483—491.

55 Nolan CM, Abernathy RD. Nephropathy associated with methicillin therapy. Arch Intern Med 1977;137:997—1000.

56 Scholand JS, Tannenbaum JF, Grilli JG. Anaphylaxis to cephalothin in a patient allergic to penicillin. J Am Med Assoc 1968;206:130—132.

57 Border WA, Lehman DH, Egan JD, *et al.* Antitubular basement-membrane antibodies in methicillin-associated interstitial nephritis. N Engl J Med 1974;291:381—384.

58 Colvin RB, Burton JR, Hyslop NE, *et al.* Penicillin-associated interstitial nephritis. Ann Intern Med 1974;81:404—405.

59 Ten RM, Torres VE, Milliner DS, *et al.* Acute interstitial nephritis: Immunologic and clinical aspects. Mayo Clin Proc 1988;63:921—930.

60 Robson M, Levi J, Dollberg L, *et al.* Acute tubulointerstitial nephritis following sulfadiazine therapy. Isr J Med Sci 1970;6:561—566.

61 Shear NH, Spielberg SP, Grant DM, *et al.* Differences in metabolism of sulfonamides predisposing to idiosyncratic toxicity. Ann Intern Med 1980;105:179—184.

62 Richmond JM, Whitworth JS, Fairley KF, *et al.* Cotrimoxasole nephrotoxicity. Lancet 1979;1:493.

63 Campese VM, Marzullo F, Schena FP, *et al.* Acute renal failure during intermittent rifampicin therapy. Nephron 1973;10:256—261.

64 Qunibi WY, Godwin J, Eknoyan G. Toxic nephropathy during continuous rifampicin therapy. South Med J 1980;73:791—792.

65 Gabriel M, Chew W. Relationship between rifampicin-dependent antibody scores, serum rifampicin concentrations and symptoms in patients with adverse reactions to intermittent rifampicin treatment. Clin Allerg 1973;3:353—362.

66 Levin ML. Patterns of tubulo-interstitial damage associated with nonsteroidal anti-inflammatory drugs. Semin Nephrol 1988;8:55—61.

67 Blackshear JL, Napier JS, Davidman M, *et al.* Renal complications of nonsteroidal anti-inflammatory drugs:

Identification and monitoring of those at risk. Semin Arthritis Rheum 1985;14:163–175.

68 Henrich WL, Blachley JD. Acute renal failure with prostaglandin inhibitors. Semin Nephrol 1981;1:57–60.

69 Clive DM, Stoff JS. Renal syndromes associated with nonsteroidal anti-inflammatory drugs. N Engl J Med 1984;310:563–572.

70 Brezin JH, Katz SM, Schwartz AB, et al. Reversible renal failure and nephrotic syndrome associated with nonsteroidal anti-inflammatory drugs. N Engl J Med 1979;301:1271–1273.

71 Abraham PA, Keane WF. Glomerular and interstitial disease induced by nonsteroidal anti-inflammatory drugs. Am J Nephrol 1984;4:1–6.

72 Handa SP. Renal effects of fenoprofen. Ann Intern Med 1980;93:508–509.

73 Fialk MA, Romankiewicz J, Perrone F, et al. Allergic interstitial nephritis with diuretics. Ann Intern Med 1974;81:403–404.

74 Lyons H, Pinn VW, Cortell S, et al. Allergic interstitial nephritis causing reversible renal failure in four patients with idiopathic nephrotic syndrome. N Engl J Med 1973;288:124–128.

75 Magil AB, Ballon HS, Cameron ES, et al. Acute interstitial nephritis associated with thiazide diuretics. Clinical and pathologic observations in three cases. Am J Med 1980;69:939–943.

76 Tolkoff-Rubin NE, Rubin RH. Urinary tract infection. Contemp Issues Nephrol 1983;10:49–82.

77 Hostetter TH, Nath KA, Hostetter MK. Infection-related chronic interstitial nephropathy. Semin Nephrol 1988;8:11–16.

78 Stamey TA, ed. *Urinary Infections.* Baltimore: Williams & Wilkins, 1972.

79 Richet G, Mayaud C. The course of acute renal failure in pyelonephritis and other types of interstitial nephritis. Nephron 1978;22:124–127.

80 Eknoyan G. The natural history of primary pyelonephritis. Contrib Nephrol 1988;75:82–89.

81 Knepshield JH, Carstens PHB, Gentile DE. Recovery from renal failure due to acute diffuse interstitial nephritis. Pediatrics 1969;43:533–539.

82 Haddon JE, Robotham JL. Acute interstitial nephritis in children. A process produced by streptococcal infection and by chemotherapeutic agents. A review. J Maine Med Assoc 1978;69:1–6.

83 Ellis D, Fried WA, Yunis EJ, et al. Acute interstitial nephritis in children: A report of 13 cases and review of the literature. Pediatrics 1981;67:862–870.

84 Foley RJ, Weinman EJ. Urate nephropathy. Am J Med Sci 1984;288:208–211.

85 Kraikipanich S, Lindeman RD, Mandal AK. Severe hyperuricemia, hypokalemic alkalosis, and tubulointerstitial nephritis. Am J Med Sci 1976;271:77–83.

86 Kjellstrand CM, Campbell DB, von Hartizsch B, et al. Hyperuricemic acute renal failure. Arch Intern Med 1974;133:349–359.

87 Benabe J, Martinez-Maldonado M. Hypercalcemic nephropathy. Arch Intern Med 1978;138:777–779.

88 Marone C, Berretta-Picoli C, Weidman P. Acute hypercalcemic hypertension in man: Role of hemodynamics, catacholamines and renin. Kidney Int 1980;20:92–96.

89 Ganote CE, Philipsborn DS, Chen E, et al. Acute calcium nephrotoxicity: An electron microscopic and semiquantitative light microscopic study. Arch Pathol Lab Med 1975;99:650–657.

90 Martinez-Maldonado M, Ramirez-Arellano GA. Renal involvement in malignant lymphoma. A survey of 49 cases. J Urol 1966;95:485–488.

91 Tsokos GC, Balow JE, Siegel RJ, et al. Renal and metabolic complications of undifferentiated and lymphoblastic lymphomas. Medicine 1980;60:218–229.

92 Suki WN. The kidney in systemic disease. Contemp Nephrol 1987;4:463–478.

93 Martinez-Maldonado M, Yium J, Suki WN, et al. Renal complications in multiple myeloma. Pathophysiology and some aspects of clinical management. J Chron Dis 1971;24:221–237.

94 Brennan S, Eknoyan G. The kidney and systemic disorders. Curr Nephrol 1990;13:49–69.

95 Graber ML, Cogan MG, Conner DG. Idiopathic acute interstitial nephritis. West J Med 1978;129:72–76.

96 Spital A, Panner BJ, Sterns RH. Acute idiopathic tubulointerstitial nephritis. Report of two cases and review of the literature. Am J Kidney Dis 1987;9:71–78.

97 Burnier M, Jaegger P, Campiche M, et al. Idiopathic acute interstitial nephritis and uveitis in the adult. Am J Nephrol 1986;6:312–315.

98 Zollinger HU, Spuhler O. Die michteitrige chronische interstitielle Nephritis. Schweiz Z Allg Pathol 1950;13:806–811.

99 Spuhler O, Zollinger HU. Die chronische interstitielle Nephritis. Z Klin Med 1953;151:1–21.

100 Eknoyan G. Analgesic nephrotoxicity and renal papillary necrosis. Semin Nephrol 1984;4:65–76.

101 Heptinstall RH. Interstitial nephritis. A brief review. Am J Pathol 1976;83:214–236.

102 Mujais SK, Quintanilla A. Chronic tubulointerstitial nephritis: Saga of the ubiquitous. Semin Nephrol 1988;8:4–10.

103 Neilson EG, Phillips SM. Cell-mediated immunity in interstitial nephritis. II. T lymphocyte effector mechanisms in nephritogenic guinea pigs: Analysis of the renotropic migration and cytotoxic response. J Immunol 1979;123:2381–2385.

104 Neilson EG, Jimenez SA, Phillips SM. Cell-mediated immunity in interstitial nephritis. III. T lymphocyte mediated fibroblast proliferation and collagen synthesis: An immune

mechanism for renal fibrogenesis. J Immunol 1980;125: 1708–1714.

105 Wilson C, Blantz R. Nephroimmunopathology and pathophysiology. Am J Physiol 1985;248:F319–F331.

106 McCluskey RT. Immunologically mediated tubulo-interstitial nephritis. Contemp Issues Nephrol 1983;10:121–149.

107 Andriole VT. The role of Tamm–Horsfall protein in the pathogenesis of reflux nephropathy and chronic pyelonephritis. Yale J Biol Med 1985;58:91–100.

108 Miller RA. The cell biology of aging: Immunological model. J Gerontol 1989;44:B4–B8.

109 Gonwa TA, Hamilton RW, Buckalew VA. Chronic renal failure and end-stage renal disease in northwest North Carolina. Arch Intern Med 1981;141:462–465.

110 Sabatini S. Analgesic-induced papillary necrosis. Semin Nephrol 1988;8:41–54.

111 Eknoyan G, Qunibi WT, Grissom RT, et al. Renal papillary necrosis. An update. Medicine 1982;61:55–73.

112 Murray TG. Drug-induced tubulo-interstitial renal disease. Contemp Issues Nephrol 1983;10:187–209.

113 Nanra RS, Stuart-Taylor J, De Leon H, et al. Analgesic nephropathy. Etiology, clinical syndrome and clinicopathologic correlations in Australia. Kidney Int 1978;13:79–92.

114 Molland EA. Experimental renal papillary necrosis. Kidney Int 1978;13:5–14.

115 Dubach UC, Rosner B, Pfister E. Epidemiologic study of abuse of analgesic containing phenacetin. Renal morbidity and mortality (1968–1979). N Engl J Med 1983;308: 357–362.

116 Murray RM. Patterns of analgesic use and abuse in medical patients. Practitioner 1973;211:639–644.

117 Wainscoat JS, Finn R. Possible role of laxatives in analgesic nephropathy. Br Med J 1974;4:697–698.

118 Bluemle LW, Goldberg M. Renal accumulation of salicylate and phenacetin: Possible mechanisms in the nephropathy of analgesic abuse. J Clin Invest 1968;47:2507–2514.

119 Duggin GG, Mudge GH. Phenacetin: Renal tubular transport and intrarenal distribution in the dog. J Pharmacol Exp Ther 1976;199:10–16.

120 Mudge GH, Gembroys MW, Duggin GG. Covalent binding of metabolites of acetaminophen to kidney protein and depletion of renal glutathione. J Pharmacol Exp Ther 1978;206:218–226.

121 McMurty RJ, Snodgrass WR, Mitchell JR. Renal necrosis, glutathione depletion, and covalent binding after acetaminophen. J Toxicol Appl Pharmacol 1978;46:87–100.

122 Zenser TV, Mattammal MB, Rapp NS, et al. Effect of aspirin on metabolism of acetaminophen and benzidine by renal inner medulla prostaglandin hydroperoxidase. J Lab Clin Med 1983;101:58–65.

123 Gonwa TA, Corbett WT, Schey HM, et al. Analgesic associated nephropathy and transitional cell carcinoma of the urinary tract. Ann Intern Med 1980;93:249–252.

124 Wilson DR. Pathophysiology of obstructive nephropathy. Kidney Int 1980;18:281–292.

125 Klahr S. Pathophysiology of obstructive nephropathy. Kidney Int 1983;23:414–426.

126 Schueter W, Battle DC. Chronic obstructive nephropathy. Semin Nephrol 1988;8:17–28.

127 Schreiner GF, Kohan DE. Regulation of renal transport processes and hemodynamics by macrophages and lymphocytes. Am J Physiol 1990;258:F761–F767.

128 Arruda JL. Obstructive uropathy. Contemp Issues Nephrol 1983;10:243–273.

129 Pridgen WR, Woodhead DM, Younger RK. Alterations in renal function produced by ureteral obstruction: Determination of critical obstruction time in relation to renal survival. J Am Med Assoc 1961;178:563–564.

130 Brunschwig A, Barger HRK, Roberts S. Return of renal function after varying periods of ureteral occlusions. J Am Med Assoc 1964;188:5–8.

131 Nelson RP, Williams A. Late return of renal function after correction of chronic obstruction. J Urol 1977;188: 462–463.

132 Bander SJ, Buerkert JE, Martin D, et al. Long-term effects of 24-hour unilateral obstruction on renal function in the rat. Kidney Int 1985;28:614–620.

133 Better OS, Arieff AI, Massry SG, et al. Studies on renal function after relief of complete unilateral obstruction of three months duration in man. Am J Med 1973;54: 234–240.

134 Battle DC, Sehy JT, Roseman MK, et al. Hyperkalemic distal renal tubular acidosis associated with obstructive uropathy. N Engl J Med 1981;304:373–380.

135 Cotran RS. Glomerulosclerosis in reflux nephropathy. Kidney Int 1982;21:528–534.

136 Talner L, Scheible W, Ellenbogen PH. How accurate is ultrasonography in detecting hydronephrosis in azotemic patients? Urol Radiol 1981;3:1–6.

137 Vaamonde CA. Renal papillary necrosis in sickle cell hemoglobinopathies. Semin Nephrol 1984;4:48–64.

138 de Jong PE, Statius van Eps LW. Sickle cell nephropathy: New insights into its pathophysiology. Kidney Int 1985; 27:711–717.

139 Hatch FE, Culbertson JW, Diggs LW. Nature of renal concentrating defect in sickle cell disease. J Clin Invest 1967; 46:336–345.

140 Battle DC, Itsarayoungyuen K, Arruda JAL, et al. Hyperkalemic hyperchloremic metabolic acidosis in sickle cell hemoglobinopathies. Am J Med 1982;72:188–192.

141 De Fronzo RA, Cooke CR, Wright JR, et al. Renal function in patients with multiple myeloma. Medicine 1978;57: 151–166.

142 Smolens P, Venkatachalam M, Stein JH. Myeloma kidney cast nephropathy in a rat model of multiple myeloma. Kidney Int 1983;24:192–204.

143 Fang LS. Light chain nephropathy. Kidney Int 1985: 27–592.

144 Zucchelli P, Pasquali S, Cagnoli L, *et al*. Controlled plasma exchange trial in acute renal failure due to multiple myeloma. Kidney Int 1988;33:1175–1180.

145 Benabe JE, Martinez-Maldonado M. Tubulointerstitial nephritis associated with systemic disease and electrolyte abnormalities. Semin Nephrol 1988;8:29–40.

17

Renal disease in diabetes mellitus in the elderly

Thomas H. Hostetter
Barbara S. Daniels

Diabetes mellitus is the most common cause of end-state renal disease in the United States. Although much of the available data do not allow distinctions between insulin-dependent (IDDM) and noninsulin-dependent (NIDDM) patients, most evidence suggests that about one-half of all diabetic end-stage diseases occurs in NIDDM [1]. Furthermore, this incidence of renal failure, at least in some populations of NIDDM, may approach that of IDDM when duration of diabetes is considered [1,2]. Because older patients with NIDDM also suffer from other serious non-renal cardiovascular disease, the crude incidence of renal disease may appear to be less than that of IDDM, likely a reflection of the competing mortality of coronary and cerebrovascular disease in the elderly NIDDM [3]. Thus because NIDDM is predominantly a disease of the older patient, diabetes is a major cause of chronic renal failure in the elderly.

Morphology

The renal lesions in NIDDM are similar if not identical to those of IDDM. Indeed, the classic description of diabetic glomerulopathy rested in a large part on material from older patients with NIDDM. Studies formally restricted to NIDDM have confirmed the near identity of the end-stage pathology results from both conditions [4]. Only modest differences have been reported. Specifically, Schmitz et al. [5] could find no glomerular enlargement in the noninsulin-dependent subjects; indeed, the mean volume for open glomeruli tended to be smaller than in age-matched, nondiabetic control subjects. Whether this lack of glomerular enlargement, seen regularly in insulin-dependent diabetes, is due to the later age of onset in noninsulin-dependent diabetes with a consequent age-induced inability to express glomerular hypertrophy or whether it is due to concurrent hypertension and vascular disease limiting the renal growth is unknown.

In advanced diabetic kidney disease four general types of glomerular lesions are classically noted. They are: the nodular intercapillary sclerosis, diffuse intercapillary sclerosis, the fibrin cap lesion, and the capsular drop lesion, the last two often collectively termed hyaline, insudative, or exudative lesions. The function implication of glomerular structural changes is considered in the section on pathogenesis below; however, it should be noted that all of the lesions described below can be regularly observed in the kidneys of patients with long-standing diabetes who have little or no clinical renal disease [6,7]. Thus, these lesions are to varying degrees indicative of chronic diabetes, but do not necessarily denote clinically significant renal dysfunction.

Nodular intercapillary sclerosis

The most specific abnormality of the four general types is the nodular lesion [6]. This is the abnormality originally described by Kimmelstiel & Wilson that bears their names [3,8] (Fig. 17.1). The nodules are oval shaped structures which vary remarkably in size as well as their number within individual glomeruli, with some glomeruli in a single specimen demonstrating one to several nodules and others none. These lesions tend to occur at the periphery of the glomerulus away from the hylus. Their ultrastructural locus is the mesangium. The nodules stain positively with *para*-aminosalicylic acid (PAS) and while generally homogenous in appearance become more lamellated with size and presumably with age. The associated

glomerular capillary in these diseased glomeruli generally becomes dilated and may even grow to microaneurysmal proportions. As with the whole kidney size, the glomerular diameter tends to remain relatively normal despite the presence of severe nodular lesions.

Even though this classic nodular lesion is the most specific for diabetes of the glomerular changes, other diseases may occasionally mimic the pattern. The lesion is relatively sparse, and the minority of diabetics are reported to manifest the lesions. First, membranoproliferative glomerulonephritis Type II may demonstrate a lobular form [9]. The nodules in that circumstance tend to be more homogeneous both in size and number than those appearing in diabetic nephropathy. In addition, electron microscopy should reveal typical changes of this type of glomerulonephritis, namely interposition of mesangial cells and the presence of dense deposits within the basement membrane. Another glomerular disease which may resemble nodular diabetic glomerulosclerosis is that arising in patients producing excess amounts of

Fig. 17.1 (a) Glomerulus from a diabetic patient demonstrating nodular intercapillary sclerosis, the Kimmelstiel–Wilson lesion. Hematoxylin and eosin, original magnification ×370. (b) Glomerulus from a diabetic patient demonstrating diffuse intercapillary sclerosis of moderate degree. Hematoxylin and eosin, ×370. (c) Glomerulus from a diabetic patient demonstrating a capsular drop (large arrow) and hyalin "fibrin" cap (small arrow). Note that these lesions are present in a glomerulus with only minimal changes of diffuse glomerulosclerosis. PAS, original magnification ×500. (From Mauer [141])

(a)   (b)   (c)

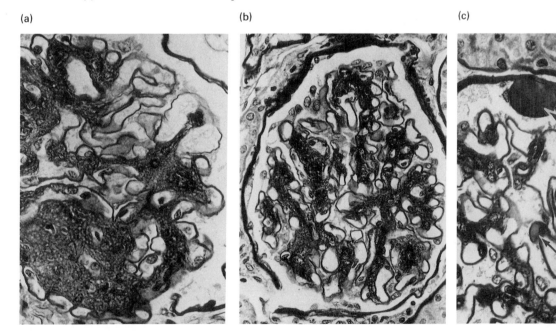

immunoglobulin light chains [10]. This nodular glomerulopathy is of particular prominence in those patients manufacturing excess light chains of the κ type. This paraproteinemic lesion is obviously attended by increased excretion of monoclonal light chain proteins type. Also, the immunofluorescence pattern of appropriately specific fluoresceinated antibody should distinguish these abnormalities from nodular diabetic glomerulosclerosis. Lastly, amyloidosis may present a diffuse to nodular glomerular pattern but appropriate stains and electron microscopic characteristics of amyloid should distinguish this disease from diabetes.

Diffuse intercapillary sclerosis

The diffuse form of diabetic intercapillary sclerosis occurs more commonly than the classic modular form and indeed is almost always seen accompanying the nodular form [11–13]. The diffuse pattern represents a range of expansion in the mesangial area from minimal to overt, conspicuous expansions which in themselves occlude capillary lumina (Fig. 17.1). The mesangial location of both the diffuse and nodular lesions are similar and their morphogenesis is generally envisioned as the same excess accumulation of matrix material, simply differing in their geometric distribution [14]. Consistent with this view is the observation that various histopathologic stains are similar for the nodular and diffuse lesions and in particular both expansions are eosinophilic and PAS positive [15].

The diffuse form of diabetic glomerulosclerosis is less specific for diabetes than is the nodular form. In its lesser degree, the diffuse expansion may be confused with thickening described in aging as well as in hypertension. Amyloid glomerulopathy may also be mistaken for the diffuse sclerotic lesion as well. Furthermore, the capillary wall thickening seen in idiopathic membranous glomerulonephritis can resemble on light microscopy that of the diffuse form of diabetic glomerulopathy.

Capsular drop lesion

This lesion appears on the parietal side of Bowman's capsule and is located between the basement membrane and the epithelial cells (Fig. 17.1). Morphologically, it is an irregularly shaped excrescence of variable size which stains intensely eosinophilic with hematoxin and eosin and indeed many of its staining characteristics are held in common with the fibrin cap lesion.

Fibrin cap lesion

Somewhat more frequent than the capsular drop lesion, the fibrin cap lesion is pathologically quite similar in its general appearance (Fig. 17.1). However, the fibrin cap lesion occurs within a glomerular capillary, where it is usually relatively smooth and its contour conforming to the wall of the capillary. This lesion is not at all specific for diabetes and has been described in several glomerulonephritides including focal segmental glomerulosclerosis, and systemic lupus erythematosus nephritis [16]. The fibrin cap has been noted as well in vascular disease of the kidney, including arteriosclerosis, and in chronic tubulointerstitial disease [17].

Tubulointerstitial lesions

With end-stage diabetic renal disease, tubules become atrophic and regularly develop thickening of the tubular basement membrane. The interstitium becomes particularly prominent in its degree of abnormalities [18,19]. Several classes of mononuclear cells, including lymphocytes and plasma cells, appear in abundance [20]. Furthermore, polymorphonuclear cells including neutrophils and eosinophils may be seen within the chronic scarring process of the end-stage diabetic kidney. Accompanying the infiltration of the inflammatory cells, increasing fibrosis is seen in the interstitium and the degree of fibrosis appears to be greatest when larger vessel disease is also present.

Immunofluorescent changes

Classic immunopathologic damage of either the immune complex type or the antiglomerular basement membrane type does not occur as a part of diabetic nephropathy. Although classic mechanisms of immune-mediated injury have not been discovered in diabetic nephropathy, deposition of a wide variety of circulating proteins can be visualized in the diabetic kidney. Westberg & Michael [21] demonstrated that about half of the kidneys taken from patients with end-state diabetic nephropathy demonstrated a thin linear staining along the glomerular basement membrane for IgG and IgM. Other circulating protein including fibrin, 1C, albumin, and ceruloplasmin were also deposited in glomerular basement membrane but less consistently than the immunoglobulins. This observation of linear deposition by a variety of plasma proteins has been extended to the tubular basement membrane where IgG and albumin have been detected in a similar linear distribution [22]. More recently Falk *et al.* [23] have emphasized the presence of the membrane attack complex of complement within end-stage diabetic and nondiabetic kidneys. Immunofluorescent studies of the nodular lesions have not resulted in consistent findings. However, the lesions appear to be occasionally positive for gamma globulin, particularly immunoglobulin types, notably IgG and IgM [23]. Exudative lesions display positive immunofluorescence for a variety of large molecular weight plasma proteins including gamma globulin, fibrinogen, and lipoproteins [23].

The glomerular content of several antigens native to the glomerulus are also increased as detected by immunofluorescent techniques. Specifically, actomyosin, collagen, laminin, and fibronectin are noted in excess quantities within the mesangium of diabetic patients [24–26].

Electron microscopic changes

Basement membrane thickening is a nonspecific but consistent feature of diabetic renal disease. Osterby [27] has demonstrated that the glomerular basement membrane is of normal thickness at the earliest stages of diabetes in humans. Detectable thickening, however, was regularly noted after 2–5 years of diabetes. Thickening tends to progress with duration of diabetes and can reach 10-times the normal dimension [23]. Its degree is greatest in the presence of nodular glomerular lesions [28]. Electron microscopy confirms that the nodular lesions, as well as the diffuse glomerular sclerosis both represent an increase in mesangial matrix material, although as noted above the increase derives from increases in several elements of that matrix [23]. Both the number and size of strands of mesangial matrix material increase in early diabetes [30]. In the late stages, collagen fibers are detected in the expanded matrix material. The number of mesangial cells does not appear to be increased to the same degree as the increase in matrix material. Glomerular epithelial cells, intially well preserved in diabetic nephropathy, eventually develop the effacement of distinct foot processes typical of proteinuric renal diseases. In addition to this "fusion" of protocytes, the epithelial cells may undergo a process of degeneration and become detached from the basement membrane, giving rise to areas stripped of epithelial cell covering [30].

Electron microscopic examination of the fibrin cap lesion reveals an electron dense material which is situated on the endothelial side of the glomerular basement membrane while its analog, the capsular drop lesion, has a similar appearance but is located in the cleft between the basement membrane of Bowman's capsule and the overlying parietal epithelium [20].

Clinical features

Course

Some evidence has suggested that the incidence of renal disease in NIDDM differs from that in IDDM. For example, in 1965 Marks studied the incidence of uremic death in diabetes, a specific, but highly insensitive, measure of diabetic renal disease [31]. He noted that 42% of patients, less than 20 years of age at the onset of diabetes (presumably IDDM), but only 2.5% of older (presumably NIDDM) patients died with uremia. There are numerous confounding variables in such a study, including coexistent vascular disease in older patients which may lead to death from myocardial infarction or stroke before the evolution of nephropathy. Furthermore, recent data have supported this impression of a lower incidence of nephropathy in NIDDM [32]. However, when the duration of diabetes was carefully considered, Pima Indians with NIDDM manifest end-stage renal disease with approximately the same incidence as IDDM patients treated at the Joslin Clinic [2]. Whether the Pima population will prove similar to others with NIDDM is uncertain, but these results suggest that as other cardiovascular complications are addressed a substantial increase in renal failure may be exposed in the elderly population with NIDDM.

Regardless of the relative rates of renal failure in NIDDM and IDDM, even a very low rate of renal failure produces a great deal of morbidity and human suffering. If 85% of all diabetics have IDDM, a 6% cumulative incidence of renal failure results in the same absolute number of patients with end-stage renal disease as a 33% cumulative incidence of renal disease in IDDM. Therefore, one cannot dismiss the overall significance of renal disease in NIDDM based on its incidence relative to that in IDDM.

The clinical course of progression renal insufficiency to failure has not been so well charted in NIDDM as in IDDM. However, no substantial qualitative differences are notable. The quantitative differences are listed in Table 17.1.

Table 17.1 The quantitative differences between insulin-dependent and noninsulin-dependent diabetes mellitus

	IDDM	NIDDM
Hypertension	Unusual except in patients with nephropathy	Common
Proteinuria at diagnosis	Same frequency as general population	More frequent than general population
Glomerular hyperfiltration	Common	Absent
Progressive proteinuria	~35%	~50%
Progressive renal dysfunction	~35%	~15–35%

IDDM, insulin-dependent diabetes mellitus; NIDDM, noninsulin-dependent diabetes mellitus.

Hypertension

Many studies in the 1940s and 1950s demonstrated an increased frequency of hypertension in patients with NIDDM compared to normal controls. However, poor study design, inadequate controls, obesity, and the presence of diabetic nephropathy, were not evaluated as potentially confounding factors in the genesis of the hypertension. One of the first controlled studies to demonstrate increased hypertension in NIDDM was reported by Pell & D'Alonzo in 1965 [33]. Using records from the employee health service at the Dupont Company, they conducted a case control study and demonstrated a 50% greater prevalence of hypertension (systolic BP > 150 mmHg or diastolic BP > 94 mmHg) in NIDDM compared to age- and sex-matched nondiabetic controls. They also demonstrated that the increased frequency of hypertension was independent of the obesity commonly observed in NIDDM, since it was present in both obese and nonobese diabetics. Hypertension also occurred more commonly in subjects with NIDDM in the absence of proteinuria or renal disease. This is in distinction to patients with IDDM where hypertension occurs with the same frequency as in the general population until renal disease becomes clinically apparent, the rise in blood pressure is temporally related to the development of diabetic nephropathy [34]. Although some IDDM patients are hypertensive in the absence of renal disease,

this is believed to represent coexistent essential hypertension which occurs at a rate which mirrors the frequency of hypertension in the general population.

It is interesting to note that Pell & D'Alonzo also demonstrated that hypertension actually preceded clinically recognizable NIDDM in some patients and was more common in patients destined to develop NIDDM [33]. That hypertension antedates NIDDM is further evidence that hypertension is not due to diabetes or to its renal or vascular complications in NIDDM and corroborates more recent findings that insulin resistance occurs with essential hypertension. Insulin resistance and hypertension occur not only in NIDDM and essential hypertension, but also in such diverse conditions as Cushing's disease, pregnancy, and cyclosporin administration [35,36]. While the relationship is interesting, its cause has not been established and the pathophysiology remain to be elucidated [37]. The possible interaction between aging and diabetes in the production of atherosclerosis may be important in augmenting the frequency of hypertension in these patients. Decreased vascular compliance due to the presence of vascular disease may increase the frequency of hypertension in NIDDM. Thus, the difference in the prevalence of hypertension in NIDDM and IDDM many reflect not only the different etiologies of the two disorders (insulin resistance vs. insulinopenia) but also the role of coexisting conditions (such as vascular disease), and emphasizes the importance of factors other than glucose in the genesis of diabetic complications.

Proteinuria

Proteinuria is usually a good marker of glomerular disease, and its presence in a patient with IDDM of more than 10 years duration strongly suggest diabetic nephropathy [34]. However, at the time of diagnosis, up to 50% of patients with NIDDM in a variety of studies, ranging from Pima Indians in New Mexico [38] to the predominantly Caucasian residents of Rochester, Minnesota, exhibited enhanced albumin or protein excretory rates, generally greater than that seen in matched populations [39].

The factors responsible for proteinuria early in the course of NIDDM have not been elucidated. Systemic hypertension is associated with increased albumin excretory rates in nondiabetic populations [40], and the high rate of hypertension in NIDDM may be the genesis of proteinuria in NIDDM. The possible presence of functional or structural abnormalities associated with classic diabetic nephropathy such as decreased glomerular proteoglycan and anionic charge sites, mesangial expansion and glomerular basement membrane thickening, have not been evaluated at an early stage of NIDDM. Recent data indicate that most overtly albuminuric patients with NIDDM will have typical diabetic lesions on renal biopsy [41]. However, about a fourth will have a different renal disease. The absence of retinopathy is an important clue suggesting nondiabetic renal disease.

The prevalence of proteinuria increases with the duration of diabetes in NIDDM as in IDDM. However, there is divergent data on the relative rates of proteinuria in NIDDM and IDDM. A predominantly Caucasian group of patients in Rochester, Minnesota with NIDDM developed proteinuria at a rate less than that seen in patients with IDDM followed for a comparable period of time. However, in Pima Indians the cumulative incidence of proteinuria after 20 years was 50% [42] which is greater than the 30–40% reported other groups in Caucasian patients with IDDM [43,44]. The reasons for these discrepant results are not apparent but could be related to either racial or other genetic differences or methodologic considerations. Race does contribute to the risk of developing nephropathy, as blacks develop diabetic nephropathy as well as other renal diseases at a higher frequency than whites.

Neither the cause or the long-term significance of proteinuria as a marker of impending diabetic nephropathy have been as well established in NIDDM as in IDDM. However, microalbuminuria (albumin excretion above the normal range but below standard detection limits) predicts progression to overt proteinuria and portends an excess mortality [45]. In a population with a high rate of proteinuria at the time of diagnosis of diabetes as occurs in NIDDM, it may not be appropriate to attribute the subsequent increase in proteinuria solely to diabetes and further studies are necessary to establish the etiolgy of proteinuria in NIDDM. Regardless of the cause of the proteinuria NIDDM patients with proteinuria have a higher mortality, usually from cardiovascular disease, than those without proteinuria.

Pathogenesis

Functional changes

The hemodynamic mechanism for the reduction in glomerular filtration rate (GFR) in established diabetic nephropathy is not completely defined. Measurements of renal plasma flow in patients with reductions in GFR to a range of 20–30 ml/min indicate proportional reductions in plasma flow such that filtration fractions remain relatively constant [46]. Therefore, the reduction in GFR can be attributed at least in part to the reduction in plasma flow. Furthermore, changes in systemic oncotic pressure clearly do not account by themselves for the fall in GFR since oncotic pressure tends to be normal or in the occasional nephrotic patient, even reduced in the face of the falling GFR [46]. Obviously, changes in the ultrafiltration coefficient are an attractive possibility for the declining GFR since falls in filtering surfacing areas due to mesangial expansion and simple capillary occlusion can be demonstrated by morphologic techniques [3,14,47]. The inverse correlations between GFR and both glomerular occlusion and mesangial expansion support such a possibility. Morphologic damage in humans with advanced diabetic renal disease is markedly heterogeneous in degree of glomerular injury. Other disease models with chronic heterogeneous damage have been investigated, and demonstrate a wide range of single-nephron filtration rates and plasma flows from nephron to nephron, a situation likely obtained in the end-stage diabetic kidney as well [48–50]. Additionally, studies of the remnant kidney model of chronic renal failure indicate that increases in the transcapillary hydraulic pressure gradient are present in the setting of progressive renal disease [51]. This increase in glomerular pressure consequent to nephron adaptation may be accentuated with concomitant diabetes. Evidence for this possibility derives from studies of diabetic rats with loss of renal mass by unilateral nephrectomy which have shown glomerular pressures greater even than the already elevated pressures seen with unilateral nephrectomy alone [52].

Pathophysiologic studies of the glomerular permselective properties during the late stages of overt proteinuria point to the emergence of a defect in size selectivity. Indeed a preliminary report concludes that size-selective glomerular defects can be discerned in new onset NIDDM when albumin excretion is still normal [54]. Studies of patients who have late diabetic nephropathy and heavy proteinuria have been conducted by Myers et al. [54]. These investigators have demonstrated that in advanced diabetic nephropathy the fractional clearance of very large molecules with molecular radii of greater than 46 Å is elevated above normal. Their mathematical analysis indicates that this elevation in the fractional clearance of such large molecules is consistent with the appearance of a very small population of large, unselective pores within the glomerular capillary wall [55]. They concluded that the development of such large pores within the glomerular filter would permit the unrestricted movement of very large plasma proteins into the urine and could account for most if not all of the proteinuria in the late stages of diabetes. Although they caution against a direct application of their pore analysis to glomerular morphology, they note that morphologic alterations have been described in the end-stage diabetic glomerulus which might lead to gross defects in size-selectivity. Specifically, the described detachment of epithelial cells from the basement membrane and defects within the glomerular basement membrane itself could provide an anatomic basis for the loss of size-selectivity [30,56,57].

Although not explored directly, changes in charge-selectivity are also probable in the late stages of diabetes. This probability arises indirectly from the observation that the major fixed negative charges within the glomerular capillary wall may be reduced in amount in diabetic nephropathy. In particular, the sialic acid component of this anionic barrier has been found to be reduced rather consistently in glomerular basement membrane of patients with long-standing diabetes [58–61]. In addition, recent reports describe a reduction in sulfated heparan within the glomerular basement membrane of rats and humans with diabetes, and reduction of negative surface charge on arterial endothelial cells from diabetic rats [62–64]. As discussed below, this glycosaminoglycan is like sialic acid, a major constituent of the glomerular capillary fixed negative charge [65]. Clinical studies of charge selectivity suggest that although an electrically dependent leak occurs it likely is more complex than a simple loss of negative charge [66,67]. Hence, reduction in negatively charged components of the glomerular capillary and/or the spatial rearrangement of charged sites engenders a charge-selective defect in evoking proteinuria. In addition, glycation of circulating proteins may enhance their permeability by effects on their charge or other molecular properties (see below). Finally, if the increased transcapillary hydraulic pressure gradients, seen with poorly controlled diabetes, are further augmented, with the loss of nephron number as seems likely from the experimental data, this increase

in pressure gradient across a glomerular capillary wall already structurally defective might provoke even greater changes in size and/or charge-selectivity [55,68]. Thus, while size-selective defects have been clearly demonstrated the potential for other permselective abnormalities to contribute to the late proteinuria clearly exists.

Glomerular lesions

Role of diabetes
The concept that some aspect(s) of the diabetic milieu leads to renal microvascular disease continues to be the dominant view. At the present time this position seems essentially certain and stands against the suggestion that diabetic microangiopathy and in particular basement membrane thickening is some extrametabolic accompaniment of diabetes due to some coinherited propensity to microvascular disease [69–71].

Many studies have provided overwhelming evidence for the casual relationship between the diabetic milieu and the presence of microvascular disease. First, diabetic lesions in the kidney can be observed in a whole variety of types of diabetes in animals and humans. That is, experimentally induced diabetes in animals leads to abnormalities in the glomerulus which in many aspects are similar to those of human diabetes [14,72,73]. Furthermore, secondary types of diabetes due to hemochromatosis, chronic pancreatitis, or acromegaly are also attended by diabetic microvascular complications. These observations certainly suggest that a genetic predisposition to IDDM or NIDDM is not necessary for the development of the renal microvascular disease of diabetes. However, genetic factors may contribute to the risk for a diabetic patient developing nephropathy. As noted, hypertension and associated erythrocyte-cation-transport abnormalities may represent such a genetic risk [74,75]. Recently, Seaquist et al. [76] have reported a familial, perhaps genetic, predisposition to nephropathy. They studied sibling pairs concordant for diabetes. One sib, the proband, was initially identified and classified as having nephropathy, not on the basis of albumin excretion. When the diabetic sibs of these probands were examined, evidence for nephropathy was found in 83% of those whose proband sibs had nephropathy but in only 17% of those whose proband sibs were free of nephropathy. These and other observations, such as the high prevalence of nephropathy among males and blacks compared to white diabetics, suggest that genetic and/or environmental factors importantly influence the risk of this complication [77–80].

While other factors appear to alter risk, diabetes itself is a necessary factor. For example, Mauer et al. [81] have firmly established that mesangial lesions of diabetes in the rat may be reversed by the transplantation of the diabetic kidney into an animal with normal β-cell function and that the transplantation of normal β-cells into the diabetic rat will lead to reversal of mesangial lesions [3,81]. The same team of investigators demonstrated that kidneys from nondiabetic human donors develop typical lesions of diabetic renal disease when they are transplanted into the diabetic [82,83]. The clinical observation that development of diabetic renal disease is strongly related to the duration of diabetes further supports the notion that the glomerulopathy is in some way related to the metabolic perturbation [85–88].

Obviously, the most compelling evidence would be studies demonstrating that control of blood sugar leads to reduced incidence of diabetic nephropathy in patients. As described below, studies which are completely scientifically satisfactory are lacking. However, the balance of information from a number of studies suggests that a correlation does exist between the degree of diabetic control and the development of late complications [74]. The strict control of blood glucose unequivocally reduces the development of diabetic renal disease in animals as manifested by prevention of both structural changes and albuminuria [88–90].

In summary, the presently available evidence compellingly argues that the diabetic's altered internal environment causes the renal disease, and strongly suggests that restoration of normal carbohydrate metabolism would prevent the appearance of diabetic renal disease. However, the particular feature of the diabetic environment which instigates glomerular injury is unknown. Moreover, other genetic and environmental factors likely influence the course of the disease and enhance or diminish risk.

Nonenzymatic glycosylation

Glucose reacts with a variety of circulating and structural proteins and the extent of this reaction is proportional to the level of blood sugar [91–93]. The best studied of these reactions is that with the amino terminal of the β-chain of hemoglobin, which occurs as a Schiff base reaction with an Amadori rearrangement to yield the glycosylated hemoglobin, HgbA1C [91]. The level of this minor hemoglobin component is proportional to the time-averaged glucose level in diabetic patients. Since this nonenzymatic glycosycated proceeds at varying rates with essentially all proteins, the glomerular basement membrane and in all likelihood, matrix components, are subjected to glycosylation [94]. In turn, the glycosycated products can undergo a complex set of chemical rearrangements to form advanced glycosycation end-product. These products constitute a variety of irreversible protein–sugar compounds [95]. Since the advanced products are irreversible, they tend to accumulate on protein, forming cross-links between tissue proteins.

Several consequences of glycosylation and its advanced products might provide a basis for further injury to the diabetic glomerulus. First, the binding of the circulating plasma proteins to glomerular basement membrane and matrix material may be enhanced by the presence of the reactive carbonyl group on the glucose attached to structural components of the diabetic glomerulus [96]. Indeed, it is more likely on this or some other nonimmune basis that circulating proteins are deposited within the glomerulus. The possibility of insulin or insulin–antibody deposition has been dispatched by the work of Westberg & Michael [21]. Of perhaps even greater significance, the advance glycosycation end-product of collagen bind greater amounts of circulating proteins such as albumin, IgG, and low-density lipoproteins [95]. This binding could clearly account for the nonspecific immunofluorescence for albumin and immunoglobulin described by Michael & Westberg [21] and Michael & Miller [22]. The long-term consequences of the accumulation of circulating proteins are unknown; however, their continued accumulation may be, in part, responsible for the expansion of both the diabetic glomerular basement membrane and the mesangial matrix. Furthermore, the binding of these proteins at these two sites of extravascular ground substance might reduce the normal mesangial mechanisms for clearing extravasated plasma protein. While more direct in vitro evidence of these mechanisms is lacking, Jeraj et al. [97] and McVerry et al. [98] produced glomerular basement membrane thickening following chronic intravenous injections of glycosylated plasma proteins in the mouse, a finding not confirmed by another study. Thus, the pathophysiologic role of glycosylation and its advanced products on glomerular protein accumulation is unsettled, but appears likely to be a contributor to this phenomenon.

Secondly, Cerami *et al.* [99] have demonstrated that in the crystalline lens of the eye, glycosylation leads to an increased oxidation of sulfhydryl groups and an increase in the degree of disulfide bridge cross-linking between the collagen components of the lens, an effect also achieved through the linking of advanced glycosycation products. Although the precise biochemical mechanism whereby glycosylation allows for this oxidative reaction is unknown, it may be related to exposure of sulfhydryl groups consequent to a molecular rearrangement occasioned by the glycosylation. A similar cross-linking by disulfide bonds might occur in glycosylated renal basement membranes or mesangial matrix. The physiologic and pathologic consequences of any such enhanced cross-linking are unknown.

Thirdly, the degradation of both trapped circulating proteins and the structural proteins native to the glomerulus may be diminished after glycosylation, since the nonenzymatic glycosylation of fibrin reduces its susceptibility to proteolytic degradation by plasmin [100]. Should this resistance to catabolism apply to glycosylated glomerular components, the observed accumulation of the mesangial matrix or glomerular basement membrane could result.

Lastly, the glycosylation of either circulating proteins or glomerular constituents might directly influence the filtration of proteins. Glycosylated proteins generally have increased anionic charge because the glucose has reacted with amino groups. This effect should enhance the repulsive charge interactions responsible for normal glomerular charge selectivity; however, increased urinary excretion of glycated albumin, increased glomerular filtration of glycosycated ferritin, and increase permanence of glycated albumin through normal basement membrane *in vitro* have all been reported [101–103]. Although simple charge effects are unlikely to account for the apparently increased permeation of glycated protein, glycosycation of albumin does alter its ligand binding properties and its conformation. Perhaps the conformational changes alter its shape or its presentation of charge sufficiently to enhance its transglomerular passage [104].

Other biochemical abnormalities of the glomerulus
Several changes in composition of diabetic basement membrane have been described, in addition to glycosylation. Since many of these findings are controversial and inconsistently found by various investigators, no general consensus exists for specific compositional changes in the diabetic glomerular basement membrane other than glycosylation. Normally, the glomerular basement membrane is composed of a collagen-like glycoprotein, which is similar in its amino acid constituents to the Clq component of complement [93,105]. The carbohydrate components of normal glomerular basement membrane are of two types. First, a disaccharide composed of glucose and galactose is attached to hydroxylsine residues along the protein. The second carbohydrate component is a complex heteropolysaccharide containing a number of carbohydrate moieties including sialic acid. These heteropolysaccharide units are present in only about one-tenth the number of the disaccharide units, but because of their greater size they have an approximately equivalent weight representation. Beisswenger & Spiro [106] described an increase in the hydroxylysine component of the glomerular basement membrane obtained from patients with long-standing diabetes [106]. The glucose and galactose disaccharides normally attaching to hydroxylysines were also elevated in this material. The mechanism for the augmentation of the disaccharide component may be found in studies of diabetic rats which demonstrated elevated activity in the renal cortex of the enzyme normally responsible for the attachment of glucose to the glycoprotein glucosyltransferase [67,107]. This finding suggested that some component of the diabetic milieu, perhaps elevated glucose levels *per se*, leads to the increased enzymatic activity and thereby accentuates the addition of disaccharide units. However, differences in content of hydroxylysine and the disaccharide subunits have not been confirmed by other studies [58,59]. Furthermore, studies of long-standing diabetes in rats also failed to demonstrate the same increments in hydroxylysine or its attached carbohydrate components [108]. Likewise, the augmentation of glucosyltransferase activity has been inconsistently detected [109]. Hence, the constancy of the abnormality in disaccharide units in diabetic glomerular basement membrane remains controversial. Moreover, the physiologic or pathologic consequences which might accrue are speculative.

A more consistent finding in studies of both humans and experimental animals with diabetes has been the reduction in sialic acid components [58,60]. A similar deficiency has been noted on the surface of diabetic erythrocytes and hepatocytes [110]. Sialic acid is believed to contribute a considerable portion of the negative charge of the glomerular capillary wall and thereby contribute to the charge selectivity for macromolecules [111,112]. Thus, a reduction in this component of the heteropolysaccharide subunit of the glomerular basement membrane might lead to increased permeability of the glomerular capillary wall to circulating anionic proteins such as albumin. The reason for the reduction in sialic acid content is unknown, but this finding suggests an intriguing link to the clinical appearance of proteinuria in long-standing diabetes.

Glomerular glycosaminoglycans are the extracellular heteropolysaccharide polymers previously termed mucopolysaccharides [113]. They subserve several functions including structural adhesion and integrity of tissues [113]. Also, their net anionic charge provides a portion of the fixed negative charge and resultant charge selectivity of the glomerular capillary [65]. This anionic charge is provided in a large part by the sulfate residues along the polymers. Cohen et al. [114] have demonstrated decreased sulfate incorporation into the glycosaminoglycan components of the glomerular basement membrane in experimental diabetes [62]. In particular, heparan sulfate undergoes reduced sulfation in both the kidney and liver of diabetic experimental animals [115,116]. The finding of diminished heparan sulfate content, recently reported for glomerular basement membrane of diabetic humans, further explains the tendency to proteinuria in diabetes [62,114]. Also, derangement in the composition of these ground substances might reduce their efficacy as an adhesive material and allow size-selective defects to arise.

The excessive accumulation of both glomerular basement membrane and mesangial matrix are structural hallmarks of diabetic glomerulopathy. The various compositional changes discussed above could contribute to this accumulation. However, independent increases in rates of synthesis or reductions in degradation of biochemically normal material might also bear a responsibility for the excess extracellular protein present in the diabetic glomerulus. In vivo studies of glomerular basement membrane turnover employing injection of tritiated amino acids have indicated that the turnover rates are extremely slow in comparison to other glomerular proteins [117]. Brownlee & Spiro [118] have studied the incorporation of radio-labelled proline into glomerular basement membrane in diabetic and normal rats; in both groups of animals the incorporation was slow, and once incorporated, the radioactive label remained in the glomerular basement membrane for a protracted period of time [118]. However, the diabetic glomerular basement membrane attained specific activities of the labelled amino acids which were twice as high as those of the control animals. These findings suggest that diabetic animals have accelerated rates of glomerular basement membrane synthesis. Using other techniques other investigators have also concluded that matrix and glomerular basement membrane synthesis is augmented in diabetic animals. For example, Cortes et al. [119,120] have demonstrated that following induction of diabetes in rats the bioavailability of uridine diphosphosugars increases within the kidney, and these substances function as donors of carbohydrate groups in the production of glycoproteins and glycosaminoglycans. Consistent with the biochemical evidence, the volume of glomerular basement membrane located along the peripheral capillary loops increases by nearly 50% in the first 4 days of experimental diabetes as measured by electron microscopic morphometry [121]. Degradation rates of glomerular basement membrane and mesangial matrix are presently uncertain, and while suggestive evidence for reduced breakdown is available, the contribution of reduced catabolism to the accumulation of these glomerular components is not yet established [93].

Tissues harboring the enzyme aldose reductase produce increased amounts of sorbitol from glucose when the latter is elevated [121]. Several indirect consequences of this reaction may include depletion of myoinositol and diminution of sodium—potassium ATPase activity. Abrogation of these biochemical alterations by pharmacologic inhibition of the aldose reductase enzyme or dietary myoinositol supplementation have ameliorated several neural and ophthalmic complications in diabetic animals [121]. The renal implications of these findings are at present uncertain. Cohen et al. [122] have reported diminutions in glomerular sorbitol accumulation in diabetic rats after aldose reductase inhibition, as well as, effects on urinary protein of such treatment [123]. Goldfarb et al. [124] reported reductions in the elevated GFR of diabetic rats by both myoinositol supplementation and aldose reductase inhibition [124]. On the other hand, Daniels & Hostetter [125] found no effect of enzyme inhibition on GFR. Thus, more study is needed to determine both the physiologic and the long-term pathologic implications of glomerular sorbitol production in diabetes.

Hemodynamics

While marked increases in GFR and renal plasma flow occur in early IDDM such changes have not been formal in NIDDM. The easy hemodynamic changes in IDDM have been incriminated in the pathogenesis of the glomerular lesions [126,127]. In particular, an elevation in glomerular capillary pressure, associated with the increase in GFR and plasma flow, has been viewed as a critical hemodynamic derangement. Unfortunately, this parameter cannot be measured directly in humans and good animal models of NIDDM are lacking. However, a genetically obese strain of rats, the Zucker rat, displays some features of NIDDM including obesity and insulin resistance but not overt hyperglycemia. Studies of this animal have failed to find notable changes in glomerular capillary hemodynamics [128]. The accelerated glomerular sclerosis exhibited by the rats may be attributable in part to hyperlipidemia [129]. Thus, lacking an overtly hyperglycemic model of NIDDM, firm conclusions for or against a prima hemodynamic cause of in the glomerulopathy of NIDDM are not possible. The clinical finding that proteinuria fell in NIDDM nephropathy with arterial pressure reduction suggests that hemodynamic factors determine the course of the disease at least in its progressive phase.

In summary, the pathogenesis of the glomerular lesions of late diabetic nephropathy is incompletely understood. However, an alteration in the metabolic hormonal milieu seems to be a necessary factor and complete normalization of the metabolic disturbances of diabetes in experimental animals appears to vitiate completely this disease process, at least when applied early in the disease. The components of the diabetic environment which produce mesangial expansion and glomerular basement membrane thickening, the hallmarks of diabetic glomerulopathy, have not been organized into a definitive pathogenetic scheme. Nevertheless, several features appear to contribute and in all likelihood interact synergistically to initiate the process of diabetic nephropathy. After the initiation of the diabetic nephropathy by some such set of events, the progression to end-stage renal disease likely follows the path(s) common to many pro-

gressive renal diseases [130,131]. In recent years considerable attention has been focused on these "final common pathways" of progressive renal insufficiency.

Treatment

Role of glycemic control in the prevention and mitigation of diabetic renal disease

Strict control of blood glucose prevents the appearance of fine diabetic microangiopathy in experimental animals [88–90]. Unfortunately, scientifically compelling evidence of this effect in humans with IDDM is difficult to obtain from the available literature and even less clear in NIDDM [84,87,132,133]. Conclusive clinical evidence proving that euglycemia prevents diabetic renal microangiopathy is lacking. This deficit probably results from the fact that clinical evidence of diabetic nephropathy requires at least 10 years of diabetes before appearing. Euglycemic control is almost impossible for large numbers of subjects for long periods, and long periods of untreated hyperglycemia often precede the diagnosis of NIDDM. Hence, euglycemic control would need to be extended over a considerable period of time to determine its value, and in the case of NIDDM, irreversible changes may have occurred even before formal diagnosis of the diabetes. Furthermore, technologic advances enabling optimal control of diabetes have only begun to appear in recent years and are still cumbersome and occasionally dangerous. Hence, the techniques to achieve euglycemia over periods of 10–20 years have not been applied, and formal clinical testing of the hypothesis that normalization of carbohydrate metabolism would abrogate the appearance of diabetic nephropathy is still awaited.

A number of retrospective studies have, in the majority, reported that patients suffering the least diabetic complications including those of the kidney, fall into groups which have achieved the best control of blood sugar even with the available insulin regimens [84,85,87,133]. Many of these studies were reviewed by Knowles approximately 25 years ago, and while he could reach no definitive conclusion regarding the value of glucose control, the balance of data favored a positive correlation between the level of glucose and the incidence of complications including nephropathy [133]. For example, a large study of the Joslin Clinic patient population revealed that in patients with clinical diabetic nephropathy, only one had been classified as having the best category of diabetic control; there was a 10-fold greater incidence of diabetic nephropathy in patients classified as having fair to poor control as compared to those within the classifications of excellent or good control [134]. In more recent prospective studies, strict diabetic control correlated with lesser amounts of proteinuria and less frequent incidences of detectable proteinuria in patients with long-standing diabetes [70,85,135,136].

After the appearance of clinically detectable proteinuria, the ability to favorably influence the progression of diabetic nephropathy by institution of careful glucose control is more doubtful. Viberti *et al.* [137] studied six insulin-dependent diabetics who had persistent clinically detectable proteinuria for as long as 4 years and a demonstrable reduction in GFR [137]. The subjects were studied for 1–2 years prior to beginning continuous subcutaneous insulin infusion, which was then carried out for up to 24 more months. During the first phase of the study, prior to the initiation of optimal glycemic control, the rate of decline of GFR was monitored and fitted the expected linear pattern of decay. Despite prompt and significant improvement in plasma glucose concentration and hemoglobin A1C levels with continuous insulin infusion, GFR continued to decline at the same rate as it had obtained prior to the institution of the subcutaneous insulin infusion. A control group of six diabetics also with clinically detectable proteinuria was studied while being maintained on conventional insulin therapy and this group behaved similarly, showing the same linear decline in GFR as those patients receiving the stricter diabetic control. The authors suggested that by the time glomerular function had begun to fail and clinically persistent proteinuria was in evidence, metabolic control of diabetes influences that progression of renal disease little, if at all. A similar result has been obtained by Tamborlane *et al.* [138], who found no reduction in proteinuria in patients with established diabetic nephropathy after a prolonged period of euglycemia maintained by continuous insulin infusion [138]. On the other hand, glycemic control as measured by glycosylated hemoglobin levels correlated with rates of progression when patients with established nephropathy were observed for 21 months [139]. Another study could find no such relation at this stage [140].

The negative findings for intentional improvement in glucose control in established nephropathy are reminiscent of the experimental observation that mesangial expansion is ameliorated with the restoration of euglycemia by transplantation of pancreatic islet cells in diabetic animals with two kidneys, or by continuous insulin infusion, but islet transplantation does not achieve this result when the diabetic animals have sustained loss of renal mass by unilateral nephrectomy [141–143]. These clinical and experimental observations give credence to the notion that once a substantial, but as yet incompletely defined, degree of functioning renal mass has been lost, the role of hyperglycemia and other metabolic abnormalities in further reducing renal function may be rather modest and that other, probably self-perpetuating (adverse hemodynamic) processes lead to the progressive decline in renal function [130,131]. Recent studies of patients at earlier stages of diabetic nephropathy suggest that some benefit may derive from rigorous insulin therapy at least in patients in whom GFR is stable and dipstick positive proteinuria is absent. In one study, patients with microalbuminuria (30–300 mg/24 hours) were treated with either continuous subcutaneous insulin or conventional insulin therapy. After 2 years, the latter group had developed more cases of progressive proteinuria but had also tended to develop more hypertension. No clearly beneficial effect on the essentially normal baseline GFR values was detected [144]. A trend toward reduction of microalbuminuria was noted in a similar shorter term trial of 8 months [145]. However, in patients at the later stage of intermittently dipstick positive urine and decreasing GFR, intensified glycemic control by insulin infusion exerted no effect on the decline in renal function [146]. Thus, glycemic control in established nephropathy does not clearly influence the course of the process although the studies supporting this statement involve small numbers of patients. It should also be borne in mind that glycemic control might still limit nonrenal complications. With microalbuminuria, but before GFR declines, strict glycemic control may be beneficial. However, studies supporting this possibility involve relatively short follow-up.

Hypertension

After demonstrating that a short course of antihypertensive treatment reduced albuminuria in patients with established diabetic nephropathy, Mogensen proposed that antihypertensive treatment might slow the progression of renal disease in such patients [147]. He later demonstrated in six insulin-dependent diabetic patients with detectable proteinuria that antihypertensive treatment reduced the rate of decline in glomerular filtration [148]. This beneficial effect of aggressive antihypertensive treatment has been confirmed and extended by Parving et al. [149] who studied insulin-dependent diabetics with established nephropathy over an average of 6 years of antihypertensive therapy. With the institution of effective antihypertensive treatment, mean arterial pressure declined from approximately 120 mmHg to less than 100 mmHg and the rate of decline of GFR fell gradually from about 1 ml/min per month prior to treatment to 0.10 ml/min per month. Concomitantly, albumin excretion rates fell. This dramatic amelioration of the progression of renal disease was achieved with diuretics, β-blockers, and vasodilators, but the excellent control of pressure must be noted, and is likely responsible for the superb results. Recently, a calcium channel blocker and a converting enzyme inhibitor have been shown to reduce proteinuria with equal efficacy in patients with nephropathy due to NIDDM.

Given the striking effects of antihypertensive therapy in hypertensive patients with established nephropathy, and the possibility that elevated glomerular capillary pressure may precede arterial hypertension, interest has attached to the possibility of lowering arterial pressure even in "normotensive" diabetics. Studies of experimental diabetes in rats have demonstrated a reduction in glomerular injury when normotensive diabetic animals were treated with a converting enzyme inhibitor [150]. Clinical studies analogous to these are not yet available; however, Marre et al. [151] treated normotensive IDDM patients at the stage of microalbuminuria with a converting enzyme inhibitor or placebo. The antihypertensive agent led to lower albumin excretion over a period of 6 months suggesting benefit.

Antihypertensive therapy mitigates established renal disease but no controlled study is available to detemine whether antihypertensive treatment would prevent or forestall the progression of diabetic retinopathy [152]. However, suggestive data obtained in Pima Indians, who have predominantly NIDDM, indicate that retinal exudates are more prevalent with elevated levels of systolic blood pressures [153]. Retrospective studies of patients with Type NIDDM diabetes also bolster the probability that systemic hypertension worsens the degree of diabetic

retinal complications [85]. Clinical case reports of preserved retinal circulations on the side of a unilateral carotid artery stenosis, despite contralateral diabetic retinopathy disease above the patient carotid system, further support a role of hemodynamic factors in promoting diabetic retinopathy [154,155].

Antihypertensive therapy in diabetes is critical and requires some special considerations. Beta-blockers carry some excess risk in the patient with insulin-requiring diabetes, principally because of the tendency to mask several of the symptoms of hypoglycemic reactions. However, these medications can be used effectively in patients with diabetes and should problems with hypoglycemia arise, presently available home glucose monitoring may offer a means of avoiding dangerous levels of undetected hypoglycemia. Diuretics, especially the thiazides, may worsen glycemic control particularly for patients with NIDDM and for those patients careful monitoring of glucose is necessary after institution of antihypertensive therapy with these agents. Also, the potassium-sparing diuretics spironolactone and triamterene should be used with caution, if at all, in any patient with renal insufficiency, but because of the increased incidence of hyperkalemia due to "hyporeninemic hypoaldosteronism" and insulinopenia in diabetics, these drugs represent a particular disadvantage in this population [156]. For the same reasons, potassium levels must also be followed when converting enzyme inhibitors are employed in these patients, particularly when GFR is depressed. Underlying autonomic dysfunction with orthostatic hypotension must be considered when treating the patient with diabetes and hypertension, since disturbing and even dangerous differences in blood pressure may occur with sitting or standing particularly after the administration of such agents as methyldopa and prazosin. Impotence developing in male patients with long-standing diabetes may pose another problem in the use of those antihypertensives which can be independently associated with impotence.

Certain types of antihypertensive drugs may be particularly beneficial in treating diabetic nephropathy. Experimental studies of the subtotal nephrectomy model have demonstrated that converting enzyme inhibition much more effectively reduced glomerular pressure and injury than a combination of thiazide, hydralazine, and reserpine which lowered arterial but not glomerular pressure, equivalently [157]. Preliminary evidence suggests a similar though less striking differential effect in experimental diabetes [158]. Whether such specific benefits accrue to converting enzyme inhibitors or other specific classes in clinical diabetic nephropathy is untested. However, several studies suggest that conventional enzyme inhibitors are beneficial. For example, Bjorck *et al.* [159] reported a decline in the rate of decline in GFR when a converting enzyme inhibitor was used. The fact that arterial pressure was only mildly reduced by the drug led the authors to speculate that glomerular pressure was preferentially improved. On the other hand, Walker *et al.* [160] have reported that use of diuretics was associated with an accelerated progression of renal disease in hypertensive diabetics [160]. Since the study only discovered a correlation, further prospective trials will be needed to determine whether diuretics are directly detrimental. Direct clinical comparisons between agents will be required to determine whether specific regimens are particularly advantageous. However, for the present it should be noted that striking improvement in the course of the disease can be achieved with conventional medications [149]. Thus, patients with diabetic nephropathy raise special considerations in the use of antihypertensive medications. Nevertheless, the clear evidence that control of blood pressure in diabetic patients slows their deterioration into renal failure, warrants careful but persistent efforts to maintain blood pressure at normal levels. The exact optimal target blood pressure is not defined but a mean arterial pressure less than 100 mmHg should be sought.

Dietary protein restriction

Protein restriction retards the progression of many experimental renal diseases including diabetes, and in many uncontrolled studies similarly salutary results in patients with a variety of renal diseases have been observed [161]. Although little controlled clinical data obtained exists, the available information supports the efficacy of protein restriction [161]. Short-term protein restriction in both diabetic and nondiabetic chronic renal disease reduced proteinuria by improving glomerular permselectivity [162,163]. While such findings suggest a diminution in glomerular injury, long-term controlled trials of protein restriction in diabetic nephropathy are few. However, at least one study in IDDM patients described a slowing of the fall in GFR with protein restriction [164]. Further trials are required to establish conclusively the value of

this therapy in generic renal disease and its value in NIDDM in particular but restriction to as low as 0.6 g of high biological value protein per kg body weight per day seems to be generally safe and may profit the patient [161,162,165].

References

1 Teutsch S, Neuman J, Eggers P. The problem of diabetic renal failure in the United States. Am J Kidney Dis 1989; 13:11−13.

2 Nelson R, Newman J, Knowler W, *et al.* End-stage renal disease in non-insulin dependent diabetes mellitus. Diabetologia 1988;31:730−736.

3 Kimmelstiel P, Wilson C. Intercapillary lesions in glomeruli of kidney. Am J Pathol 1936;12:83.

4 Kamenetzky SA, Bennett PH, Dippe SE, *et al.* A clinical and histologic study of diabetic nephropathy in the Pima Indians. Diabetes 1974;37:405−412.

5 Schmitz A, Gundersen HJG, Osterby R. Glomerular morphology by light microscopy in noninsulin dependent diabetes mellitus. Lack of glomerular hypertrophy. Diabetes 1988;37:38.

6 Hostetter TH, Daniels BS. Natural history of renal structural abnormalities in diabetes mellitus. In Brenner BM, Stein JH, eds. *The Kidney in Diabetes Mellitus. Contemporary Issues in Nephrology.* New York: Churchill Livingstone, 1989:51−66.

7 Thomsen OF, Andersen AR, Sandahl Christiansen J, *et al.* Renal changes in long-term type I (insulin-dependent) diabetic patients with and without clinical nephropathy: a light microscopic, morphometric study of autopsy material. Diabetologia 1984;26:361.

8 Honey GE, Pryse-Davies J, Roberts DM. A survey of nephropathy in young diabetics. Q J Med, New Series 31, 1962.

9 Seymour AE, Spargo BH, Penksa R. Contributions of renal biopsy studies to the understanding of disease. Am J Pathol 1971;65:550.

10 Smithline N, Kassirer JP, Cohen JJ. Light chain nephropathy. N Engl J Med 1976;294:71.

11 Bell ET. Renal vascular disease in diabetes mellitus. Diabetes 1953;2:376.

12 Gellman DD, Pirani CI, Soothill JE, *et al.* Diabetic nephropathy: A clinical and pathologic study based on renal biopsies. Medicine 1959;38:321.

13 Hatch FE, Watt MF, Kramer NC, *et al.* Diabetic glomerulosclerosis: a long-term follow-up study based on renal biopsies. Am J Med 1961;31:216.

14 Mauer SM, Steffes MW, Brown DM. The kidney in diabetes. Am J Med 1981;70:603.

15 Muirhead EE, Montgomery PO, Booth E. The glomerular lesions of diabetes mellitus: Cellular hyaline and acellular

hyaline lesions of "intercapillary glomerulosclerosis" as depicted by histochemical studies. Arch Intern Med 1956;98:146.

16 Bloodworth JH Jr, Hamwi GJ. Experimental diabetic glomerulosclerosis. Diabetes 1956;5:37.

17 Laufer A, Stein O. The exudative lesion in diabetic glomerulosclerosis. Am J Clin Pathol 1959;32:56.

18 Wilson JL, Root HF, Marble A. Diabetic nephropathy a clinical syndrome. N Engl J Med 1951;245:513.

19 Bader R, Bader H, Grund KE, et al. Structure and function of the kidney in diabetic glomerulosclerosis: correlations between morphologic and functional parameters. Path Res Pract 1980;167−204.

20 Jarrett RJ, Keen H, Chakrabarti R. Diabetes, hyperglycemia, and arterial disease. In Keen H, Harrett J, eds. Complications of Diabetes, 2nd edn. London: Edward Arnold, 1982:179.

21 Westberg NG, Michael AF. Immunohistopathology of diabetic glomerulosclerosis. Diabetes 1972;21:163.

22 Michael AF, Miller K. Immunopathology of renal extracellular membranes in diabetes mellitus: Specificity of tubular basement-membrane immunofluorescent. Diabetes 1976;25:701.

23 Falk RJ, Dalmasso AP, Kim Y, et al. Neoantigen of the polymerized ninth component of complement. J Clin Invest 1983;72:560.

24 Heptinstall RH. Diabetes mellitus and gout. In Pathology of the Kidney, 3rd edn. Boston: Little Brown & Co., 1983:1397.

25 Scheinman JI, Steffes MW, Brown DM, et al. The immunohistopathology of glomerular antigens; increased mesangial actomyosin in experimental diabetes in the rat. Diabetes 1978;27:632.

26 Falk RJ, Scheinman JI, Mauer SM, et al. Polyantigenic expansion of basement membrane constituents in diabetic nephropathy. Diabetes 1983;32:34.

27 Osterby R. Early phases in the development of diabetic glomerulopathy. Acta Med Scand 1975;574(Suppl.):1.

28 Kimmelstiel P, Osawa G, Beres J. Glomerular basement membrane in diabetics. Am J Clin Pathol 1966;45:21.

29 Dachs S, Churg J, Mautner W, et al. Diabetic nephropathy. Am J Pathol 1964;44:155.

30 Cohen A, Mampaso F, Zamboni L. Glomerular podocyte degeneration in human renal disease. An ultrastructural study. Lab Invest 1977;37:40.

31 Marks HH. Longevity and mortality of diabetes. Am J Public Health 1965;55:416−428.

32 Rettig B, Teutsch SM. The incidence of end-stage renal disease in Type I and Type II diabetes mellitus. Diabetic Nephropathy 1984;3:26−27.

33 Pell S, D'Alonzo CA. Some aspects of hypertension in diabetes mellitus. J Am Med Assoc 1967;202:10−16.

34 Hostetter TH. Diabetic nephropathy. In Brenner B, Rector F, eds. The Kidney, 3rd edn. Philadelphia: WB Saunders Co., 1986.

35 Modan M, Halkin H, Almog S, et al. Hyperinsulinemia.

J Clin Invest 1985;75:809−817.

36 O'Hare JA. The enigma of insulin resistance and hypertension. Am J Med 1988;84:505−510.

37 Reaven GM. Role of insulin resistance in human disease. Diabetes 1988;37:1595−1607.

38 Kamenetzky SA, Bennett PH, Dippe SE, et al. A clinical and histologic study of diabetic nephropathy in the Pima Indians. Diabetes 1974;23:61−68.

39 Ballard DJ, Humphrey LL, Melton LJ III, et al. Epidemiology of persistent proteinuria in type II diabetes mellitus. Diabetes 1988;37:405−412.

40 Mogensen CE, Gjode P, Christensen CK. Albumin excretion in operating surgeons and in hypertension. Lancet 1979;i:774.

41 Parving H-H, Gall M-A, Scott P, et al. Prevalence and causes of albuminuria in noninsulin diabetic patients. Am Soc Nephrol 1989, 22nd meeting, SSA.

42 Kunzelman CI, Knowler WC, Pettitt DJ, et al. Incidence of proteinuria in Type 2 diabetes mellitus in the Pima Indians. Kidney Int 1989;35:681−687.

43 Krolewski AS, Warram JH, Christlieb AR, et al. The changing natural history of nephropathy in Type I diabetes. Am J Med 1985;78:785−794.

44 Andersen AR, Christiansen JS, Andersen JH, et al. Diabetic nephropathy in Type I (insulin-dependent) diabetes: An epidemiological study. Diabetologia 1983;25:496−501.

45 Mogensen CE. Microalbuminuria predicts clinical proteinuria and early mortality in maturity onset diabetes. N Engl J Med 1984;310:356−360.

46 Winetz JA, Golbetz HV, Spencer RJ, et al. Glomerular function in advanced human diabetic nephropathy. Kidney Int 1982;21:750.

47 Gundersen HJG, Osterby R. Glomerular size and structure in diabetes mellitus. II. Late abnormalities. Diabetologia 1977;13:43.

48 Allison MEM, Wilson CB, Gottschalk CW. Pathophysiology of experimental glomerulonephritis in rats. J Clin Invest 1974;53:1402.

49 Bank H, Aynedjian HS. Individual function in experimental pyelonephritis. I. Glomerular filtration rate and proximal tubular sodium, potassium and water reabsorption. J Lab Clin Med 1966;68:713.

50 Ichikawa I, Hoyer JR, Seiler MW, et al. Mechanism of glomerulotubular balance in the setting of heterogeneous glomerular injury. J Clin Invest 1982;69:185.

51 Hostetter TH, Olson JL, Rennke HD, et al. Hyperfiltration in remnant nephrons: a potentially adverse response to renal ablation. Am J Physiol 1981;241:F85.

52 Hostetter TH, Meyer TW, Rennke HG, et al. Influence of strict control of diabetes on intrarenal hemodynamics. Kidney Int 1983;23:215.

53 Loon N, Nelson R, Myers BD. Glomerular barrier abnormality in new onset NIDDM in Pima Indians. Am Soc Nephrol 1989; 22nd Meeting: 325A.

54 Myers BD, Winetz JA, Chui F, *et al.* Mechanisms of proteinuria in diabetic nephropathy: A study of glomerular barrier function. Kidney Int 1982;21:633.

55 Deen WM, Bridges CR, Brenner BM, *et al.* Hetero-porous model of glomerular size-selectivity: application to normal and nephrotic humans. Am J Physiol 1985; 249: F374.

56 Stalder G, Schmid R. Severe functional disorders of glomerular capillaries and renal hemodynamics in treated diabetes mellitus during childhood. Ann Pediatr 1959;193:129.

57 Osterby-Hansen R. The basement membrane morphology in diabetes mellitus. In Ellenberg M, Rifkin J, eds. *Diabetes Mellitus: Theory and Practice.* New York: McGraw-Hill, 1970:178.

58 Westberg MG, Michael AF. Human glomerular basement membrane: Chemical composition in diabetes mellitus. Acta Med Scand 1973;194:39.

59 Kefalides NA. Biochemical properties of human glomerular basement membrane in normal and diabetic kidneys. J Clin Invest 1974;53:403.

60 Cruz A, Moreau-Lalande H. Biochemical studies on glomerular basement membrane in human diabetic microangiopathy. Pathol Biol 1978;26:411.

61 Wahl P, Deppermann D, Hasslacher C. Biochemistry of glomerular basement membrane of the normal and diabetic human. Kidney Int 1982;21:744.

62 Cohen MP, Surma ML. Sulfate incorporation into glomerular basement membrane is decreased in experimental diabetes. J Lab Clin Med 1981;78:715.

63 Parthasarathy N, Spiro RG. Effect of diabetes on the glycosaminoglycan component of the human glomerular basement membrane. Diabetes 1982;31:738.

64 Raz I, Havivi Y, Yarom R. Reduced negative surface charge on arterial endothelium of diabetic rats. Diabetologic 1988; 31:618.

65 Farquhar MG. The glomerular basement membrane: A selective macromolecular filter. In Hay ED, ed. *Cell Biology of the Extra-cellular Matrix.* New York: Plenum Press, 1982:335.

66 Michels LD, Davidman M, Keane WF. Glomerular permeability to neutral and anionic dextrans in experimental diabetes. Kidney Int 1982;21:669-705.

67 Mogensen CE. Microalbuminuria as a predictor of clinical diabetic nephropathy. Kidney Int 1987;31:673-689.

68 Hostetter TH, Troy JL, Brenner BM. Glomerular hemodynamics in experimental diabetes mellitus. Kidney Int 1981;19:410-415.

69 McMillan DE. The microcirculation: Changes in diabetes mellitus. Mayo Clin Proc 1988;63:517-520.

70 Winegrad AI. Does a common mechanism induce the diverse complications of diabetes? Diabetes 1987;36: 396-406.

71 Williamson JR, Kilo C. Current status of capillary basement membrane disease in diabetes mellitus. Diabetes 1977;26: 65-73.

72 Hostetter TH. Diabetic nephropathy. New Engl J Med 1985; 312:642-644.

73 Steffes MW, Mauer SM. Diabetic glomerulopathy in man and experimental animal models. Int Rev Exp Pathol 1984; 26:147-175.

74 Mangili R, Bending JJ, Scott G, *et al.* Increased sodium-lithium countertransport activity in red cells of patients with insulin-dependent diabetes and nephropathy. New Engl J Med 1988;318:146-150.

75 Krolewski AS, Canessa M, Warram JH, *et al.* Predisposition to hypertension and susceptibility to renal disease in insulin-dependent diabetes mellitus. New Engl J Med 1988; 318:140-145.

76 Seaquist ER, Goetz FC, Rich S, *et al.* Familial clustering of diabetic kidney disease, evidence of genetic susceptibility to diabetic nephropathy. New Engl J Med 1989;320: 1161-1166.

77 Reddi AS, Camerini-Davalos RA. Diabetic nephropathy. An update. Arch Intern Med 1990;150:31-43.

78 Weller JM, Wu SH, Ferguson W. *et al.* End-stage renal disease in Michigan. Am J Nephrol 1985;5:84-95.

79 Cowie CC, Port FK, Wolfe RA, *et al.* Disparities in incidence of diabetic end-stage renal disease according to race and type of diabetes. New Engl J Med 1989;321:1074-1079.

80 Easterling RE. Racial factors in the incidence and causation of end-stage renal disease (ESRD). Trans Am Soc Artif Intern Organs 1977;23:28-33.

81 Mauer SM, Steffes MW, Brown DM, *et al.* Amelioration of mesangial volume and surface alterations following islet transplantation in diabetic rats. Diabetes 1980; 29:509.

82 Mauer SM, Barbosa J, Vernier RL, *et al.* Development of diabetic vascular lesions in normal kidneys transplanted into patients with diabetes mellitus. N Engl J Med 1976; 295:916.

83 Mauer SM, Steffes MW, Connett J, *et al.* The development of lesions in the glomerular basement membrane and mesangium after transplantation of normal kidneys to diabetic patients. Diabetes 1983;32:948.

84 Raskin P, Rosenstock J. Blood glucose control and diabetic complications. Ann Intern Med 1986;105:254.

85 Krolewski AS, Warram JH, Rand LI, *et al.* Epidemiologic approach to the etiology of Type I diabetes mellitus and its complications. N Engl J Med 1987;317:1390.

86 Pirart J. Diabetes mellitus and its degenerative complications: a prospective study of 4400 patients observed between 1947 and 1973. Diabetes Care 1978;1:168-252.

87 Brownlee M, Cahill GF Jr. Diabetic control and vascular complications. Atherosclerosis Rev 1979;4:29.

88 Mauer SM, Steffes MW, Sutherland DER, *et al.* Studies of the rate of regression of the glomerular lesions in diabetic rats treated with pancreatic islet transplantation. Diabetes 1974;24:280.

89 Rasch R. Prevention of diabetic glomerulopathy in strepto-

zotocin diabetic rats. Diabetologia 1979;16:319.

90 Rasch R. Prevention of diabetic glomerulopathy in streptozotocin diabetic rats. Diabetologia 1980;18:413.

91 Bunn HF, Gabbay KH, Gallop PM. The glycosylation of hemoglobin: relevance to diabetes mellitus. Science 1978; 200:21.

92 Miller JA, Gravallese E, Bunn HF. Nonenzymatic glycosylation of erythrocyte membrane proteins. J Clin Invest 1980;65:896.

93 Brownlee M, Cerami A. The biochemistry of the complications of diabetes mellitus. Ann Rev Biochem 1981;50:385.

94 Schober E, Pollak A, Coradello, et al. Glycosylation of glomerular basement membrane in Type I (insulin-dependent) diabetic children. Diabetologia 1982;23:485.

95 Brownlee M, Cerami A, Vlassara H. Advanced glycosylation end products in tissue and the biochemical basis of diabetic complications. N Engl J Med 1988;318:1315.

96 Brownlee M, Pongor S, Cerami A. Covalent attachment of soluble proteins by nonenzymatically glycosylated collagen. J Exp Med 1983;158:1739.

97 Jeraj KP, Michael AF, Mauer SM, et al. Glucosylated and normal human or rat albumin do not bind to renal basement membranes of diabetic and control rats. Diabetes 1983;32:380.

98 McVerry BA, Hopp A, Fischer C, et al. Production of pseudodiabetic renal glomerular changes in mice after repeated injections of glucosylated proteins. Lancet 1980; 1:738.

99 Cerami A, Stevens VJ, Rouzer CA, et al. Diabetic cataract formation: potential role of glycosylation of lens crystallins. Proc Natl Acad Sci USA 1978;75:2918.

100 Brownlee M, Vlassara H, Cerami A. Nonenzymatic glycosylation reduces the susceptibility of fibrin to degradation by plasmin. Diabetes 1983;32:680.

101 Ghiggeri GM, Candiano G, Delfino G, et al. Electrical charge of serum and urinary albumin in normal and diabetic humans. Kidney Int 1985;28:168.

102 Williams SK, Siegal RK. Preferential transport of nonenzymatically glucosylated ferritin across the kidney glomerulus. Kidney Int 1985;28:146.

103 Hauser E, Hostetter TH, Daniels BS. Nonenzymatic glycation of albumin enhances its permeability through glomerular basement membrane. Am Soc Nephrol 1989; 22nd Meeting; 319A.

104 Shaklai N, Garlick RL, Bunn HF. Nonenzymatic glycosylation of human serum albumin alters its conformation and function. J Biol Chem 1984;259:3812.

105 Spiro RG. Search for a biochemical basis of diabetic microangiopathy. Diabetologia 1976;12:1.

106 Beisswenger PJ, Spiro RG. Studies on the human glomerular basement membrane. Composition, nature of the carbohydrate units and chemical changes in diabetes mellitus. Diabetes 1972;22:180.

107 Spiro RG, Spiro MJ. Effect of diabetes on the biosynthesis of the renal glomerular basement membrane. Studies on the glucosyltransferase. Diabetes 1971;20:164.

108 Beisswenger P. Glomerular basement membrane. Biosynthesis and chemical composition in the streptozotocin diabetic rat. J Clin Invest 1976;58:844.

109 Risteli J, Koivisto VA, Akerblom HK, et al. Intracellular enzymes of collagen biosynthesis in rat kidney in streptozotocin diabetes. Diabetes 1976;25:1066.

110 Chandramouli V, Carter JR. Cell membrane changes in chronically diabetic rats. Diabetes 1975;24:257.

111 Brenner BM, Hostetter TH, Humes HD. Molecular basis of proteinuria of glomerular origin. N Engl J Med 1978; 298:826.

112 Mohos SC, Skoza L. Glomerular sialoprotein. Science 1969; 164:1519.

113 Alberts B, Bray D, Lewis J, et al. Cell–cell adhesion and the extracellular matrix. In Molecular Biology of the Cell. New York: Garland Publishing, 1983:674.

114 Cohen MP, Wu VY, Wilson B. Disturbances in glomerular basement membrane glycosaminoglycans in experimental diabetes. Diabetes 1987;36:679.

115 Rohrbach DH, Hassell HR, Kleinman HK, et al. Alterations in the basement membrane (heparan sulfate) proteoglycan in diabetic mice. Diabetes 1982;31:185.

116 Kjellen L, Bielefeld D, Hook M. Reduced sulfation of liver heparan sulfate in experimentally diabetic rats. Diabetes 1983;32:337.

117 Price RG, Spiro RG. Studies on the metabolism of the renal glomerular basement membrane. Turnover measurements in the rat with the use of radiolabeled amino acids. J Biol Chem 1977;252:8597.

118 Brownlee M, Spiro RG. Glomerular basement membrane metabolism in the diabetic rat. Diabetes 1979;28:121.

119 Cortes P, Dumler F, Sury Sastry KS, et al. Effects of early diabetes on uridine diphosphosugar synthesis in the rat renal cortex. Kidney Int 1982;21:676.

120 Cortes P, Dumler F, Paielli DL, et al. Glomerular uracil nucleotide synthesis: effects of diabetes and protein intake. Am J Physiol 1988;255:F647.

121 Greene DA, Lattimer SA, Sima AF. Sorbitol, phosphoinositides, and sodium-potassium-ATPase in the pathogenesis of diabetic complications. N Engl J Med 1987; 316:599.

122 Cohen MP, Beyer-Mears A, Ku L. Glomerular polyol accumulation in diabetes and its prevention by oral sorbinil. Diabetes 1984;33:604.

123 Beyer-Mears A. The polyol pathway, sorbinil, and renal dysfunction. Metabolism 1986;35(Suppl. 1):46.

124 Goldfarb S, Simmons A, Kern GFO. Amelioration of glomerular hyperfiltration in acute experimental diabetes mellitus by dietary myoinositol supplementation and aldose reductase inhibition. Trans Assoc Am Physicians 1986; 99:67.

125 Daniels BS, Hostetter TH. Aldose reductase inhibition does

not ameliorate glomerular abnormalities in diabetic rats. Clin Res 1988;36:A594.

126 Hostetter TH, Rennke HG, Brenner BM. The case for intra-renal hypertension in the initiation and progression of diabetic and other glomerulopathies. Am J Med 1982; 72:375.

127 Zatz R, Brenner BM. Pathogenesis of diabetic microangiopathy. Am J Med 1986;80:443.

128 Kasiske BL, Cleary MP, O'Donell MP, et al. Effects of genetic obesity on renal structure and function in the Zucker rat I and II. J Lab Clin Med 1985;106:598−610.

129 Kasiske BL, O'Donell MP, Cleary MP, et al. Effects of reduced renal mass on tissue lipids and renal injury in hyperlipidemic rats. Kidney Int 1989;35:40−47.

130 Brenner BM, Meyer TW, Hostetter TH. Dietary protein intake and the progressive nature of kidney disease: the role of hemodynamically mediated glomerular injury in the pathogenesis of progressive glomerular sclerosis in aging, renal ablation, and intrinsic renal disease. N Engl J Med 1982;307:652.

131 Klahr S, Schreiner G, Ichikawa I. The progression of renal disease. N Engl J Med 1988;318:1657.

132 Raskin P. Diabetic regulation and its relationship to micro-angiopathy. Metabolism 1978;27:235.

133 Knowles HC. The problem of the relation of the control of diabetes to the development of vascular disease. Trans Am Clin Climatol Assoc 1964;76:142.

134 Keiding NR, Root HD, Marble A. Importance of control of diabetes in prevention of vascular complications. J Am Med Assoc 1952;150:964.

135 Tshobroutsky G. Relation of diabetes control to development of microvascular complications. Diabetologia 1978; 15:143.

136 Takazakura E, Nakamoto Y, Hayakawa H. Onset and progression of diabetic glomerulopathy. Diabetes 1975;24:1.

137 Viberti GC, Bilous RW, Mackintoch D, et al. Long-term correction of hyperglycaemia and progression of renal failure in insulin dependent diabetes. Br Med J 1983;286:598.

138 Tamborlane WV, Puklin JE, Bergman M, et al. Long-term improvement of metabolic control with the insulin pump does not reverse diabetic microangiopathy. Diabetes Care 1982;5:58.

139 Nyberg G, Blohme G, Norden G. Impact of metabolic control in progression of clinical diabetic nephropathy. Diabetologia 1987;30:82.

140 Hasslacher C, Stech W, Wahl P, et al. Blood pressure and metabolic control as risk factors for nephropathy in Type I diabetes. Diabetologia 1985;28:6.

141 Mauer SM. Diabetic glomerulopathy in the urinephrectomized rat resists amelioration following islet transplantation. Diabetologia 1982;23:347.

142 Petersen J, Ross J, Rabkin R. Effect of insulin therapy on established diabetic nephropathy in rats. Diabetes 1988; 37:1346.

143 Orloff MJ, Yamanaka N, Greenlead GE, et al. Reversal of mesangial enlargement in rats with long-standing diabetes by whole pancreas transplantation. Diabetes 1986; 35:347.

144 Feldt-Rasmussen B, Mathiesen ER, Deckert T. Effect of two years of strict metabolic control. Progression of incipient nephropathy in IDDM. Lancet 1986;2:1300.

145 The Kroc Collaborative Study Group. Blood glucose control and the evolution of diabetic retinopathy and albuminuria. N Engl J Med 1984;311:365.

146 Bending JJ, Viberti GC, Watkins PJ, et al. Intermittent clinical proteinuria and renal function in diabetes: evaluation and the effect of glycaemic control. Br Med J 1986; 292:83.

147 Mogensen CE. Progression of nephropathy in long-term diabetes with proteinuria and effect of initial antihypertensive treatment. Scand J Clin Invest 1976;36:383.

148 Mogensen CE. Long-term antihypertensive treatment inhibiting progression of diabetic nephropathy. Br Med J 1982; 285:685.

149 Parving H-H, Andersen AR, Smidt UM, et al. Effect of antihypertensive treatment on kidney function in diabetic nephropathy. Br Med J 1987;294:1443.

150 Zatz R, Rentz Dunn B, Meyer TW, et al. Prevention of diabetic glomerulopathy by pharmacological amelioration of glomerular capillary hypertension. J Clin Invest 1986; 77:1925.

151 Marre M, Leblanc H, Suarez L, et al. Converting enzyme inhibition and kidney function in normotensive diabetic patients with persistent microalbuminuria. Br Med J 1987; 294:1448.

152 Drury PL. Diabetes and arterial hypertension. Diabetologia 1983;24:1.

153 Knowles WC, Bennett PH, Ballintin EJ. Increased incidence of retinopathy in diabetics with elevated blood pressure. N Engl J Med 1980;302:645.

154 Yoshida A, Feke GT, Morales-Stoppello J, et al. Retinal blood flow determinations during progression of diabetic retinopathy. Arch Ophthalmol 1983;101:225.

155 Gay AM, Rosenbaum AL. Retinal artery pressure in asymmetric diabetic retinopathy. Arch Ophthalmol 1966;75:758.

156 DeFronzo RA. Hyperkalemia and hyporeninemic hypoaldosteronism. Kidney Int 1980;17:118.

157 Anderson S, Rennke HG, Brenner BM. Therapeutic advantage of converting enzyme inhibitors in arresting progressive renal disease associated with systemic hypertension in the rat. J Clin Invest 1986;77:1993.

158 Anderson S, Riley SL, Rennke HG, et al. Superiority of captopril over combination triple therapy in arresting diabetic glomerulopathy in the rat. Kidney Int 1989;35:422.

159 Bjorck S, Nyberg G, Mulec H, et al. Beneficial effects of angiotensin-converting enzyme inhibition on renal function in patients with diabetic nephropathy. Br Med J 1986; 293:471.

160 Walker WG, Herman J, Yin DP, *et al.* Diuretics accelerate diabetic nephropathy in hypertensive insulin dependent and noninsulin dependent subjects. Trans Assoc Am Physicians 1987;100:305.

161 Hostetter TH. Dietary protein restriction in control of progressive renal failure. In Davison AM, ed. *Nephrology.* Philadelphia: Balliere Tindall, 1988:1196.

162 Rosenberg ME, Swanson JE, Thomas BL, *et al.* Glomerular and hormonal responses to dietary protein intake in human renal disease. Am J Physiol 1987;253:F1083.

163 Bending JJ, Dodds RA, Keen H, *et al.* Renal response to restricted protein intake in diabetic nephropathy. Diabetes 1988;37:1641.

164 Evanoff G, Thompson C, Brown J, *et al.* Prolonged dietary protein restriction in diabetic nephropathy. Arch Intern Med 1989;149:1129–1133.

165 Levine SE, D'Elia JA, Bistrian B, *et al.* Protein-restricted diets in diabetic nephropathy. Nephron 1989;52:55–61.

18

Cholesterol embolization

William J. Stone
Agnes Fogo

Introduction

Much like a nation in the atomic age, the atherosclerotic aorta lies ready to launch missiles when foreign intruders disturb its quiescence. Tragically, the intruders (surgeons and vascular catheters) mean well, but the ensuing conflagration is self-destructive.

Advances in vascular surgery and interventional radiology have greatly increased the incidence of cholesterol embolization (CE) and reacquainted us with its many clinical presentations. Clinicians are often misled by the varied signs and symptoms of CE so that alternative diagnoses are erroneously made, and inappropriate treatment plans are instituted. The syndrome also eludes detection by conventional roentgenography, computed tomography, magnetic resonance imaging, ultrasound, radionuclide scans, and an array of blood tests. A simple biopsy of involved tissue is diagnostic. However, even well-trained pathologists may overlook subtle cholesterol emboli and be fooled by mistaking the characteristic clefts, left by cholesterol crystals washed out during tissue fixation, for vascular lumina. Although there is no current treatment of CE beyond supportive care and therapy of organ failure (dialysis, infarcted bowel resection, amputation, etc.), it is important to recognize the syndrome and to prevent its recurrence. Furthermore, clinicians must realize that arteriograms and other procedures utilizing intraaortic catheters are potentially hazardous to patients with atherosclerosis. Therefore these tests must have a high therapeutic yield in the individual situation or they should not be scheduled.

We wish to illustrate the many faces of CE and bring about a better understanding of its natural history.

Pathogenesis

There is a single cause of the CE syndrome. Advanced atherosclerosis of major arteries, especially the aorta, is responsible [1,2]. Microemboli to distal organs occur when cholesterol crystals are released from ulcerated or abraded atherosclerotic plaque. Although spontaneous CE is well documented, currently it is responsible for less than half of cases [3]. More commonly, the patient described in Table 18.1 has undergone a procedure. Typically, an arteriogram, balloon angioplasty or vascular surgical reconstruction/endarterectomy has just taken place [4,5]. In some cases the patient has been anti-

Table 18.1 The typical patient with cholesterol embolism. Any or all of the following may apply

---

Coronary artery disease
Angina pectoris, myocardial infarction, previous coronary artery bypass surgery

Distal aortic disease
Claudication, abdominal and femoral bruits, renovascular hypertension, ischemic renal disease, abdominal aortic aneurysm

Carotid artery disease
Transient ischemic attacks, stroke, retinal emboli, amaurosis fugax, carotid bruits

Smoker

Chronic hyperlipidemia
Aged 50−70 years, usually male caucasian

---

coagulated, probably making the atheromas more susceptible to disruption by trauma [2]. Because the syndrome of CE is still insufficiently considered in the patient with atherosclerosis who deteriorates spontaneously or after a procedure, we wish to outline its pathology first and then its clinical features.

Pathology

Atherosclerosis is a disease of the intima of blood vessels of undetermined pathogenesis. Lipid-laden areas of the intima may be precursors of the atheromatous plaque lesions. Yellowish, flat fatty streaks, up to 1−2 mm in width and 10 mm in length, are found distributed throughout the entire aorta after age 1 [6,7]. In the first decade of life, approximately 10% of the surface of the aorta may be involved with fatty streaks, increasing to 30−50% by the third decade. Later in life, atherosclerotic plaque lesions predominate, and the fatty streaks appear to regress. This progression is illustrated in Figure 18.1. Clearly, since these lesions do not correlate, either in their extent or location, with the development of atherosclerosis, it is thought that additional factors contribute to the development of atheromatous lesions. Current research has focused on the inflammatory hypothesis, which attributes the major pathogenetic role in atherosclerosis to monocyte influx, and the response-to-injury hypothesis, which has centered on growth factors, notably platelet-derived growth factor (PDGF), and activated platelets as early events leading to atheromas [7].

Common risk factors are advanced age, male gender, familial predisposition, hyperlipidemia, hypertension, cigarette smoking, and diabetes mellitus. The atheroma,

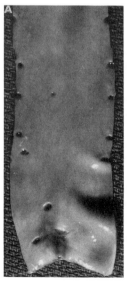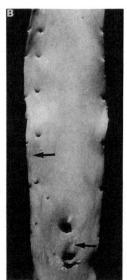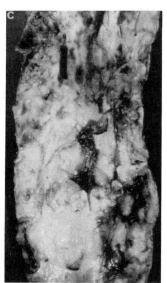

Fig. 18.1 (A−C) Progression of atherosclerosis. The normal intimal surface of the abdominal aorta of a 15-year-old is illustrated in A. The surface is smooth with minimal fatty streaks. By age 25 years (B) early atherosclerotic lesions appear, seen here as a slightly irregular intimal surface (arrows). In severe cases, atherosclerosis may progress to the extent seen in a 60-year-old woman (C). The intimal surface is virtually destroyed by the presence of nearly confluent ulcerated atherosclerotic plaques.

or fibrofatty plaque, is the central lesion and consists of focal raised areas within the intima. Grossly, atheromas have a whitish-yellowish appearance and are 0.3–1.5 cm in diameter. In severe cases, lesions may become confluent and cover larger areas, and may also involve and thereby weaken the media, leading to aneurysm formation. The plaques are much more common in the abdominal aorta (especially beyond the renal arteries) than in the thoracic aorta, and have a particular propensity for areas adjacent to or surrounding the ostia of branch vessels. The distal location of aortic plaque also places the deposits of cholesterol crystals directly in the path of angiographic catheters. The surface of the atheromatous plaque is covered by endothelial cells with an underlying fibrous cap, consisting of smooth-muscle cells, macrophages, and extracellular matrix proteins. When the plaque is sectioned, grumous fluid extrudes; thus the term "atheroma" from the Greek word "athere", meaning "gruel". Atheroembolism is another term used for the CE syndrome. The center of the plaque contains necrotic cellular debris, crystals of cholesterol (in the form of cholesterol bound to proteins and cholesteryl esters), macrophages, and foam cells. Calcium may be present in varying amounts (Fig. 18.2).

The time course to develop the plaque lesion may extend 20–40 years after the initial pathologic events.

Often the extent and severity of atheromatous disease may not be clinically apparent, and may only be discovered at autopsy. However, if the atheromas evolve into so-called complicated plaques, the consequences can be catastrophic with substantial morbidity and mortality. The complicated plaque has undergone one or more of the following changes: calcification, ulceration, hemorrhage within the plaque, aneurysm formation, and perhaps the most serious change, thrombosis. Cholesterol embolization occurs when an atheromatous plaque becomes ulcerated or traumatized by a catheter or at surgery. This allows discharge of the contents of its necrotic center, including cholesterol crystals. Thus, atherosclerotic disease is a prerequisite for CE.

In one autopsy series of 267 consecutive adult patients, CE was present in 12.3% of patients with severe aortic atheroclerotic disease, in 1.3% of those with moderate aortic involvement, and in none of those patients without ulcerated plaques [1]. However, Kealy [8] found CE only in 0.79% of 2126 routine autopsies, with the kidney involved most frequently (81.2%). In other studies there was up to a 4% incidence of CE in patients with mild atherosclerosis of the aorta vs. 7–30% in patients with severe disease including abdominal aortic aneurysms [9–12]. In an autopsy series of patients over the age of 50 years, CE was detected in 4.7% of males and 2.7%

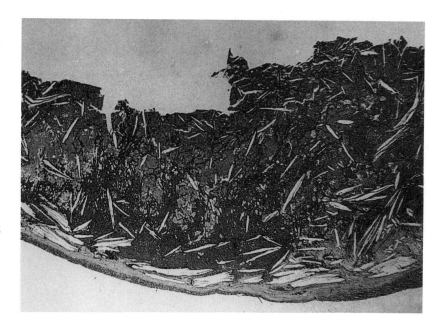

Fig. 18.2 Microscopic appearance of atherosclerotic ulcerated plaque. This cross-section of a portion of the aorta pictured in Figure 18.1C, illustrates the lack of overlying endothelium. The underlying plaque has ruptured, allowing escape of its contents, namely grumous cellular debris and cholesterol crystals. The cholesterol is dissolved by tissue processing and is seen here as needle-shaped clefts. Hematoxylin and eosin, original magnification ×40.

of females [13], while an incidence of 9% in routine autopsies has also been reported [12]. In patients who had undergone aortography, the incidence at autopsy was 25.5% [10], while in patients who had undergone resection of an abdominal aneurysm, CE was present in 77% [12]. As can be deduced from the clinical picture, CE most often involves multiple organs, and has been reported in virtually all tissues. In a review of 221 reported cases, autopsy data were available from 173 patients [2]. The kidney was the most commonly affected organ at autopsy (75%) (Fig. 18.3), followed by spleen (55%), pancreas (52%), gastrointestinal tract (31%), and the adrenals (20%). Ante-mortem diagnosis was made in only 68 of these 221 patients (31%). This was accomplished by single or multiple tissue biopsy of muscle (19 patients), skin (19 patients), kidney (17 patients), and gastrointestinal tract/intestinal resection (five patients). In four patients diagnosis was made on prostate biopsy obtained at transurethral resection of the prostate. Individual patients were diagnosed based on lymph node biopsy, resected ureteral stricture, splenectomy due to hemolytic anemia, and bone marrow, respectively. In

seven patients the diagnosis was made upon examination of an amputated toe or extremity.

The histologic diagnosis of CE is based on the finding of the characteristic needle-shaped slits of dissolved cholesterol crystals in the lumina of arterial blood vessels (Fig. 18.4). The crystals are dissolved by routine tissue processing, but are birefringent and stain positive for fat on frozen section. The crystals may dislodge spontaneously from the complicated atheromatous plaques, or more commonly (see above) shower into the distal vessels after instrumentation or trauma to the fragile ulcerated plaques. The cholesterol crystals usually lodge in arteries of 150−300 μm diameter. In the kidney the lesions are most common in arcuate and interlobular arteries, although glomeruli may also be involved (Fig. 18.5). When there is massive CE, an acute decline in renal function is frequent along with patchy cortical necrosis and tubular necrosis. If the process is more gradual, there may be a mixture of necrosis due to acute local ischemia from occluded vessels, and more chronic ischemic changes, such as glomerular scarring, tubular atrophy, and interstitial fibrosis. The early response, based on animal models, consists of mononuclear cell infiltration in the vessel and foreign body giant cell reaction surrounding the crystals. Polymorphonuclear leukocytes and eosinophils may also be seen transiently in the vascular lumen in the first 24 hours after embolization [13]. The vessel may then become thrombosed in the subacute stage from 24−72 hours. After the initial acute phase of injury, there is endothelial cell proliferation and intravascular fibrosis. Cholesterol crystals may remain detectable for as long as 9 months after the acute event [13].

Although muscle and skin biopsies may be useful in patients with livedo reticularis (19 out of 21 skin biopsies and 13 out of 14 muscle biopsies were diagnostic in one review) [2], many patients may not present with such dramatic cutaneous manifestations. Renal biopsy may then provide an ante-mortem diagnosis. In one series of 755 consecutive renal biopsies, CE was detected in eight cases. All were men aged 49−72 years [14]. The clinical indication for biopsy in each of these eight patients was a newly detected decline in renal function. Ultrastructural examination of the initial phase revealed cholesterol crystals within the lumen without tissue reaction. In slightly more advanced lesions, histiocytes surrounded the surface of the crystal with deposition of myelin-body-

Fig. 18.3 Segmental renal infarcts secondary to cholesterol emboli. The upper pole of a kidney with multiple small wedge-shaped infarcts (arrows) is shown. Microscopic examination revealed numerous arteries and arterioles occluded by cholesterol emboli (Fig. 18.4). The renal parenchyma showed patchy acute tubular necrosis and interstitial fibrosis in the areas adjacent to the infarcts.

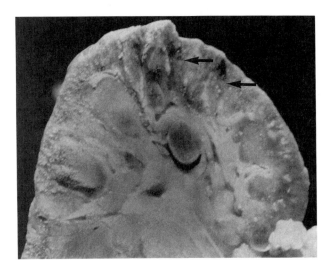

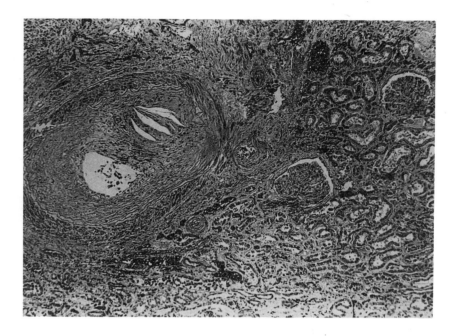

Fig. 18.4 Cholesterol embolus in a medium-sized arteriole. The slit-shaped clefts pathognomonic of cholesterol crystal embolization are seen. There is fibrous intimal hyperplasia with recanalization (rounded lumen). The glomeruli appear intact in this field, but there is interstitial fibrosis and tubular atrophy accompanying the cholesterol embolization. Hematoxylin and eosin, original magnification ×90.

like material on the crystal. In the intermediate phase, crystals within the lumen were associated with acute endothelial injury, evidenced by endothelial cell blebbing and focal platelet aggregation. At this stage, crystals were

Fig. 18.5 Glomerulus with cholesterol embolization. Although cholesterol crystals most commonly lodge in vessels of 150–300 μ diameter as illustrated, they may affect the glomerulus. This patient also had numerous cholesterol emboli in arteries and arterioles. Periodic acid Schiff, original magnification ×510.

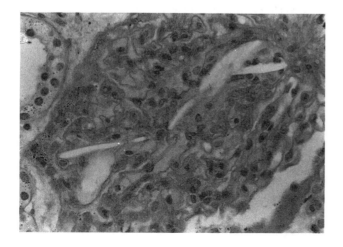

surrounded by giant cells or aggregated histiocytes. The later stages were characterized by intimal proliferation, with rare crystals seen outside the subendothelial basement membrane, still surrounded by giant cells [14].

Although sequential time course data are rare in humans, in one patient an open renal biopsy was performed 4 weeks after renal arteriography, due to a decline in renal function [15]. The biopsy demonstrated occlusion of two-thirds of the medium-sized arteries (150–300 μm) by CE with surrounding foreign body giant cell reaction. There was also patchy cortical necrosis. At autopsy 3 weeks after biopsy, widespread ulcerated atherosclerosis of the aorta was found. The kidneys showed organized atheromatous emboli with some recanalization of vessels. The foreign body giant cell reaction was no longer apparent, and there was cortical atrophy, glomerular sclerosis, and also atherosclerosis of the renal arteries.

At our institutions, we have seen a similar incidence of CE in renal biopsy material. In 1219 consecutive native kidney biopsies, 10 (0.8%) diagnoses of CE have been made. In the Veterans Administration Medical Center population of mainly middle-aged to elderly men, five out of 91 (5.5%) native kidney biopsies demonstrated CE. Although CE was suspected clinically in five cases, in five other renal biopsies the atheroemboli were unexpected. In the latter cases CE was found superimposed on other, more chronic changes of arteriolar nephrosclerosis or a variety of renal diseases. Six out of 10 (60%) patients had undergone angiography or aortic surgery just prior to biopsy.

Clinical setting

Acute cholesterol embolization

A typical scenario follows. A 65-year-old patient was returned to the ward following a balloon angioplasty of an isolated coronary artery stenosis. Although he became hypertensive after a cardiac catheterization a few days beforehand, and his serum creatinine and blood urea nitrogen increased by approximately 50%, these findings were attributed to the volume load and contrast nephropathy, respectively. Because the hypertension responded to additional medication and the renal insufficiency was believed to be reversible, it was decided to proceed with the balloon angioplasty to ameliorate angina pectoris and prevent future myocardial infarction.

Within a few hours after cardiac catheterization, the patient was again noted to be hypertensive. A low-grade fever was found. Antihypertensive medication was given and blood cultures taken. It was assumed that the patient became bacteremic from the intravascular catheter or was developing an allergic reaction to the radiologic contrast material. Parenteral antimicrobials were administered along with analgesic injections for back and leg pain. The latter symptoms were dismissed as related to the procedure and to the patient's smoking habit and "poor circulation." His legs and back were not examined so that the livedo pattern of skin discoloration remained undetected. When routine laboratory tests returned the next afternoon, the following abnormalities were discovered. There was peripheral blood leukocytosis with a mildly elevated eosinophil count. The blood urea nitrogen and serum creatinine were further increased. His serum aspartate aminotransferase and creatinine kinase levels were elevated, but the serum bilirubin and alkaline phosphatase were not. Myocardial infarction was suspected. Petechial lesions were discovered over the feet leading to the diagnosis of a drug-induced vasculitis. Studies were ordered pertaining to the diagnosis of "vasculitis." The sedimentation rate was elevated but antinuclear antibodies and rheumatoid factor were not. The serum complement was depressed, prompting in-

Table 18.2 Syndrome of acute CE — major features

Sudden exacerbation or new appearance of hypertension
Progressive renal insufficiency with differing course from acute tubular necrosis

Cutaneous findings (trunk, legs)
    Livedo reticularis
    Gangrene
    Cyanosis, purpura

Fever
Pain in back, abdomen, legs, and feet

itiation of corticosteroid therapy. Hepatitis serologies were returned on the next day and were negative. It was decided to biopsy the pedal skin lesions, hoping to confirm the diagnosis of vasculitis. Only then was the correct diagnosis of CE reached. This syndrome is summarized in Table 18.2.

Chronic cholesterol embolization

When the disease is chronic, the diagnosis is less obvious. Nevertheless, the same patient groups described in Table 18.1 apply. Usually, there is also a history of multiple arteriograms and vascular surgical procedures, although not necessarily in the immediate past. Anticoagulation and vasodilator therapy may be ongoing. The diagnosis is most often made as follows: a renal biopsy is performed to delineate the cause of progressive nephron loss, an ulcerative lesion in the gastrointestinal tract is sampled, a skin lesion is biopsied, a necrotic digit is amputated, or a cholesterol embolus is seen in the retina. The patient will have signs and symptoms referrable to multiple organ systems as in Table 18.1, leading to a variety of misdiagnoses (Table 18.3).

Diagnosis

Laboratory tests

The laboratory results, accumulated mainly by Fine *et al.* [2] in a review of 221 cases of CE in the English literature from 1965—1985, are shown in Table 18.4 [16,17]. All results are nonspecific but may be helpful when taken as a whole. Eosinophilia and hypocomplementia are transient and may be absent at the time of evaluation [16,17].

Table 18.3 Common misdiagnoses in patients with CE

Acute CE

Systemic vasculitis/allergic reaction

Bacteremia, including endocarditis

Hypertensive crisis

Contrast nephropathy

Cardiac mural thrombus/myxoma with peripheral emboli

Chronic CE

Ischemia/infarction of multiple organs due to progressive obliterative atherosclerosis

Accelerated hypertension

Systemic vasculitis

End-stage renal disease

Table 18.4 Laboratory tests in CE. (From Fine *et al.* [2], Meyrier *et al.* [16], and Kasinath & Lewis [17])

	%
Blood	
Elevated sedimentation rate	97
Leukocytosis	57
Eosinophilia	57
Anemia	46
Blood urea nitrogen (>20 mg/dl)	91
Serum creatinine (>2.0 mg/dl)	83
Serum creatinine kinase (>80 units/liter)	38
Serum aspartate aminotransferase (>30 units/liter)	60
Serum amylase (>100 Somogyi units)	60
Serum complement decreased	25–70
Urine	
Proteinuria	54
Cylindruria	41
Microscopic hematuria	31
Microscopic pyuria	16
Eosinophiluria	Unknown

Biopsy/resection

The series of Fine *et al.* [2] gives the broadest view of the ante-mortem diagnosis of CE by biopsy or resection of involved tissue. Of 75 sites in 68 patients which involved 11 different tissues, the highest yield was obtained from skeletal muscle (19), skin (19), kidney (17), amputated toe (6), gastrointestinal mucosa (5), and prostate (4).

Organ system involvement

Kidneys

Because of proximity to the main site of aortic atherosclerosis and the high rate of renal blood flow (RBF), the kidneys are frequently damaged in the syndrome of CE. Although spontaneous renal CE may occur in a relatively asymptomatic state, more commonly acute renal insufficiency is discovered after angiography, angioplasty, or aortic surgery. The differential diagnosis in such a situation is broad (Table 18.5). However, usually a high index of suspicion can be reached if any of the features listed in Table 18.2 accompany the loss of renal function.

Vidt *et al.* [18] reviewed 24 patients with CE proven by renal biopsy. Risk factors included coronary artery disease (67%), cigarette smoking (92%), hypertension (100%), aortic atherosclerosis by angiography (100%), carotid occlusive disease (63%), stroke (33%), renal artery stenosis (79%), and ileofemoral atherosclerosis (75%). In two-thirds of the patients there was a definite or probable causal relationship between CE and an aortic surgical or angiographic procedure. All 24 had received arteriograms in the past. Accompanying organ involvement included skin changes (50%), gastrointestinal bleeding (25%), retinal emboli (17%), abdominal pain (25%), and pancreatitis (4%). Although a rapid decline in renal function was seen in 7 out of 24 patients and suggested CE as the main cause of the decrease, in 19 out of 24 the progressive nature of the renal failure was felt to be a combination of renal artery stenosis and CE. Results of surgical and medical therapy were variable.

A group of 32 French patients with renal failure related to various aspects of atheromatous disease was reported in 1988 [16]. Ten had CE, with coexistent major renal artery atheromata in eight out of the 10. Laboratory results demonstrated peripheral blood eosinophilia in 50% and hypocomplementia in 25%. Renal biopsies were diagnostic in all six patients in whom they were done. Triggering factors were angiography in 70%, vascular surgery in 20%, and apparent spontaneous CE in 10%. A poor outcome (dialysis/death) was seen in six out of 10 patients.

We have seen several patients develop an acute loss of

Table 18.5 Differential diagnosis of acute renal insufficiency after angiography, angioplasty, or aortic surgery

Acute tubular necrosis
  Hemorrhage/hypovolemia
  Contrast nephropathy
  Bacteremia

Therapeutic drug nephrotoxicity*

Hypersensitivity phenomena
  Anaphylactoid reactions
  Vasculitis

Obstructive uropathy†

Thrombosis or dissection causing renal artery occlusion

CE

* Patients requiring these procedures are often receiving antimicrobials, angiotensin-converting enzyme inhibitors, calcium channel antagonists, diuretics, nonsteroidals, and other nephrotoxic agents.
† Older males may have urinary obstruction after aortic surgery or go into urinary retention from prostatic hypertrophy.

Table 18.6 Procedures prone to cause CE

Abdominal aortic surgery
Balloon angioplasty (arterial)
Arteriography
Left heart catheterization without angiography

renal function following angiography, often to a creatinine clearance of 10 ml/min or less. Some required dialysis. Renal biopsy proved CE in each case. One patient has been reported [19]. After a period of several weeks of azotemia, a very slow recovery of renal function has ensued in some patients. However, a return to baseline renal function has never been achieved in our experience. One patient required more than 1 year after CE to reach his lowest serum creatinine concentration. Two similar patients were reported by Siemons *et al.* in Belgium [20]. They employed peritoneal dialysis for 3 days and 10 months, respectively. Remarkably, the latter patient eventually attained his baseline serum creatinine value. McGowan & Greenberg [21] described three patients who developed acute renal failure in the setting of CE. Diagnosis was made by skin biopsy. Two survived the immediate insult, although one had to be dialyzed for 2 months. Recovery of renal function was incomplete in each patient. Finally, Smith *et al.* [22] also found renal failure to be reversible in four of their five patients with CE, although one required dialysis for 4 months. The rate of recovery of renal function was much slower (months) than for acute tubular necrosis (ATN) (1–2 weeks) and never normalized as happens post-ATN. Permanent renal

failure with requirement for maintenance dialysis has also resulted [5,18]. Cholesterol emboli can even involve renal allografts, with origin either in donor or recipient aortas [23].

The diagnosis of CE should be sought in any patient with loss of renal function in the setting of known or suspected atheromatous disease, especially following anticoagulation or a procedure involving a major artery (Table 18.6). Suspicion of CE should be heightened by compatible skin findings, fever, exacerbated hypertension, and signs and symptoms referrable to skeletal muscle and the gastrointestinal tract. If there is not a likely skin lesion to biopsy, percutaneous renal biopsy should be considered. Pathologists processing the samples should be alerted to the possibility of CE beforehand. In the follow-up period after a renal insult from CE, recovery of some renal function is frequent although delayed (Fig. 18.6). Return of renal function even after months of dialysis has been observed [20,22].

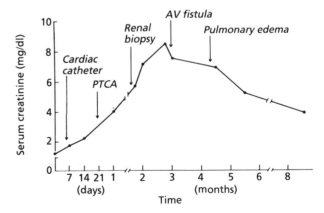

Fig. 18.6 Time course of the serum creatinine concentration of a 58-year-old man who developed cholesterol embolization (documented by renal biopsy) following a cardiac catheterization and percutaneous transluminal coronary angioplasty (PTCA). While partial recovery of renal function ensued, the patient remained prone to pulmonary edema.

Skin

Cutaneous manifestations of CE have been documented in 35−75% of patients [18,24]. In our experience it is even more common but often goes undetected. Livedo reticularis is the most frequent finding. This consists of a net-like mottling of the skin distal to the origin of the CE. The legs, feet, back, buttocks, and abdominal wall are characteristic sites. Dermal vessels are occluded or in spasm. Petechiae and larger areas of dermal necrosis may be found (Fig. 18.7). Blue or purple toes occurred in 17% of patients with renal CE in one study while 33% had livedo reticularis [18]. Colt *et al.* [4] found 75% of their patients with CE had livedo reticularis and 50% developed cyanotic toes. Larger areas of necrosis may progress to dermal ulceration and gangrene. Livedo reticularis may persist for many days and mimics the cutaneous changes of shock, but often is accompanied by good arterial pulses and normal to high arterial blood pressure. Biopsy of an involved area of skin which is not necrotic will lead to the diagnosis in at least 92% of cases of confirmed CE [24].

> Chest pain struck an old man from Paris.
> "It's angina" said Doctor Harris.
> In the cath lab he froze.
> He came back with blue toes
> And livedo reticularis.

Gastrointestinal tract

Approximately one-third of patients with CE have gastrointestinal involvement [2]. Portions of the gut from esophagus to anus have been embolized. Clinical findings include abdominal pain, nausea, vomiting, hemorrhage, ileus, pseudopolyps, ulceration, perforation, diffuse necrosis, and stricture formation. Anderson *et al.* [25] described three autopsied patients with gastrointestinal necrosis and bleeding from multiple cholesterol emboli in submucosal small arteries. They emphasized that these ulcerative lesions are easy to overlook and may re-epithelialize. Perforation of CE-related ulcers in the jejunum and colon has been reported [26]. A focal superficial infarct of the cecum due to CE has mimicked a carcinoma and resulted in an unnecessary hemicolectomy [27]. Inflammatory polypoid lesions (pseudopolyps) in the small intestine with associated, presumably causal, CE on histologic section have also caused gastrointestinal hemorrhage [28]. Finally, an aggressive surgical approach to extensive bowel infarction as a result of CE has salvaged two patients [29]. Since gastrointestinal tract lesions are

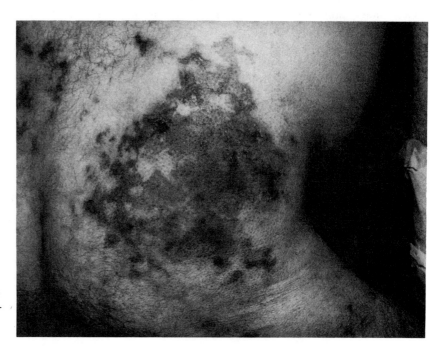

Fig. 18.7 Livedo reticularis and extensive areas of infarction in the skin of a 62-year-old man immediately following a renal arteriogram.

not rare in CE, they need to be sought in patients with the CE syndrome and complaints referrable to the digestive system.

Nervous system

Since atherosclerosis is most pronounced in the abdominal aorta, the brain and retina are spared in many cases of systemic CE. However, thoracic aortic and carotid plaques can release emboli to both sites. In a series of 85 patients with visible retinal emboli, 69 (80%) these were found to be CE [30]. Carotid atheromatous disease was discovered in over 80% at arteriography. Patients with retinal CE had a greatly reduced survival curve compared to age- and sex-matched controls, chiefly due to fatal stroke. Cholesterol embolization was single in 79% and most often in the temporal field. The degree of visual loss was unpredictable and ranged from none to permanent field defects associated with CE lodged at vessel bifurcations.

Brain involvement is usually clinically deduced but can only be proven at autopsy. The minute emboli and subsequent infarctions often escape detection by radiologic tests. Confusional states and gradual deterioration in neurologic function without focal deficits have been attributed to CE [4]. Spinal cord infarction is uncommon but may follow abdominal angiography or aortic surgery [8,31]. Slowly progressive spinal cord syndromes in the elderly may be related to CE [32].

Other organs involved

At autopsy the spleen and pancreas are embolized in more than 50% of cases of CE [2]. However, symptomatic pancreatitis and splenic infarction are unusual [2,4,18]. Similarly, hepatic CE has been found in 17% of autopsies but probably has no clinical consequences [2]. Adrenal involvement by CE is common but acute adrenal insufficiency is rare [2,4]. Rhabdomyolysis sufficient to cause ATN is unusual but myalgias are common [2,33]. Muscle biopsy may be used to make the diagnosis of CE [2]. Non-Q wave myocardial infarction due to diffuse CE has followed balloon angioplasty of the coronary arteries (percutaneous transluminal coronary angioplasty, PTCA). Cholesterol embolization may be more prevalent (2.5−3.0%) when saphenous vein grafts are dilated than when PTCA is performed on native coronary arteries [34]. However, since the mortality rate after PTCA is only about 1% [35] and the diagnosis of myocardial CE can only be made with confidence at autopsy, these figures are likely to be underestimates. Complications in the lower genitourinary tract have included penile and scrotal necrosis as well as rupture of the urinary bladder [24,36].

Treatment

There is no specific treatment of CE, and the prognosis is often poor [2,4,5]. Prevention of further insults by avoidance of anticoagulation, angiography, or arterial surgery is counseled. However, this is often impossible because of the diffuse nature of atherosclerosis. The need to diagnose and bypass or endarterectomize arterial lesions is an ongoing clinical problem. There may be a risk of myocardial infarction, the patient may have an aortic aneurysm, the brain may be threatened, and the patient can be having disabling claudification. A complicated decision will have to be reached weighing the confounding variables. Certainly, Doppler ultrasonography can be helpful in obviating arteriography in some circumstances. Use of the brachial rather than the femoral artery for angiography seems to carry less risk of CE, probably because the bulk of atheromatous disease is in the abdominal rather than thoracic aorta. Following infarction of the gastrointestinal tract, digits, or extensive areas of skin, corrective surgical procedures can be lifesaving or prevent further complications such as infection. Resection of large atheromata, especially in the abdominal aorta, is of theoretical benefit but often not feasible. We have not undertaken this in any of our patients unless an aneurysm was present. Renal failure can be treated with dialysis, which may only be needed transiently. Probably the best therapy of CE is through the prevention of atherosclerosis in future generations. In the interim much physician education is necessary so that this common condition is not misdiagnosed and mistreated.

Acknowledgment

Dr Agnes Fogo is a recipient of a Clinician−Scientist Award from the American Heart Association.

References

1 Flory CM. Arterial occlusions produced by emboli from eroded aortic atheromatous plaques. Am J Pathol 1945; 21:549−565.

2 Fine MJ, Kapoor W, Falanga V. Cholesterol crystal embolization: a review of 221 cases in the English literature. Angiology 1987;38:769–784.

3 Jennings WC, Corder CN, Jarolim DR, et al. Atheromatous embolism: varied clinical presentation and prognosis. South Med J 1989;82:849–852.

4 Colt HG, Begg RJ, Saporito JJ, et al. Cholesterol emboli after cardiac catheterization. Eight cases and a review of the literature. Medicine 1988;67:389–400.

5 Drost H, Buis B, Haan D, et al. Cholesterol embolism as a complication of left heart catheterisation. Report of seven cases. Br Heart J 1984;52:339–342.

6 Berenson GS, Srinivasan SR, Freedman DS, et al. Review: atherosclerosis and its evolution in childhood. Am J Med Sci 1987;294:429–440.

7 Ross R. The pathogenesis of atherosclerosis—an update. N Engl J Med 1986;314:488–500.

8 Kealy WF. Atheroembolism. J Clin Pathol 1978;31:984–989.

9 Greendyke RM, Akamatsu Y. Atheromatous embolism as a cause of renal failure. J Urol 1960;83:231–237.

10 Ramirez G, O'Neill WM, Lambert R, et al. Cholesterol embolization. A complication of angiography. Arch Intern Med 1978;138:1430–1432.

11 Rosansky SJ, Deschamps EG. Multiple cholesterol emboli syndrome after angiography. Am J Med Sci 1984;288:45–48.

12 Thurlbeck WM, Castleman B. Atheromatous emboli to the kidneys after aortic surgery. N Engl J Med 1957; 257: 442–447.

13 Gore I, McCombs HL, Lindquist RL. Observations on the fate of cholesterol emboli. J Atherosclerosis Res 1964;4:527–535.

14 Jones DB, Iannacone PM. Atheromatous emboli in renal biopsies. An ultrastructural study. Am J Pathol 1975; 78:261–276.

15 Harrington JT, Sommers SC, Kassirer JP. Atheromatous emboli with progressive renal failure. Renal arteriography as the probable inciting factor. Ann Intern Med 1968; 68:152–160.

16 Meyrier A, Buchet P, Simon P, et al. Atheromatous renal disease. Am J Med 1988;85:139–146.

17 Kasinath BS, Lewis EJ. Eosinophilia as a clue to the diagnosis of atheroembolic renal disease. Arch Intern Med 1987; 147:1384–1385.

18 Vidt DG, Eisele G, Gephardt GN, et al. Atheroembolic renal disease: association with renal artery stenosis. Cleve Clin J Med 1989;56:407–413.

19 Tilley WS, Harston WE, Siami G, et al. Renal failure due to cholesterol emboli following PTCA. Am Heart J 1985; 110:1301–1302.

20 Siemons L, van den Heuvel P, Parizel G, et al. Peritoneal dialysis in acute renal failure due to cholesterol embolization:

two cases of recovery of renal function and extended survival. Clin Nephrol 1987;28:205–208.

21 McGowan JA, Greenberg A. Cholesterol atheroembolic renal disease. Report of 3 cases with emphasis on diagnosis by skin biopsy and extended survival. Am J Nephrol 1986; 6:135–139.

22 Smith MC, Ghose MK, Henry AR. The clinical spectrum of renal cholesterol embolization. Am J Med 1981;71:174–180.

23 Aujla ND, Greenberg A, Banner BF, et al. Atheroembolic involvement of renal allografts. Am J Kidney Dis 1989;13: 329–332.

24 Falanga V, Fine MJ, Kapoor WN. The cutaneous manifestations of cholesterol crystal embolization. Arch Dermatol 1986;122:1194–1198.

25 Anderson WR, Richards AM, Weiss L. Hemorrhage and necrosis of the stomach and bowel due to atheroembolism. Am J Clin Pathol 1967;48:30–38.

26 Rushovich AM. Perforation of the jejunum: a complication of atheromatous embolization. Am J Gastroenterol 1983; 78:77–82.

27 Chan T, Levine MS, Park Y. Cholesterol embolization as a cause of cecal infarct mimicking carcinoma. Am J Roentgenol 1988;150:1315–1316.

28 Francis J, Kapoor WN. Intestinal pseudopolyps and gastrointestinal hemorrhage due to cholesterol crystal embolization. Am J Med 1988;85:269–271.

29 Hendel RC, Cuenoud HF, Giansiracusa DF, et al. Multiple cholesterol emboli syndrome. Bowel infarction after retrograde angiography. Arch Intern Med 1989; 149:2371–2374.

30 Howard RS, Ross Russell RW. Prognosis of patients with retinal embolism. J Neurol Neurosurg Psychiatry 1987; 50:1142–1147.

31 Harrington D, Amplatz K. Cholesterol embolization and spinal infarction following aortic catheterization. Am J Roentgenol 1972;115:171–174.

32 Slavin RE, Gonzalez-Vitale JC, Marin OSM. Atheromatous emboli to the lumbosacral spinal cord. Stroke 1975; 6:411–416.

33 Palmer FJ, Warren BA. Multiple cholesterol emboli syndrome complicating angiographic techniques. Clin Radiol 1988; 39:519–522.

34 Trono R, Sutton C, Hollman J, et al. Multiple myocardial infarctions associated with atheromatous emboli after PTCA of saphenous vein grafts. Cleve Clin J Med 1989;56:581–584.

35 Kent KM. Coronary angioplasty. A decade of experience. N Engl J Med 1987;316:1148–1150.

36 Piser JA, Kamer M, Rowland RG. Spontaneous bladder rupture owing to atherosclerotic emboli: a case report. J Urol 1986;136:1068–1070.

19

Obstructive urinary tract disease in the elderly

William E. Yarger

Introduction

This chapter is devoted to understanding the effects of urinary tract obstruction, particularly as it affects elderly patients. It will be limited to discussing the causes, presentations, potential for recovery, and the diagnosis of urinary tract obstructive disease. It will not discuss treatment which is discussed in Chapter 20.

Definition of terms

Obstruction of the urinary tract is one of the most common preventable causes of renal insufficiency and renal failure, particularly in the elderly. Several terms are used in the literature to describe the occurrence of urinary tract obstruction and its consequences. These terms include hydronephrosis, obstructive nephropathy, obstructive uropathy, and pelvicaliectasis. Unfortunately, there is a lack of consistency in the use of these terms. For example, the term "hydronephrosis" often means something quite different to the radiologist than it means to the pathologist. In this chapter the author will use these terms as previously defined [1]:

1 hydronephrosis—distention of the renal pelvis and calyces with urine as a result of obstruction of urine flow at some point beyond the ducts of Bellini accompanied by atrophy of the renal parenchyma;

2 obstructive uropathy—any change in the structure or function of the urinary collecting system from the renal pelvis to the tip of the urethra that either causes or results from obstruction;

3 obstructive nephropathy—any alteration in renal function that results from obstruction, irrespective of whether gross loss of parenchyma is present or not;

4 pelvicaliectasis—distention of the renal pelvis and calyces without demonstrable loss of renal parenchymal tissue.

Thus hydronephrosis is essentially an anatomic term referring to the combination of pelvicaliceal dilation of sufficient duration so that loss of renal parenchyma has resulted. Obstruction uropathy refers to changes in the structure or function of the collecting system. Obstructive nephropathy refers to the effects of obstruction on renal function. Pelvicaliectasis refers to demonstrable dilatation of the pelvis and calyces as seen, usually, by various radiographic or ultrasonographic means.

Etiology of urinary tract obstruction

The causes of urinary tract obstruction can be grouped in many ways, but the one the author will use here separates these various etiologies by the primary organ system whose disease leads to the obstruction. In this way, the likelihood of obstruction in patients with known or suspected disease of other organ systems can most easily be identified.

Primary diseases of the urinary system causing obstruction

Although congenital or developmental abnormalities of the urinary tract most commonly present in infants and young children [1], they may be detected in later life if the degree of obstruction is mild [2–5], thus unexplained unilateral asymptomatic hydronephrosis, even in adults, should prompt one to consider a congenital cause. The possibility of congenital obstructive uropathy not withstanding, however, the most common causes of urinary tract obstruction in western societies are prostatic hypertrophy (Fig. 19.1A) [6], nephrolithiasis (Fig. 19.1C) [7], and cancer (see Fig. 19.2) [8]. In elderly males benign or

Fig. 19.1 A, Incidence (per 100 000 males per year) of benign prostatic obstruction. (From Lytton et al. [6].) B, The incidence (per 100 000 females per year) of procidentia (uterine prolapse). (From Steensberg et al. [7].) C, The prevalence of nephrolithiasis (per 100 000 males or females). (The data for 40–49, 50–59, and 60–69 are taken from Ljunghall [16]. The data for the 70+ age group are estimated from the data of Johnson et al. [17] and Fetter et al. [11].)

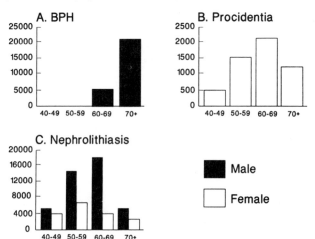

malignant disease of the prostate, and in females genital malignancy are the most frequent causes.

Prostatic hyperplasia

Hyperplasia of the prostate is the commonest form of benign hyperplasia to affect males (Fig. 19.1A) and results in some degree of bladder neck outlet obstruction in 75% of men over 50 years of age [9] and leads to the performance of over 350 000 prostatectomies every year [10,11]. Generally, the effects of prostatic obstruction are easily recognized because of their common constellation of symptoms, discussed below. However, on occasion, the symptoms and changes in micturition can be so mild as to escape detection by either the patient or physician even though progressive damage to the kidney may have resulted [12]. This more silent and insidious form of prostatic obstruction occurs predominantly in the older age group. Although the incidence of some degree of bladder neck obstruction resulting from prostatic hypertrophy is high there is some disagreement as to the incidence of hydronephrosis which results. Abrams et al. [13] have suggested that 5% of patients with prostatic hypertrophy will develop hydronephrosis. George et al. [14], however, feel that is much less common, and is limited to only those patients who have "high pressure" chronic retention. Both of these estimates of the frequency of hydronephrosis in patients with prostatic hyperplasia are largely derived from the use of intravenous pyelography. As discussed below, when more sensitive tests of abnormal upper tract function are used to determine the presence of abnormal function, the incidence is much higher.

Unfortunately, intravenous urography, the most common tool used to assess the effects of prostatic hypertrophy on the kidney, may underestimate the degree of damage. Meyhoff et al. [15] studied randomly selected patients who were going to be operated on for prostatic obstruction. Only 15% of these patients had anatomically demonstrable dilation of the upper urinary collecting system by routine intravenous pyelography. But 54% had abnormal upper urinary tract drainage when studied by gamma camera renography after the injection of 51Cr-EDTA. Of these, 6% had reduced glomerular filtration rates (GFRs) when compared with age-matched normals. As a group, patients with abnormal emptying of the upper urinary tract demonstrated with 51Cr-EDTA had lower GFRs than those whose upper tracts were functionally normal. Although prostatectomy restored upper tract size and emptying time, GFR decreased even further. In addition to benign hypertrophy, prostatic carcinoma, discussed below, is the next most common cause of obstructive urinary tract disease in men.

Nephrolithiasis
Although the prevalence of nephrolithiasis varies widely from one region of the world to another, there was a peak in the population studied by Ljunghall [16] in the fifth through seventh decades (see Fig. 19.1C). In general, approximately 20% of patients will present for the first time at the age of 60 years and 4−10% in patients over the age of 70 [17]. Although males as a group predominate by approximately three to one, in the elderly the rates are nearly equal [17,18]. The prevalence of nephrolithiasis can vary from a low of 1% in males less than 30 years to a level of 21% in males between 50 and 65 years of age [19]. In the older patient, there is a tendency for the stones to be composed of either uric acid or a combination of calcium oxalate and calcium phosphate as contrasted with pure calcium oxalate stones in younger age groups [20].

Other nonmalignant conditions of the urogenital system
Urinomas are pathologic peripelvic collections of extravasated urine that can both cause and result from obstructive uropathy. They most commonly result from acute ureteral obstruction due to an impacted stone, from tumoral obstruction of the ureter, or from prostatic hypertrophy [21]. A nonneoplastic gynecologic condition commonly associated with obstructive uropathy is uterine prolapse, the incidence of which increases with age (see Fig. 19.1B). Hydronephrosis is reported to occur in 4−7% of women with procidentia [22].

Neoplasia as a cause of obstructive uropathy
Obstructive uropathy resulting from local or distal metastasis of various neoplasms is common. Because the overall age-adjusted incidence of many cancers increase with age [23] as shown in Figure 19.2(a), the link between neoplasia and obstructive uropathy also increases. This is particularly true for cancers of the prostate, colon, breast, and bladder, which, along with cervical cancer, are among the more common neoplastic causes of obstructive uropathy, as shown in Figure 19.2(b). The exact incidence of obstruction resulting from neoplastic disease is

not known, but Cohen *et al.* [24] reported that approximately 1% of all patients with cancer, excluding only dermal squamous cell tumors, may develop urinary obstruction. The data in Figure 19.2(b) that relate the incidence of obstructive uropathy observed in several common neoplasms have been constructed from several sources [24−29].

Primary urogenital cancer
It is not surprising that primary cancer of the urogenital tract is the most common neoplastic cause of obstruction. Although the incidence for cervical cancer remains relatively stable as women age (Fig. 19.2a) the importance of this tumor in the causation of urinary obstruction derives from two facts. Firstly, it is the most common neoplastic cause of obstruction with approximately 30% of patients with cervical cancer being effected [30,31]. Second, the uremia that results is one of the major causes of death in such patients [32]. In addition, as we will see below, hysterectomy, for whatever reason, is also the surgical

Table 19.1 Obstructive uropathy resulting as a complication of surgery. (From Sieben *et al.* [33], Zinman *et al.* [34], Gangai *et al.* [35], Higgins [36], Ihse *et al.* [37], and Dowling *et al.* [38])

Surgical specialty	Percentage within group	Group percentage of total
Urology		
Ureteral surgery	48.8%	15.5%
Transurethral resection	21.33%	
Pyelolithotomy	6.1%	
Other urologic	24.0%	
Gynecology		
Hysterectomy	87.3%	62.5%
Oophorectomy	6.1%	
Vaginal surgery	5.5%	
Other	1.1%	
General Surgery		
Colon resection	57.7%	19.3%
Aortic surgery	15.5%	
Retroperitoneal surgery	13.3%	
Other	13.5%	
Neurosurgical or orthopedic surgery		
Sympathectomy	57.2%	2.7%
Spinal fusion	14.2%	
Other	28.6%	

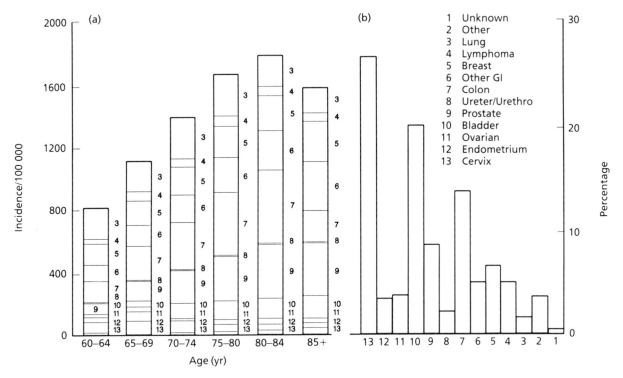

Fig. 19.2 (a) Age-adjusted incidence (per 100 000 per year) of several cancers associated with obstructive uropathy. (From Young *et al.* [8].) There are no data in the columns of Fig. 19.2(a) to represent the categories of unknown or other because these refer to categories in Fig. 19.2(b) only. Note also that the age-adjusted incidence for ureteral/urethral carcinomas is too small to be seen in this graph. The values are (per 100 000): 60–64, 2.0; 65–69, 3.1; 70–74, 3.3; 75–79, 4.0; 80–84, 5.7; 85+, 3.1. (b) Percentage estimate frequency of obstructive uropathy due to various tumors. (From Cohen *et al.* [24], Meyer *et al.* [25], Brin *et al.* [26], Grabstald & McPhee [27], Scott & McDonald [28], and Presman & Ehrlich [29].)

procedure most often associated with iatrogenic obstructive uropathy (Table 19.1) [33–38].

Cancer of the prostate is the second leading cause of death due to cancer death in American men. There are more than 75 000 new cases diagnosed annually [39]. The most common finding leading to the diagnosis is the discovery of a suspicious nodule in the prostate. The work-up of such a finding should include the measurement of acid phosphatase and a needle biopsy of the suspicious nodule [40]. As shown in the bottom of Figure 19.2, prostatic carcinoma is the third most common tumor of the urologic system to cause obstructive uropathy. Obstruction by prostatic cancer can occur at several levels. The bladder neck can be obstructed by the bulk of the tumor itself. The ureteral outlets can become obstructed as the tumor invades the bladder wall. In addition, metastasis to pelvic nodes or to the ureter can also cause obstruction [41].

Bladder cancer is the most common urothelial neoplasm associated with obstructive uropathy and the incidence of this condition is highest in the over 70 age group. Cancer of the ureter or urethra also accounts for slightly over 2% of neoplastic-induced obstructive uropathy. The relative frequency with which various urothelial neoplasms were observed at the Memorial Sloan Kettering Cancer center over a 26-year period were reported by Batala *et al.* [42] to be: bladder, 2251; urethral, 182; renal pelvic, 70; ureteral, 63. Thus, including cervical, prostatic, and these other urogenital tumors, neoplasia of the male and female urinary and genital system account for roughly 60% of all cases of obstruction which arise as a result of cancer.

Nonurogenital cancer as a cause of obstruction
Of tumors outside of the urogenital system that commonly cause obstruction, those of colon (see Fig. 19.2) and breast are the cancers most commonly associated with obstruction. The incidence of both of these tumors increases logarithmically with age so that the rate in the seventh decade is 10−100 times greater than it is in the fourth decade [43]. Therefore, although these tumors account for 13.4% and 6.5% of the malignant causes of obstruction when all patients are considered, they are particularly important in the elderly.

Retroperitoneal fibrosis as a cause of obstructive uropathy
Neoplastic disease often results in ureteral obstruction due to metastasis to the retroperitoneal nodes. However, retroperitoneal fibrosis unrelated to neoplasia often presents as unilateral or bilateral ureteral obstruction [1]. Retroperitoneal fibrosis can result from many conditions. Wagneknecht & Hardy [44] collected 430 cases shown in Figure 19.3 by surveying over 2000 physicians in eight western European countries over a 5-year period. Of these 430 cases, 185 (43.0%) were felt to be idiopathic, 30 (7.0%) were due to neighboring inflammation (terminal ileitis, 9; ulcerative colitis, 4; diverticulitis, 7; appendicitis, 7; and pancreatitis, 3). Sixty-six were posttraumatic (15.3%). Of these, 55 were associated with previous surgery, seven with extravasation of urine, and four with

retroperitoneal hematoma. One of the more interesting conditions, discussed below, was 36 (8.4%) cases that were associated with arterial aneurysms. Fifty-two (12.1%) cases followed radiation therapy and 48 (11.2%) were associated with malignancies. Although almost all physicians are aware of the association of retroperitoneal fibrosis with chronic ingestion of the drug methysergide [45], this is a relatively rare condition, being associated with only 13 (3%) of cases.

Idiopathic retroperitoneal fibrosis
Idiopathic retroperitoneal fibrosis, the most common form of the condition, characteristically occurs in later life. Baker *et al.* [46] reported on 60 cases seen in two British institutions over a 20-year period. The mean age at presentation of their patients was 56 years. Flank pain, backache, polyuria, nocturia, and oliguria, were common presenting complaints. The condition was three times more likely to occur in men than in women, and 87% presented with an increased erythrocyte sedimentation rate. The likelihood of death increased sharply with increasing age, with the majority of deaths occurring in patients in the seventh and eighth decades. Uremia due to bilateral ureteral obstruction, or associated conditions, such as peritoneal dialysis with peritonitis, was the most common cause of death.

Retroperitoneal fibrosis associated with inflammatory aneurysms of the aorta
There is an interesting and perhaps related form of retroperitoneal fibrosis that is associated with abdominal aortic aneurysms [47], which represented 8.4% of Wagneknecht's patients [44]. Others [48] have also reported a similar percentage in patients with retroperitoneal fibrosis. This is a peculiar condition because it occurs almost exclusively in men, and because the vast majority exhibit elevated erythrocyte sedimentation rates [49−52]. The cause is not known. Although there has been much speculation that perianeurysmal blood leak into the retroperitoneal space sets up the condition, efforts to find hemosiderin-laden macrophages or other evidence of bleeding has usually been unsuccessful [53]. Rather, one generally finds evidence of chronic inflammation, and, occasionally medium-sized vessel vasculitis [51]. Such aneurysms have been called "inflammatory" [54] and may differ significantly from the more common atherosclerotic abdominal aneurysms. The frequency of

Fig. 19.3 The percentage of the various etiologies that have been reported to cause retroperitoneal fibrosis. (From Wagneknecht & Hardy [44].)

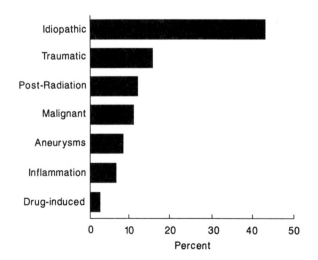

such inflammatory aneurysms in unknown, but they may account for as much as one quarter of all aneurysms in some series [55]. They are of interest because there are several reports of successful corticosteroid treatment of the ureteral obstruction that frequently accompanies these aneurysms when surgery was not an option [48,50,52,56]. This process of perianeurysmal entrapment of the ureters is not limited to abdominal aneurysms. Aneurysms of the internal and common iliac arteries have also been reported to cause obstruction [57].

Hematologic causes of obstructive uropathy and nephropathy

The incidence of both myeloma [58] and non-Hodgkin's lymphoma [59] increases progressively with age, reaching a peak in patients over the age of 80, and both conditions can be associated with obstructive uropathy. As many as 8% of patients with lymphosarcoma or histiocytic lymphoma may have urinary tract obstruction [60] due principally to involvement of retroperitoneal nodes. The precipitation of paraproteins, most commonly within the nephron [61], but occasionally within the renal pelvis itself [62,63] can lead to either intrarenal obstruction or extrarenal obstruction, which, in the latter case, may be unilateral. For whatever reason, renal failure, in myeloma, is a major cause of morbidity and mortality.

Acute uric acid nephropathy

Acute renal failure due to the precipitation of uric acid during chemotherapy, particularly of lymphomas [64] is another cause of obstructive nephropathy seen in hematologic patients. Polycythemia vera, another hematologic condition of older people [65] can also result in acute uric acid nephropathy. Although acute uric acid nephropathy most characteristically presents during the treatment of hematologic malignancies, it can occur prior to treatment in other conditions including hemolytic anemia [66] and disseminated carcinoma [67].

The syndrome of acute uric acid nephropathy is thought to result from the precipitation of uric acid in the acidic environment of the distal nephron [68,69]. Increased uric acid production during the treatment of hematologic malignancies may also cause acute renal failure by the formation of multiple stones in the renal pelvis and ureter [70]. The diagnosis of acute uric acid nephropathy is generally not difficult because it so characteristically presents during initial treatment of a

select number of conditions. However, such patients are often ill and may have other causes for acute renal failure. Kelton et al. [71] have shown that in such patients, a uric acid/creatinine ratio greater than one is diagnostic of acute uric acid nephropathy.

The prevention of acute uric acid nephropathy requires an increase in the volume and alkalinity of the urine [72], and the prophylactic use of allopurinol to decrease uric acid levels. Although the combination of acetazolamide (Diamox) and intravenous sodium bicarbonate may be required to adequately alkalinize the urine in the treatment of established acute uric acid nephropathy, elderly patients may be overly susceptible to the development of congestive heart failure under such conditions. Therefore, in the face of any significant decrease in cardiac reserve, or evidence of extracellular fluid (ECF) volume overload, acute hemodialysis can be used to treat both the excess volume and excess load of uric acid [72].

Gastrointestinal, vasculitic, and granulomatous causes of obstructive uropathy

Gastrointestinal diseases that can produce urinary tract obstruction include inflammatory bowel disease [73], due either to the primary inflammatory process or, secondarily, due to associated increase in nephrolithiasis [74]. The nephrolithiasis which results from inflammatory bowel disease has a much higher incidence that is seen in the general population. Approximately 0.1% of general hospital admissions are due to de novo nephrolithiasis, while 8–19% of patients with inflammatory bowel disease may be so afflicted, although even here it appears to be limited to patients with Crohn's disease, particularly those with small bowel involvement. Diverticulitis, which is more common in the elderly can also result in obstruction, which is frequently unilateral involving predominantly the left side [75].

A wide variety of other conditions has also been associated with obstructive uropathy. These include systemic lupus erythematosus [76], polyarteritis nodosa [77], Wegeners granulomatosis [78], allergic vasculitis [79], and sarcoidosis [80]. There have also been over 100 cases of ureteral obstruction due to nodular amyloid deposits [81], the frequency of which increases with age [82].

Neurologic causes of obstructive uropathy

Although obstructive uropathy can result from tumors of neuroendocrine origin, the predominant neurologic cause of obstruction is any condition that produces a neurogenic bladder. In adults, the most common causes are trauma, neoplasia impinging on the spinal cord, diabetes, tabes dorsalis, multiple sclerosis, and pernicious anemia [83]. In patients with a neurogenic bladder the occurrence of urinary obstruction is most closely linked to whether the patient can be maintained without an indwelling catheter [84]. If the chord is traumatized above the level of S1−S4 a spastic neurogenic bladder will result. A spastic bladder acts as a good reservoir and is responsive to external stimulating devices, thus, such patients may be maintained without a catheter 80−90% of the time. However, if the sacral micturition centers are damaged, a flaccid neurogenic bladder results which generally necessitates the use of catheter drainage, although some patients may remain catheter-free by the use of the Crede maneuver along with increasing abdominal pressure.

Iatrogenic causes of obstructive uropathy

Surgery performed by gynecologists and general surgeons

Surgical complications are the most common iatrogenic cause of obstructive uropathy. The most common operations causing obstruction are shown in Table 19.1 collected from several different reports in the literature [33−38]. Gynecologic surgery is most commonly associated with obstruction. St Martin et al. [85] reviewed all patients undergoing gynecologic surgery at the Shreveport Charity Hospital from 1949−1951. They found evidence of hydronephrosis in 36 out of 332 patients (10.8%) undergoing gynecologic surgery prior to operation, of which three demonstrated a return to normal after operation. However, evidence of obstruction due to intraoperative damage developed in eight (2.4%) of the patients. Three of these had no symptoms of obstruction and might have gone undetected but for the nature of the study. During 1950−1952, 20 patients were studied while undergoing radical hysterectomy for carcinoma of the cervix. Although six of these patients (30%) suffered ureteral damage during the procedure, it should be stressed that carcinoma of the cervix itself, not the operation, remains the most common cause of obstructive uropathy in these patients, even after undergoing radical surgery. The occurrence of ureteral damage during hysterectomy is 3−10 times [38] more likely [34] in abdominal than in vaginal procedures for treatment of cervical cancer [38].

Resection of the colon, particularly associated with an abdominal−perineal resection [36] and resection of an abdominal aortic aneurysm are the two most common causes of iatrogenic ureteral injury in procedures performed by general surgeons.

Obstruction as a result of urologic treatments

In patients treated by urologists, ureteral surgery, ureteroscopy, and transurethral resection of either prostatic or bladder pathology are the most common causes of ureteral damage [38]. Although ileal conduits are frequently performed to relieve obstruction, some degree of obstruction associated with the conduit itself may occur in as much as one-third of cases [86]. Previously, surgical removal of an obstructing stone was a common cause of ureteral injury leading to ureteral stenosis and obstruction, but the advent of shockwave lithotripsy may eventually reduce the number of cases of obstruction due to surgical removal of a stone.

Percutaneous lithotripsy has become a preferred method of treating nephrolithiasis, but the procedure is not without obstructive complications of its own. In fact, in some reports using first generation lithotripters, the incidence of complications was actually somewhat higher than that observed with conventional percutaneous technique [87]. Complications are more likely if the patient has previous ureteral stenosis [88] or if the stones are large. Complications result in more than 20% of patients with stones greater than 20 mm in size [89], although the success rate of second generation lithotripters are somewhat better [90]. Unfortunately, the ureteral obstruction that follows lithotripsy is not invariably symptomatic, and has been reported to cause irreversible renal damage because the lack of symptoms failed to alert either the patient or the physician [91].

The incidence of postprocedure ureteral obstruction of both large [92] and staghorn [93,94] stones treated by lithotripsy can be further reduced by the prophylactic placement of double pigtail ureteral stents. It was initially through this that such stents could work by allowing the passage of stone fragments through the stent. However, it has recently been suggested [95] that the stents actually allow the reflux of urine from the bladder into the renal pelvis during micturition which facilitates the passage of the fragments around, not through, the stent. If this hypotheses is correct, it is obvious that smaller, not larger stents would be more useful. Such prophylactic stent placement can reduce the incidence of complications of large stones from 26% to less than 10% [92].

However, there are some cases (e.g., upper ureteral stones, particularly large stones), and occasions when the collecting system is filled with stone fragments (steinstrasse), which do not respond well to extracorporeal shockwave lithotripsy [96], but are amenable to transurethral ultrasonic ureterolithotripsy utilizing a solid-wire probe [97]. Thus, the various modalities of lithotripsy represent a significant advance in our ability to care for patients with renal stones, and in particular, the elderly [98]. The advent of second generation lithotripters, which employ ultrasound imaging and piezoelectric shockwave generation, will become increasingly important to the treatment of nephrolithiasis in the elderly, because they do not require routine analgesia or sedation, and in the majority of cases the procedure can be performed on outpatients [90].

Obstruction as a result of drugs
In addition to surgical iatrogenic causes of obstruction, drugs can also cause obstructive uropathy. Those which have been implicated include sulfa drugs [99], intravesicular or intrapelvic infusions of a hemiacidrin solution [100] to dissolve struvite stones, or a formalin solution [101] to treat hemorrhagic cystitis. Of drugs used by internists, anticholinergics [102], levodopa, used to treat Parkinson's disease [103], and epsilon aminocaproic acid, used to treat uncontrollable hemorrhage [104] have all been implicated in the causation or obstruction. Aspirin and other cyclo-oxygenase inhibitors are also important. Although interstitial nephritis is the most common renal disease to result from abuse of analgesic preparations containing aspirin and phenacetin, papillary necrosis as well as an increased incidence of carcinomas of the renal pelvis and increased numbers of ureteral strictures, all of which may cause obstruction, are also observed in these analgesic abusers [105].

Signs and symptoms of urinary tract obstruction

Bladder outlet obstruction and bladder hyperreflexia
The symptoms associated with obstruction of the bladder neck and any resulting changes in bladder function are generally divided into those of obstruction and those of bladder irritation [34,106]. Obstructive symptoms include hesitancy, straining, incomplete bladder emptying, de-

creased size and force of stream, and prolonged and intermittent voiding. Irritative symptoms include dysuria, frequency, nocturia, and urgency [106]. Irritative symptoms, in the absence of infection, suggest detrusor hyperreflexia [107]. Work-up of the patient with prostatic disease should look for these symptoms. The physical examination of these patients includes rectal examination to assess the size and consistency of the prostate. The prostate of patients with benign hypertrophy is enlarged and firmer than normal. The consistency of the prostate of those with benign hypertrophy is frequently described as feeling like the tip of the nose, as opposed to the tactile sensation of a knuckle described in patients with prostatic carcinoma. Measurement of residual volume is helpful, but it is essential to stress that patients with bladder hyperreflexia, may actually have rather small volumes as compared to those with normoreflexia [108]. It is important to realize that age plays an important role in the symptomatology of prostatic obstruction. In general, irritative symptoms tend to increase with age, while obstructive symptoms tend to diminish [106]. This decrease in obstructive symptomatology probably reflects adaptation or acceptance rather than any diminution of the obstruction because bladder trabeculation actually increases with age [106]. Urodynamic evaluation has added a quantitative dimension to the evaluation of these symptoms, but there has been great debate as to whether symptoms correlate with these urodynamic findings or not. Thus, whether routine urodynamic evaluation is necessary in the work-up of patients with prostatic disease remains problematic [109].

This is a relatively important question, because patients exhibiting irritative symptoms are much more likely to have a poor symptomatic response to surgery to decrease the size of the prostate. Cote *et al.* [108] reported that 28% of patients with bladder hyperreflexia reported a worsening of symptoms 4 weeks after surgery. By 3 months, although 60% of patients who were hyperreflexic preoperatively became normoreflexic, of the 40% who remained hyperreflexic, seven out of 10 had urgency or stress incontinence and four out of 10 were actually symptomatically worse than preoperatively. All of those who were or who became normoreflexic had no residual symptoms.

It is clear then, that it is important to identify patients with hyperreflexia, and to warn them of possible poor outcome, at least in the immediate postoperative period. Jones & Schoenberg [110] and others [108] report that

50% of patients with significant bladder outlet obstruction have urodynamic evidence of bladder hyperreflexia. The importance of this finding may be questioned because Andersen & Nordling [109] reported a similar incidence in healthy elderly males. One explanation may be that the vast majority of elderly males will have prostatic enlargement [8] but the effects may not cause symptomatic disease, even though more sensitive urodynamic testing will detect changes in bladder function.

An alternative hypothesis is that bladder hyperreflexia is a normal consequence of aging. To test this hypothesis, Jones & Schoenberg [110] compared bladder hyperreflexia in patients with benign prostatic hypertrophy with age-matched female controls who had no evidence of neurologic or other diseases known to produce a hyperreflexic bladder. They found that approximately 10% of aged female patients (without neurologic bladder) had urodynamic evidence of bladder hyperreflexia. Thus some of the residual symptomatology in men operated on for prostatic hypertrophy may be due to the aging process and these symptomatic patients may require pharmacologic therapy to control their symptoms.

In summary, in dealing with patients with prostatic hypertrophy, the absolute indications for surgical correction are: (1) compromised renal function; (2) hydronephrosis; (3) recurrent urinary tract infection; (4) urinary retention; and (5) bladder calculi [34]. Relative indications include: (1) nocturia; (2) decreased force of stream; (3) urinary frequency; and (4) postvoid residual >150 ml [34].

Abnormalities of urine concentration and flow rate

Causative factors
An almost invariant response to urinary tract obstruction of almost any degree or duration is an alteration in the kidney's ability to concentrate the urine. These changes may be mild and restricted to a slight impairment in maximal urine concentration or they may occasionally result in impressive diuretic states during which urine may be either isosmotic to plasma (a solute diuresis) or markedly hypotonic to plasma (a water diuresis). These changes in the kidney's concentrating ability arise from several interacting mechanisms.

Damage to the medullary solute gradient. The osmolality of interstitial fluid in the medulla normally increases in a progressive fashion from the corticomedullary junction to the tip of the papilla. This continually increasing solute gradient is essential to the function of the counter current multiplier of the loop of Henle, which generates the gradient; the counter current exchanger of the vasa recta blood flow, which protects the gradient; and the medullary and papillary collecting ducts which use this gradient to extract water from the tubular fluid so that the urine becomes concentrated. The medullary solute gradient can be disrupted in several ways:

1 active solute reabsorption by the cells of the ascending limb of Henle's loop can be decreased due to damage or by the presence of local or systemic inhibitors of transport;
2 solutes can be removed from the medulla via vasa recta blood flow faster than active reabsorption can replenish them;
3 the effect of vasopressin to increase the permeability of the collecting duct epithelium to water may be blocked by increased local production of counterregulatory hormones such as prostaglandin E_2 (PGE_2) or because the collecting duct cells are unable to respond to vasopressin.

As we will see, all of these occur to some degree at various times after obstruction and will occur irrespective of whether one or both kidneys are obstructed. Thus any type of impairment leads to the most common effect of obstruction—a decrease in maximal urine osmolality. However, most of these changes, in the absence of severe structural damage, will ultimately be corrected if the obstruction is removed.

Alterations of the extracellular environment. Obstruction-induced change to the medullary solute gradient that can decrease maximal urine concentration can be unilateral or bilateral. In contrast, changes in the extracellular environment that affect urine concentration after the obstruction is released require that both kidneys be obstructed. One of the consequences of bilateral or total obstruction is the accumulation of nitrogenous waste products such as urea, leading to uremia. Obstructions may be present for some time before the development of uremia leads to anorexia. During this period there may be continued ingestion of salt and water, such that expansion of the extracellular volume can occur. Finally, factors such as atrial natriuretic peptides or other natriuretic hormonal substances may accumulate. Retention of natriuretic hormonal substances may not be unique to the azotemia of urinary tract obstruction. Nevertheless, release of obstruction before irreversible severe structural damage has occurred to the kidney will permit an effect of those natriuretic/diuretic factors and may lead to a unique and impressively intense rate of urine excretion called postobstructive diuresis (POD).

Damage to the collecting duct epithelium. It is rare that if obstruction is sufficiently prolonged, the epithelium of the collecting tubules in the cortex and the collecting ducts in the papilla may be damaged and become incapable of responding to the action of vasopressin, making them relatively impermeable to water. As a consequence, nephrogenic diabetes insipidus (NDI) results. This type of impairment differs from the very common effect of obstruction to decrease maximal urine concentration. In NDI, the concentration of urine is significantly less than that of plasma; by contrast, alteration of maximal urinary osmolality, as a result of obstruction, leads to urine that is slightly more concentrated than blood.

Decreased maximal urinary concentration
A decreased ability to elaborate maximally concentrated urine occurs in almost all obstructed kidneys. It is rarely a serious problem for the patient although it is probably responsible for the frequency and nocturia which occur quite commonly in patients with chronic, partial urinary tract obstruction. This defect in the concentrating mechanism has been demonstrated in men with unilateral obstruction [111] provided that urine from the two kidneys can be collected separately. Gillenwater *et al.* [111] collected urine from each kidney of 10 adult patients 1 week after surgical repair of unilateral obstructive uropathy, due predominantly to congenital ureteropelvic junction obstruction (UPJ). Urine from the previously obstructed kidney became hypertonic to plasma after administration of exogenous vasopressin, but it was only two-thirds as concentrated as urine from the contralateral normal kidney.

The mechanisms of this defect were explored by studying the ability of the kidney to reabsorb solute-free water ($T^C_{H_2O}$) during a solute diuresis in the presence of exogenous vasopressin, and to excrete solute-free water (C_{H_2O}) during a water diuresis [111]. The previously obstructed kidney reabsorbed significantly less free water at all levels of solute excretion (solute excretion is a measure of the amount of sodium chloride presented to the loop of Henle (i.e., the substrate the kidney uses to

build the medullary concentration gradient)), even when the reabsorption rates were corrected for the decrease in GFR. In fact, some of the samples collected from these previously obstructed kidneys were actually hypotonic to plasma despite the presence of pharmacologic amounts of vasopressin. In contrast, the previously obstructed kidneys excreted essentially identical amounts of free water after correcting for the decrease in their GFRs.

The medullary concentration gradient that enables the kidney to reabsorb solute-free water, is created by solute reabsorption to the exclusion of water in the medullary portions of the loop of Henle. Sodium chloride reabsorption that generates solute-free water excretion in the absence of vasopressin takes place predominantly in the cortical segments of the loop. These data of Gillenwater *et al.* [111] do not allow us to determine precisely whether the concentrating defect occurs because of defective reabsorption of solute in the medullary portions of the loop, because of an inability of the medulla to conserve the reabsorbed solute, or a combination of both. Nevertheless, normal C_{H_2O}, after correction for falls in GFR, suggest that loop solute reabsorption is normal.

Increase in pressure within the nephron does not seem to be the cause of defective reabsorption by the loop since the more distal cortical segments of the loop of Henle do not appear to be more damaged than the more proximal segments within the medulla. Thus, it seems that the decreased concentrating capacity of obstructed kidneys is most likely due to some change in the medullary environment rather than increased pressure. Nevertheless, some studies in experimental animals suggest that relatively brief periods of ureteral obstruction do indeed directly damage the transport mechanism of the collecting tubules [112].

At least two changes in the medullary environment could impair maximal concentration. First, medullary blood flow is increased relative to the delivery of solute from the outer cortical glomeruli. This can be observed immediately after obstruction is produced [113,114] and also when it is corrected, even within 24 hours [115]. This results in a continuous washout of the medullary concentration gradient [116,117] without which the urine cannot be concentrated.

Second, it is well known that the renal medulla is an extremely rich source of PGE_2 and it has been shown that papillary PGE_2 production is increased by an increase in hydrostatic pressure [118]. Stokes has shown [119] that

PGE_2 inhibits chloride reabsorption in the ascending thick limb of Henle's loop. Grantham & Orloff [120] demonstrated that PGE_2 blocks the effect of vasopressin to increase the water permeability of the distal nephron. Thus the effect of obstruction to cause a relative increase in medullary blood flow vs. solute delivery and to increase production of PGE_2 may act in concert to decrease the medullary solute gradient and to subsequently decrease maximal urine concentration.

Postobstructive diuresis (POD)

Clinical characteristics of POD. Postobstructive diuresis is an impressive diuretic and natriuretic state which, unlike the decrease in maximal urine concentration discussed above, is of concern to both the patient and physician. Postobstructive diuresis was first described by Wilson *et al.* in 1951 [121] as a condition which resulted when total, or near total obstruction of both kidneys is first released. This early report described three patients all of whom experienced an impressive diuresis upon release of total obstruction, which was superimposed on a background history of long-standing partial obstruction. Because these patients developed changes in consciousness ranging from drowsiness to coma, flaccid paralysis, acidosis, or other relatively alarming clinical complications during the POD, this condition came to be appreciated as one which could lead to dire consequences. In addition, because "severe salt depletion" was implicated as the cause of these complications, many subsequent patients with this syndrome have been vigorously, or even over-vigorously, treated with replacement fluids in an effort to prevent such dire consequences. Unfortunately, this early report antedated the ability of physicians to routinely measure plasma electrolytes so we do not know the exact reason why the patients described by Wilson *et al.* [121] suffered such alarming complications.

Six years later, Bricker *et al.* [122] gave a complete description of four patients with POD. Several key observations about this condition were noted for the first time. It was noted that it is possible to develop a POD if a single kidney is obstructed, provided that it is the only kidney or if the opposite kidney is so damaged that it contributes little to total renal function. Because obstruction of a single functioning kidney or both functioning kidneys will cause azotemia, this observation clearly

established urinary tract obstruction as a cause of acute azotemia.

Bricker *et al.* [122] also noted that although these patients may present with edema, venous congestive state, or other evidence of ECF volume expansion (two of their four cases), that this is not invariably the case. One of their patients actually presented with clinical evidence of ECF volume contraction. In spite of this, a POD developed when this patient's obstruction was released.

A new observation made in this seminal study was that although POD generally abates in less than a week, an occasional patient will experience a salt-losing state that can last for many months.

Much of our subsequent understanding of this condition has evolved from this study. Because POD occurs after the release of complete, or nearly complete, bilateral obstruction, it has most commonly been described in patients with bladder outlet obstruction due to prostatic disease. The patients usually have a history which suggests partial obstruction for many months, but often relate complete cessation of urination for a period of several days to a week before presentation to their physician. Because of lack of urination, most of these patients will present with azotemia. The retention of urea during the period of obstruction was suggested to be the cause of POD [122] so that, upon release of the obstruction urea excretion leads to an osmotic diuresis. The relation between elevated plasma urea and the onset of POD as well as its diminution as urea levels fall can be seen in a patient described by Peterson *et al.* [123] shown in Figure 19.4(a).

Edema and a venous congestive state have been common factors in patients undergoing POD [122,123]. Because these signs frequently clear up after the cessation of the POD [122–124], postobstructive excretion of retained salt has also been suggested to be important in the causation of the syndrome. Because most of these patients generally continued to ingest food and water during the period of obstruction, even though their urine output is markedly diminished or absent, abnormal sodium retention is not a surprising finding.

Partial chronic urinary tract obstruction can also cause sodium retention. Muldowney *et al.* [124] studied patients with acute or chronic partial urinary tract obstruction. Only one of these patients had a blood urea nitrogen higher than 60, and none had a POD when the obstruction was relieved. Nevertheless, when their total

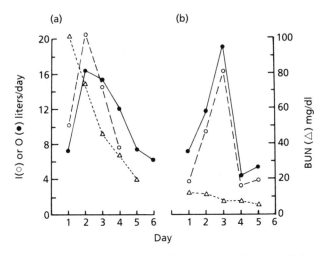

Fig. 19.4 A 76-year-old man with benign prostatic hyperplasia who presented with a normal central venous pressure (2–7 cm H$_2$O) and no evidence of edema. Fluid intake is noted by open circles, urine output by closed circles, and blood urea nitrogen (BUN) by open triangles. The BUN in this patient was initially quite elevated. Note also that for several days his fluid intake originally exceeded output. The BUN concentration decreased during the course of the diuresis; the diuresis abated as the urea concentration fell, suggesting that the postobstructive diuresis (POD) was related to an urea diuresis. In this case the POD may have been aggravated by initial excessive fluid replacement therapy. (b) A 77-year-old man with benign prostatic hypertrophy without edema and a initial BUN concentration which was normal. Note also that fluid intake was always less than urine output. Thus the POD in this patient seems unrelated to either the level of BUN, or to iatrogenic fluid therapy. (From Peterson *et al.* [123].)

extracellular sodium content ([Na]e) was measured using radioactive sodium, and the patients were segregated into acute or chronic groups depending on the duration of their symptoms, two-thirds of the chronic, but none of the acute, patients had significantly increased amounts of extracellular sodium. Despite a normal value for [Na]e, several of the acute patients, as well as all of the chronic patients with increased values, went into negative sodium balance for several days after the relief of their obstructive process. Thus the acute retention of sodium during the anuric phase, added to an already expanded total body burden from the preceding partial obstructed phase, leads to significant sodium accumulation in many of these POD patients. It is important to note that the significant

natriuresis during the POD probably represents a needed readjustment of this excess salt burden.

Although retained urea and sodium play a major, perhaps preponderant, role in the production of POD in most cases, there are some clinical cases which suggest that other factors must also be important. One of these is shown in Figure 19.4(b) [123]. Although this patient's initial blood urea concentration was normal (12 mg/dl), he nevertheless underwent a marked POD with a maximal urine excretion rate of almost 20 liter/day. This case suggests the importance of some other natriuretic factor or factors (other than urea or extracellular volume expansion); but as discussed below, studies in experimental animals are necessary to confirm their importance.

Normally, most patients with a POD will taper off to relatively normal values for urine excretion in a week or less [123]. However, there are well-described cases in both adults [122] and children [125,126] where excessive salt loss can continue for months. As discussed below, POD results largely from the interaction of an abnormal extracellular environment on the postobstructive kidney, and abates as the extracellular environment returns to normal. These relative rare cases of continuing inability to appropriately conserve sodium, or "salt-losing nephritis" (sic), however, occur in the setting of a normal or even salt-depleted environment, and must be due to damage to the tubular epithelium itself.

Management of POD. Although POD is generally a self-limited condition, it can be magnified and prolonged by injudicious fluid and electrolyte replacement therapy. Unfortunately, the first patients with POD, described by Wilson *et al.* [121], not only excreted enormous quantities of urine but several also suffered some acute catastrophic illness. Fortunately, similar catastrophic findings are extraordinarily rare today. There have been attempts to prevent these relatively rare catastrophic changes by the infusion of large volumes of fluids containing salt or glucose, in an attempt to prevent cardiovascular collapse. This results in an iatrogenic-induced osmotic diuresis superimposed on the POD. Because these patients are most often elderly and often have a limited cardiovascular reserve, this unnecessary excessive fluid replacement can not only cause amplification and prolongation of the POD, but may provoke the development of congestive heart failure as well.

There are several reports of dramatically amplified

POD in the literature. Peterson *et al.* [123] describe a patient whose urine output was 36 liters/day due to excessive volume replacement of lost urine with half-normal and normal saline. Even more dramatic is the diuresis described by Witte *et al.* [127] in which the rate of urine loss exceeded 100 liters/day due to use of glucose containing replacement fluids.

The patients reported by Peterson *et al.* [123] and Witte *et al.* [127] were treated in the era prior to the use of balloon-directed catheters to measure pulmonary capillary wedge pressures, and replacement therapy was guided by the physical examination or central venous pressure, both of which may give quite misleading clues as to fluid volume status. In general, most of these patients can be managed without resorting to invasive monitoring techniques. However, if the diuresis appears to be unusually excessive or prolonged, or if the patient appears to be unstable or to have an unknown ECF volume status or limited cardiovascular reserve, then monitoring of the replacement therapy by the measurement of pulmonary capillary wedge pressure is appropriate.

Because the initial isosthenuric urine usually has a sodium concentration in the range of 80 mmol/liter [123] half-normal sodium chloride solution in amounts slightly less than the rate of diuresis is an appropriate starting therapy. It is necessary to continually monitor serum electrolytes because large amounts of univalent and divalent cations such as potassium, calcium, and magnesium may be lost and must be replaced if needed. In addition, prolonged treatment with half-normal saline may result in profound hyponatremia as well as metabolic acidosis due to the loss of bicarbonate. Thus, as the diuresis abates, it may be necessary to switch to isotonic saline in which bicarbonate constitutes at least part of the infused anions. During the height of the POD various workers have attempted to treat patients with either vasopressin or mineralocorticoids. Although these have uniformly proven to be useless during the diuresis [123] they may lead to unwanted salt and water retention after the diuresis has abated, and should be avoided. In the absence of any cardiovascular instability, administration of replacement fluids in amounts somewhat less than excreted will generally produce a smooth and controlled end to the POD provided that the biochemical constituents of the patients' extracellular fluids are carefully monitored and replaced as needed.

Pathogenesis of POD. The pathogenesis of POD has been the subject of intense study. The factors that lead to its production are, as a consequence, fairly well understood. We have knowledge of how conditions within the kidney, particularly changes in renal hemodynamics and local hormone production, are involved. In addition, we have information on the effects of various systemic factors — urea, sodium, and various "natriuretic" hormonal substances in the pathogenesis of POD.

Renal hemodynamic: renal vascular resistance (RVR), renal blood flow (RBF), and GFR are changed in animals undergoing a POD. These changes contribute to causing POD because they decrease the amount of fluid reabsorbed in the nephron, and because they occur in an uneven fashion in different parts of the cortex. The best model for studying these changes in RVR, RBF, and GFR is the release of bilateral ureteral obstruction (BUO) induced in rats, which is always followed by a POD. The contribution of the hemodynamic factors to POD can best be understood by comparing changes in renal hemodynamics in normal rats to those rats studied after the release of BUO and after the release of unilateral ureteral obstruction (UUO). Study of UUO provides a useful comparison to BUO because these animals, although obstructed, do not undergo a POD when the obstruction is released.

Renal hemodynamics influence POD by:
1 changes in the peritubular hydraulic and oncotic pressure; and
2 by redistribution of filtration throughout the superficial and juxtamedullary cortex.

The effects of BUO and UUO on peritubular physical forces are seen in Figure 19.5 [115,128–130]. The balance between peritubular capillary hydraulic pressure, which impedes reabsorption, and peritubular capillary oncotic pressure, which favors it, somehow regulates reabsorption from the nephron. The nature of hydraulic and oncotic pressures in the peritubular capillaries is dependent on the resistance to blood flow in the afferent and efferent arteriole. Because resistances are higher after UUO (see Fig. 19.5a), hydraulic pressure is reduced much more than oncotic pressure and this favors increased reabsorption in UUO vs. BUO (see Fig. 19.5b). Because GFR is also decreased (Fig. 19.6a), the transit time, which reflects the time that tubule fluid is in contact with the reabsorbing epithelium, is markedly prolonged in UUO (see Fig. 19.5c), also favoring increased reabsorption.

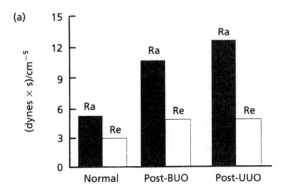

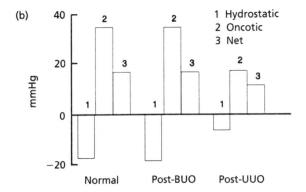

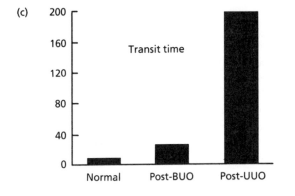

Fig. 19.5 (a) Afferent (Ra) and efferent (Re) arteriolar resistances in normal rats, and in rats following the release of 24 hours of either bilateral ureteral obstruction (BUO) or 24 hours of unilateral ureteral obstruction (UUO). Both afferent and efferent resistances are increased after either BUO or UUO, but Ra is highest after UUO. (b) Pressures in peritubular capillaries favoring reabsorption in normal rats, and in rats following the release of BUO or UUO. Hydrostatic pressure acts to impede fluid reabsorption, while oncotic pressure favors it. The net pressure is the difference between the two and in UUO rats is nearly normal, while that in BUO rats is markedly reduced. (c) Transit times to the end of the proximal tubule in normal, BUO, and UUO rats. These values, obtained in micropuncture studies after the injection of a colored dye which is filtered, are measured from the time the dye first appears in the kidney blood vessels until it reaches the end of the visable portion of the proximal convoluted tubule. Thus it reflects the time that tubule fluid is in contact with the tubular epithelium. The value for UUO rats is an approximation, values ranging from 100 to over 400 seconds have been reported. (From Yarger & Griffith [115], Yarger et al. [128], and Dal Canton et al. [129,130].)

The effect of these changes in RVR and peritubular factors on reabsorption of salt and water in nephrons in the superficial (S) and juxtamedullary (J) cortex are seen in Figure 19.6 [115,129–139]. Much of the water and almost all of the sodium filtered by superficial nephrons in UUO animals is reabsorbed by the end of the distal tubule. This is partially offset by relatively decreased reabsorption in juxtamedullary nephrons. The result is that the volume of urine and the amount of sodium excreted by UUO rats is not markedly different from normal.

In contrast, less sodium and water are reabsorbed by

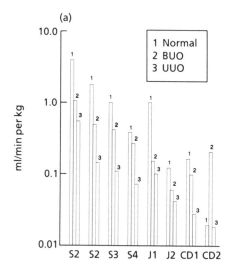

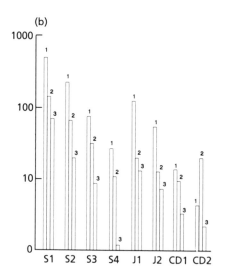

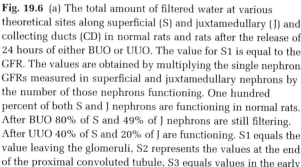

Fig. 19.6 (a) The total amount of filtered water at various theoretical sites along superficial (S) and juxtamedullary (J) and collecting ducts (CD) in normal rats and rats after the release of 24 hours of either BUO or UUO. The value for S1 is equal to the GFR. The values are obtained by multiplying the single nephron GFRs measured in superficial and juxtamedullary nephrons by the number of those nephrons functioning. One hundred percent of both S and J nephrons are functioning in normal rats. After BUO 80% of S and 49% of J nephrons are still filtering. After UUO 40% of S and 20% of J are functioning. S1 equals the value leaving the glomeruli, S2 represents the values at the end of the proximal convoluted tubule, S3 equals values in the early distal tubule, and S4 the end of the distal tubule. J1 equals the filtrate leaving the glomeruli of J nephrons, J2 equals the amount left at the tip of the loop of Henle. CD1 equals values from the collecting duct at the base of the papilla, and CD2 equals the amount of urine flowing into the renal pelvis. (b) The total amount of sodium remaining at various theoretical sites along the nephrons. The symbols are the same as those used in Fig. 19.6(a). (From Yarger & Griffith [115], Dal Canton *et al.* [129−131], Buerkert *et al.* [132], Jaenike [133], Buerkert *et al.* [134], McDougal & Wright [135], Wilson [136], Buerkert *et al.* [137,138], and Sonnenberg [139].)

superficial and juxtamedullary nephrons of BUO rats. The greatest change, however, is the net addition of sodium and water as urine flows through the collecting ducts. These changes in the collecting duct are probably unrelated to hemodynamics, but may relate to the effect of obstruction on the tubular epithelium and to some circulating natriuretic hormonal factor(s) [139].

The decrease in reabsorption of fluid by juxtamedullary nephrons probably results from both altered hemodynamic forces and changes in intrarenal PGE_2 production. Prostaglandin E_2 production by the renal medullar is increased during obstruction [118]. The hydronephrotic kidney also produces an increased amount of this eicosanoid vasodilator after the obstruction is released [140−142]. This eicosanoid could effect postobstructive renal salt and water excretion in two ways. Firstly, it could lead to vasodilatation of the efferent arterioles of juxtamedullary nephrons as it is carried up into the cortex by fluid in the ascending limb of the loop of Henle [143]. Secondly, PGE_2 can inhibit NaCl reabsorption in the ascending limb of Henle's loop [119].

The potential effect of PGE_2 on juxtamedullary resistance has been studied by Harris & Yarger [144] in two ways (Figs 19.7 and 19.8). Firstly, as seen in Figures 19.7A−D, normal and obstructed kidneys are studied after ferrocyanide injection. Ferrocyanide is a compound which the kidney excretes in a fashion essentially identically to inulin and thus can be used to reflect GFR. If the kidney is snap frozen several seconds after the intravenous injection of a bolus of ferrocyanide, and then treated with ferric chloride, both the filtered ferrocyanide as well as the ferrocyanide remaining in peritubular blood is converted to an insoluble colored product, prussian blue (PB). The appearance of PB throughout the kidney reflects the distribution of filtered tubule fluid and peritubular blood at the moment when the ferro-

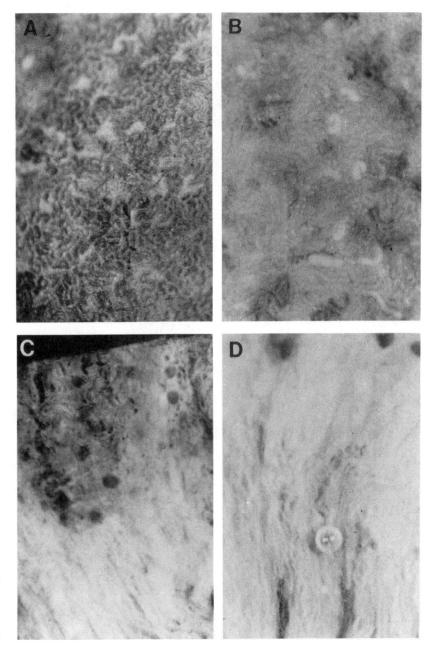

Fig. 19.7 Injection of sodium ferrocyanide into normal (A and C) and UUO (B and D) rats. The kidneys are frozen and treated with alcoholic ferric chloride, which converts the ferrocyanide to an insoluble blue precipitate, prussian blue (PB). A, Capsular surface of a normal rat kidney; PB is visible in nearly all superficial nephrons. B, Capsular surface of UUO kidneys; note absence on PB in most tubules. C, Sagittal surface of normal rat kidney. Cortex is at the top and the medulla at the bottom. Prussian blue is present in nearly all nephrons and peritubular capillaries in the juxtamedullary cortex, as well as in the vasa recta. D, Sagittal surface of UUO kidneys. Prussian blue is virtually absent in juxtamedullary proximal tubules and their peritubular capillaries, but is present in juxtamedullary glomeruli and vasa recta. C and D are nonplanar fracture surfaces; as a consequence some areas are out of focus. (From Harris & Yarger [144].)

cyanide was injected. As shown in Figure 19.7 the distribution of GFR and RBF through normal and obstructed kidneys can be visualized. The second method, shown in Figure 19.8 involves filling the renal vasculature with a silicone rubber compound which has a viscosity close to

that of blood and which, upon polymerization, will mark the vascular space. The kidneys are then fixed, clarified, and sectioned so that a definition of RBF distribution at the time of injection can be seen.

Examination of Figures 19.7D and 19.8B demonstrates

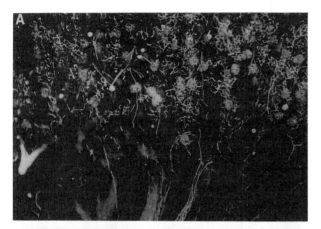

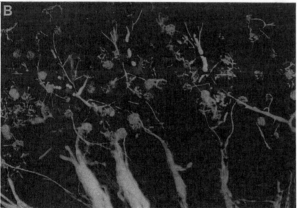

Fig. 19.8 Arterial tree of a normal right kidney (A) and a previously obstructed left kidney (B) of a rat injected with silicone rubber. The cortical tissue was clarified by dehydration with alcohol and treatment with methylsalicylate. The previously obstructed kidney demonstrates multiple areas of poorly filled, or unfilled capillaries in the outer cortex. There is virtually no filling of the peritubular capillaries in the juxtamedullary cortex, although the juxtamedullary glomeruli and vasa recta are well filled. (From Harris & Yarger [144].)

that most of the blood leaving the juxtamedullary glomeruli enters the vasa recta, and not the peritubular capillaries in the inner cortex. This probably decreases reabsorption by the proximal tubules of these deep nephrons because there is less blood around the convoluted segment of the proximal tubules to reabsorb the filtrate.

Natriuretic factors in the extracellular fluid: although the effects of renal hemodynamics just discussed un-

doubtedly help to cause POD, the major factors responsible for POD do not originate within the kidney. The primary effectors of POD are several natriuretic factors found in the extracellular fluid. There are three natriuretic factors which have been clearly linked to POD; these are urea, sodium, and atrial natriuretic peptides. In addition, a fourth, as yet uncharacterized natriuretic hormone also appears to be important.

Urea: as noted above, studies of patients [122] were the first to suggest that urea was important in POD. However, early attempts to establish the importance of urea in POD using experimental animals, were confusing. It was hypothesized that elevated blood urea concentrations interacted with a previously obstructed kidney to cause a POD. Infusions of urea into experimental animals with renal obstruction [128] led to the excretion of large amounts of urine with a high urea concentration from the normal kidney, but the previously obstructed kidney did not undergo a POD, despite the presence of elevated plasma urea concentrations. It was subsequently learned that RBF of the previously obstructed kidney is exquisitely sensitive to the effects of intravascular volume contraction [145,146]. Thus, these early studies of urea infusion and elevated blood urea concentrations failed to produce a POD from a single previously obstructed kidney, because RBF and GFR of that kidney were markedly decreased. These severe hemodynamic changes resulted because the urea-induced osmotic diuresis by the normal kidney contracted the ECV. Harris & Yarger [146] subjected UUO rats to a continuous urea infusion during the 24 hours of obstruction, but they prevented volume contraction by continually infusing a quantity of water, salt, and urea equal to that lost in the urine of the normal contralateral kidney (see Fig. 19.9). Under these conditions, after release of the UUO, the previously obstructed kidney underwent a massive POD similar in all ways to that seen in bilaterally obstructed animals. In other rats, these workers prevented extracellular volume contraction by the reinfusion of the actual urine excreted by the normal kidney during the period of obstruction. Here too, they observed a POD when the UUO was released. These studies demonstrate that urea is an important cause of POD, provided the ECF volume does not become contracted. However, as we will see shortly, these latter experiments where urine was reinfused, led to some surprising results.

Sodium: in addition to urea, sodium has also been

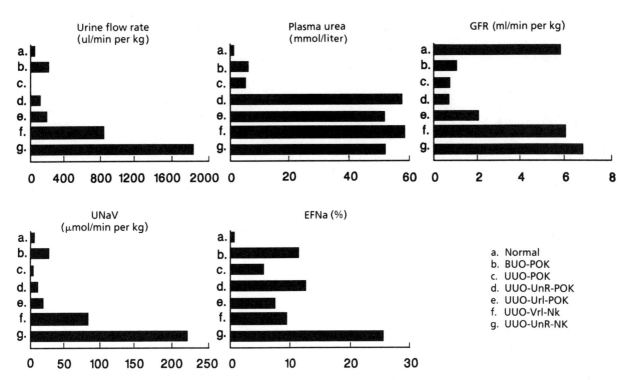

Fig. 19.9 (a) Urine flow rate from: (a) the kidneys of normal rats (Normal); (b) one of the previously obstructed kidney (POK) of rats which had been subjected to 24 hours of bilateral ureteral obstruction (BUO−POK); (c) the POK of rats previously subjected to 24 hours of unilateral ureteral obstruction (UUO), but without any infusions administered during the 24 hours of obstruction (UUO−POK); (d) the POK of rats subjected to UUO which had the urine from its unobstructed kidney continuously reinfused (UnR) during the 24 hours of the obstructive period (UUO−UnR−POK); (e) the POK of rats subjected to UUO who received a continuous infusion of a solution of urea, sodium, and potassium (UrI) equal to urinary losses from the normal kidney during the 24 hours of the obstructive period (UUO−UrI−POK); (f) the normal unobstructed kidney (NK) of the rats in Group 4 which were subjected to urine reinfusion (UUO−UnR−NK); and (g) the NK of the rats in Group 5 which received the urea infusion (UUO−UrI−NK). Note the significant POD in the BUO−POK kidneys as compared with either the Normal or UUO−POK kidneys. The urine flow rate in the UUO−POK rats is very small. Note also that the POD from the POK of both the UUO−UnR−POK and the UUO−UrI−POK rats is comparable to that of the BUO−POK rats, i.e., a POD. Finally, note that the diuresis from the NK of the UUO−UnR−NK rats, which underwent urine reinfusion, is enormous and is much greater than that from the NK of the UUO−UrI−NK rats which received the urea solution infusion. (b) Plasma urea concentrations in these same groups of rats as in (a) above. Note that plasma urea concentration is similar in the BUO rats and the UUO rats which receiver underwent urine reinfusion (UnR) or infusion of a urea solution (UrI). (c) Glomerular filtration rate in the same groups of rats. Note the significant reductions of GFR in the BUO−POK, UUO−POK rats and the UUO−UnR−POK rats which underwent urine reinfusion. The GFR of the UUO−UrI−POK rats which received the urea infusion is greater than that of any of the other UUO−POK groups. Note that in contrast to its lack of effect on the POK, urine reinfusion increases GFR in the NK of the UUO−UnR−NK rats above that seen in Normal rats, although urea infusion to the UUO−UrI−NK rats does not. (d) Absolute sodium excretion ($U_{Na}V$) in the kidneys of these different groups of rats. (e) Fraction of filtered sodium excreted in the urine (EF_{Na}). Note that although both urea infusion (UrI) and urine reinfusion (UnR) increase absolute and fractional excretion of sodium by both the POK and the NK, that there is an enormous natriuresis from the NK of UnR rats (UUO−UnR−NK), even though the plasma urea concentrations, and presumably the urea osmotic diuresis, are comparable to that of the UUO−NrI−NK kidneys.

implicated in the production of a POD [124]. Wilson [147] infused hypotonic saline solution into rats previously subjected to chronic partial UUO. He observed that the previously obstructed kidney excreted almost twice as much urine under these conditions as the contralateral kidney which had not been obstructed, even though its GFR was 40% lower than that of the normal kidney. These data suggest that the previously obstructed kidney is also quite sensitive to the effects of volume expansion, so that patients with bilateral obstruction, who present with evidence of excess total body sodium, may undergo an increased rate of POD in response to extracellular volume expansion.

The data of Wilson [147], Huguenin et al. [145], and Harris & Yarger [146] suggest that the postobstructive kidney is extraordinarily sensitive to the effects of both ECF volume contraction and expansion. Two clinically relevant points can be derived. Firstly, the treating physician can take some comfort from the tendency of the obstructed kidney to markedly decrease its rate of filtration and excretion under conditions of intravascular volume contraction, because it is likely that renal function will slow before serious volume depletion can affect other parts of the cardiovascular system. Thus, excessive fluid replacement therapy to prevent cardiovascular collapse is rarely needed and fluids can thus be given more judiciously.

Secondly, the astonishing rates of urine excretion that can occasionally be achieved in patients undergoing a POD almost certainly represent the sensitivity of those kidneys to the effects of volume expansion. This heightened response to increased ECF volume is probably mediated in part by the third known natriuretic factor, atrial natriuretic peptide.

Atrial natriuretic peptide (ANP): a role of ANP in POD was first suggested by Fried et al. [148]. These workers measured plasma ANP levels in normal rats, and in rats previously subjected to 24 hours of either unilateral or bilateral ureteral obstruction. Atrial natriuretic peptide levels in UUO rats who do not undergo a POD (see Fig. 19.9a) were not different from normal, but levels in BUO rats were significantly greater than normal.

A further link between ANP and POD was made by Olsen et al. [149] who demonstrated that the previously obstructed kidney of rats subjected to UUO is unusually sensitive to the natriuretic effects of ANP. They showed

that ANP infused into rats previously subjected to UUO increased urinary salt and water losses by 600%. Excretion of sodium and water by the normal kidney also increased, but by a different mechanism. While part of the POD from the previously obstructed kidney (POK) was due to a 300% increase in GFR of that kidney in response to ANP, GFR of the normal kidney did not increase, even though the excretion of salt and water did. Thus GFR of the POK seems particularly responsive to ANP.

A probable corollary of this sensitivity of POKs to ANP in humans was observed by Peterson et al. [123]. One of their patients, a 64-year-old man, presented with a blood urea nitrogen of 144 mg/dl. Injudicious fluid replacement in this patient with sodium-containing fluids caused him to excrete almost 36 liters or urine per day for 2 days. Despite the level of azotemia on admission, inulin and *P*-aminohippurate clearances measured during the height of the diuresis were supranormal (157 and 633 ml/min, respectively). Clearly, this man had some stimulus to increase, not only urinary salt and water losses, but also GFR and RBF. In light of the work of Olsen et al. [149] the most likely explanation is that ANP is stimulated by the massive levels of fluid infused.

These studies of Olsen et al. [149] perhaps explain massive iatrogenic POD in some patients, but they do not shed light on the mechanisms of increased ANP levels in BUO. The rats in the study of Fried et al. [148] were deprived of food and water during the obstructive period and thus were ECF volume contracted. Extracellular fluid volume expansion is the usual stimulus to endogenous ANP secretion therefore increased levels of the peptide in these BUO rats may relate to some other factor, such as decreased degradation. Condra et al. [150] have demonstrated that 85% of infused ANP is cleared within a few seconds by an undefined mechanism. The remainder is slowly degraded enzymatically, principally by the kidney.

Another mechanism by which ANP may mediate POD is through the natriuretic eicosanoid PGE_2 and PGI_2 [142]. Himmelstein et al. [151] have shown that ANP infused into hydronephrotic kidneys increases the production of these vasodilator and natriuretic eicosanoids. Thus, bilateral obstruction may lead to the accumulation of undegraded ANP that causes increased release of vasodilator prostaglandin, which increases GFR and RBF after the obstruction is released. These eicosanoids may also act by inhibiting sodium reabsorption in the ascending limb of Henle's loop. Finally, ANP itself may also act to block solute reabsorption.

Uncharacterized natriuretic hormone: in addition to urea, sodium, and ANP a fourth factor may be involved in POD. The urine reinfusion studies of Harris & Yarger [146] noted above have provided direct evidence for the existance of a natiuretic hormone unrelated to ANP. These workers noted that a comparable POD from the previously obstructed kidney was seen when plasma urea levels were maintained by infusion of an artificial solution to replace lost urea, water, and salt, or when plasma urea was maintained by simply reinfusing the urine from the opposite kidney (see Fig. 19.9). Thus the previously obstructed kidney responded to elevated urea from any source provided ECF volume contraction was prevented. But the response of the normal kidney was markedly different.

The rate of salt and water excretion by the normal contralateral kidney of rats infused with either the urea/salt solution or urine was quite increased, as might be expected from a kidney undergoing an osmotic diuresis of urea. Yet, despite comparably normal ECF volumes and plasma sodium concentrations, and despite comparably elevated plasma urea concentrations, sodium excretion by the normal kidney in animals infused with their own urine was two to three times as much as that by the kidney of rats receiving a salt/urea solution. This observation suggests that a potent natriuretic factor(s), is retained in the circulation when falls in urine flow, such as those seen in acute renal failure and BUO occur. When the substances are returned to the circulation by urine reinfusion they are capable of producing an intense diuresis particularly from normal kidneys.

There are several reasons to believe that this substance is neither ANP nor urea nor sodium. Firstly, ANP is a peptide, and is destroyed as it passes through the kidney. Secondly, ANP and sodium (or perhaps volume expansion) appear to have their main effect on the previously obstructed, not the normal kidney. Finally the effect of urea on the normal kidney cannot explain this phenomenon since urea infusion would have been expected to duplicate the natriuresis of urine reinfusion. In summary, there appears to be a natriuretic substance which survives passage through the kidney, which is intensely natriuretic and which, if retained in blood as a result of complete urinary obstruction, may contribute to the production of a POD.

Nephrogenic diabetes insipidus (NDI)

While a decrease in maximal urinary concentration is almost universal in obstructed patients and common in POD, NDI is very uncommon. It has been noted by studies in both man [111,152] and experimental animals [147] that although the ability of the previously obstructed kidney to reabsorb free water is markedly deranged, the ability to excrete free water in dilute urine is either normal, or even supranormal. Several factors are required for the kidney to be able to excrete urine of an osmolality significantly less than that of plasma. First, the ability of the ascending limb of Henle's loop and of the collecting ducts to reabsorb sodium chloride against a gradient is required to lower the osmolality of tubular fluid. Secondly, antidiuretic hormone (vasopressin) must be absent, or the kidney must be resistant to its effects. This latter condition is referred to as a NDI.

As has already been mentioned, NDI following urinary tract obstruction is very rare [153–157]. Roussak & Oleesky [154] first described NDI in patients with chronic urinary tract obstruction. Taken together [153–157], the cases of NDI differ from POD is several ways. Firstly, urine specific gravity ranges from 1.000 to 1.004, unlike POD where urine is characteristically isothermic (1.010). Secondly, urine flow rates range from 3–6 liters/day, which is significantly less than seen in POD. Thirdly, these patients rarely present with acute renal failure but, like patients who present with POD, often have a prolonged history of obstructive symptoms. Finally, unlike POD which generally abates in a few days, patients with NDI will continue to excrete an inappropriately dilute urine for many months.

In vitro perfusion of isolated cortical collecting tubule of UUO rats [112] demonstrate that the normal ability of vasopressin to increase hydro-osmotic conductivity is impaired in this segment of the nephron at a biochemical locus beyond the point of cAMP generation.

In summary, POD appears to be a response of the kidney to expansion of the extracellular fluid and abates as correction of this abnormality is achieved. Nephrogenic diabetes insipidus, however, develops after longer periods of symptomatic obstruction and takes much longer to correct itself than POD after the obstruction is relieved. These observations suggest that NDI results not from changes in the ECF but from damage to the epithelium of the distal nephron, as shown in animal studies [112].

Defects of urinary acidification

A number of integrated actions must occur before the kidney can accomplish the two main objectives of renal hydrogen ion excretion:

1 reclamation of filtered bicarbonate;
2 excretion of protons equal to the acid ingested in the normal human diet.

In the proximal tubules these functions are accomplished by hydrogen ion secretions sufficient to reclaim most of the filtered bicarbonate. It remains for the distal tubule to reclaim the small amount of remaining bicarbonate, titrate divalent anions, principally phosphate ("titratable acidity"), convert uncharged ammonia (NH_3) to charged ammonium ions (NH_4^+), and lower the pH of the urine to a level substantially lower than blood. The amount of hydrogen ion excreted as titratable acidity and ammonium ion, minus any unreclaimed bicarbonate represents net acid excretion and over time should equal the excess of metabolic acids ingested in the diet. Because the amount of phosphate in the urine is limited by the diet and GFR, the main renal defense against chronic acidosis, is the kidney's ability to increase ammonia production when stimulated by an acidic environment.

In the cortical collecting tubule (CCT) segment of the distal nephron, hydrogen ion secretion is linked to the reabsorption of sodium and to intraluminal negativity. Aldosterone acts on the distal nephron to facilitate sodium reabsorption as well as bulk proton and potassium secretion. In the medullary collecting duct, protons are secreted in even greater amounts than in the CCT and also move against an electrical gradient [158].

Obstructive nephropathy can alter all of the acidification functions, although, in general, derangement of distal acidification is more common than decreased proximal tubule function. Proximal RTA (Type II), or bicarbonate wasting RTA, is relatively uncommon, but has been reported in association with renal salt wasting in infants [126,159], and temporarily during POD in adults [160].

Several different types of distal RTA have been described in patients with obstructive nephropathy; these include classic (Type I) distal RTA as well as a variety of distal acidification failures which differ from Type I RTA in that the latter is generally associated with hypokalemia, while those most commonly seen in obstructive nephropathy are generally associated with hyperkalemia. These hyperkalemic forms of RTA can be produced by several mechanisms including:

1 aldosterone deficiency of 10 associated with absolute or relative hyporeninemia;
2 tubular resistance to the effects of aldosterone;
3 a distal defect in the ability to reabsorb sodium, linked to impaired hydrogen ion secretion against the pH gradient normally present in the distal nephron.

There are several tests for investigating the mechanism of distal RTA. The most common is performed with an infusion of either excess bicarbonate or phosphate, during which the partial pressure of CO_2 in the urine is measured [161]. When hydrogen ions are secreted in the distal nephron, the dehydration of H_2CO_3 to CO_2 and H_2O is not enzymatically catalyzed and proceeds sufficiently slowly so that the CO_2 formed is trapped in the urine in the collecting ducts by the counter current exchanger action of the vasa recta. If distal delivery of either bicarbonate or phosphate is sufficient and the distal nephron is capable of secreting hydrogen ions normally, then the urinary P_{CO_2} will be significantly higher than blood. Erricsson et al. [159] first described distal RTA in children with urinary tract obstruction, who were hyperchloremic and who exhibited features of classic distal RTA since they could not acidify their urine, even in the presence of a systemic acidosis. Later, Hutchenson et al. [161] studied nine patients with various degrees of renal hydronephrotic changes. Six of these presented with acidosis and mild renal insufficiency, but three had normal pH and filtration on admission. When urine P_{CO_2} was compared to blood P_{CO_2} during bicarbonate loading, all of the acidotic and two of the nonacidotic patients had very low urine–blood P_{CO_2} comparable to those seen in patients with Classic (Type I) distal RTA (DRTA). Kurtzman [158] demonstrated that periods of ureteral obstruction in the dog as short as 24 hours are capable of inducing this defect in distal hydrogen ion secretion.

Although the classic form of distal RTA can be observed in patients with obstructive nephropathy, it is much more common to observe a hyperkalemic form of distal RTA. Obstructive hyperkalemic RTA in children is frequently associated with aldosterone resistance [125, 126,162]. These children often present with alarming degrees of hyperkalemia, markedly elevated aldosterone concentrations, and plasma renin activity. This type of aldosterone resistance in children is often associated with both obstructive nephropathy and pyelonephritis, and the exact contribution of each is in some doubt because the acidosis occasionally responds to antibiotic treatment.

In adults, hyperkalemic distal RTA has been seen both with aldosterone resistance [163] and deficiency [164, 163]. Although the patients described by Pelleya et al. [163] presented with decreased aldosterone levels and hyperkalemic acidosis in association with urinary tract obstruction, they did not respond to treatment with supraphysiologic levels of mineralocorticoid, thereby demonstrating both aldosterone deficiency and resistance.

Battle et al. [164] described an interesting group of 13 adult patients, ranging in age from 51–73 years, who presented with unexplained hyperkalemia. All were known to have obstructive nephropathy or it was discovered during the work-up of their hyperkalemia. Because of the age of the patients involved, it is not surprising that prostatic obstruction was the most common cause of obstruction in these patients. After induction of a systemic metabolic acidosis, five of these patients were able to lower their urine pH below 5.5, and thus did not have Type I distal RTA. The plasma aldosterone concentrations in these five patients were reduced along with low or inappropriately normal renin levels, even after volume contraction induced by furosemide administration. These patients are thus similar to patients with Type IV (hyporenin–hypoaldosterone) RTA originally described by Sebastian et al. [165]. The acidosis in these cases appears to be caused by inhibition of ammoniagenesis by the hyperkalemia, since the acidosis can frequently be corrected by the use of potassium/sodium exchange resin [166].

The other eight patients were unable to lower the urine pH to less than 5.5, and hence had distal RTA. Three of these had hypoaldosteronism, indicating that lack of mineraldocorticoid was a contributory factor in these patients. In addition the mechanism of hyperkalemia in these patients was investigated by infusing sodium sulfate. When the sodium moiety is reabsorbed in the CCT, the negatively charged sulfate remains, leading to intense intraluminal electronegativity. In normal people, this intraluminal negativity greatly increases the secretion of protons and potassium ions and, as a result, urine pH

is often less than 5.0 and potassium excretion is greatly augmented. However, sulfate infusions in the obstructed patients did not lower urine pH or increase potassium secretion, suggesting a primary defect in the secretory process in the distal nephron. Kurtzman [158] produced a very similar type of acidosis in dogs by the use of amiloride, a diuretic which blocks sodium entry into cells of the distal nephron. This suggests that impaired distal-sodium reabsorption may be the final common pathway which causes both the hyperkalemia and acidosis in this group of patients. Thus urinary tract obstruction can lead to a variety of different types of renal tubular acidosis, most of which are associated with hyperkalemia.

Urinary tract obstruction can often be occult since several patients have been discovered to have obstructive uropathy only after undergoing a work-up for unexplained hyperkalemia [164]. We have seen two cases of hyperkalemia in renal transplant recipients with new onset azotemia in which the hyperkalemia seemed out of proportion to the degree of impairment of GFR. Both of these patients failed to respond to antirejection therapy but had significant decreases in plasma potassium when a partially obstructed ureter was stented. Thus the presence of unexplained hyperkalemia, particularly in the elderly with prostatic disease, should always prompt an exploration for silent obstruction.

Recovery of function after relief of obstruction

Relation between duration of obstruction and recovery of function

Physicians caring for a patient with unilateral renal obstruction must determine whether an attempt should be made to correct the cause, and if so, how rapidly recovery may occur. Studies in experimental animals often suggest that irreversible hydronephrosis and functional loss of the kidney can occur rapidly. Although GFR and urine flow are almost unmeasurable in the rat after 7 days of complete UUO, GFR can increase to about 40% of normal 2 weeks after release of UUO [167]. If the normal contralateral kidney is removed when the ureter is deligated, recovery approaches 60%. However, if the kidney is obstructed for 3 weeks in this model less than 10% of function returns [167]. The effect of semiacute UUO on dogs is less severe. After 7 days of obstruction, the GFR immediately after release is approximately 25% of normal and approaches 65% at the time of maximal recovery [168]. After 2 weeks of obstruction in dogs maximal recovery peaks at 45% of normal at 4 months [169].

These data in animals, however, are not strictly comparable to man. Shapiro & Bennett [170] report three patients who had been obstructed, two patients for 28 days and one patient for 150 days. All of these patients demonstrated some return of function within a week, and the patient who was obstructed for 150 days showed even further return 6 months later. The obstruction was due to a stone (two cases) or blood clot lodged in a ureter. The degree of ureteral obstruction could not be determined, and thus may not be comparable to animal models with complete obstruction. Nevertheless, Lewis & Pierce [171] report the case of a woman whose ureter was completely occluded during an emergency hysterectomy and freed 69 days later. Despite this prolonged period of total obstruction, her renal function as assessed by a radioactive hippuran scan 19 months later demonstrated essentially normal function. Better *et al.* [152] reported a similar case of ureteral ligation during emergency surgery to control uterine bleeding. In this case the ureter was not deligated for 3 months. Glomerular filtration rate from the previously obstructed kidney was 2.6 ml/min shortly after deligation and rose to a maximum value of 11.3 ml/min 25 days later, without further improvement.

Time for maximum return of function after release of obstruction

Kerr [172] studied dogs after 4 weeks of unilateral ureteral ligation. They showed that functional improvement was never complete and ceased at about 40 days. Reports of the effects of acute obstruction in patients, however, are somewhat more encouraging. Nelson & Williams [173] reported a patient with renal failure due to severe right interstitial nephritis and severe left hydronephrosis resulting from stone-induced renal pelvis obstruction. Despite a well-draining nephrostomy tube, no urine was excreted by the previously obstructed kidney for up to 9 days after pyelolithotomy and dialysis was instituted. Ten weeks later, however, the kidney began to excrete copious amounts of urine and GFR rose to 25 ml/min allowing the discontinuation of dialysis, suggesting that significant recovery can occur after more prolonged times of obstruction. However, it should be noted that Kerr

[172] as well as Provoost & Molenaar [167] have shown that removal of the normal contralateral kidney in experimental animals can cause further functional improvement of the previously obstructed kidney, as late as 1 year after deligation. Removal of the normal kidney causes severe azotemia, which seems to facilitate the increase in GFR of the previously hydronephrotic kidney, even though the functional impairment appeared to have stabilized. Thus, the time course of recovery, as well as its degree, can be modulated by a uremic environment, which may explain the prolonged recovery period of the patient reported by Nelson & Williams [173].

Prediction of recovery

Attempts to assess anatomic integrity of the kidney to decide, by various imaging techniques, whether to repair or remove a seriously damaged kidney are often confusing. Ibrahim and Fahal [174] used urine pH from the affected kidney of patients with unilateral hydronephrosis to predict recoverability. All patients who could acidify their urine to a pH less than 6.0 had good evidence of radiologic recovery of function, 25% with urine pH in the range of 6.0−7.1 demonstrated good recovery and 50% showed some recovery. Recovery did not occur in patients with urine pH greater than 7.1. McDougal & Flanigan [175] used technetium-labeled dimercaptosuccinic acid to predict recovery in experimental animals subjected to UUO, and demonstrated that increased uptake of the nucleotide correlated with improved chance of recovery.

Diagnosis of urinary tract obstruction

There is a wide variety of imaging techniques available to assist in the diagnosis of obstructive uropathy and nephropathy. Their usefulness depends on the stage of the disease and its relationship to the diagnostic procedure. Each technique should be considered on the basis of several important qualities as shown in Table 19.2.

Renal ultrasound (US)

Gray-scale ultrasonography has become the preferred screening method in the diagnosis of urinary tract obstruction. Its preferred position as a screening tool derives from its ease of use, its safety—neither ionizing radiation nor nephrotoxic contrast agents are used—and its high

Table 19.2 The characteristics of various imaging modalities in patients with renal obstruction

Characteristic/test	US	IVU	RP	AP	CT	RNI	MRI
Ease of use	++++	+++	+	++	++	+++	−−
Safety	++++	++	+	+	+++	+++	++++
Cost	++++	+++	+	+	++	++	−−
Spatial resolution	+	++++	++++	++++	++++	−−	+++
Assess function	−−	+++	−−	−−	+	++++	?+
Sensitivity	+	+++	+++	++++	++++	++	?
Specificity	++++	++++	+++	+++	++	+++	?
Assist therapy	−	−	−	++++	−	−	−
Use in azotemia	++++	+	++	++++	++	++	?

US, renal ultrasound; IVU, intravenous urogram; RP, retrograde pyelogram; AP, antegrade pyelogram; CT, computerized tomogram; RNI, radionuclide imaging techniques (there are several different techniques used as discussed in the text); MRI, magnetic resonance imaging (at the present time this is essentially a research tool).
++++ to +, very beneficial or useful to only modestly beneficial; −, neutral or of little or no benefit; −−, negative impact or ill-advised for this purpose.

degree of specificity. A test with a high degree of specificity, that is, true negative test results divided by all of the patients without the disease, is important in a screening test. The specificity of renal ultrasound has been reported to range from 93−100% [176,177] depending on what "gold standard" was used to diagnose obstruction. Stated another way, only 0−7% of patients who are not obstructed will be misdiagnosed as being obstructed by ultrasound. Although this is an acceptably high level of specificity for a screening test, obviously some obstructed patients will be missed. Thus, the treating physician should retain some skepticism even in the face of an apparently negative test. This is particularly true if the patient is known to have staghorn calculi or nephrocalcinosis [178], retroperitoneal fibrosis [179], or intravascular volume contraction, particularly in patients with bilateral obstruction, because these conditions are most often associated with a false negative renal sonogram.

Although renal ultrasound is an acceptable screening tool to rule out the presence of obstruction in most cases, it is not particularly useful for showing that obstruction is present. Reports of its sensitivity (true positive tests divided by all the patients with the disease) have been reported to range from 80−92% [180], meaning that 8−20% of patients will be falsely identified as having disease. Such false positive tests can arise because of anatomic variants of kidney structure, such as an extrarenal pelvis, from failure to empty the bladder before

testing, or from any drug or condition which causes the patient to undergo a diuresis [181].

Renal ultrasound also fails to identify the site of obstruction in most cases because of its poor spatial resolution. It also gives no information about the functional capacity (degree of function during obstruction) or reserve (degree of anticipated return of function after release of obstruction).

Thus, renal ultrasound is a good screening tool given the previously expressed caveats. However, once a patient is suspected of having obstruction, other tests are required to establish the exact site of obstruction, its cause, and the resultant effect on renal function and capacity to recover.

Intravenous urography (IVU) retrograde (RP), and antegrade pyelography (AP)

Once the possibility of obstructive uropathy has been suggested, techniques with good spatial resolution are required to determine the site of obstruction, as well as to help diagnose the cause. Intravenous urography is frequently used to better define the anatomy of the obstructive process in the absence of significant degrees of azotemia or other disease processes, such as multiple myeloma or diabetes, known to increase the risk of intravenous contrast-agent-induced nephropathy [182]. Some workers have suggested that high-dose intravenous urography can reveal renal anatomy even in the presence of severe azotemia, but more recent work suggests that this is true less than half of the time [182]. In the absence of azotemia, however, intravenous urography is a good method for identifying the site and often the cause of obstruction. In addition, the nephrogram phase of the study and the speed with which dye appears in the collecting system gives a reasonable estimate of renal function.

If azotemia or other diseases preclude the use of IVU, either RP or AP can be used to define the anatomy of the urinary collecting system. Retrograde pyelography is useful, particularly in unilateral obstruction if the ureters can be successfully catheterized from below. However, in the presence of total or near total obstruction of the ureter, this technique may not adequately define the degree of pelvocaliectasis of the upper collecting system because dye cannot pass the point of obstruction. Under such circumstances, and perhaps in most patients whose level of renal function precludes IVU, antegrade pyelography is the preferred method of outlining the upper tract. Fluoroscopic or ultrasonographic placement of catheters percutaneously into the renal pelvis has several advantages. Firstly, if fine needles are used, the risk of significant bleeding or other complications are probably less than 5% [183]. Excellent definition of the renal pelvis and calyces as well as the ureter down to the point of obstruction are obtained. Finally, in the presence of a totally obstructed ureter, antegrade pyelography can be the initial step in the placement of percutaneous nephrostomy tubes to provide adequate drainage to an obstructed kidney, thereby stopping obstructive damage. Unfortunately, neither type of pyelography provides any estimate or renal function.

Computed tomography (CT)

Computed tomograms of the abdomen also have excellent spatial resolution. If sufficient cuts are obtained, the site and often the cause of obstruction can be determined. In the presence of azotemia, the dilated renal pelvis and calyces can be visualized without contrast media. Thus CT is a sensitive technique for diagnosing the site and cause of obstruction [184]. However, even when contrast agents are given, less functional information is derived than with standard intravenous urography; thus CT plays little role in functional assessment.

Radionuclide imaging (RNI)

Techniques utilizing agents labeled with radioisotopes excreted by or concentrated in the kidney have an important role in the assessment of obstructive uropathy and nephropathy. In general, these techniques have very poor spatial resolution, and thus are generally useless in the diagnosis of the site or cause of obstruction [185]. They do, however, provide excellent information about renal functional capacity and reserve of the obstructed kidney. McAfee et al. [185] demonstrated that radionuclide scans were one and one-half times more efficient in demonstrating reduced RBF as contrasted with standard IVU.

Three types of isotopically labeled compounds are used. Agents such as ^{99m}-Technetium labeled diethylenetriamine pentaacetic acid (DTPA) are predominantly excreted by glomerular filtration. As such, they are generally less effective in reflecting RBF than agents such as ^{131}-I labeled hippuran which are excreted by both filtration and tubular secretion. Finally, ^{99m}-Technetium labeled dimercaptosuccenic acid (DMSA) is not excreted to any appreciable degree, but is taken up and concentrated in renal tubular cells. Because counts arising from the parenchyma of the kidney are not confused with counts coming from isotopes concentrated in the pelvis and calyces, DMSA scans are particularly useful in assessing the degree of cortex remaining after a prolonged period of obstruction, and hence are helpful is assessing functional recovery after the obstruction is released [186].

Radionuclide imaging techniques have also proven particularly useful in distinguishing true obstruction from mere dilatation of the renal pelvis and calyces. O'Reilly et al. [187] first showed that the sequential administration of a secreted radionuclide followed by a loop diuretic, the so-called diuresis renogram compared very favorably with the much more invasive Whitaker test [188] in distinguishing true obstruction from mere dilatation. The logic of the test is as follows: excreted isotope accumulating in the pelvic region of the kidney could be due to either true obstruction, or merely to a dilated but unobstructed collecting system. If after most of the radioactivity has been cleared from the blood a powerful loop diuretic is administered, then a large bolus of nonradioactive urine will be excreted and flush the isotope from the dilated but unobstructed kidney, but not from the kidney with true obstruction. Although the diuresis renogram and Whitaker test were originally devised to rule out true ureteropelvic junction obstruction in children, the use of the diuresis renogram is becoming popular in adult nephrology and serves essentially the same purpose.

Nuclear magnetic resonance imaging (MRI)

This technique has both excellent spatial resolution and, when used with paramagnetic agents such a gadolinium-labeled DTPA, the ability to detect changes in renal function [189]. Its cost and relative lack of general availability makes it, at the present time, essentially a research tool, but a potential useful technique for the future.

References

1 Yarger WE. Urinary tract obstruction. In Brenner BM, Rector FC, eds. *The Kidney*, 4th edn. Philadelphia: WB Saunders Co., 1991:1768–1808.

2 Lowe FC, Marshall FF. Ureteropelvic junction obstruction in adults. Urology 1984;23:331.

3 Clark WR, Malek RS. Ureteropelvic junction obstruction. I. Observations on the classic type in adults. J Urol 1987; 138:276.

4 Frohneberg D, Walz PH, Hohenfellner R. Primary megaureter in adults. Eur Urol 1983;9:321.

5 Martin J, Anderson J, Raz S. Posterior urethral valves in adults: a report of 2 cases. J Urol 1977;118:978.

6 Lytton B, Emery JM, Harvard BM. The incidence of benign prostatic obstruction. J Urol 1968;99:639–645.

7 Steensberg J, Bartels ED, Bay-Nielsen H, *et al.* Br Med J 1969;4:390–394.

8 Young JL, Percy CL, Asire AJ, eds. Cancer incidence and mortality in the United States, 1973–77. NCI Monographs 1981;57:1–187.

9 Peters CA, Walsh PC. The effect of nafarelin acetate, a luteinizing-hormone-releasing agonist, on benign prostatic hyperplasia. N Engl J Med 1987;317:559.

10 Walsh PC. Human benign prostatic hyperplasia: etiologic considerations. In Kimball FA, Buhl AE, Carter DB, eds. *New Approaches to the Study of Benign Prostatic Hyperplasia: Proceedings of the Ninth Brook Lodge Workshop on Problems in Reproductive Physiology.* New York: Alan R Liss, 1984:1.

11 Fetter TR, Zimskind PD, Graham RH, *et al.* Statistical analysis of patients with ureteral calculi. J Am Med Assoc 1963;186:127–129.

12 Mukamel E, Nissenkorn I, Boner G, *et al.* Occultu progressive renal damage in the elderly male due to benign prostatic hypertrophy. J Am Geriat Soc 1979;27:403–406.

13 Abrams PH, Roylance J, Feneley RCL. Excretion urography in treatment of prostatism. Br J Urol 1976;48:681.

14 George NJR, Feneley RCL, Roberts JMB. Identification of the poor risk patient with "Prostatism" and detrusor failure. Br J Urol 1986;58:290.

15 Meyhoff HH, Munck O, Juul C, *et al.* The effect of prostatectomy on upper urinary tract function. Scand J Urol Nephrol 1982;16:97.

16 Ljunghall S. Incidence of renal stones in western countries. In Schwille PO, Smith LH, Robertson WG, *et al.* eds. *Urolithiasis and Related Clinical Research.* New York: Plenum Press, 1985:31–37.

17 Johnson CM, Wilson DM, O'Fallon WM, *et al.* Renal stone epidemiology: A 25 year study in Rochester, Minnesota. Kidney Int 1979;16:624–631.

18 Hiatt RA, Dales LG, Friedman GD, *et al.* Frequency of urolithiasis in a prepaid medical care program. Am J Epidemiol 1982;115:255–265.

19 Ahlstrand C, Tiselius HG. Renal stone disease in a Swedish district during one year. Scand J Urol Nephrol 1981;15: 143–146.

20 Scholz D, Schwille PO, Ulbrich D, *et al.* Composition of renal stones and their frequency in a stone clinic: relationship to parameters of mineral metabolism in serum and urine. Urol Res 1979;7:161–170.

21 Urbain D, Vanderauwera J, Dewitt S, *et al.* Perirenal urinoma secondary to prostatic obstruction. J Urol 1985;134:967.

22 Kontogeorgos L, Vassilopoulos P, Tentes A. Bilateral severe hydroureteronephrosis due to uterine prolapse. Br J Urol 1985;57:360.

23 Cohen HJ, Crawford J. Cancer. In *Practical Geriatric Medicine.* Edinburgh: Churchill Livingstone, 1985:57–65.

24 Cohen WM, Freed SZ, Hasson J. Metastatic cancer to the ureter: A review of the literature and case presentations. J Urol 1974;112:188.

25 Meyer JE, Yatsuhashi M, Green LAH. Palliating urinary diversion in patients with advanced pelvic malignancy. Cancer 1980;45:2689.

26 Brin EN, Schiff M, Weiss RM. Palliative urinary diversion for pelvic malignancy. J Urol 1975;113:619.

27 Grabstald H, McPhee M. Nephrostomy and the cancer patient. South Med J 1973;66:217.

28 Scott WW, McDonald DF. Tumors of the ureter. In Campbell MF, Harrison JH, eds. *Urology*, 3rd edn. Philadelphia: WB Saunders Co., 1970:977.

29 Presman D, Ehrlich L. Metastatic tumors of the ureter. J Urol 1948;59:312.

30 Goldman SM, Fishman EK, Rosenshin NB, *et al.* Excretory urography and computed tomography in the initial evaluation of patients with cervical carcinoma: Are both examinations necessary? Am J Roentgenol 1984;143:991.

31 Jones CR, Woodhouse CRJ, Hendry WF. Urologic problems following treatment of carcinoma of the cervix. Br J Urol 1984;56:609.

32 Sakkas JL, Androulakes J, Pisidis A. Ureteral obstruction due to carcinoma of the cervix uteri: A study by means of intravenous pyelography and lymphography of the cervix. Am Surgeon 1979;45:569.

33 Sieben DM, Howerton L, Amin M, et al. The role of the ureteral stenting in the management of surgical injuries of the ureter. J Urol 1978;119:330.

34 Zinman LM, Libertino JA, Roth RA. Management of ureteral injuries. Urology 1978;12:290.

35 Gangai MP, Agee RE, Spence CR. Surgical injuries to the ureter. Urology 1976;8:22.

36 Higgins CC. Ureteral injuries during surgery. J Am Med Assoc 1967;199:82.

37 Ihse I, Arnesjp B, Jonsson G. Surgical injuries of the ureter: A review of 42 cases. Scand J Urol Nephrol 1975;9:39.

38 Dowling RA, Corrier JN, Sandler CM. Iatrogenic ureteral injury. J Urol 1986;135:912.

39 Silverberg E, Lubera JA. A review of American Cancer Society estimates of cancer cases and deaths. Cancer J Clin 1983;33:2.

40 Loughlin KR, Whitmore WF. Managing prostate disorders in middle age and beyond. Geriatrics 1987;42:45−56.

41 Marks LS, Gallo DA. Ureteral obstruction in the patient with prostatic carcinoma. Br J Urol 1972;44:411.

42 Batala MA, Whitmore WF, Hilaris BS, et al. Primary carcinoma of the ureter, a prognostic study. Cancer 1975; 35:1626.

43 Pike MC. Age-related factors in cancers of the breast, ovary, and endometrium. J Chron Dis 1987;40(Suppl. 2):S59−S69.

44 Wagneknecht LV, Hardy JC. Value of various treatments for retroperitoneal fibrosis. Eur Urol 1981;7:193.

45 Graham JR, Suby HI, LeCompte PR, et al. Fibrotic disorders associated with methysergide therapy for headache. N Engl J Med 1966;274:359−3099.

46 Baker LRI, Mallinson WJW, Gregory MC, et al. Idiopathic retroperitoneal fibrosis. A retrospective analysis of 60 cases. Br J Urol 1988;60:497−503.

47 Clyne CA, Abercrombie GF. Perianeurysmal retroperitoneal fibrosis: two cases responding to steroids. Br J Urol 1977; 49:463.

48 Littlejohn GO, Keystone EC. The association of retroperitoneal fibrosis with systemic vasculitis and HLA-B27: a case report and review of the literature. J Rheumatol 1981; 8:665−669.

49 Allibone GW, Saxton HM. The association of aortoilliac aneurysms with ureteral obstruction. Urol Radiol 1980; 1:205−210.

50 Bainbridge ET, Woodward DAK. Inflammatory aneurysms of the abdominal aorta with associated ureteric obstruction or medial deviation. J Cardiovasc Surg 1982;23:365−370.

51 Lindell OI, Sariola HV, Lehtonen TA. The occurrence of vasculitis in perianeurysmal fibrosis. J Urol 1987; 138:727−729.

52 Baskerville PA, Browse NL. Periaortic fibrosis: progression and regression. J Cardiovasc Surg 1987;28:30−31.

53 Parira JJ, Win AH, Barker CF, et al. Bilateral complete ureteral obstruction secondary to an abdominal aortic aneurysm with perianeurysmal fibrosis: Diagnosed by computed tomography. J Urol 1979;121:103−106.

54 Walker DI, Bloor K, Williams G, et al. Inflammatory aneurysms of the abdominal aorta. Br J Surg 1972;59: 609−614.

55 Bloor K, Humphreys WV. Aneurysms of the abdominal aorta. Br J Hosp Med 1979;21:568−583.

56 Feldberg MAM, van Waes PFMG, ten Haken GB. CT diagnosis of perianeurysmal fibrotic reactions in aortoiliac aneurysms. J Comput Assist Tomograph 1982;6:465−471.

57 Safran R, Sklenicka R, Kay H. Iliac artery aneurysms: A common cause of ureteral obstruction. J Urol 1975; 113:605.

58 Bergsagel DE, Bailey AJ, Langley GR, et al. The chemotherapy of plasma cell myeloma and the incidence of acute leukemia. N Engl J Med 1979;301:743−748.

59 Cantor KP, Fraumeni JF. Distribution of non-Hodgkins lymphoma in the United States between 1950 and 1975. Cancer Res 1980;40:2645−2652.

60 Abeloff MD, Lenhard RE. Clinical management of ureteral obstruction secondary to malignant lymphoma. John Hopkins Med J 1974;134:34.

61 DeFronzo RA, Humphries RL, Wright JR, et al. Acute renal failure in multiple myeloma. Medicine 1975;54:209.

62 Waugh DA, Ibels LS. Multiple myeloma presenting as obstructive uropathy. Aust NZ J Med 1980;10:555.

63 Roth RM, Glovsky MM, Cooper JF, et al. Gamma A myeloma with hyperviscosity and obstructive uropathy. J Urol 1977;117:527.

64 Muggia FM, Chia GA, Mickley DW. Hyperphosphatemic hypocalcemia in neoplastic disorders. N Engl J Med 1974;290:857.

65 Modan B. Polycythemia: A review of epidemiological and clinical data. J Chron Dis 1965;18:605.

66 Schroder LE, Vilter RW. Bilteral ureteral obstruction due to uric acid stones in association with immune hemolytic anemia. Arch Intern Med 1983;143:1020.

67 Crittenden DR, Ackerman GL. Hyperuricemic acute renal failure in disseminated carcinoma. Arch Intern Med 1977; 137:97.

68 Rieselbach RE, Bentzel CJ, Cotlov E, et al. Uric acid excretion and renal function in acute hyperuricemia of leukemia. Am J Med 1964;37:872.

69 Spencer HW, Yarger WE, Robinson RR. Alterations of renal function during dietary-induced hyperuricemia in the rat. Kidney Int 1976;9:4890.

70 Schroder LE, Viltar RW. Bilateral ureteral obstruction due to uric acid stones in association with immune hemolytic anemia. Arch Intern Med 1983;143:1020.

71 Kelton J, Kelly WM, Holmes EW. A rapid method for the diagnosis of acute uric acid nephropathy. Arch Intern Med 1978;138:612.

72 Kjellstrand CW, Campbell DC, Von Hartitzsch B. Hyperuricemic acute renal failure. Arch Intern Med 1974;133:349.

73 Banner MO. Genitourinary complications of inflammatory bowel disease. Radiol Clin North Am 1987;25:199.

74 Shields DE, Lytton B, Weiss RM, et al. Urologic complications of inflammatory bowel disease. J Urol 1976;115:701.

75 Ney C, Cruz FS, Carvajal S, et al. Ureteral involvement secondary to diverticulitis of the colon. Surg Gynecol Obstet 1986;163:215.

76 Weisman MH, McDonald EC, Wilson CB. Studies of the pathogenesis of interstitial cystitis, obstructive uropathy, and intestinal malabsorption in a patient with systemic lupus erythematosus. Am J Med 1981;70:875.

77 Melin JP, Lemaire P, Biembaut P, et al. Polyarteritis nodosa with bilateral ureteral involvement. Nephron 1982;32:87.

78 Adelizzi RA, Shockley FK, Pietras JR. Wegener's granulomatosis with ureteric obstruction. J Rheumatol 1980;13:448.

79 Yonker RA, Katz P. Necrotizing granulomatous vasculitis with eosinophilic infiltrates limited to the prostate. Am J Med 1984;77:362.

80 Schoenfeld RH, Belville WD, Buck A, et al. Unilateral ureteral obstruction secondary to sarcoidosis. Urology 1985;25:57.

81 Robinson CR, Fowler JE. Localized amyloidosis of the ureter. J Urol 1984;131:112.

82 Glenner GG. Amyloid deposits and amyloidosis: The beta fibrilloses. N Engl J Med 1980;302:1283–1292, 1333–1343.

83 Sherman RL, Schneider M. Obstructive uropathy as seen by the internist: The role of ultrasound and CT scanning. DM 1984;1–41.

84 Hackler RH. Spinal cord injuries. Urologic care. Urology 1973;2:13.

85 St Martin EC, Trichel BE, Campbell JH, et al. Ureteral injuries in gynecologic surgery. J Urol 1953;70:51.

86 Cronan JJ, Amis ES, Scola FH, et al. Renal obstruction in patients with ileal loops: US evaluation. Radiology 1988; 158:647.

87 Leroy AJ, Segura JW, Williams HJ, et al. Percutaneous renal calculus removal in an extracorporeal shock wave lithotripsy practice. J Urol 1987;138:703–706.

88 Green DF, Lytton B, Glickman M. Ureteropelvic junction obstruction after percutaneous nephrolithotripsy. J Urol 1987;138:599–602.

89 Neerhut GJ, Ritchie AW, Tolley DA. Extracorporeal piezoelectric lithotripsy for all renal stones: effectiveness and limitations. Br J Urol 1989;64:5–9.

90 Kiely EA, Ryan PC, McDermott TE, et al. Extracorporeal shockwave lithotripsy using ultrasonic imaging: urologists' experience. Br J Urol 1989;64:1–4.

91 Hardy MR, McLeod DG. Silent renal obstruction with severe functional loss after extracorporeal shock wave lithotripsy: a report of 2 cases. J Urol 1987;137:91–92.

92 Libby JM, Meacham RB, Griffith DP. The role of silicone ureteral stents in extracorporeal shock wave lithotripsy of large renal calculi. J Urol 1988;139:15–17.

93 Pode D, Verstandig A, Shapiro AR, et al. Treatment of complete staghorn calculi by extracorporeal shock wave lithotripsy monotherapy with special reference to internal stenting. J Urol 1988;140:260–265.

94 Pode D, Shapiro AR, Verstandig A, et al. Use of internal polyethylene ureteral stents in extracorporeal shock-wave lithotripsy of staghorn calculi. Eur Urol 1987;13:174–175.

95 Fine H, Gordon RL, Lebensart PD. Extracorporeal shock wave lithotripsy and stents: fluoroscopic observations and a hypothesis on the mechanisms of stent function. Urol Radiol 1989;11:37–41.

96 Tegtmeyer CJ, Kellum CD, Jenkins A, et al. Extracorporeal shock wave lithotripsy: interventional radiologic solutions to associated problems. Radiology 1986;161:587–592.

97 Chaussy C, Fuchs G, Kahn R, et al. Transurethral ultrasonic ureterolithotripsy using a solid-wire probe. Urology 1987; 29:531–532.

98 Kramolowsky EV, Quinlan SM, Loening SA. Extracorporeal shock wave lithotripsy for the treatment of urinary calculi in the elderly. J Am Geriatr Soc 1987;35:251–254.

99 Schaimuch LJ, Hano JE. Bilateral ureteral obstruction following sulfamethoxazole. J Urol 1967;98:466.

100 Kline RS, Cattolica EV, Rankin KN. Hemiacidrin renal irrigations: Complications and successful renal management. J Urol 1982;128:241–242.

101 Melman A, Lavelle K, Ludwig J. Bilateral renal loss resulting from intravessicular formalin instillation. South Med J 1978;71:1152.

102 Novicki DE, Willscher MK. Case-Profile, Anticholinergic-induced hydronephrosis. Urology 1979;13:324.

103 Murdock MI, Olsson CS, Sac DS, et al. Effects of levodopa on the bladder outlet. J Urol 1975;113:803.

104 Hilgartner MW. Intrarenal obstruction in haemophilia. Lancet 1966;1:486.

105 McGregor B, Saker BM, England EJ. Ureteric stricture associated with analgesic nephropathy. Med J Aust 1979;1:287.

106 Simonsen S, Moller-Madsen B, Dorflinger T, et al. The significance of age on symptoms and urodynamic- and cystoscopic findings in benign prostatic hypertrophy. Urol Res 1987;15:355–358.

107 Frimodt-Miller PC, Jensen KM, Iversen P, et al. Analysis of presenting symptoms in prostatism. J Urol 1984;132: 272–276.

108 Cote RJ, Burke H, Schoenberg HW. Prediction of unusual postoperative results by urodynamic testing in benign prostatic hyperplasia. J Urol 1981;125:690–692.

109 Andersen JT, Nordling J. Prostatism. II. The correlation between cysto-urethroscopic, cystometric and urodynamic

findings. Scand J Urol Nephrol 1980;14:23.

110 Jones KW, Schoenberg HW. Comparison of the incidence of bladder hyperreflexia in patients with benign prostatic hypertrophy and age-matched female controls. J Urol 1984; 133:425.

111 Gillenwater JY, Westervelt J, Vaughan ED, *et al.* Renal function after release of chronic unilateral hydronephrosis in man. Kidney Int 1975;7:179.

112 Hanley MJ, Davidson K. Isolated nephron segments from rabbit models of obstructive nephropathy. J Clin Invest 1982;69:165.

113 Bay WH, Stein JH, Rector JB, *et al.* Redistribution of renal cortical blood flow during elevated ureteral pressure. Am J Physiol 1972;222:33.

114 Abe Y, Kishimoto T, Yamamoto K, *et al.* Intrarenal distribution of blood flow during ureteral and venous pressure elevation. Am J Physiol 1973;224:746.

115 Yarger WE, Griffith LD. Intrarenal hemodynamics following chronic unilateral ureteral obstruction in the dog. Am J Physiol 1974;227:816.

116 Kessler RH. Acute effects of brief ureteral stasis on urinary and renal papillary chloride concentration. Am J Physiol 1960;199:1215−1218.

117 Honda N, Aizawa C, Morikawa A, *et al.* Effect of elevated ureteral pressure on renal medullary osmolal concentration in hydropenic rabbits. Am J Physiol 1971;221:698−703.

118 Anggard E, Bohman SO, Griffin JE, *et al.* Subcellular localization of the prostaglandin system in the rabbit papilla. Acta Physiol Scand 1972;84:231.

119 Stokes JB. Effect of prostaglandin E2 on chloride transport across the rabbit thick ascending limb of Henle. Selective inhibition of the medullary portion. J Clin Invest 1979; 64:495.

120 Grantham JJ, Orloff J. Effect of prostaglandin E1 on the permeability response of the isolated collecting tubule to vasopressin, adenosine 3′,5′-monophosphate, and theophylline. J Clin Invest 1968;47:1154−1161.

121 Wilson B, Reisman DD, Moyer CA. Fluid balance in the urological patient: Disturbances in the renal regulation of the excretion of water and sodium salts following decompression of the urinary bladder. J Urol 1951;66:805.

122 Bricker NS, Shwayru EI, Reardan JB, *et al.* An abnormality in renal function resulting from urinary tract obstruction. Am J Med 1957;23:554.

123 Peterson LJ, Yarger WE, Schocken DD, *et al.* Postobstructive diuresis: A varied syndrome. J Urol 1975; 113:190.

124 Muldowney FP, Duffy GJ, Kelly DG, *et al.* Sodium diuresis after relief of obstructive uropathy. N Engl J Med 1966; 274:1294.

125 Rodriguez-Soriano J, Vallo A, Oliveros R, *et al.* Transient pseudohypoaldosteronism secondary to obstructive uropathy in infancy. J Pediatr 1983;103:375.

126 v d Heijden AJ, Versteegh FGA, Wolff ED, *et al.* Acute tubular dysfunction in infants with obstructive uropathy. Acta Paediatr Scand 1985;74:589.

127 Witte MH, Short FA, Hollander J. Massive polyuria and natriuresis following relief of urinary tract obstruction. Am J Med 1964;37:320.

128 Yarger WE, Aynedjian HS, Bank N. A micropuncture study of postobstructive diuresis in the rat. J Clin Invest 1972; 51:625.

129 Dal Canton A, Corradi A, Stanziale R, *et al.* Effects of 24-hour unilateral ureteral obstruction on glomerular hemodynamics in rat kidney. Kidney Int 1979;15:457.

130 Dal Canton A, Corradi A, Stanziale R, *et al.* Glomerular hemodynamics before and after release of 24-hour bilateral ureteral obstruction. Kidney Int 1980;17:491.

131 Dal Canton A, Stanziale R, Corradi A, *et al.* Effects of acute ureteral obstruction on glomerular hemodynamics in rat kidneys. Kidney Int 1977;12:403.

132 Buerkert J, Martin D, Head M, *et al.* Deep nephron function after release of acute unilateral ureteral obstruction in the young rat. J Clin Invest 1978;62:1228.

133 Jaenike JR. The renal functional defect of postobstructive nephropathy: The effects of bilateral ureteral obstruction in the rat. J Clin Invest 1972;51:2999.

134 Buerkert J, Head M, Klahr S. Effects of acute bilateral ureteral obstruction on deep nephron and terminal collecting duct function in the young rat. J Clin Invest 1977; 59:1055.

135 McDougal WS, Wright FS. Defect in proximal and distal sodium transport in postobstructive diuresis. Kidney Int 1972;2:304.

136 Wilson DR. Nephron functional heterogeneity in the postobstructive kidney. Kidney Int 1974;7:19.

137 Buerkert J, Martin D, Head M. Effect of acute ureteral obstruction on terminal collecting duct function in the weanling rat. Am J Physiol 1979;236:F260.

138 Buerkert J, Alexander E, Purkerson M, *et al.* On the site of decreased fluid reabsorption after release of ureteral obstruction in the rat. J Lab Clin Med 1976;87:397.

139 Sonnenberg H, Wilson DR. The role of the medullary collecting ducts in postobstructive diuresis. J Clin Invest 1976; 57:1564.

140 Yarger WE, Schocken DD, Harris RH. Obstructive nephropathy in the rat. Possible roles for the renin−angiotensin system, prostaglandins, and thromboxanes in postobstructive renal function. J Clin Invest 1980;65:400−412.

141 Reingold DF, Watters K, Holmberf S, *et al.* Differential biosynthesis of prostaglandins by hydronephrotic rabbit and cat kidneys. J Pharmacol Exp Ther 1981;216:510−515.

142 Klotman PE, Smith SR, Volpp BD, *et al.* Thromboxane synthetase inhibition improves function of hydronephrotic rat kidneys. Am J Physiol 1986;250:F282−F287.

143 Williams WM, Frolich JC, Nies AS, *et al.* Urinary

prostaglandins: Site of entry into the renal tubular fluid. Kidney Int 1977;11:256.

144 Harris RH, Yarger WE. Renal function after release of unilateral ureteral obstruction in rats. Am J Physiol 1974; 227:806.

145 Huguenin M, Ott CE, Romero JC, et al. Influence of renin depletion on renal function after release of 24-hour ureteral obstruction. J Lab Clin Med 1976;87:58.

146 Harris RH, Yarger WE. The pathogenesis of postobstructive diuresis: The role of circulating natriuretic and diuretic factors, including urea. J Clin Invest 1975;56:880.

147 Wilson DR. The influence of volume expansion on renal function after relief of chronic unilateral ureteral obstruction. Kidney Int 1974;5:402−410.

148 Fried TA, Lau AT, Ayon MA, et al. Elevation of ANP levels in ureteral obstruction in the rat. Clin Res 1986; 34:A204.

149 Olsen UB, Weis JU, Diness V, et al. Atriopeptin III improves renal functions in a ureterobstructed rat kidney model. Eur J Pharmacol 1986;122:191.

150 Condra CL, Leidy EA, Bunting P, et al. Clearance and early hydrolysis of atrial natriuretic factor in vivo: Structural analysis of cleavage sites and design of an analogue that inhibits hormone cleavage. J Clin Invest 1988;81:1348.

151 Himmelstein SI, Yarger WE, Klotman PE. Atrial natriuretic peptide increases PGE2 and 6-keto PGF1a production in normal and hydronephrotic kidneys. Kidney Int 1987; 31:272.

152 Better OS, Arieff AI, Massry SG, et al. Studies on renal function after relief of complete unilateral ureteral obstruction of three months' duration in man. Am J Med 1973;54: 234−240.

153 Berlyne GM. Distal tubular function in chronic hydronephrosis. Q J Med 1961;30:339.

154 Roussak NJ, Oleesky S. Water-losing nephritis. Q J Med 1954;23:147.

155 Winberg J. Renal function in water losing syndrome due to lower urinary tract obstruction before and after treatment. Acta Paediatr Scand 1959;48:149.

156 Earley LE. Extreme polyuria in obstructive uropathy: Report of a case of "Water-losing nephritis" in an infant, with a discussion of polyuria. N Engl J Med 1956;255:600.

157 Knowland D, Corrado M, Schreiner GE. Periureteral fibrosis, with a diabetes insipidus-like syndrome occurring with progressive partial obstruction of a ureter unilaterally. Am J Med 1960;31:22−31.

158 Kurtzman NA. Acquired distal renal tubular acidosis. Kidney Int 1983;24:807−819.

159 Ericsson NO, Winberg J, Zetterstrom R. Renal function in infantile obstructive uropathy. Acta Paediatr Scand 1955; 44:444.

160 Falls WF, Stacy WK. Postobstructive diuresis: Studies in dialyzed patient with a solitary kidney. Am J Med 1973;

54:404−412.

161 Hutchenson RA, Kaplan BS, Drummond KN. Distal renal tubular acidosis in children with chronic hydronephrosis. J Pediatr 1976;89:372.

162 Marra G, Goj V, Appiani AC, et al. Persistent tubular resistance to aldosterone in infants with congenital hydronephrosis corrected neonatally. J Pediatr 1987;110:868.

163 Pelleya R, Oster JR, Perez GO. Hyporeninemic hypoaldosteronism, sodium wasting and mineralocorticoid-resistant hyperkalemia in two patients with obstructive uropathy. Am J Nephrol 1983;3:223−227.

164 Battle DC, Arruda JA, Kurtzman NA. Hyperkalemic distal renal tubular acidosis associated with obstructive uropathy. N Engl J Med 1981;304:373−380.

165 Sebastian A, Schambelan M, Lindfeld S, et al. Amelioration of metabolic acidosis with fludrocortisone therapy in hyporeninemic hypoaldosteronism. N Engl J Med 1977;297:576−583.

166 Szylman P, Better OS, Chaimowitz C, et al. Role of hyperkalemia in the metabolic acidosis of isolated hypoaldosteronism. N Engl J Med 1976;294:361−365.

167 Provoost AP, Molenaar JC. Renal function during and after a temporary complete unilateral ureter obstruction in rats. Invest Urol 1981;18:242−246.

168 Kerr WS. Effect of complete ureteral obstruction for one week on kidney function. J Appl Physiol 1954;6:762−772.

169 Vaughan ED, Sweet RE, Gillenwater JY. Unilateral ureteral occlusion; Pattern of nephron repair and compensatory response. J Urol 1973;109:979−982.

170 Shapiro AR, Bennett AH. Recovery of renal function after prolonged unilateral ureteral obstruction. J Urol 1976; 115:136−140.

171 Lewis HY, Pierce JM. Return of function after relief of complete ureteral obstruction of 69 days duration. J Urol 1962;88:377−379.

172 Kerr WS. Effects of complete ureteral obstruction in dogs on kidney function. Am J Physiol 1956;184:521−526.

173 Nelson RP, Williams A. Late return of renal function after correction of chronic obstruction. J Urol 1977;118:462−463.

174 Ibrahim A, Fahal AH. Recovery of radiologically functionless obstructed kidneys. Br J Urol 1984;56:113−115.

175 McDougal WS, Flanigan RC. Renal functional recovery of the hydronephrotic kidney predicted before relief of the obstruction. Invest Radiol 1981;18:440−442.

176 Rao KG, Hackler RH, Woodlief RM, et al. Real-time renal sonography in spinal cord injury patients: Prospective comparison with excretory urography. J Urol 1986;135:72.

177 Sanders RC, Jeck DL. Ultrasound in the evaluation of renal failure. Radiology 1976;119:199.

178 Talner LB, Scheible W, Ellenbogen PH, et al. How accurate is ultrasound in detecting hydronephrosis in azotemic patients? Urol Radiol 1981;3:1.

179 Lalli AF. Retroperitoneal fibrosis and inapparent obstruc-

tive uropathy. Radiology 1977;122:339.

180 Scheible W, Talner LB. Gray-scale ultrasound and the genitourinary tract: A review of clinical applications. Radiol Clin North Am 1979;17:281.

181 Amis ES, Cronan JJ, Pfister RC, *et al.* Ultrasonic inaccuracies in diagnosing renal obstruction. Urology 1982; 19:101.

182 McClennan BL. Current approaches to the azotemic patient. Radiol Clin North Am 1979;17:197.

183 Maillet PJ, Pelle-Francoz D, Laville M, *et al.* Nondilated obstructive acute renal failure: Diagnostic procedures and therapeutic management. Radiology 1986;160:659.

184 Sherman RL, Schneider M. Obstructive uropathy as seen by the internist: The role of ultrasound and CT scanning. DM 1984;11.

185 McAfee JG, Singh A, O'Callaghan JP. Nuclear imaging supplementary to urography in obstructive uropathy. Radiology 1980;137:487.

186 Schelfhout W, Simons M, Oosterlinch W, *et al.* Evaluation of 99mTc-Dimercaptosuccinic acid renal uptake as an index of individual kidney function after acute ureteral obstruction and deobstruction. Eur Urol 1983; 9:221–226.

187 O'Reilly PH, Testa HJ, Lawson RS, *et al.* Diuresis renography in equivocal urinary tract obstruction. Br J Urol 1978;50:76.

188 Whitaker RH. Methods of assessing obstruction in dilated ureters. Br J Urol 1973;45:15.

189 Kikinis R, von Schulthess GK, Jager P, *et al.* Normal and hydronephrotic kidney: Evaluation of renal function with contrast-enhanced MR Imaging. Radiology 1987;165:837.

20

Urologic aspects of obstructive disease in the elderly

W. Scott McDougal

The clinical aspects of obstructive uropathy may be conveniently divided into two groups: obstructions of the upper urinary tract; and those of the lower urinary tract. Obstructions of the upper urinary tract are caused by diseases which result in impairment of urine flow from the level of the ureterovesicle junction cephalad, whereas lower urinary tract obstruction involves disease entities which effect either the bladder, the bladder outlet, or the urethra. The division is not arbitrary as each group shares many similarities irrespective of the primary disease. The symptoms of presentation, the effect on the physiologic alterations and impairment of renal function, and the likelihood of renal failure differ depending upon whether the obstruction is in the lower or upper urinary tract. Thus, obstructions of the lower urinary tract are generally manifested by disorders of micturition. Such obstructions, when prolonged, are more likely to result in uremia as the entire nephrogenic mass is obstructed by the disease entity, usually at the bladder outlet. Conversely, partial obstructs of the lower urinary tract are more likely to result in preservation of individual renal function rather than partial obstructions of the upper urinary tract as the destructive effects of obstruction are initially visited upon the bladder. Provided the antireflux mechanism of the ureterovesicle junction is intact, the pressure effects of lower urinary obstruction are blunted in the upper urinary tract. Diseases of the upper urinary tract generally manifest themselves by symptoms of renal colic. Since there are two kidneys, an obstruction of the upper urinary tract rarely results in uremia unless the obstruction is bilateral. For these reasons, a discussion of lower urinary tract obstruction will be followed by a discussion of upper urinary tract obstruction.

Lower urinary tract obstruction

Diseases which result in lower urinary tract obstruction may be conveniently divided into three groups: (1) neurogenic; (2) anatomic obstructions of the bladder outlet; and (3) anatomic obstructions of the urethra (Table 20.1). The incidence of lower urinary tract obstruction increases with age. In the male there is a significant increase from the fifth to ninth decade. The main cause of obstruction in these decades involves prostatic hypertrophy, and less commonly, prostatic cancer. In the female, urinary tract obstruction also increases with age but is more likely due to neurogenic causes and/or loss of anatomic integrity with loss of the urethral vesicle angle.

Table 20.1 Etiology of lower urinary tract obstruction

Neurogenic
Vesical dysfunction
  Motor
  Sensory
Urethral sphincter dysfunction

Anatomic obstructions of the bladder outlet
Benign prostatic hypertrophy
Adenocarcinoma of the prostate
Inflammation of the prostate
Cancer of the bladder
Ureteroceles
Vesical calculi
Stricture
Loss of the urethravesical angle

Anatomic obstructions of the urethra
Stricture
Valves
Cancer
Calculi
Trauma with periurethral hematoma
Urethral diverticulae

Neurogenic outlet obstruction

Obstruction of urinary flow from bladder to urethral meatus may be due to a variety of neurogenic lesions. The bladder muscle (detrusor) may be injured to such a degree that the bladder is incapable of contracting or the detrusor muscle innervation (parasympathetic) may be impaired so that the bladder does not respond to the stimuli to void. This type of neurogenic bladder is referred to as a motor neurogenic bladder. In other circumstances, patients have a sensory neurogenic bladder in which the patient is incapable of determining when the bladder is full. This may result in overdistention of the bladder with disruption of the capability of muscular contraction. Thus, a sensory neurogenic bladder, although classified as a neurogenic bladder, may in fact result in inability of the bladder to contract due to a direct injury to the muscle itself [1]. This abnormality is not uncommonly found in diabetics. Neurogenic disease may not only effect the bladder and result in outlet obstruction, but may effect the urethral internal and external sphincters as well. In a coordinated voiding response, as the detrusor or bladder muscle contracts, the urethral sphincters, both internal and external, relax. The internal sphincter is controlled by the sympathetic nervous system; the external sphincter is innervated by the somatic nervous system and receives its innervation by way of the pudendal nerve. If the urethral sphincters, either internal or external, do not relax as the detrusor muscle contracts then a functional obstruction results. This is not uncommonly found in spinal cord injury patients and patients with multiple sclerosis. These patients are generally treated with pharmacologic agents to achieve a coordinated micturition response. If this is not possible pharmacologically, such patients are then placed on self-intermittent catheterization.

The diagnosis of neurogenic bladder is confirmed by urodynamic evaluation. Urodynamic evaluation is divided into four parts: (1) cystometrogram; (2) electromyography; (3) urethral pressure profile; and (4) uroflowmetry. A cystometrogram is a pressure volume curve. The bladder is generally filled with water and the pressure recorded. Electromyography determines the activity of the external sphincter. The myographic activity of the external sphincter is generally recorded simultaneously with the cystometrogram. The patient is asked to indicate when the bladder is full and then voluntarily void. A normal cystometrogram reveals a low filling pressure and a first urge to void of 150−250 ml. At that point when the patient is asked to void, the electromyogram should become silent indicating relaxation of the external sphincter and the pressure in the bladder should rise indicating a contraction of the detrusor muscle.

Uroflowmetry measures the velocity at which the urine is expelled. If there is no outlet obstruction, the sphincters relax correctly and the detrusor muscle has adequate strength; a male should be able to achieve a 25 ml/s voiding velocity and a female should be able to achieve a 15−20 ml/s voiding velocity. Urethral pressure profilemetry measures the resistance along the urethra. This indicates the level of the sphincter and its activity. At rest or when the patient is not voiding, the male shows two sphincter spikes; one at the outlet and the second at the apex of the prostate. These are relatively narrow spikes. The female, on the other hand, demonstrates a broadened increased resistance along the proximal and middle third of the urethra. These pressures exceed the pressure in the bladder. If they do not, then incontinence results [2].

Anatomic bladder outlet obstruction

Anatomic causes of bladder outlet obstruction in the

male include benign prostatic hyperplasia, carcinoma of the prostate, acute and chronic prostatitis, bladder neoplasms, bladder neck contracture, vesicle calculi, and ectopic ureteroceles. In the female, bladder neck contracture, bladder descensus, and ureteroceles, along with vesicle calculi may be etiologic. Symptoms of bladder outlet obstruction include those which suggest an obstructive nature and those which suggest an irritative etiology. Symptoms suggesting an obstructive etiology include decreased force and caliber of the urinary stream, difficulty beginning and stopping the stream, postmicturition dribbling, urinary retention, and overflow urinary incontinence. Irritative symptoms include dysuria, frequency, nocturia, urgency, and urgency incontinence. The diagnosis of bladder outlet obstruction is suggested by the history and confirmed by a physical examination along with roentgenologic and cystoscopic examination. Signs which suggest outlet obstruction on physical examination include a distended and percussable bladder above the symphysis pubis, an enlarged prostate (if soft, this suggests benign prostatic hypertrophy; if rock hard, carcinoma of the prostate is suggested; and if boggy and tender, acute prostatitis should be suspected) and in the female, bladder descensus with a cystourethrocele. Examination of the urine is generally nondiagnostic since pure outlet obstruction due to benign prostatic hypertrophy and carcinoma of the prostate in the male and cytourethroceles and neurogenic bladder in the female, the most common causes, generally reveal a normal urinalysis. However, inflammatory lesions such as acute prostatitis and vesicle calculi may result in hematuria and pyuria. Laboratory examination may reveal normal serum electrolytes, creatinine, and urea provided the outlet obstruction has not caused deterioration of renal function and/or the patient is not in retention. On the other hand, should complete urinary retention occur or if the chronic obstruction has caused deterioration of renal function then an elevated blood urea nitrogen (BUN) and creatinine may be in evidence. As in parenchymal renal failure (intrarenal failure) the BUN/creatinine ratio is 10:1. If the creatinine is above 4 mg/dl, the chance of complete renal recovery is not likely whereas if it is less than 4 mg/dl at the time of relief of obstruction, complete recovery of normal renal function is the rule [3].

Roentgenologic examination includes intravenous urography, voiding cystourethrography, and computerized axial tomography of the pelvis. On intravenous

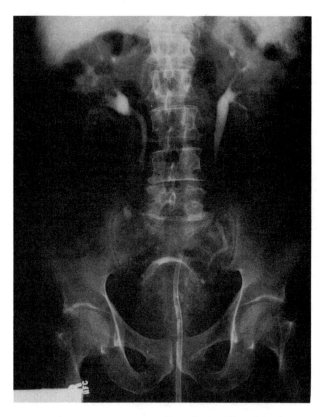

Fig. 20.1 Intravenous urogram of a patient with outlet obstruction due to benign prostatic hypertrophy. Notice "J hooking" of the ureter and enlarged prostate impression at the base of the bladder.

urography, one may note bilateral hydroureteronephrosis suggestive of obstruction at the bladder, "J hooking" of the ureters suggestive of an enlarged prostate, and a prostatic impression on the base of the bladder (Fig. 20.1). Diverticula and trabeculation noted on the bladder films and an increased postvoid residual on the postvoid film are also helpful clues. Voiding cystourethrography for outlet obstruction is generally not helpful and usually demonstrates an increased postvoid residual. Computerized axial tomography may be helpful in showing an enlarged prostate and in circumstances of carcinoma of the prostate, evidence of extension of the tumor locally or pelvic lymphadenopathy. Ultrasonography has also been utilized to demonstrate an enlarged prostate as well as suggest malignant disease as evidenced by hyper- and hypoechoic nodularity of the prostate. Urodynamic evaluation is helpful in determining the significance of the outlet obstruction. A cystometrogram is generally normal. Uroflowmetry which measures the velocity at which the urine is voided shows a reduced velocity of flow [4]. In the male, significant outlet obstruction generally results in a uroflow of 15 ml/s or less (normal is about 25 ml/s) and in the female, 10 ml/s or less (normal is >15 ml/s). Electromyography of the external sphincter should show relaxation at the time the detrusor muscle contracts. The diagnosis of outlet obstruction is confirmed by endoscopic examination of the bladder. Urethroscopy reveals occlusion of the prostate or vesicle calculi, ureterocele, or the other causes of outlet obstruction.

In the older population, the most common cause of outlet obstruction is benign prostatic hypertrophy. There is an increase in the size of the prostate from birth until puberty at which time the prostate achieves a weight of approximately 20–25 g. After the age of 30, the prostate begins to show evidence of benign prostatic hyperplasia such that by age 50 approximately 20–30% of men have significant benign prostatic hypertrophy. About 5% of patients will have what is called "silent prostatism" in which renal deterioration occurs without the patient having significant symptoms. Cancer of the prostate is also a common cause of outlet obstruction in the elderly since cancer of the prostate is the second most common cancer in the adult male and the third leading cause of cancer death in the adult male. Its frequency is illustrated by the fact that at age 60 approximately 20–40% of adult males at autopsy will have foci of adenocarcinoma of the prostate. The other causes of bladder outlet obstruction in the United States, i.e., vesicle calculi, ureterocele, and bladder neck contracture, are relatively rare causes of anatomic outlet obstruction in the elderly population.

The treatment of outlet obstruction due to benign prostatic hypertrophy is directed at relieving the outlet obstruction. This may be accomplished by: (1) transurethral resection of the prostate or open prostatectomy; (2) hormonal manipulation of the prostate; (3) balloon dilatation of the prostate; and (4) hyperthermia of the prostate. Standard therapy for benign prostatic hypertrophy which causes significant symptoms and/or deterioration of renal function is a transurethral resection of the prostate. However, other modalities of treatment have recently come to the fore. It is to transurethral resection of the prostate that these modalities must be compared. The

mortality for transurethral resection of the prostate is less than 0.2% and the relief of symptoms is approximately 80–85%. Transurethral resection is a useful modality for glands of limited size. However, exceedingly enlarged glands require an open surgical procedure in which the adenoma is enucleated. In either case, the prostate adenoma is removed from the outlet, thus relieving the outlet obstruction. The complications of prostatectomy may be divided into early and late. Early complications which are associated with transurethral resection of the prostate include hematuria, sepsis, postoperative epididymitis, and pulmonary emboli. Their incidence is relatively rare. Late complications include bladder neck contracture in up to 10% of patients, urethral stricture in 3–10%, urinary incontinence in less than 2%, impotence in approximately 6–30%, and retrograde ejaculation in the majority. Other modalities have recently been tried to treat prostatic obstruction due to benign disease. Balloon dilatation which involves placing a balloon under fluoroscopic guidance in the prostatic fossa and dilating the area for approximately 30 min has had limited success. In preliminary studies in which this has been tried, approximately 30–40% of patients have subjective improvement; however, objective improvement as determined by urodynamic parameters is generally difficult to document. Moreover, long-term follow-up suggests that those patients who would normally require a transurethral resection will eventually require it at a later date [5]. The advantage of balloon dilatation is that some patients gain relief and their surgery may be delayed for a period of time. Medical manipulation of the prostate includes suppression of circulating testosterone through luteinizing hormone releasing hormone (LHRH) agonist and/or antiandrogen compounds. When administered, these compounds result in about a 25% reduction in the size of the prostate with subjective signs of improvement in about 60% of patients [6,7]. Other drugs which relax the sphincters have also been tried such as the α-blockers. These have met with variable results and again, the objective findings of improvement cannot be documented, whereas subjective improvement is variable [8]. Hyperthermia is just beginning to be utilized and it is too early at this time to determine its efficacy.

The treatment of cancer of the prostate provided it is confined to the prostate and the patient has a 5–10 year survival is radical surgical extirpation. However, in the elderly age group, usually cancer of the prostate does not present confined to the prostate but rather is locally extensive or regional lymph nodes are involved [9]. Under these circumstances, hormonal manipulation utilizing estrogens and LHRH agonists in an attempt to depress serum testosterone, antiandrogen compounds, or castration are generally helpful in relieving the symptoms [10,11]. Those patients who are obstructed or who are in retention will respond to a transurethral resection of the prostate followed by hormonal manipulation.

Urethral obstruction

Anatomic urethral obstruction may be due to meatal stenosis, urethral strictures, urethral tumors, urethral diverticula, trauma, or cystourethrocele. Meatal stenosis is perhaps the most common cause of urethral stricture following transurethral manipulation in the male. In the female, it may occur primarily. It is diagnosed by calibrating the meatus in both sexes. Both the male and female meatus should easily accommodate a 16−20 Foley catheter. Urethral strictures may be either congenital (and as such would have been discovered long before the patient reaches the elderly population), or acquired. Acquired strictures are caused by infections usually due to sexually transmitted diseases such as gonorrhea, blunt trauma such as pelvic crush injuries, or the injuries sustained during delivery through the birth canal, and iatrogenic trauma due to manipulation. Neoplasms may rarely cause obstruction of the urethra (the most common pathologic type being squamous cell carcinoma). In the female, urethral diverticula or a cystourethrocele may be etiologic. The diagnosis is made by urethroscopy and urethrography. It may also be suggested by poor uroflowmetry on urodynamic evaluation. The treatment of strictures involves incision of the stricture by visual internal urethrotomy and in situations where the stricture is extensive, an on-lay graft with reconstruction may be required. Urethral diverticulae are excised and descensus with cystourethrocele requires surgical repositioning of the bladder into its normal anatomic position. Tumors require extirpation.

Upper urinary tract

Obstruction of the upper urinary tract is not an uncommon event in the elderly patient; however, when compared to lower urinary tract obstruction, it certainly has a lesser incidence. Obstructions of the upper urinary tract may be conveniently divided into those which occur at the level of the ureterovesicle junction, those which occur along the course of the ureter, and those which occur at the ureteropelvic junction. As mentioned above, patients with acute obstructions of the upper collecting system generally present with signs and symptoms of renal colic. Depending on the etiology, the urinalysis may show red cells, white cells, or crystals. If the obstruction is unilateral, generally there is no deterioration in renal function provided the contralateral kidney is relatively normal. However, certain diseases cause bilateral obstruction of the upper urinary tract and such patients may present with signs and symptoms of uremia. More chronic obstructions generally present silently and are discovered when the disease causing them is discovered, or incidently when a patient is being evaluated for another problem. The etiology for obstruction of the upper urinary tract at the ureterovesicle junction includes cancer of the prostate which has infiltrated to the ureteral orifices, cancer of the bladder obstructing the ureteral orifice, ureteroceles, or periureteral diverticula. Calculi may lodge at the ureterovesicle junction and also cause obstructions of the upper urinary tract — calculi are often arrested at the narrowest portions of the ureter/ureteropelvic junction, where the ureter crosses the great vessels, and at the ureterovesical junction. Diseases which cause obstruction of the ureter itself include those which are intrinsic and include ureteral calculi, inflammatory diseases of the ureter including tuberculosis, as well as common urinary pathogens, primary tumors of the ureter which pathologically are generally transitional cell cancer in type, bleeding from the kidney which results in clots and sloughed renal papillae. Sloughed renal papillae may occur in patients who have pyelonephritis or who have obstruction for other reasons: those with sickle cell anemia, analgesic abuse, cirrhosis, diabetes, or tuberculosis. Lesions which are extrinsic to the ureter and cause obstruction include retroperitoneal fibrosis which may be idiopathic or may be secondary to cancer, crossing vessels particularly the vena cava, ovarian vein, and iliac vessels, and tumors which are not primarily ureteral. These include tumors of adjacent visceral organs including the rectosigmoid and colon, the ovary, uterus, and cervix. Metastatic lesions from the breast, lungs, and testes may result in ureteral obstruction and primary retroperitoneal tumors including liposarcoma, fibrosarcoma, lymphoma, and rhabdomyosarcoma have all resulted in obstruction of the ureter. The diagnosis of ureteral obstruction is suspected by the symptoms of renal colic or by discovery of an elevated BUN and creatinine when the obstruction is bilateral. The diagnosis may be made roentgenographically by intravenous urography which shows delay in excretion of the contrast material on the side of obstruction and columnization of the contrast to the level of the obstruction. Rarely, when the obstruction has been long term, contrast will not be picked up by the kidney at all. Calculi may be seen as radio dense lesions or on occasion if uric acid in composition they will be radiolucent. Retrograde pyelography is the definitive procedure for defining the nature and level of ureteral obstruction. Computerized axial tomography has revolutionized the diagnosis of ureteral obstruction due to extrinsic lesions. This modality is exceedingly helpful for determining secondary tumor implantation and tumors of adjacent visceral organs causing obstruction. Magnetic resonance imaging is an excellent modality for determining obstructions due to the vena cava, ovarian vein, or iliac vessels. Ultrasonography may be helpful in demonstrating a hydroureteronephrosis but often it is not particularly helpful in discovering the primary etiology particularly when it is in the lower third of the ureter. The treatment of upper ureteral obstruction depends upon the etiology. Perhaps the most common cause in the elderly patient is either calculi or cancers which are either intrinsic or extrinsic to the urinary collecting system. Calculi may be extracted, pushed back into the kidney and then treated with extracorporeal shock wave lithotripsy, directly fractured with either laser, ultrasound, or electrohydrolic energy [12]. Calculi are generally removed but if they cannot be removed, their obstruction may be bypassed either by placing a nephrostomy, usually done percutaneously under fluoroscopic or ultrasonographic guidance, or by placing an internal stent cystoscopically. The internal stent, called a double J catheter, is a soft silastic catheter placed up the ureter with one loop in the renal pelvis and the second loop in the bladder. This is done under fluoroscopic control. This method of bypassing obstruction is particularly helpful for lesions which are external to the collecting system and cause compression of the ureter. This type of bypass is particularly helpful in relieving obstruction, returning renal function to normal so that such patients can have their therapy directed to the full extent at the primary tumor. Obstructions due to inflammatory lesions such as tuberculosis or enteric organisms require therapy with an antibiotic and during that therapy, generally require placement of a double J catheter so that the ureter does not stricture. Retroperitoneal fibrosis may be treated with internal indwelling double J catheters or by surgical translocation of the ureters from the retroperitoneal mass.

References

1 Resnick NM, Yalla SV. Detursor hyperactivity with impaired contractile functions: an unrecognized but common cause of incontinence in elderly patients. J Am Med Assoc 1987;257:3076–3081.

2 Diokno AC, Wells TJ, Brink CA. Urinary incontinence in elderly women: urodynamic evaluation. J Am Geriatr Soc 1987;35:940–946.

3 Sarmina I, Resnick MI. Risk factors in the development of renal dysfunction in patients with benign prostatic hyperplasia. Abst Am Urol Assoc 1988:445.

4 Jensen KME, Jorgensen JB, Mogensen P, et al. Some clinical aspects of uroflowmetry in elderly males: a population survey. Scand J Urol Nephrol 1986;20:93–99.

5 Castaneda F, Reddy P, Wasserman W, et al. Benign prostatic hypertrophy: retrograde transurethral dilatation of the prostatic urethra in humans: work in progress. Radiology 1987;163:649–654.

6 Peters CA, Walsh PC. The effect of nafarelin acetate, a luteinizing-hormone-releasing hormone agonist, on benign prostatic hyperplasia. N Engl J Med 1987;317:599–604.

7 Bosch RJLH, Derek J, Griffiths JHMB, et al. Treatment of benign prostatic hyperplasia by androgen deprivation: effects on prostate size and urodynamic parameters. J Urol 1989; 141:68–72.

8 Ferrie BG, Paterson PJ. Phenoxybenzamine in prostatic hypertrophy. A double-blind study. Br J Urol 1987;59: 63–65.

9 McNeal JE, Bostwick DG, Kindrachuk RS, et al. Patterns of progression in prostate cancer. Lancet 1986;1:60–63.

10 Grant JBF, Ahmed SR, Chalet SM, et al. Testosterone and gonadotropic profiles in patients on daily or monthly LHRH analogue ICI 118630 (Zoladex) compared with orchiectomy. Br J Urol 1986;58:539–544.

11 Henriksson P, Johansson S. Predictions of cardiovascular complications in patients with prostatic cancer treated with estrogen. Am J Epidemiol 1987;125:970–978.

12 Drach GW, Dretler S, Fair W, et al. Report of the United States cooperative study of extracorporeal shock wave lithotripsy. J Urol 1986;135:1127–1133.

21

Urinary tract infections in the elderly

John W. Warren

Introduction

Urinary tract infections are comprised of a series of clinical presentations, the common denominator of which is almost always bacteria in the urine [1]. Bacteriuria is very common among the aged with prevalence in women averaging about 20% and in men 10% [2]. In the great majority of cases and for the greater proportion of its duration, this bacteriuria is asymptomatic in both men and women. However, certain symptomatic clinical presentations can develop including the syndromes of dysuria/frequency, acute pyelonephritis, and bacteremia. This chapter will discuss the epidemiology, pathogenesis, clinical manifestations, diagnosis, and treatment of bacteriuria in its asymptomatic and symptomatic presentations. Because of the differing pathogeneses and presentations of urinary tract infection in men and women, these syndromes in each sex will be discussed separately.

Certain definitions will pertain throughout the chapter. *Bacteriuria* literally means bacteria in the urine. Careful specimen collection and bacteriologic culture methods have allowed quantitation of bacteria in order to distinguish organisms actually within bladder urine from urethral and periurethral organisms contaminating the urine at the time of collection. *Cystitis* is the symptom complex of burning upon urination with or without frequency and urgency of urination; although clinically interpreted as lower tract infection, a proportion of these cases actually have organisms in the upper tract as well. *Acute pyelonephritis* refers to the triad of flank pain, fever, and bacteriuria; while usually clinically interpreted as renal infection, localization studies have demonstrated a proportion of such cases to have no organisms in the upper tract. *Relapse* of urinary tract infections is the reappearance after antibiotic treatment of the same bacterial strain causing the original infection. *Re-infection*, on the other hand, is the appearance after antibiotic treatment of a bacterial strain in the urine different from that eliciting the original treatment.

Pathogenesis

In order to cause urinary tract infection, microorganisms have to enter the urinary tract. There have been two methods by which this can be accomplished:

1 hematogenous, from a nonurinary site in the body;
2 far more commonly, ascending through the urethra.

Hematogenous seeding of the kidney may be recognized as the isolation of organisms from the urine following bacteremia (or candidemia), particularly with certain pathogens including *Staphylococcus aureus*, Salmonella species, *Pseudomonas aeruginosa*, and *Candida* species [3]. The isolation of these organisms, in the absence of a foreign body in the urinary tract such as a urethral catheter, should suggest a hematogenous source. Rubin *et al.* [3] estimate that less than 3% of infections of the kidneys are via the hematogenous route.

The great proportion of urinary tract infections develop from an ascending route through the urethra. Studies examining this route of infection usually have been of young adult women, and usually of those with recurrent bacteriuria. These studies have indicated that periurethral colonization with uropathogenic organisms have often preceded the onset of symptomatic or asymptomatic bacteriuria. The proximity of the urethral orifice to the vagina and to the anus in women and thus the greater potential for periurethral colonization (as well as the shorter urethra of women) have often been postulated as reasons for the greater incidence and prevalence of bacteriuria in women than in men. To explain the increased prevalence of bacteriuria among the aged, this reasoning led to studies examining the ability of uropathogenic bacteria to colonize the genital areas of aged compared to younger patients. Marrie *et al.* [4] found that normal flora of the urethra more commonly included Gram-negative facultative aerobic organisms in aged women than in younger women; these species are those which commonly cause bacteriuria. To examine whether this prominence of urogenital colonization in the aged was because of changes in the ability of epithelial cells to allow adherence of micro-organisms, Sobel & Muller [5] examined vaginal epithelial cells from 30 aged and 20 young women. These investigators did not find greater adherence of uropathogenic *Escherichia coli* to the cells from the elderly individuals. In two of the four bacterial strains studied, there was no difference in their ability to adhere to cells of the young and elderly women; the two other strains adhered in significantly greater numbers to cells from the younger women. Subsequent studies by these investigators helped to explain the enhanced adherence to the younger women's cells. They showed with animal studies (which corroborated observations of other investigators of women during menstrual cycles) that estrogen tends to stimulate adherence of

E. coli to vaginal epithelial cells as well as to exfoliated bladder epithelial cells [6].

These relatively subtle distinctions of the ease of colonization between younger and elderly women regularly may be overwhelmed by fecal contamination from bowel incontinence experienced by some aged women. Brocklehurst *et al.* [7] have demonstrated that bacteriuria in elderly women is significantly associated with fecal incontinence.

Once in the periurethral area, organisms may be able to traverse the urethra to the bladder. This passage may take place during vaginal intercourse or medical instrumentation, such as urethral catheterization [8]. It seems reasonable to conclude that the greater incidence and duration of hospitalization among the elderly with often attendant instrumentation may result in entry and subsequent residence of bacteria in the urinary tract.

Although one can speculate that organisms via these means may enter the bladder, sustained bacteriuria rarely results in the normally functioning urinary tract. This may be due to several protective mechanisms, one or more of which may be defective in elderly people. For instance, voiding will flush from the urinary tract perhaps 99% of recently entered bacteria. Most *E. coli* possess Type 1 fimbriae which adhere to Tamm–Horsfall protein, the major component of urinary mucous [9]. This mucous, suspended in bladder urine and laden with organisms, thus may prevent adherence of the bacteria to bladder mucosa while facilitating their excretion in the next voiding. Sobel & Kaye [10] compared urinary mucous in younger and elderly men and women and found that the elderly group excreted significantly less uromucoid in the urine. To the extent that Tamm–Horsfall protein is protective, these investigators speculated that this lower production and excretion of Tamm–Horsfall protein may be related to the increased prevalence of asymptomatic bacteriuria in aged individuals.

Furthermore, incomplete bladder emptying is common among the aged [7]. For women the presence of vaginal descensus, uterine prolapse, cystocele, or urethrocele [11]; for men, prostatic hypertrophy or carcinoma [12]; and for both sexes bladder diverticulae, bladder tumor, or neurogenic bladder may lead to residual bladder urine. Moreover, diabetes mellitus is relatively common in the aged population and may result in autonomic neuropathy and urine retention [13–15]. Furthermore, it is interesting to note that Sawers *et al.* [16] found that autonomic dysfunction, as demonstrated by certain cardiovascular maneuvers, was associated with bacteriuria in aged diabetics even in the absence of urinary retention.

Even if the flushing mechanism of urination is effective, invariably a few bacteria will be left clinging to the mucosa of the bladder in the 1 or 2 ml of urine which remains after a normal voiding. These bacteria in the normal urinary tract are killed by still poorly understood bladder defense mechanisms which appear to be physically associated with the mucosa. Bacteria adherent to or internalized by bladder epithelial cells will be effectively removed by the shedding of these cells into the urine and subsequent voiding. The importance of this mechanism has not been delineated and its relative role in aged as compared with young individuals has likewise not been explored.

Indeed, adherence to uroepithelial cells (as observed of those voided in the urine) has been associated with urinary tract infection in children and young women. Such adherence has also been examined in aged patients and reports of such studies offer conflicting information. Sobel & Kaye [17] found that voided uroepithelial cells from young women allowed the adherence of more E. coli than those from older women. Reid et al. [18], on the other hand, found an increased adherence of several species of organisms to cells of elderly women as compared to young women. The reason for these differences are not clear but may be related to the different donors as well as to different bacteria studied. Additionally, the situation in men may be different. Sobel & Kaye [17] examined cells from young and elderly men and found that those from older men appeared to allow the adherence of greater numbers of bacteria than those from younger men.

Unless and until bacteria invade the uroepithelium, they will be bathed in urine. While most bacteria grow in this medium, the composition of urine changes dependent upon hydration, diet, and metabolic processes. Therefore, at times, urine may actually inhibit bacteria because of low pH, high osmolality, or certain constituents such as urea and hippuric acid. Whether these bacteriostatic mechanisms change with age has not been studied.

While bacteria may be able to sustain themselves in the lumen of the urinary tract and multiply, they still must move to the kidney in order to cause acute pyelonephritis. The means by which bacteria move from the bladder to the kidney in the aged are unknown. Vesicoureteral reflux appears not to be a common finding in this population but may be important in the presence of prostatic hypertrophy or other types of bladder outflow obstruction. By whatever mechanisms, once bacteria gain entry to the renal pelvis and possibly the tubular system of the kidney, the steps of pathogenesis remain unclear. It does appear reasonable to assume that bacteria must reach an epithelium beyond which is the renal interstitium, cross that epithelium by going through or between or by killing epithelial cells, and enter the interstitium where an accumulating population of polymorphonuclear leukocytes defines what pathologically can be termed acute pyelonephritis.

Women

Asymptomatic bacteriuria

Diagnosis
Asymptomatic bacteriuria is usually defined as the presence of 100 000 colony-forming units (CFU)/ml of urine or more on two separate urine specimens. A finding on one specimen is about 80% specific, on two this specificity increases to 95% [1]. While the bacterial culture serves as the gold standard for diagnosis of bacteriuria, other more rapid tests can be used to estimate the presence of a concentration of 10^5 CFU/ml or more. Microscopy of voided urine is a useful test. The presence of at least one bacterium per high power field in centrifuged but unstained urine suggests 10^5 CFU/ml or more as does one organism per oil immersion field in uncentrifuged but Gram-stained urine [1].

A recent study of 418 elderly people (322 women and 96 men) is useful to assess several other rapid screening tests for bacteriuria [19]. One of the tests studied was a venerable one: observation of the urine for turbidity when viewed against a white background. The finding of turbidity was 90% sensitive in detecting bacteriuria although only 66% specific. Additional analyses revealed that the combination of turbidity plus nitrite and leukocyte esterase (as measured by dipsticks) was 96% sensitive with a negative predictive value of 95%. In other words, these three tests being negative in an aged individual would indicate that urine does not contain bacteriuria of 10^5 or more and thus may not require culturing. This type of screening procedure would save perhaps 30% of the urine specimens submitted to a hospital laboratory [19].

Epidemiology

Beginning in puberty, the prevalence of asymptomatic bacteriuria in women increases about 1% point per decade. However, during the seventh decade, this increase in prevalence accelerates, reaching 14% in the 1960s, 19% in the 1970s and 1980s, and 22% in the 1990s [20]. Aged individuals in hospitals or nursing homes have higher prevalences of bacteriuria than those living at home (Table 21.1). Bacteriuria, in the ambulatory aged at least, appears to be a dynamic process with few individuals being continously bacteriuric. Most community-living bacteriuric individuals have spontaneous appearance and disappearance of the bacteriuria. Boscia *et al.* [20] demonstrated this in a longitudinal study in which 16−20% of women were bacteriuric on each of three surveys performed at 6 month intervals. However, those comprising the bacteriuric women differed on each survey. For instance, by the third survey, a total of 30% of all women had been identified as bacteriuric. But only 6% of women were bacteriuric on all three surveys; the additional 24% had experienced spontaneous appearance or disappearance of bacteriuria on one or more of the surveys. Almost all asymptomatic bacteriuria in aged women is a monomicrobial infection. Gram-negative rods are the most common organisms [20−23]. Boscia *et al.* [20] found 93% of episodes were caused by gram-negative rods. *Escherichia coli* was the most common pathogen, comprising 79% of the total organisms. Other bacteriuric organisms included *Klebsiella pneumoniae*, *Proteus mirabilis*, *Enterococcus*, and non-enterococcus *Streptococcus*.

This "asymptomatic" bacteriuria is truly asymptomatic.

Boscia *et al.* [24] studied 72 subjects who were bacteriuric on one survey and not bacteriuric on another. At the time each urine specimen was collected, a questionaire was completed about symptoms. Whether the participants were bacteriuric or not, there was no difference in the following symptoms: urinary symptoms including suprapubic pain, flank pain, fever, incontinence (separately assessed as while awake, while asleep, or during a cough or sneeze), frequency or urgency; or more generalized including anorexia, difficulty in falling asleep or in staying asleep, fatigue, malaise, or weakness.

Even though asymptomatic, this bacteriuria commonly is accompanied by evidence of acute inflammation in the urinary tract. Boscia *et al.* [24] examined first morning voided urine for leukocytes, defining pyuria as 10 leukocytes/mm^3 of uncentrifuged urine [25]. Of 317 women studied, 46 had bacteriuria of 10^5 CFU/ml or greater; of these, 94% had pyuria. Fourteen women had bacteriuria of 10^2−10^4 CFU/ml; 64% of their specimens demonstrated pyuria. It is interesting to note that while the prevalence of pyuria in the nonbacteriuric women was significantly less than that in the bacteriuric women, it was not zero. Of the 257 women without bacteriuria (i.e., less than 10^2 CFU/ml), 32% had pyuria. The authors conclude that while pyuria is not specific for urinary tract infection it is quite sensitive; a screening test which demonstrates no pyuria would be suitable for estimating the absence of bacteriuria of 10^5 CFU/ml or more in an asymptomatic aged women.

One-third to two-thirds of women with asymptomatic bacteriuria may have bacteria in their upper tract, presumably in one or both pelvices or kidneys. Boscia *et al.* [20] demonstrated this with the use of antibody-coated bacteria, a finding initially reported to imply upper tract infection. In women with asymptomatic bacteriuria, one-third had antibody-coated bacteria in their urine [26,27]. Those with such findings were more likely to be bacteriuric on subsequent surveys than those without antibody-coated bacteria in the urine. Nicolle *et al.* [28], using a bladder washout technique developed by Fairley *et al.* [29], found that two-thirds of institutionalized women with asymptomatic bacteriuria had an upper tract infection. Others have found similar results [30]. Using the washout technique as the standard, Nicolle *et al.* [28] found that the antibody-coated technique was only 58% sensitive and 71% specific in identifying upper tract bacteria. Indeed, high concentration pyuria was

Table 21.1 Prevalence of bacteriuria in subjects older than 65 years of age. (From Boscia & Kaye [2])

Living situation	Percentage with bacteriuria	
	Women	Men
Living at home	17−33	6−13
Nursing home	23−27	17−26
Hospital	32−50	30−34

better in estimating upper tract disease than was the antibody-coated bacteria test [28].

Consequences

Asymptomatic bacteriuria may be quite prevalent among aged women but what are the sequelae of this infection? During the 1950s and 1960s merely the identification of bacteria 10^5/ml or more in the urine over several examinations was enough for clinicians and investigators to assume that the patient had chronic renal infection. As longitudinal studies in young, middle-aged, and aged women were performed, however, it became clear that the two most discussed consequences, hypertension and renal failure, did not develop as a consequence of bacteriuria, at least in the absence of obstruction or functional abnormalities of the urinary tract [31–34]. Indeed, it appeared that the only consequence of asymptomatic bacteriuria in the otherwise normal urinary tract was an increased incidence of symptomatic episodes of urinary tract infection [34]. Consequently, during the 1970s, students of urinary tract infections became comfortable in suggesting that asymptomatic bacteriuria in adult women with normal urinary tracts did not require treatment [35], recommending that only the appearance of the occasional symptomatic urinary tract infection should elicit antibiotic therapy.

However, this posture became increasingly uncomfortable with three reports in the 1970s and early 1980s of longitudinal studies of individuals who at study outset had been categorized as bacteriuric or nonbacteriuric [36–38]. All three studies demonstrated an increased mortality rate among the bacteriuric individuals over a follow-up period of 5, 10, and 15 years, respectively. However, these studies elicited at least two concerns. The first was that bacteriuria was not causally related to mortality but merely was a marker for sicker or more debilitated patients who were likely to die of causes unrelated to urinary tract infection. For instance, dementia and other neurologic diseases have been associated with asymptomatic bacteriuria in the aged [7]. This cognitive impairment may result in frequent hospitalizations and urinary instrumentation, fecal incontinence with perineal contamination [7], and urinary incontinence [7] with possible urethral catheterization. Each of these situations may result in entry of organisms into the urinary tract. Ineffective voiding mechanisms and residual urine, common in aged patients [7], may then

result in persistance of the bacteriuria. The second concern was that bacteriuria was a marker for another characteristic associated with increased mortality, i.e., older age. The prevalence of bacteriuria increases with age; clearly, the incidence of mortality increases with age. Consequently, the connection observed in these studies may not have been a causal one between bacteriuria and mortality but between age and mortality. A Swedish study, for instance, noted that in the elderly an age difference of 2 years resulted in a 20% difference in mortality [39]. The data as presented in these three studies were of age groupings of 5 years, 10 years, and variable years (less than 45, 45–54, and more than 54 years of age). Both bacteriuria and mortality could have been clustered towards the end of each of these age groupings.

In 1986, a 9-year study was reported from Sweden which clarified these issues [39]. This study examined women who at the time of entering the study were within 2 months of their 70th birthday. The diagnosis of bacteriuria on entry was established by two positive cultures with at least 10^5 bacteria/ml of urine. A total of 1079 women participated of whom 97 (9%) were bacteriuric. Findings significantly different among the bacteriuric women were reports of previous urinary tract infection (58% vs. 43%), pain upon voiding (7% vs. 2%), urgency (25% vs. 17%), and use of a catheter (5% vs. 0.2%). There were no differences in the prevalence of diabetes mellitus, myocardial infarction, hypertension, or cancer. At follow-up 5 years and 9 years later, there was no difference in mortality rates between women with bacteriuria and those without. By this methodology, these investigators removed the heterogeneity of age which hampered conclusions of the earlier studies of bacteriuria and mortality. This design clarifies the association of bacteriuria and mortality which appears to be more of an epiphenomenon rather than a causal relationship.

A subsequent study in Sweden of institutionalized women over the age of 85 similarly revealed no difference in mortality rates between those who were bacteriuric or nonbacteriuric at entry into a 5-year study [40].

Of concern in all these investigations is that patients were assigned to the bacteriuric or nonbacteriuric groups based upon their status at initiation of the study. The ongoing investigations by Boscia et al. [20] indicate that bacteriuria often is a transient phenomenon in the ambulatory elderly. The ideal study of bacteriuria and mortality would be one of individuals of identical ages in whom periodic urine cultures divided into groups defined as never bacteriuric, one or more gradings of intermittently bacteriuric, and continuously bacteriuric, with a rigorous effort to identify underlying diseases and causes of death.

Treatment

At present, can we make some assessments as to the usefulness of antibiotic therapy in asymptomatic bacteriuria? As noted, Boscia *et al.* [24] have demonstrated that at any given time asymptomatic bacteriuria is indeed just that. However, in studies of young women, Asscher *et al.* [34] demonstrated that the incidence of symptomatic urinary tract infection was higher in women who earlier had had asymptomatic bacteriuria than in women who had not. Boscia *et al.* [41] studied the incidence of symptomatic disease in women with asymptomatic bacteriuria over time. This was in a controlled trial of antibiotic therapy in which the treatment group received up to two courses of antibiotics at the outset of the study; the placebo group received no antibiotics. At the end of 6 months, 36% of the treatment group were bacteriuric compared with 65% of the placebo group. The incidence of symptomatic infection was 8% in the treatment and 16% in the placebo group (nonsignificant) over the 6-month period. In a subsequent editorial, these investigators noted that the beneficial effects of antibiotic therapy of asymptomatic bacteriuria in the short-term were minimal; that adverse drug effects occur, particularly in the aged; that screening of the aged for bacteriuria would be costly; and that "at present, in the absence of obstructed uropathy (which is rare in women), no evidence exists to support the routine use of antimicrobial therapy for asymptomatic bacteriuria in elderly persons" [42].

Nicolle *et al.* [43,44] came to the same conclusion following a randomized trial of antibiotic therapy in institutionalized noncatheterized women with asymptomatic bacteriuria. In this study, their treatment group received single-dose antibiotic therapy; then, if relapse occurred, a 2-week course; and with a subsequent relapse, a final 6-week course of antibiotics. In the placebo group, these investigators found that bacteriuria in this institutionalized population of women tended to be persistent; this is contrary to the findings of Boscia *et al.* [41,42] in ambulatory patients. Nicolle *et al.* [43,44] found

that there was a lower prevalence of bacteriuria over the 12-month period in the treatment group as compared with the placebo group. However, this lower prevalence was relatively minor and most patients in the therapy group did not maintain prolonged bacteriuria-free intervals because of frequent reinfections. The women in the treatment group experienced a number of adverse effects of the antibiotic therapy, particularly during the 2- and 6-week courses. Additionally, an increased incidence of antibiotic-resistant organisms tended to be found in the treatment group. These investigators concluded from their trial that asymptomatic bacteriuria of institutionalized elderly women was not treated. Other investigators have similarly been discouraged following single-dose therapy [45,46] or serial courses with different antibiotic groups [47].

Overall, most students of asymptomatic bacteriuria in the elderly feel at present that therapy is not warranted [2–3,7,42,43,47,48]. An ongoing controlled trial of recurrent treatment of asymptomatic bacteriuria in ambulatory elderly individuals [20,24,25,41] when completed may or may not modify this recommendation.

Symptomatic bacteriuria

Cystitis-like symptoms (dysuria, frequency, urgency, etc.) occur in aged women [30,41,49]. What proportion of such symptom complexes are preceded by periods of asymptomatic bacteriuria is unclear. As noted, Boscia *et al.* [41] in their prospective trial of antibiotic treatment of asymptomatic bacteriuria found that over a 6-month period 16% of the women receiving placebo developed symptomatic urinary tract infection with 10^5 CFU/ml bacteria or more in their urine. That lower concentrations of bacteriuria may cause similar symptoms in aged females, as has been found in younger women, is possible but has not been adequately explored.

While short course antibiotic therapy (single dose or 3 days) for cystitis symptoms have been shown to be effective in younger women, this therapy has not been well tested in aged women. At least two studies have demonstrated the relative ineffectiveness of short courses of antibiotics for, mostly, asymptomatic bacteriuria in older women. One-day therapy of asymptomatic bacteriuric elderly women with trimethoprim resulted in immediate clearance of the bacteriuria in all women but, at 6-weeks follow-up, 70% of the women were bacteriuric. Two-thirds of these recurrent infections were relapses with the same organisms [45]. Another study compared single dose with 5-days therapy with trimethoprim [46]. Most of the aged women treated were asymptomatic although apparently some had "relevant symptoms and signs." Two weeks following therapy (the longest follow-up) 67% of the patients receiving the single dose were still bacteriuric as compared to 39% of those receiving the 5-day course (P less than 0.01). At present, the usefulness of short course antibiotic therapy in the aged women with symptomatic (or asymptomatic) bacteriuria is unclear. The prudent practice seems to be to treat aged women with cystitis-type symptoms with antibiotics for 10–14 days. The role of prolapse syndromes, diabetic neuropathy, and other causes of residual urine in this population in the hindrance of successful therapy requires exploration.

Parsons & Schmidt [49] have treated a group of women with frequent recurrent symptomatic bacteriuria with intravaginal estrogen as well as antibiotics. They demonstrated a change in vaginal pH associated with diminished vaginal colonization of facultative anaerobic gram-negative rods. This was associated with a diminished vaginal incidence of symptomatic urinary tract infection in these women.

Acute pyelonephritis and bacteremia

The incidence of acute pyelonephritis in elderly women is difficult to judge. However, studies of aged women being admitted to a hospital have demonstrated that the urinary tract is the most common source of community-acquired bacteremia [50]. A study specifically looking at acute pyelonephritis is that of 23 women 65 years or older with "fewer, constitutional symptoms, and bacteriuria of greater than 10^5 CFU/ml or more" [51]. Pyuria was present in 22 (95%) of the women and *E. coli* was the pathogen in 16 (69%). Blood cultures were performed in 20 of the women and in 12 demonstrated bacteria (52% of the total with acute pyelonephritis). Radiologic assessments of 15 women demonstrated postvoid bladder residual urine in 5, renal calculus in 2, hydronephrosis in 2, ureteral calculus in 1, chronic pyelonephritis in 1, and renal abscess in 1. Six women had normal intravenous pyelograms. All but one of the women defervesed within 48 hours of hospitalization with antibiotic and supportive therapy. (These data regarding women with acute pyelonephritis were calculated from data available in [51,73]).

The authors compared this very high incidence of bacteremia in elderly women (52%) to studies in the literature in which 19 out of 120 (15%) young women with acute symptomatic pyelonephritis had bacteremia. This difference between the aged and younger women was significant at P less than 0.001. Similarly, five out of 23 (22%) of the elderly women had septic shock compared to three out of 99 (3%) young women reported in the literature, also a significant difference. Gleckman *et al.* [52] subsequently conducted a prospective survey of women being admitted with acute pyelonephritis to a hospital. (In this study, the authors removed from analysis nine patients 50 years of age or older who had renal calculi or, in one, a rectovesicular fistula.) Of 20 younger women (18–44 years) 17 had blood cultures of which none showed bacteria. However, of 34 elderly women, 33 had blood cultures obtained of which 16 (48%) had organisms present. This was significant at P less than 0.005. The authors further demonstrated that among patients who by intravenous pyelography had no obstruction, 0 out of seven young women were bacteremic as compared with 12 out of 18 (67%) elderly women; P less than 0.025.

The urinary tract appears to be the most frequent source of bacteremia in the elderly whether they are in the community, the hospital, or the nursing home [50,53, 54]. Esposito *et al.* [50] found that of 100 consecutive bacteremias in aged people admitted to a hospital, 34 were from the urinary tract. Meyers *et al.* [54] reviewed 100 elderly bacteremic patients admitted to a hospital; 27% were from the urinary tract. In each case, the urinary tract was the most common source.

Gleckman *et al.* [55] examined duration of therapy of acute pyelonephritis in women with median ages in the 10-day and 21-day groups of 65 and 70 years, respectively. Patients with urinary catheters, obstructions, and fistulae were excluded from study. All women received 2 or 3 days of intravenous aminoglycoside therapy. Half the women were randomly assigned to then receive the balance of a 10-day course of oral antibiotics active against the urinary pathogens; the other half to receive the balance of a 21-day course. Of those treated for 10 days, 21 were cured of their initial infection (although four experienced reinfection) and none had a relapse. Of those treated for 21 days, 17 were cured of their initial infection (five experienced reinfection) and three had a relapse. There was no significant difference between these two groups. The authors suggest that 10 days of antibiotics, with the first 2 or 3 days being intravenous administration, is equivalent to 3 weeks of therapy and probably satisfactory for women with acute pyelonephritis not complicated by structural abnormalities.

Men

Microbiologic diagnosis

In men, studies of asymptomatic bacteriuria and of acute pyelonephritis have used the criterion of 10^5 CFU/ml urine or more to diagnose bacteriuria [19,20,22,23,36, 37,39,40,51]. However, this microbiologic criterion was developed, mostly in women, to distinguish periurethral contamination from bladder bacteriuria. Anatomic differences between men and women suggest that periurethral contamination is less common among men. Lipsky et al. [56] have examined this by comparing voided urines with either suprapubic or catheterized urines in 76 sets of specimens from 66 men. Of these men 34 (52%) had "irritative" symptoms of burning, etc., 20 (30%) had obstructive symptoms, and 12 (18%) apparently had no symptoms but were undergoing other types of urologic work-up. These investigators found that bladder bacteriuria (suprapubic or urethral catheter specimens) was present in 36 (47%) of these pairs of specimens; using these as the standards, they found that clean catch midstream voided specimens were 97% specific and 97% sensitive if the criterion of 10^3 CFU/ml of urine or more was used. They demonstrated that uncleansed first voided specimen was as sensitive (97%) as the midstream voided specimen although somewhat less specific (91%). They also found that both bladder bacteriuria and pyuria were significantly more frequent in patients with irritative symptoms (76% and 69%, respectively) than in those with other urinary problems (37% and 31%, respectively).

Asymptomatic bacteriuria

Epidemiology

Notwithstanding the above, in men just as in women, the microbiologic criterion for asymptomatic bacteriuria to date has been 10^5/ml urine. Boscia et al. [20] studied 150 aged men (mean age 84.6 years) using this criterion for diagnosis. Of men in their 70s, the prevalence of bacteriuria was zero out of 31 (0%); in their 80s, seven out of 82

(8.5%); and in their 90s, two out of 37 (5.4%). Although these prevalences are much higher than the essentially zero prevalence found in males between their neonatal years and their aged years [1,57], they were significantly lower than those in women of the same ages who were studied. Seventy-six of these men had three urine surveys 6 months apart. The prevalence of bacteriuria on each survey was similar, between 4 and 6%. However, like asymptomatic bacteriuria in women, in men this syndrome was dynamic. By the third survey, 11% of the men had had bacteriuria on at least one survey. However, only one man (1.3%) had persistence of the same species over all three surveys [20].

As opposed to the women, in whom gram-negative rods predominated, among the men in this study the monomicrobial bacteriuria consisted about equally of gram-negative rods and gram-positive organisms including enterococcus and *Staphylococcus epidermidis*. Others have found that gram-positive organisms are more prominent among elderly men than among elderly women [56]. Although most authors feel that the development of prostatic disease, particularly benign prostatic hypertrophy, is responsible for the marked increased in prevalence of asymptomatic bacteriuria in men of old age [57], symptoms of obstruction either were not noted or not inquired about in this study.

Pyuria is common in men with asymptomatic bacteriuria. Norman et al. [58] found that 68% of elderly men with asymptomatic bacteriuria demonstrated pyuria. Indeed, they found that the absence of pyuria was an excellent screening device suggesting the absence of bacteriuria. They found the negative predictive value was 97% for ambulatory elderly men. A study of institutionalized men, most of whom were wearing condom catheters, found that pyuria was present in 91% of bacteriuric patients [59].

Consequences

Several of the studies between association of asymptomatic bacteriuria and mortality discussed above in regard to women also included men. In the report by Dontas et al. [37], the association between mortality and bacteriuria in men was not quite significant ($P = 0.07$). Similarly, the study by Sourander & Kasanen [36] showed no increase in mortality of the men that were bacteriuric. The same criticisms of these studies regarding women can be applied to assessments of the association of bacteriuria and mortality in men. The best study to date of bacteriuria and mortality is that of Nordenstam *et al.* [39] in which age was kept as a constant (70 years ± 2 months at entry). These investigators found that the 70-year-old men with bacteriuria had a significantly increased prevalence of cancer at entry into the study (27% vs. 6%). Although the data are not presented, the authors indicate that the difference was statistically significant for "urogenital (including prostatic) cancer but not for cancer at other sites." After excluding men with cancer, 5-year mortality was 15% vs. 13%. Thus, like women, bacteriuria in aged men does not appear to be associated with increased mortality, at least in the absence of certain concomitant fatal diseases.

Nicolle *et al.* [60] classified elderly institutionalized men by periodic urine cultures into continuously, intermittently, or nonbacteriuric over a 3-year period. They followed these men for a total of 6 years and found no difference in survival among the three population groups even though the continuously and intermittent bacteriuric patients were more often demented and incontinent of urine and stool.

Treatment

Should asymptomatic bacteriuria in elderly men be treated? There are little data to assist in answering this question. Nicolle *et al.* [59] studied institutionalized males, 70% of whom wore condom catheters. Using successively longer courses of therapy, they found that by the end of the study (mean of 10½ months), 94% of men in the therapy group compared to 100% of men in the placebo group were bacteriuric. Their conclusion was "thus, therapy for eradication of bacteriuria in this population appears to be futile" [59].

Symptomatic bacteriuria

In men, symptoms of urinary tract infection can usually be classified into two major syndromes. The first is similar to that of "cystitis" in women and includes dysuria, frequency, and urgency of urination [56,61]. The second is more common to men and includes hesitancy, nocturia, slow stream, and dribbing, usually related to benign prostatic hypertrophy [12] or, alternatively, to inflammation of the prostate itself [62]. Lipsky *et al.* [56] found that about three-quarters of men with primarily irritative symptoms and about one-third with primarily obstructive symptoms had bacteriuria.

In elderly male patients, the understanding of bacterial infections requires an understanding of prostatic syndromes. Unfortunately, the latter are themselves not fully understood.

Benign prostatic hypertrophy is a nearly universal accompaniment of aging in men and results from proliferation of the periurethral glands of the prostate. Enlargement of the medial portion of the prostate compresses the enclosed urethra as well as the outer prostatic glands. This obstruction of bladder outflow leads to diminished ability of normal voiding processes to rid the bladder of bacteria which have entered. With increasing obstruction, increased volumes and pressures can lead to not only bladder mucosal infections but also entry (possibly through vesicoureteral reflux) of bacteria into one or both kidneys with subsequent acute pyelonephritis. Indications for surgical therapy are essentially two:

1 urinary tract obstruction resulting in dilatation of the ureters, calyces, and hydronephrosis;
2 intolerable symptoms of obstruction.

The most common surgery is transurethral prostatectomy in which the hypertrophied medial periurethral gland tissue is resected from the thick rind formed by compression of the outer prostatic glands [12].

In addition to benign prostatic hypertrophy, several prostatitis syndromes may present in aged men. Perhaps 50% of men will experience symptoms of prostatitis sometime during their lives [63]. A useful method of classification of prostatitis syndromes is the following [64]:

1 acute prostatitis;
2 chronic bacterial prostatitis;
3 "nonbacterial" prostatitis;
4 prostatodynia.

The first two syndromes are bacterial infections; the latter two, comprising by far the greater proportion of men presenting with prostatitis-type symptoms, are not associated with bacteriuria and are of unknown etiology. Consequently, in order to understand and treat these syndromes properly, appropriate bacteriologic studies are necessary.

Acute prostatitis

This is not a subtle diagnosis. The patient presents commonly with urinary frequency and dysuria and often with systemic toxicity including fever and myalgias. The rectal examination reveals an exquisitly tender prostate.

Evaluation of urine shows pyuria and high concentrations of uropathogens such as *E. coli*, Klebsiella, etc. Blood cultures may be positive with the same organism, before or after prostatic examination which should be performed gingerly [62].

Chronic bacterial prostatitis

This may be the most common cause of recurrent urinary tract infection in men, usually by relapses of the same organism [62]. The diagnosis is made by establishing the presence of a bacterial species in the prostate which has been implicated in prior episodes of bacteriuria. The method of Meares & Stamey [65] is that most commonly used to localize infection of the prostate (Table 21.2). This procedure is not useful if all specimens show bacteria at high concentration. Consequently, it is sometimes necessary to clear bacteriuria with antibiotics that do not localize to the prostate, for example, nitrofurantoin. The procedure is useful if it demonstrates a step-up of bacterial concentration either in prostatic secretions or in the voided urine following prostatic massage. Gram-negative rods are the usual etiologic agents; gram-positive cocci have been implicated in a few cases [66]. Patients generally present with a history of recurring urinary tract infection with dysuria and urgency, thought to be caused by periodic multiplication of organisms within the urinary tract outside the prostate. Patients also may have chronic or recurrent perineal, lower back, and/or lower abdominal pain. Prostatic stones may be present and contribute to the chronicity of prostatic infections.

Stamey *et al.* [67] in 1968 identified in dogs and in humans the presence in prostatic secretions of a factor which was bacteriocidal for a variety of gram-negative and positive organisms. They found that the fraction containing this effect was heat stable, of low molecular weight, and was inactivated by human serum. Fair *et al.* [68] subsequently demonstrated that this factor was a zinc-containing compound. They noted that others had decades earlier determined that the prostate contained more zinc than any organ in the body and that in the mid-1950s investigators had noted that some patients with chronic bacterial prostatitis had decreased prostate levels of zinc. These investigators demonstrated, indeed, that patients with chronic bacterial prostatitis had markedly diminished or absent antibacterial activity and zinc concentrations.

Because 40–50% of men with recurrent bacteriuria

Table 21.2 Procedure for localization of infection in the male lower urinary tract by use of segmented urine cultures. (From Meares & Stamey [65], and Krieger [62])

Specimen	Symbol	Description
Voided bladder 1	VB_1	Initial 5–10 ml of urinary stream
Voided bladder 2	VB_2	Midstream specimen
Expressed prostatic secretions	EPS	Secretions expressed from prostate by digital massage after midstream specimen
Voided bladder 3	VB_3	First 5–10 ml of urinary stream immediately after prostatic massage

will have localization of infection to the prostate [61] the treatment of recurrent infection will be discussed in this section. Trimethoprim and the quinolones diffuse into the prostate and thus are good candidates for treatment of chronic bacterial prostatitis. Two studies have compared therapy with trimethoprim–sulfamethoxazole of 10 days with 12 weeks and of 2 weeks with 6 weeks, respectively, in men with recurrent urinary infections [61,69]. The median ages of patients in these studies were 69 and 60 years, respectively. Both studies found that the shorter course was significantly less useful than the longer course at 12- and 6-week follow-up, respectively. However, even the longer therapies were associated with only 60 and 68% success rates. Of those patients whose infections were recurrent, most were relapses occurring within 4 weeks of discontinuation of the antibiotic. A recent study of a quinolone (norfloxacin) was compared to trimethoprim–sulfamethoxazole in a randomized trial of 4–6 weeks treatment of men with recurrent urinary tract infections. Follow-up specimens were obtained 4–6 weeks after therapy was completed. Norfloxacin was effective at follow-up in eradicating bacteriuria in 56 out of 60 (93%) compared with 39 out of 49 (80%) of those treated with trimethoprim–sulfamethoxazole. Of men who had organisms isolated from prostatic secretions, the eradication rates were 92% and 67% [70].

"Nonbacterial" prostatitis

Most men presenting with symptoms such as those noted for chronic bacterial prostatitis will not have bacteriuria recurrently nor will they have bacteria demonstrated to be in the prostate. However, examination of prostatic fluid does reveal polymorphonuclear leukocytes, i.e., inflammation apparently in the prostate. The etiology of this syndrome is unknown [71,72].

Prostatodynia

Complaints are similar to those of chronic bacterial or nonbacterial prostatitis. In this case, however, neither bacteria nor leukocytes are present in the expressed prostatic secretions. Although also very common, this, like the "nonbacterial" prostatitis, is of unknown etiology; furthermore, its relationship to infection is unclear [62].

Acute pyelonephritis and bacteremia

Gleckman et al. [73] identified 12 men with acute pyelonephritis; those with Foley and condom catheters, acute prostatitis, and epididymitis were excluded from study. As with the women, E. coli was prominent causing six of the episodes; Klebsiella pneumoniae and Pseudomonas aeruginosa each caused two. Blood cultures were performed in 11, and seven (64%) grew organisms reflective of the urinary isolates. Radiologic assessments were conducted in 10 of the men and demonstrated postvoid bladder residual urine in six, renal calculus in three, chronic pyelonephritis in one, and a perinephric phlegmon in one; in one man the intravenous pyelography was normal. Eleven of the 12 patients' fevers defervesced within 48 hours of antibiotic therapy.

Urologic imaging

The role of imaging procedures in men with urinary tract infections is a controversial one. Some authors suggest that one episode of bacteriuria merits a urologic evaluation. Studies demonstrate that 50–80% of elderly men with recurrent bacteriuria have abnormalities in the upper tract [57,61,69,73–75]. Uncertainty remains, however, as to what proportion of such findings would change the therapeutic approach to the patient. However, many students would suggest that recurrent infections, acute pyelonephritis, failure to respond to treatment, or any other situation suggesting a complicated presentation should elicit urologic studies [57]. Which study(ies) should be performed however, remain unclear. The role of ultrasonography, intravenous pyelography, cystography, or cystoscopy should be individualized to the patient's situation [57].

Nosocomial urinary tract infections

Catheter-associated bacteriuria

Each year millions of urinary catheters are placed in aged patients in acute care hospitals, rehabilitation units, and chronic care facilities [76]. With the exception of occasional nonbacterial urethritis [77] and mechanical trauma [78], virtually all complications of urinary catheterization are results of consequent bacteriuria. The majority of these bacteria are from the patients own colonic flora [79] and may be native inhabitants or new immigrants, i.e., exogenous organisms from the hospital environment [80]. Just as with the pathogenesis of urinary tract infection in noncatheterized patients, these colonic bacteria may migrate across the perinium to colonize the periurethral area. Additionally, exogenous organisms may colonize directly the periurethral area or catheter equipment [81]. Organisms may be transferred to the patient by the hands of healthcare personnel [81] or infrequently by contaminated products or containers.

Once in or on the patient or on the catheter system surface, organisms may enter the bladder through one of three ways:

1 at the time of catheter insertion;
2 through the catheter lumen;
3 along the catheter–mucosal interface.

Furthermore, the risk of bacteriuria may persist in the hours or days after catheter removal [82].

Although univariate analyses suggest that the aged patient is at higher risk for catheter-associated bacteriuria than the younger patient, multivariate analyses show that age is not independently associated with the development of bacteriuria once the catheter is put in place. It appears that aged patients in hospitals are overrepresented among catheterized patients; additionally, they may have catheters in place for longer durations than younger patients. Indeed, the duration of catheterization is the most important risk factor for the development of catheter-associated bacteriuria [82–86]. It depends upon the indications for catheterization which may be grouped into four main categories:

1 urine output measurement;
2 surgical operation;
3 urine retention;
4 urinary incontinence.

Short-term catheterization

Between 15–25% of patients in acute care hospitals may have a catheter in place sometime during their stay [87]. Most are in place for only a short time: up to one-third for less than a day [85,88] and both the mean and median durations are between 2 and 4 days [84,85,87]. Nevertheless, between 10–30% of these catheterized patients develop bacteriuria [84,85,87], significantly greater than the 1% found among noncatheterized patients [87]. Because of the large number of patients catheterized, catheter-associated bacteriuria is the most common hospital-acquired infection, representing about 40% of such infections and constituting the majority of the 900 000 patients with nosocomial bacteriuria in American hospitals each year [89].

Among short-term catheterized patients, *E. coli* is the most frequent bacteriuric species isolated. Other common organisms are *Pseudomonas aeruginosa*, *Klebsiella pneumoniae*, *Proteus mirabilis*, *Staphylococcus epidermidis*, and enterococci [76,84,86,90,91] (Table 21.2). Particularly when antibiotics are in use, yeast may be isolated as well [91]. To establish a diagnosis many investigators have required organism concentrations of at least 100 000 CFU/ml of urine; others have selected lower concentrations. Most bacteria first identified at low concentrations in a catheterized urinary tract will over succeeding days reach a density of 100 000 CFU/ml or more [92]. Thus, identifying the onset of bacteriuria even in small numbers is of epidemiologic significance.

The majority of episodes of short-term catheter-associated bacteriuria are asymptomatic. However, fevers or other symptoms of urinary tract infection occur in 10–30% of patients with catheter-associated bacteriuria [82,87,88]; daily cultures of urine indicate that many symptomatic urinary tract infections occur on the first day of bacteriuria [88]. Of catheter-associated bacteriuric patients, only 1–5% will develop clinical bacteremia [88,93–95] and bacteremias from nosocomial urinary tract infections represent 6–15% of the total nosocomial bacteremias [94,95]. Men with catheter-associated bacteriuria are at greater risk than women for the development of bacteremia [94]. In some reports, certain bacteriuric organisms, for example, *Serratia marcescens*, may be more likely than others to cause bacteremia [93,94]. The mortality directly attributed to bacteremia from nosocomial bacteriuria is 13%; most deaths are in patients with severe underlying diseases [95]. At autopsy,

patients with catheter-associated bacteriuria dying in a hospital may have acute pyelonephritis, urinary stones, or perinephric abscesses [95,96]. Additionally, even without overt evidence of systemic infection, catheter-associated bacteriuria may be related to an increased risk of death [97].

Long-term catheterization

Although the magnitude of long-term urethral catheter use has not been directly measured, extrapolations from several studies [98–100] suggest that at any given time more than 100 000 elderly patients in American nursing homes have urethral catheters in place. Many of these patients have been catheterized for months and in some cases years. The two most frequent indications are:

1 urinary incontinence (mostly women);
2 bladder outlet obstruction (mostly men).

Urinary incontinence is by far the more common; women constitute up to 80% of long-term catheterized patients [100]. In nursing homes, the prevalence of patients with urinary incontinence ranges up to 50% [101]. Because a common perception is that continually wet skin may become macerated and lead to decubitus ulcers, a catheter is often used as a preventive or management technique. Of nursing-home patients with long-term urethral catheters, 34–69% have decubitus ulcers [101–103].

Even with excellent care, all patients eventually become bacteriuric if catheterized long enough. This universal prevalence of bacteriuria in long-term catheterized patients [104,105] is a function of two related phenomena. The first is an incidence of new episodes of bacteriuria similar to that seen in short-term catheterized patients [104] and, over time, caused by a wide variety of gram-negative and gram-positive bacterial species. The second is the ability of some of these strains to persist for weeks and months in the catheterized urinary tract [104]. These phenomena result in polymicrobial bacteriuria in 75–95% of urine specimens from long-term catheterized patients. Such specimens commonly have 2–4 bacterial species, each at concentrations of 10^5 CFU/ml or more [103–105]; some may have up to 6–8 species at that concentration [103]. These are not only common uropathogens such as *E. coli*, *P. aeruginosa*, and *P. mirabilis*, but also less familiar species such as *P. stuartii* and *Morganella morganii* [98,103,104,106].

Complications of long-term catheter-associated bacteriuria fall into two categories. The first includes symptomatic urinary tract infections such as seen with short-term catheterization, i.e., fever, acute pyelonephritis, and bacteremia; as in short-term catheterized patients, some of these episodes may result in death. The second group encompasses those occurring during long-term catheterization: obstruction, urinary tract stones, chronic renal inflammation, and especially among men, local periurinary infections.

Although two-thirds of febrile episodes in aged long-term catheterized patients may arise from the urinary tract [103], the incidence is low, about one febrile episode per 100 days of catheterization [103,107]. In women at least, most such episodes are of low-grade fever, last for 1 day or less, and resolve without antibiotic therapy [103]. However, bacteremia may occur during some of these fevers, even by "nonuropathogens" such as *P. stuartii* or *M. morganii* [103,108]. Bacteremia and death are more frequent during episodes of fever of more than 102°F [103]. Autopsies have revealed acute pyelonephritis in more than one-third of patients dying with long-term catheters in place [109].

In long-term catheterized patients a catheter obstruction may be a problem and, in some patients, a recurrent one [110,111]. The complex material that obstructs urinary catheters is composed of bacteria, glycocalyx, Tamm–Horsfall protein, and precipitated crystals [112–114]. *Proteus mirabilis* bacteriuria is associated with catheter obstruction [113], probably because of its potent urease [115,116] which hydrolyzes urea to ammonia, increasing urine pH and causing crystalization of struvite and apatite in the catheter lumen.

A similar bacterial process can occur in the urinary tract itself resulting in the crystallization of struvite and apatite in the form of "infection stones," a common problem in long-term catheterized patients [117]. Such stones in the bladder, often crusting around the catheter balloon and tip, are relatively benign. However, renal stones may be more serious, leading to chronic pyelonephritis and renal dysfunction [118].

Chronic renal inflammation, common in long-term catheterized persons [106,118,119], is related directly to the duration of catheterization [106]. However, chronic pyelonephritis, i.e., chronic renal inflammation with the additional components of deformed calyces and overlying parenchymal scarring, is found in only a minority of chronically inflamed kidneys and is often associated with the presence of pelvic or renal stones [118].

Prevention of catheterization

Obviously, the most direct method to prevent catheter-associated bacteriuria is to prevent catheterization. The last several decades have seen major advances in understanding complications of catheterization, in weighing its risks and benefits, and in determining appropriate indications for catheter insertion [1,76,120–123]. This understanding has prompted the use of alternatives to the urethral catheter. For instance, for incontinent patients, healthcare providers have encouraged a greater use of patient training, biofeedback, medications, surgery, and special clothes and bedclothes as management techniques. Additionally, several devices have been further explored as options to the urethral catheter; none, however, have been compared to urethral catheters in controlled trials of long-term use.

For men with urinary incontinence, external collectors applied about the penis which empty through a collection tube into a drainage bag have been widely used. Although these avoid problems of a tube in the urinary tract, urine within the condom catheters may have high concentrations of organisms, the urethra and skin may be colonized with uropathogens, and bladder bacteriuria may develop particularly in patients who frequently manipulate the condom [124,125]. Careful collection of urine in a new condom by well-trained individuals is necessary to distinguish bladder bacteriuria from skin or condom contamination [126,127].

For chronic urine retention, intermittent catheterization is useful. Many spinal injured patients or others with neurogenic bladders can use their bladders as containers for urine storage yet cannot initiate urination. Insertion of a sterile or clean catheter every 3–6 hours by caregivers or the patient, drainage of urine, and immediate removal of the catheter provide periodic bladder emptying [128]. However, bacteriuria develops in 27–100% of such patients within the first month [129,130]. Incidences of bacteriuria range from 21–27 new episodes per 100 patient-weeks [131,132]. These rates in spinal injured patients are less than half that of patients with long-term indwelling catheters [104].

Short-term suprapubic catheterization has been used in gynecologic, urologic, and other types of surgery [133]. The concept supporting its use is that the lower density of bacteria on the anterior abdominal skin will yield lower rates of bacteriuria than that associated with catheters in the urethra. Another feature is that clamping of the suprapubic catheter allows testing of voiding per urethra, obviously an advantage not shared with the urethral catheter. For comfort and convenience, patients and caregivers usually prefer suprapubic over indwelling catheters. Suprapubic catheterization appears promising and deserves well-designed trials to evaluate its effectiveness in different patient populations now requiring short-term and long-term urethral catheters.

Prevention of bacteriuria and its complications

Once a urethral catheter is in place, only two principles are universally recommended for prevention of bacteriuria:
1 maintain the closed catheter system;
2 minimize the duration of catheterization.

These and associated catheter hygiene practices have been well described [1,120−123]. If the catheter can be removed before bacteriuria develops, postponement becomes prevention. Hartstein *et al.* [82], using a predetermined list of durations appropriate for each indication, found that more than a third of catheterization days were unnecessary. Importantly, the majority of bacteriurias occurred after the catheter would have been removed had the appropriate catheter durations been observed.

Up to 80% of catheterized patients, because of underlying diseases and/or procedures, are administered antibiotics during but (usually) not because of catheterization. Comparisons of these patients with those not receiving antibiotics have consistently shown that antibiotic use is associated with a lower incidence of bacteriuria [82,85,86,88,106,134]. Nevertheless, the studies which have followed patients for a sufficient period of time have revealed that antibiotics are effective in postponement but not prevention of bacteriuria [82,85,86, 106,134]. Antibiotics appear to be effective for the first several days of use and then resistant organisms begin to appear in the urine [106,135]. Most authorities feel that the use of antibiotics to postpone bacteriuria is not indicated because of side-effects, cost, and emergence of antibiotic-resistant bacteria in the patient and the medical unit [1,136−138].

A low proportion of fevers are associated with catheter obstruction [103,107] and, in at least one study in women, a relatively low proportion of obstructions are associated with fever [103]. However, certain patients have recurrent obstructions [110,111] and for these, measures to prevent recurrences might be useful. Unfortunately, the very simple technique of once daily catheter irrigation with normal saline has been demonstrated in a crossover randomized trial to be ineffective in diminishing obstructions or fevers [139]. Methenamine preparations may diminish the incidence of catheter obstruction [140], apparently not because of antimicrobial activity but because of biochemical alteration of salt solubility.

Treatment

In general, clinicians should not be compelled to treat asymptomatic bacteriuria in catheterized patients [82,136−138]. However, because of the study by Platt *et al.* [97] which reported excess mortality related to short-term catheter-associated bacteriuria, often without apparent evidence of systemic infection, this stance may be modified as further data accumulate. Additionally, specific exceptions may pertain if certain bacterial strains in the institution are known to cause a high incidence of bacteremia. For instance, some investigators have reported that *Serr. marcescens* may be such an organism [93,94].

For the patient who develops fever and/or signs of bacteremia, the clinician should rule out sources outside the urinary tract, catheter obstruction and, especially among men, periurethral infection; cultures of urine and blood should be obtained. Many clinicians would empirically treat such patients with parenteral antibiotics at doses high enough to achieve concentrations in the serum adequate to treat bacteremia. The selection of antibiotics should be based upon knowledge of organisms common in the medical unit and Gram stain of the patient's urine at the time of the fever. Not surprisingly, survival of patients with bacteremia from nosocomial urinary tract infections is related to the administration of antibiotics active against the bacteremic strain [95].

The catheterized patient with lower abdominal pain, dysuria, and/or urgency, and without fever or other evidence of systemic infection may benefit from an oral antibiotic active *in vitro* in the same doses used for noncatheterized urinary tract infections.

Appropriate durations of parenteral or oral therapies have not been well established. For patients with increasing renal dysfunction or evidence of recalcitrant or recurring bacteremia, a search for urinary stones may be helpful [95] in anticipation of direct intervention.

Nosocomial bacteriuria not associated with a catheter

The pathogenesis of the 10−20% of nosocomial urinary tract infections not associated with catheterization or any instrumentation is not well understood. A partial explanation may be that the natural history of asymptomatic bacteriuria in these patients simply has continued and an episode has occurred in-hospital rather than in the community. A study in American hospitals revealed that hospital-acquired urinary tract infections occurring in the absence of instrumentation were significantly associated with age, female sex, and history of previous urinary tract infections [83]. These characteristics define a population group, hospitalized or not, that has a relatively high incidence of asymptomatic bacteriuria, as described above. Rates of bacteriuria are higher in debilitated than in healthy individuals [7,20,60] and hospitalization appears to enhance colonization of the skin with potential pathogens [141]; these findings suggest that hospitalized patients may have higher incidence of asymptomatic bacteriuria than nonhospitalized patients.

Summary

Bacteriuria is very common among the aged. This may be related to several factors. One is that there appears to be an increased periurethral colonization which is compounded by the relatively high frequency of fecal incontinence in older individuals. Entry of periurethral organisms may be prompted by urethral catheterizations attendant upon frequent hospitalizations for acute and chronic diseases. Elderly individuals may have diminished excretion of Tamm−Horsfall protein; to the extent that this suspended mucous binds planktonic bacteria and facilitates their clearance by urination, the elderly may be more susceptible to maintenance of bacteriuria. Additionally, residual urine is a common problem in the elderly because of prolapse syndromes, neurogenic bladders, diabetes mellitus, or benign prostatic hypertrophy; this too results in inefficient clearing of bacteria from the bladder urine.

Among men, benign prostatic hypertrophy may lead to bladder outflow obstruction, increased intravesicular pressure, maintenance of bacteriuria, and encouragement of the organisms' ascent to the kidneys. Additionally, the mere presence of the prostate allows the development of chronic bacterial prostatitis, likely the most common cause of recurrent urinary tract infections in men.

These phenomena, and perhaps others that have not been elucidated, result in prevalences of bacteriuria averaging 20% in women and 10% in men 65 years of age or more. Although hypertension, renal failure, and mortality have been in the past considered to be associated with asymptomatic bacteriuria, in the absence of anatomic or functional abnormalities of the urinary tract, these do not appear to be common consequences. These observations, coupled with low incidences of symptomatic manifestations, high cost of screening the elderly, high incidence of adverse drug reactions in this population, and frequent development of antibiotic-resistant organisms upon reinfection, lead most experts to believe that treatment of asymptomatic bacteriuria in aged people with normal urinary tracts is not necessary. This stance may be changed based upon data from ongoing studies.

Symptomatic infections do occur, however, and should be treated. Cystitis-type symptoms develop in aged women. Although more data are required, this symptom complex may not respond to single-dose antibiotic therapy as frequently as do similar infections in younger women; 5-day to 2-week courses are probably appropriate. Among men with symptomatic urinary tract infection, the prostate in the form of hypertrophy or of chronic bacterial prostatitis is frequently involved making cure of bacterial infection difficult. Surgery for the former and prolonged bacterial therapy for the latter are often indicated.

Acute pyelonephritis appears more commonly to cause bacteremia in the aged than in the younger adult patient. Indeed, the urinary tract is the most common source of bacteremia in aged people in the community, hospital, and nursing home. Treatment of acute pyelonephritis in the elderly should be that of an acute bacteremia but, if an otherwise normal urinary tract is infected, usually can be achieved with 2 or 3 days of intravenous antibiotics followed by oral antibiotics for a total of 2 weeks therapy.

Urinary catheters are often used in the aged both for short-term management in hospitals and for long-term (months to years) in nursing homes. Catheter-associated bacteriuria is invariable after several months of catheterization and is usually polymicrobial. Fevers, acute pyelonephritis, urinary stones, and death are associated with the use of this device. Although treatment of asymptomatic catheter-associated bacteriuria is not indicated, the clinician should be alert to signs of bacteremia and be prepared to treat patients with such findings with parentenal antibiotics active against the often antibiotic-resistant organisms found in the urine and blood of these patients. Prevention of catheter use would diminish catheter-associated bacteriuria and its complications.

References

1 Kunin CM. *Detection, Prevention and Management of Urinary Tract Infections*, 4th edn. Philadelphia: Lea & Febiger, 1987.

2 Boscia JA, Kaye D. Asymptomatic bacteriuria in the elderly. Clin Geriatr Med 1988;4:57−70.

3 Rubin RH, Tolkoff-Rubin NE, Cotran RS. Urinary tract infection, pyelonephritis, and reflux nephropathy. In Brenner BM, Rector FC Jr, eds. *The Kidney*, 3rd edn. Philadelphia: WB Saunders Co., 1986.

4 Marrie TJ, Swantee CA, Hartien M. Aerobic and anaerobic urethral flora of healthy females in various physiologic age groups and of females with urinary tract infections. J Clin Microbiol 1980;11:654−659.

5 Sobel JD, Muller G. Pathogenesis of bacteriuria in elderly women: the role of *Escherichia coli* adherence to vaginal epithelial cells. J Gerontol 1984;39:682−685.

6 Sobel JD, Kaye D. Enhancement of *Escherichia coli* adherence to epithelial cells derived from estrogen-stimulated rats. Infect Immun 1986;53:53−56.

7 Brocklehurst JC, Bee P, Jones D, *et al*. Bacteriuria in geriatric hospital patients: its correlates and management. Age Ageing 1977;6:240−245.

8 Turck M, Goffe B, Petersdorf RG. The urethral catheter and urinary tract infection. J Urol 1962;88:834−837.

9 Orskov I, Ferencz A, Orskov F. Tamm−Horsfall protein or uromucoid is the normal urinary slime that traps Type 1 fimbriated *Escherichia coli*. Lancet 1980;i:887.

10 Sobel JD, Kaye D. Reduced uromucoid excretion in the elderly. J Infect Dis 1985;152:653.

11 Sourander LB, Ruikka I, Gronroos M. Correlation between urinary tract infection, prolapse conditions and function of the bladder in aged female hospital patients. Gerontol Clin 1965;7:179−184.

12 Whitmore WF III. Benign prostatic hyperplasia: widespread and sometimes worrisome. Geratrics 1981;36:119−132.

13 Buck AC, Reed PI, Siddiq YK, *et al*. Bladder dysfunction and neuropathy in diabetes. Diabetologia 1976;12:251−258.

14 Zincke H, Campbell JT, Palumbo PJ, *et al*. Neurogenic vesical dysfunction in diabetes mellitus: another look at vesical neck resection. J Urol 1974;111:488−490.

15 Ellenberg M. Diabetic neurogenic vesical dysfunction. Arch Intern Med 1966;117:348−354.

16 Sawers JS, Todd WA, Kellett HA, *et al*. Bacteriuria and autonomic nerve function in diabetic women. Diabetes Care 1986;9:460−464.

17 Sobel JD, Kaye D. The role of bacterial adherence in urinary tract infections in elderly adults. J Gerontol 1987;42:29−32.

18 Reid G, Zorzitto ML, Bruce AW, *et al*. Pathogenesis of urinary tract infection in the elderly: the role of bacterial adherence to uroepithelial cells. Current Microbiol 1984; 11:67−72.

19 Flanagan PG, Davies EA, Rooney PG, *et al*. Evaluation of four screening tests for bacteriuria in elderly people. Lancet 1989; i: 1117−1119.

20 Boscia JA, Kobasa WD, Knight RA, *et al*. Epidemiology of bacteriuria in an elderly ambulatory population. Am J Med 1986;80:208−213.

21 Kaye D. Urinary tract infections in the elderly. Bull NY Acad Med 1980:56:209−220.

22 Akhtar AJ, Andrews GR, Caird FI, *et al*. Urinary tract infections in the elderly: A population study. Age Ageing 1:48−54.

23 Brocklehurst JC, Dillane JB, Griffiths L, *et al*. The prevalence of urinary tract infection in an aged population. Gerontol Clin 1968;10:242−253.

24 Boscia JA, Kobasa WD, Abrutyn E, *et al*. Lack of association between bacteriuria and symptoms in the elderly. Am J Med 1986;81:979−982.

25 Boscia JA, Abrutyn E, Levison ME, *et al*. Pyuria and asymptomatic bacteriuria in elderly ambulatory women. Ann Intern Med 1989;110:404−405.

26 Thomas V, Shelokov A, Forland M. Antibody-coated bacteria in the urine and the site of urinary tract infection. N Engl J Med 1974;290:588−590.

27 Jones SR, Smith JW, Sanford JP. Localization of urinary tract infections by detection of antibody-coated bacteria in urine sediment. N Engl J Med 290:591−593.

28 Nicolle LE, Muir P, Harding GKM, *et al*. Localization of urinary tract infection in elderly, institutionalized women with asymptomatic bacteriuria. J Infect Dis 1988;157:65−70.

29 Fairley KF, Bond AG, Brown RB, *et al*. Simple test to determine the site of urinary tract infection. Lancet 1967;ii: 427−428.

30 Suntharalingam M, Seth V, Moore-Smith B. Site of urinary tract infection in elderly women admitted to an acute geriatric assessment unit. Age Ageing 1983;12:317−322.

31 Murray T, Goldberg M. Chronic interstitial nephritis: etiologic factors. Ann Intern Med 1975;82:453.

32 Johnson CW, Smyth CM. Renal function in patients with chronic bacteriuria: a longitudinal study. South Med J 1969;62:81.

33 Freedman LR, Andriole V. The long-term follow-up of women with urinary tract infections. In *Proceedings of the 5th International Congress of Nephrology*. Mexico 1972;3:230−235.

34 Asscher AW, Chick S, Radford N. Natural history of asymptomatic bacteriuria (ASB) in non-pregnant women. In

Brumfitt W, Asscher AW, eds. *Urinary Tract Infection.* London: Oxford University Press, 1973:51−60.

35 Gleckman R. The controversy of treatment of asymptomatic bacteriuria in non-pregnant women-resolved. J Urol 1976;116:776−777.

36 Sourander LB, Kasanen A. A 5-year follow-up of bacteriuria in the aged. Gerontol Clin 1972;14:274−281.

37 Dontas AS, Kasviki-Charvati P, Papanayiotou PC, *et al.* Bacteriuria and survival in old age. N Engl J Med 1981;304: 939−943.

38 Evans DA, Hennekens CH, Miao L, *et al.* Bacteriuria and subsequent mortality in women. Lancet 1982;i:156−158.

39 Nordenstam GR, Brandberg CA, Oden AS, *et al.* Bacteriuria and mortality in an elderly population. N Engl J Med 1986;314:1152−1156.

40 Heinamaki P, Haavisto M, Hakulinen T, *et al.* Mortality in relation to urinary characteristics in the very aged. Gerontology 1986;32:167−171.

41 Boscia JA, Kobasa WD, Knight RA, *et al.* Therapy vs no therapy for bacteriuria in elderly ambulatory non-hospitalized women. J Am Med Assoc 1987;257: 1067−1071.

42 Boscia JA, Abrutyn E, Kaye D. Asymptomatic bacteriuria in elderly persons: treat or do not treat? Ann Intern Med 1987;106:764−766.

43 Nicolle LE, Mayhew WJ, Bryan L. Prospective randomized comparison of therapy and no therapy for asymptomatic bacteriuria in institutionalized elderly women. Am J Med 1987;83:27−33.

44 Nicolle LE, Mayhew JW, Bryan L. Outcome following anti-microbial therapy for asymptomatic bacteriuria in elderly resident in an institution. Age Ageing 1988;17:187−192.

45 Renneberg J, Paerregaard A. Single-day treatment with trimethoprim for asymptomatic bacteriuria in the elderly patient. J Urol 1984;132:934−935.

46 Lacey RW, Simpson MHC, Lord VL, *et al.* Comparison of single-dose trimethoprim with a five-day course for the treatment of urinary tract infections in the elderly. Age Ageing 1981;10:179−185.

47 Alling B, Brandberg A, Seeberg S, *et al.* Effect of consecutive antibacterial therapy on bacteriuria in hospitalized geriatric patients. Scand J Infect Dis 1975;7:201−207.

48 Abrutyn E, Boscia JA, Kaye D. The treatment of asymptomatic bacteriuria in the elderly. J Am Geriatr Soc 1988;36:473−475.

49 Parsons CL, Schmidt JD. Control of recurrent lower urinary tract infection in the postmenopausal woman. J Urol 1982;128:1224−1226.

50 Esposito AL, Gleckman RA, Cram S, *et al.* Community-acquired bacteremia in the elderly: analysis of one hundred consecutive episodes. J Am Geriatr Soc 1980;28:315−319.

51 Gleckman RA, Blagg N, Hibert D, *et al.* Acute pyelonephritis in the elderly. South Med J 1982;75:551−554.

52 Gleckman RA, Bradley PJ, Roth RM, *et al.* Bacteremic urosepsis: a phenomenon unique to elderly women. J Urol 1985;133:174−175.

53 McCue JD. Gram-negative bacillary bacteremia in the elderly: incidence, ecology, etiology, and mortality. J Am Geriatr Soc 1987;35:213−218.

54 Meyers BR, Sherman E, Mendelson MH, *et al.* Bloodstream infections in the elderly. Am J Med 1989;86:379−384.

55 Gleckman RA, Bradley PJ, Roth RM, *et al.* Therapy of symptomatic pyelonephritis in women. J Urol 1985;133: 176−178.

56 Lipsky BA, Ireton RC, Fihn SD, *et al.* Diagnosis of bacteriuria in men: specimen collection and culture interpretation. J Infect Dis 1987;155:847−854.

57 Lipsky BA. Urinary tract infections in men: epidemiology, pathophysiology, diagnosis, and treatment. Ann Intern Med 1989;110:138−150.

58 Norman DC, Yamamura R, Yoshikawa TT. Pyuria: its predictive value of asymptomatic bacteriuria in ambulatory elderly men. J Urol 1986;135:520−522.

59 Nicolle LE, Bjornson J, Harding GKM, *et al.* Bacteriuria in elderly institutionalized men. N Engl J Med 1983;309: 1392−1420.

60 Nicolle LE, Henderson E, Bjornson J, *et al.* The association of bacteriuria with resident characteristics and survival in elderly institutionalized men. Ann Intern Med 1987;106: 682−686.

61 Smith JW, Jones SR, Reed WP, *et al.* Recurrent urinary tract infections in men. Ann Intern Med 1979;91:544−548.

62 Krieger JN. Prostatitis syndromes: pathophysiology, differential diagnosis, and treatment. Sex Transm Dis 1984;11:100−112.

63 Stamey TA. *Pathogenesis and Treatment of Urinary Tract Infections.* Baltimore: Williams & Wilkins, 1980.

64 Drach GW, Meares EM Jr, Fair WR, *et al.* Classification of benign disease associated with prostatic pain: prostatitis or prostatodynia? J Urol 1978;120:266.

65 Meares EM Jr, Stamey TA. Bacteriologic localization patterns in bacterial prostatitis and urethritis. Invest Urol 1968;5:492−518.

66 Krieger JN, McGonagle LA. Diagnostic considerations and interpretation of microbiological findings for evaluation of chronic prostatitis. J Clin Microbiol 1989;27:2240−2244.

67 Stamey TA, Fair WR, Timothy MM, *et al.* Antibacterial nature of prostatic fluid. Nature 1968;218:444−447.

68 Fair WR, Couch J, Wehner N. Prostatic antibacterial factor: identity and significance. Urology 1976;7:169−177.

69 Gleckman RA, Crowley M, Natsios GA. Therapy of recurrent invasive urinary tract infections of men. N Engl J Med 1979;301:878−880.

70 Sabbaj J, Hoagland VL, Cook T. Norfloxacin versus co-trimoxazole in the treatment of recurring urinary tract infections in men. Scand J Infect Dis 1986;48(Suppl.):48−53.

71 Berger RE, Krieger JN, Kessler D, *et al.* Case-control study of men with suspected chronic idiopathic prostatitis. J Urol 1989;141:328–331.

72 Uehling DT. Abacterial prostatitis: more about what it isn't but what is it? J Urol 1989;141:367–368.

73 Gleckman RA, Blagg N, Hibert D, *et al.* Symptomatic pyelonephritis in elderly men. J Am Geriatr Soc 1982;30:690–693.

74 Wolfson SA, Kalmanson GM, Rubini ME, *et al.* Epidemiology of bacteriuria in a predominantly geriatric male population. Am J Med Sci 1965;250:168–173.

75 Freeman RB, McFate Smith W, Richardson JA. Long-term therapy for chronic bacteriuria in men. US Public Health Service cooperative study. Ann Intern Med 1975;83:133–148.

76 Garibaldi RA. Hospital acquired urinary tract infection. In Wenzel RP, ed. *CRC Handbook of Hospital Acquired Infections.* Florida: CRC Press Inc., 1981:513–537.

77 Syme R. Epidemic of acute urethral stricture after prostate surgery. Lancet 1982;2:1925.

78 Freed J, Krespi Y. Urologic catheter: Unusual complications. NY State J Med 1979;1892–1893.

79 Daifuku R, Stamm W. Association of rectal and urethral colonization with urinary tract infection in patients with indwelling catheters. J Am Med Assoc 1984;252:2028–2030.

80 Shooter RA, Walker KA, Williams VR, *et al.* Faecal carriage of *Pseudomonas aeruginosa* in hospital patients: possible spread from patient to patient. Lancet 1966;ii:1331–1334.

81 Rutala WA, Kennedy VA, Loflin HB, *et al. Serratia marcescens* nosocomial infections of the urinary tract associated with urine measuring containers and urinometers. Am J Med 1981;70:659–663.

82 Hartstein AI, Garber SB, Ward TT, *et al.* Nosocomial urinary tract infection: a prospective evaluation of 108 catheterized patients. Infect Control 1981;2:380–386.

83 Hooton TM, Haley RW, Culver DH, *et al.* The joint associations of multiple risk factors with the occurrence of nosocomial infection. Am J Med 1981;70:960–970.

84 Kunin CM, McCormack RC. Prevention of catheter-induced urinary-tract infections by sterile closed drainage. N Engl J Med 1966;274:1155.

85 Garibaldi RA, Burke JP, Dickman ML, *et al.* Factors predisposing to bacteriuria during indwelling urethral catheterization. N Engl J Med 1974;291:215.

86 Platt R, Polk BF, Murdock B, *et al.* Risk factors for nosocomial urinary tract infection. Am J Epidemiol 1986;124:977–985.

87 Haley RW, Hooton TM, Culver DH, *et al.* Nosocomial infections in U.S. hospitals, 1975–1976: estimated frequency by selected characteristics of patients. Am J Med 1981;70:947–959.

88 Garibaldi RA, Mooney BR, Epstein BJ, *et al.* An evaluation of daily bacteriologic monitoring to identify preventable episodes of catheter-associated urinary tract infection. Infect Control 1982;3:466–470.

89 Haley R, Culver D, White J, *et al.* The nationwide nosocomial infection rate: a new need for vital statistics. Am J Epidemiol 1985;121:159–167.

90 Morrison AJ, Wenzel RP. Nosocomial urinary tract infections due to enterococcus. Arch Intern Med 1986;146:1549–1551.

91 Warren JW, Platt R, Thomas RJ, *et al.* Antibiotic irrigation and catheter-associated urinary-tract infections. N Engl J Med 1978;299:570.

92 Stark RP, Maki DG. Bacteriuria in the catheterized patient. What quantitative level of bacteriuria is relevant? N Engl J Med 1984;311:560–564.

93 Stamm WE, Martin SM, Bennett JV. Epidemiology of nosocomial infections due to gram-negative bacilli: aspects relevant to development and use of vaccines. J Infect Dis 1977;136S:S151–S160.

94 Krieger JN, Kaiser DL, Wenzel RP. Urinary tract etiology of bloodstream infections in hospitalized patients. J Infect Dis 1983;148:57–62.

95 Bryan C, Reynolds K. Hospital-acquired bacteremic urinary tract infection: epidemiology and outcome. J Urol 1984;132:494–498.

96 Gordon D, Bune A, Grime B, *et al.* Diagnostic criteria and natural history of catheter-associated urinary tract infections after prostatectomy. Lancet 1983;1:1269–1271.

97 Platt R, Polk BF, Murdock B, *et al.* Mortality associated with nosocomial urinary tract infection. N Engl J Med 1982;307:637.

98 Garibaldi RA, Brodine S, Matsumiya S. Infections among patients in nursing homes. Policies, prevalence and problems. N Engl J Med 1981;305:731–735.

99 Kunin CM, Chin QF, Chambers S. Indwelling urinary catheters in the elderly. Am J Med 1987;82:405–411.

100 Warren JW, Steinberg L, Hebel JR, *et al.* The prevalence of urethral catheterization in Maryland nursing homes. Arch Intern Med 1989;149:1535–1537.

101 Ouslander JG, Kane RL, Abrass IB. Urinary incontinence in elderly nursing home patients. J Am Med Assoc 1982;94:661–666.

102 Marron KR, Fillit U, Peskowitz M, *et al.* The non-use of urethral catheterization in the management of urinary incontinence in the teaching nursing home. J Am Geriatr Soc 1983;31:278–281.

103 Warren JW, Damron D, Tenney JH, *et al.* Fever, bacteremia, and death as complications of bacteriuria in women with long-term urethral catheters. J Infect Dis 1987;155:1151–1158.

104 Warren JW, Tenney JH, Hoopes JM, *et al.* A prospective microbiologic study of bacteriuria in patients with chronic

indwelling urethral catheters. J Infect Dis 1982;146:719−723.

105 Steward DK, Wood GL, Cohen RL, *et al.* Failure of the urinalysis and quantitative urine culture in diagnosing symptomatic urinary tract infections in patients with long-term urinary catheters. Am J Infect Control 1985;13:154−160.

106 Nyren P, Runeberg L, Kostiala AI, *et al.* Prophylactic methenamine hippurate or nitrofurantoin in patients with an indwelling urinary catheter. Ann Clin Res 1981;13:16−21.

107 Ouslander JG, Greengold B, Chen S. Complications of chronic indwelling urinary catheters among male nursing home patients: a prospective study. J Urol 1987;138:1191−1195.

108 Warren JW. *Providencia stuartii*: A common cause of antibiotic-resistant bacteriuria in patients with long-term indwelling catheters. Rev Infect Dis 1986;8:61−67.

109 Warren JW, Muncie HL Jr, Hall-Craggs M. Acute pyelonephritis associated with the bacteriuria of long-term catheterization: a prospective clinico-pathological study. J Infect Dis 1988;158:1341−1346.

110 Kunin CM, Chin QF, Chambers S. Formation of encrustations on indwelling urinary catheters in the elderly: a comparison of different types of catheter materials in "blockers" and "nonblockers." J Urol 1987;138:899−902.

111 Muncie HL Jr, Warren JW. Reasons for replacement of long-term urethral catheters: implications for randomized trials. J Urol 1990;143:507−509.

112 Hedelin H, Eddeland A, Larsson L, *et al.* The composition of catheter encrustations, including the effects of allopurinol treatment. Br J Urol 1984;56:250−254.

113 Mobley HLT, Warren JW. Urease-positive bacteriuria and obstruction of long-term urinary catheters. J Clin Microbiol 1987;25:2216−2217.

114 Bruce AW, Sira SS, Clark AF, *et al.* The problem of catheter encrustation. Can Med Assoc J 1974;111:238−239.

115 Jones B, Mobley H. Genetic and biochemical diversity of ureases of *Proteus*, *Providencia* and *Morganella* species isolated from urinary tract infection. Infect Immun 1987;55:2198−2203.

116 Mobley HLT, Jones B, Jerse AE. Cloning of urease gene sequences from *Providencia stuartii*. Infect Immun 1986;54:161−169.

117 Nikakhtar B, Vaziri ND, Khonsari F, *et al.* Urolithiasis in patients with spinal cord injury. Paraplegia 1981;19:363−366.

118 Tribe CR, Silver JR. *Renal Failure in Paraplegia.* London: Pitman Medical Publishing Co., 1969.

119 Carty M, Brocklehurst J, Carty J. Bacteriuria and its correlates in old age. Gerontology 1981;27:72−75.

120 Stamm WE. Guidelines for prevention of catheter-associated urinary tract infections. Ann Intern Med 1975;82:386−390.

121 Wong ES. Guidelines for prevention of catheter-associated urinary tract infections. Am J Infect Control 1983;11:28−36.

122 Schaeffer AJ. Catheter-associated bacteriuria. Urol Clin North Am 1986;13:735−747.

123 Schaberg DR, Zervos MJ. Nosocomial urinary tract infection. Compr Ther 1986;12:8−11.

124 Fierer J, Ekstrom M. An outbreak of *Providencia stuartii* urinary tract infections. Patients with condom catheters are a reservoir of the bacteria. J Am Med Assoc 1981;245:1553−1555.

125 Hirsh DD, Fainstein V, Musher DM. Do condom catheter collecting systems cause urinary tract infection? J Am Med Assoc 1979;242:340−341.

126 Ouslander JG, Greengold BA, Silverblatt FJ, *et al.* An accurate method to obtain urine for culture in men with external catheters. Arch Intern Med 1987;147:286−288.

127 Nicolle LE, Harding GKM, Kennedy J, *et al.* Urine specimen collection with external devices for diagnosis of bacteriuria in elderly incontinent men. J Clin Microbiol 1988;26:1115−1119.

128 Guttmann L, Frankel H. The value of intermittent catheterization in the early management of traumatic paraplegia and tetraplegia. Paraplegia 1966;4:63.

129 Kuhlemeier K, Stover S, Lloyd L. Prophylactic antibacterial therapy for preventing urinary tract infections in spinal cord injury patients. J Urol 1985;134:514−517.

130 Kevorkian CG, Merritt JL, Ilstrup DM. Methenamine mandelate with acidification: an effective urinary antiseptic in patients with neurogenic bladder. Mayo Clin Proc 1984;59:523−529.

131 Anderson RU. Prophylaxis of bacteriuria during intermittent catheterization of the acute neurogenic bladder. J Urol 1980;123:364−366.

132 Mohler JL, Cowen DL, Flanigan RC. Suppression and treatment of urinary tract infection in patients with an intermittently catheterized neurogenic bladder. J Urol 1987;138:336−340.

133 Frymire LJ. Comparison of suprapubic versus Foley drains. Obstet Gynecol 1971;38:239−244.

134 Polk BF, Tager IB, Shapiro M, *et al.* Randomized clinical trial of perioperative cefazolin in preventing infection after hysterectomy. Lancet 1980;1:437−440.

135 Warren JW, Anthony WC, Hoopes JM, *et al.* Cephalexin for susceptible bacteriuria in afebrile, long-term catheterized patients. J Am Med Assoc 1982;248:454−458.

136 Slade N, Gillespie WA, eds. *The Urinary Tract and the Catheter: Infection and Other Problems.* New York: John Wiley & Sons, 1985.

137 Garibaldi RA. Hospital-acquired urinary tract infections: epidemiology and prevention. In Wenzel RP, ed. *Prevention and Control of Nosocomial Infections.* Baltimore: Williams & Wilkins, 1987:335−343.

138 Warren JW. Catheter-associated urinary tract infections. In *Infectious Disease Clinics of North America*. Philadelphia: WB Saunders Co., 1987;1:823–854.

139 Hoopes JM, Muncie HL Jr, Warren JW, *et al*. Once-daily irrigation of long-term urethral catheters with normal saline: lack of benefit. Arch Intern Med 1989;149:441–443.

140 Norberg A, Norberg B, Parikhede U, *et al*. Randomized double-blind study of prophylactic methenamine hippurate treatment of patients with indwelling catheters. Eur J Clin Pharmacol 1980;18:497–500.

141 Stratford B, Gallus AS, Mattiesson AM, *et al*. Alteration of superficial bacterial flora in severely ill patients. Lancet 1968;i:68.

22

Hemodynamic alterations in aged patients during hemodialysis, other dialysis procedures, and transplantation

Pietro Zucchelli
Alessandro Zuccala
Antonio Santoro

Introduction

Over the past two decades, dialysis has become a routine therapy for the overwhelming majority of patients with end-stage renal failure (ESRF). In addition, increasingly high numbers of elderly people with ESRF have been submitted to renal replacement therapy in most of the economically developed countries. This growing proportion of aged patients undergoing renal replacement therapy (RRT) is due to the fact that elderly people are particularly prone to renal insufficiency and also to the more liberal access of elderly patients to life-saving treatments. In fact, epidemiologic data indicate an exponential increase with age in the number of deaths due to uremia [1], while preventive care and therapeutic measures seem to have significantly reduced the incidence of ESRF in young people. Systemic diseases such as vasculitidis, myeloma and diabetes mellitus, and renal vascular diseases are particularly frequent over the age of 60 years. Moreover, the more widespread acceptance of elderly people on RRT has been made possible by the continued growth and diversification of the recently available therapeutic procedures [2]. The high proportion of elderly patients with a high-risk clinical status, at times not self-sufficient, has definitely brought to the forefront many new issues in RRT that involve ethical, psychologic, socioeconomic, and clinical aspects. In this chapter, we will give an analysis of the hemodynamic implications of RRT in elderly patients.

Patient demography

Numerous reports from various registries on elderly patients (over age 60 years) have documented a progressive growth both in acceptance rates at the start of treatment and in survival rates of patients on RRT. The 17th Combined Report of the EDTA−ERA Registry that covered 624 million inhabitants in Europe during 1986, demonstrated that the number of patients per million population (p.m.p.) alive on a known method of RRT increased progressively from 23 p.m.p in 1971, to 100 p.m.p in 1980, and to approximately 200 p.m.p in 1986, being more than 300 p.m.p in Belgium, France, Germany, Israel, Italy, Spain, Sweden, and Switzerland. The highest rate of acceptance in the world has been reported in Japan, where 604 p.m.p were on dialysis by the end of 1986 [3].

The number of elderly patients at the start of treatment has progressively increased in Europe: the newly accepted patients who were over 60 years of age totalled 23.2% (of 14 886) in 1980, 25% (of 16 394) in 1981, and 27.1% (of 17 242) in 1982 [4]. Moreover, demographic trends in the United States patient population are similar to those reported in Europe. By 1986, patients aged over 60 accounted for 52% of the 26 654 new enrolments under the Health Care Financing Administration (HCFA) [3]. From 1977 to 1984, the number of 60 years plus patients admitted to RRT yearly in Languedoc-Roussillon varied from 35.8−45.9% of the total flow of new patients [5]. Thirty-eight per cent of the 690 new patients accepted in Lombardy, Italy, during 1986 were over age 65 years [6]. In our region, Emilia-Romagna, with its 4.5 million inhabitants, we have observed the same overall world trend regarding new patients accepted over the last couple of decades, as reported in Figure 22.1. Thus, there is no doubt that a progressive growth in elderly patients on RRT has been documented during the last decade in developed countries.

Age represents one of the major adverse factors for the survival rate in RRT, given a four-fold rise in the risk ratio as the starting age increases from 25−65 years [7]. In the EDTA−ERA Registry [4], the survival rate at 5 years of patients over 60 years, with nonsystemic renal disease when commencing hemodialysis, was 41.2% in comparison to 82.9% of patients aged below 60.

In many reports the overall survival of patients over 70 years of age when starting dialysis varied from 55−47% at 2 years while it was approximately 25% at 5 years [4,8,9]. Although older patients have a higher mortality rate, their overall survival has significantly improved over the last few years thanks to high-performance blood purification techniques. Increased survival rates, and especially the high acceptance rates, have determined a progressive increase in the median age of RRT patients. The median age of dialysis patients at North Shore University Hospital, in fact, rose from 47 years in 1970−1973, to 54 years in 1978−1981, and to 60 years in 1982−1985 [7]. Similar results have been found in the Emilia-Romagna region of Northern Italy (Fig. 22.1). In Italy by the end of 1987 the vast majority of elderly uremic patients were being treated by hemodialysis in hospital centers, 7% were in limited care centers, while 9% were undergoing peritoneal dialysis [10]. Hospital center hemodialysis has been the most commonly used method of therapy for older patients in the rest of Europe; however, peritoneal dialysis has also begun to offer an attractive alternative. The relative distribution of elderly people treated with peritoneal dialysis varied from 0−40% of the total RRT population depending on the hospital set-up, facilities, and policy. In both the short and long term, however, continuous ambulatory peritoneal dialysis (CAPD) has indeed proven to be

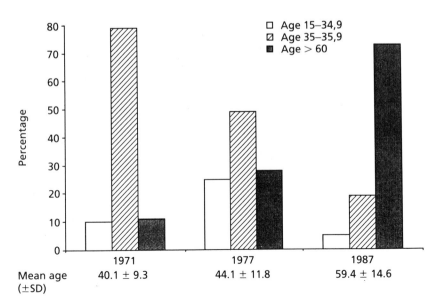

Fig. 22.1 Age at the start of renal replacement therapy in the Emilia-Romagna region.

an efficient and reliable alternative to hemodialysis. It has been thought to be the preferred treatment for high-risk patients over the age of 65 [11].

In the past, patients aged over 50 have been considered to be at high risk in renal transplantation, particularly when the kidney was obtained from cadaveric donors. In recent years, with growing experience in renal transplantation and the introduction of cyclosporine A, the outcome of such a treatment has significantly improved. A recently published paper suggests that transplantation should be the preferred treatment modality for ESRF patients aged from 50–64 [12]. The United States, the Scandinavian countries, and the United Kingdom have used transplantation liberally in the >55 year age group. In Italy, France, and Germany, however, where transplantation is less popular, renal grafts in patients >55 years contribute less than 1% of the total number of transplants performed in these countries [13]. As the number of transplanted patients aged over 60–65 years still represents a very small proportion of the total number of transplants performed worldwide, this problem will not be analysed at any great length.

Clinical aspects

The aetiology of primary renal disease in patients aged over 60 at the start of RRT shows a tendency towards a substantial increase in renal vascular diseases. In patients aged over 60, glomerulonephritis is reported to vary from 19.2–38.8% [5,14], with an average of 26.1% in Europe [4]. Nephrosclerosis varies from 29.3–8.5% [5,14] with an average of 21% in the EDTA−ERA Registry [4]. Moreover, the proportion of patients with undetermined nephropathy has been reported to be significantly elevated in elderly patients over the last few years.

Elderly patients usually need as much dialysis as younger patients when taking into account body size and residual renal function [14]. Indeed, almost 60% of patients on hemodialysis in Europe were reported as having three 4-hour weekly sessions [3] with virtually no difference in the average duration of the dialysis session between young and elderly patients [4].

Artheriosclerosis in the limb vessels may be responsible for some problems in creating the vascular access. Moreover, skin atrophy and the reduction of the patent vein must be taken into account when constructing blood accesses for geriatric patients. In actual fact, no significant difference can be seen in the overall distribution of the various types of vascular access used in different patient age groups, whilst the single-needle technique was more frequently used in elderly people in Europe during 1984 [4].

Hypotensive episodes, angina, and arrhythmia have a significantly higher incidence in older patients than in younger ones, as can be seen in Table 22.1. It reports the main intradialytic side-effects recorded in our hemodialysis patients (standard acetate hemodialysis) in two different age groups. Moreover, in our study, therapeutic intradialytic treatments, usually intravenous infusion of saline solution or plasma expander, were significantly higher in older than in younger patients. Similar percentages are reported by other authors [4,5].

The French Diaphane Registry [4] has recorded cardiovascular complications as well as clinical symptoms of peripheral arteriopathy in a significantly high proportion of elderly patients treated by hemodialysis. The same results were obtained in a survey of the Emilia-Romagna region performed in 1986. Lastly, the overall cardio- and cerebrovascular death rate was 43% of all the deaths recorded in patients aged over 60 years at start of hemodialysis in the period 1980–1982, for the countries reporting to the EDTA−ERA Registry [4]. These fatal cerebrovascular and cardiac accidents were of similar frequency in patients aged less than or over 60 years despite the higher frequency of cardiovascular nonfatal complications in elderly patients [4]. Only myocardial infarction seems to account for a smaller proportion of deaths in patients aged over 70 years [4,7].

Hemodynamic abnormalities in elderly uremic patients

As a result of aging, a variety of structural and functional changes may occur in the cardiovascular system [15]. These changes are the consequence of a number of alterations involving arterial walls [15], cardiac performance [16], intravascular volume and plasma renin activity [17], baroreceptor reflexes and noradrenaline kinetics [18,19]. In addition, uremia is also a well-known cause of cardiovascular dysfunction. In fact, accelerated atherosclerosis due to uremia alone [20] and to alterations in lipoprotein and lipids [21], has been suggested. Moreover, abnormalities in baroreflex sensitivity [22], a reduced responsiveness to noradrenaline [23], parasympathetic dysfunction

Table 22.1 Incidence of intradialytic complications (%)

	Group I (young pts) Mean ± SD	Group II (aged pts) Mean ± SD	P
Headache	3.1 ± 2.1	3.1 ± 1.7	NS
Vomiting	3.1 ± 1.6	2.8 ± 1.1	NS
Cramps	6.0 ± 3.0	5.1 ± 3.1	NS
Angina	0.09 ± 0.1	0.9 ± 0.8	<0.05
Arrhythmia	2.7 ± 1.4	8.0 ± 4.9	<0.05
Hypotension (sys <90 mmHg)	12.5 ± 6.1	22.5 ± 7.9	<0.05

NS, not significant.
Group I, patients below 55 years.
Group II, patients above 64 years.

[24] and alterations in cardiac performance [25] have also been documented. Last but not least, dialysis treatment itself may be highly burdensome for the cardiovascular system. In fact, as reported in Table 22.1 intratreatment cardiovascular symptoms very frequently occur in elderly dialysis patients.

Therefore, given the progressive increase in the median age of the dialysis population, we shall explore hemodynamic problems deriving from aging and uremia, and last of all, from dialytic treatment.

Age-related causes

These causes involve structural changes in the arterial wall and impairment of the autonomic nervous control of circulation.

Anatomic alterations in the arterial wall associated to aging include collagen degeneration, loss of elastine, fatty streaks, calcium deposition, hyaline thickening of the intima and media, and an increased number of smooth-muscle cells [15,26], as described in other chapters. Two other pathologic processes, both of which worsen with age, may accelerate the development of the foregoing alterations; hypertension and atherosclerosis [26]. The net effect of aging and atherosclerosis together may be cumulative resulting in a significant loss of arterial wall elasticity. The hemodynamic consequence of the increased arterial wall stiffness in an increased left ventricular afterload, a decreased cardiac output at rest and during exercise, a higher total peripheral resistance

and a reduced perfusion of critical vascular beds, particularly cerebral and coronary ones [16,17]. Consequently, blood pressure (BP) tends to exhibit greater variability. Factors such as sleep or bed-resting tend to sharply reduce BP [27], whereas factors such as physical exercise or emotional events may suddenly raise it [15,16].

A number of autonomic nervous dysfunctions have been reported in elderly subjects. For instance, a reduced baroreflex response to both phenilephrine and nitro-prusside has been documented [18]. Heart rate variability, which results from changing levels of parasympathetic and sympathetic cardiac drive, is also reduced in older people [28]. Moreover, elderly individuals exhibit a lower recruitment of baroreceptor activity following postural change, thus explaining why erect heart rate decreases with age and why BP may fall after a meal [29]. Postural hypotension is very frequent in elderly people, with an incidence of 30−50% in individuals over 74 years old [30]. Several cross-sectional and longitudinal studies have indicated that plasma noradrenaline (NA) increases with age in humans [31], in part due to an elevation of the NA appearance rate [32]. The main consequence of the high plasma NA levels is the down-regulation of adrenergic receptors. Indeed, a diminished adreno-receptors responsiveness has been demonstrated in elderly human volunteers [31−33].

We can therefore conclude that a striking and selective age-associated decreased response to autonomic nervous system (ANS) stimulation may occur. As the main role of the ANS is to keep tissue perfusion constant during sudden variations in circulating volume [31,33], then the greater susceptibility of elderly patients to volume contraction and dehydration may become clear. Figure 22.2 summarizes the various mechanisms likely to be involved in the greater cardiovascular lability of elderly patients.

Uremia-related causes

These causes, as in the age-related ones, involve structural changes in the arterial wall and the impairment of the autonomic nervous control of circulation.

Numerous risk factors such as hypertension, hyperuricemia, and glucose intolerance are commonly associated to the development of atherosclerosis in uremic patients [21]. Moreover, there are many reports of an increased concentration in very low-density lipoprotein (VLDL) with cholesterol enrichment, an increase in the size and triglyceride content of low-density lipoprotein

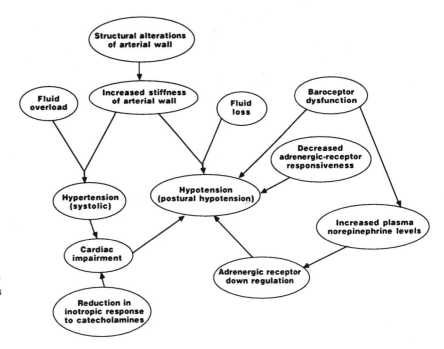

Fig. 22.2 Schematic representation of the mechanisms involved in the pathogenesis of hypertension and hypotension in elderly patients on maintenance dialysis treatment.

(LDL) particles, a prevalence of electrophoretic subclass (late pre-β-lipoprotein) of VLDL, an abnormally low content of linoleic acid, and plasma cholesterol esters [21,34].

Another important cause of arterial stiffness in uremia may be secondary hyperparathyroidism [35]. Finally, other mechanisms have been suggested as being involved in uremic atherosclerosis, such as membrane-plasticizer exposure with time in hemodialysis, aluminum intoxication from phosphate binders, and so on [36,37]. All the above factors may, along with aging, contribute to the low vascular tree adaptation to sharp variations in circulating volume.

Autonomic neuropathy has been thought to be one of the major ESRF complications [23]. Indeed, several abnormalities in the ANS, such as an abnormal response to the Valsalva maneuver, a reduced baroreceptor sensitivity, increased plasma NA levels, and adrenoreceptor hyporesponsiveness have been reported in such patients [22–24,38]. According to our study [38,39], a parasympathetic dysfunction associated to an increased plasma NA level and a reduced adrenoceptor responsiveness is frequently encountered in ESRF patients. The severity and importance of such defects seems to have become reduced during RRT. It is, however, possible that uremic

autonomic dysfunction may add to those age-related problems of elderly patients. Figure 22.3 aims to summarize the various alterations that uremic patients undergo.

Renal replacement therapy

Arterial hypertension

In the preceding pages we have reported that cardiovascular diseases are the major causes of morbidity and mortality in aged uremic patients. It is also known that hypertensive people run great risks of coronary artery disease and stroke [40]; hypertension is also considered the most important risk factor for cardiac and cerebrovascular complications in ESRF patients [41,42]. Although large multicenter trials on essential hypertension have failed to document a reduction in coronary mortality [40] and controlled trials on RRT patients are not yet available, the elimination of hypertension both during the predialytic phase and during long-term RRT is judged to be a key factor in the long-term survival of RRT patients [41,42]. The pathogenesis of hypertension in these patients is thought to be a multifactorial process that includes sodium retention and volume expansion, renin–angiotensin and adrenergic nervous system hyper-

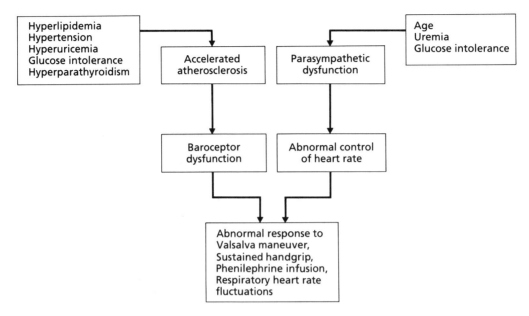

Fig. 22.3 Autonomic dysfunction in elderly uremic patients: the role of various mechanisms in its genesis.

activity, divalent ion derangement, and parathyroid hormone hyperactivity [43,44].

To provide a description of hypertension in aged uremic patients, we shall report BP behaviour throughout the first year of dialysis in 100 consecutive unselected ESRF patients treated at our Dialysis Unit, between January 1984 and December 1986. At the start of RRT, 61 patients were aged below 64 and 39 above the age of 64. The percentage of hypertensive patients (i.e., BP ≥ 160/95) was 70% in the older patient group in comparison to 78.7% in the younger uremic group (Fig. 22.4). Hypertension was particularly severe and even resistant to various antihypertensive drugs in patients with renal vascular diseases, some of whom were later found to have renal artery stenosis.

We have studied the possible mechanisms underlying high BP in ESRF patients undergoing conservative treatment by measuring plasma renin activity (PRA), exchangeable sodium (NaE), plasma catecholamines, plasma volume, and so on [43,45]. Multiple regression analysis, using mean blood pressure (MBP) as the dependent variable, demonstrated that the combined effect of NaE and PRA accounted for over 50% of the MBP levels. No significant differences were found when comparing the younger and older patient groups. These data confirm that volume-dependent hypertension is widely encountered in ESRF patients at any age before beginning RRT and that body sodium—fluid state emerges as the dominant BP modulating factor. The precise mechanisms by which sodium retention and volume expansion might lead to increases in total peripheral resistence remain unknown. However, various mechanisms may be pointed to, such as:

1 an abnormal relation between the renin—angiotensin system and volume state [46];

2 myogenic response to flow-dependent dilation [47];

3 derangement in endothelium vasoactive modulation with an increased release of endothelin [48];

4 an increased production of natriuretic hormone with digitalis-like properties which may increase intracellular Na and Ca concentrations leading to vasoconstriction [49]; and

5 a reduced compliance of the interstitial space [50].

Maintenance hemodialysis has achieved both a satisfactory and progressive control of BP in many of our elderly uremic patients. Indeed, approximately 50% of aged patients had normal and stable BP without the use of antihypertensive drugs after 6 months of hemodialysis.

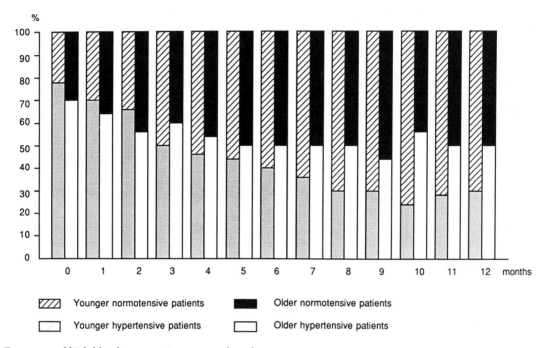

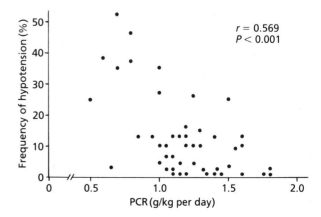

Fig. 22.4 Frequency of high blood pressure in young and aged patients during the first year of maintenance hemodialysis.

This figure is significantly lower than that of younger patients who reached normal BP in approximately 70% of cases (Fig. 22.4). The other 50% of elderly patients showed supine BP levels $\geq 160/95$ mmHg (or MBP $>$ 110 mmHg) on two or more occasions in a month, prior to the dialysis session, and were classified as hypertensive patients. It is interesting to note that while the incidence of hypertension increases with age in the general western population, the opposite seems to be true in hemodialysis patients who have a progressive reduction in the frequency of hypertension [51].

So-called "dialysis-refractory hypertension" is usually considered to be renin-dependent hypertension [52]. In our opinion, many subsets of dialysis-uncontrollable hypertension can be identified. Table 22.2 summarizes our ideas on this topic [43]. We have studied our hemodialysis patients after 6–12 months of maintenance treatment. All antihypertensive therapies were discontinued at least 2 weeks before the study. The main clinical findings of hemodialysis patients are shown in Table 22.3. Elderly patients had mean systolic BP values higher than younger patients. However, the difference

did not reach the level of significance owing to the high interpatient variability. In addition, the mean heart rate was significantly lower in elderly than in younger patients.

Fig. 22.5 Relationship between protein catabolic rate (PCR) and the frequency of hypotension during standard acetate hemodialysis in elderly uremic patients.

Table 22.2 Hypertension during maintenance hemodialysis

Subsets	Clinical picture	Pathogenesis
Malignant hypertension	Weight loss, hyponatriemia, thirst, ortostatic hypotension	Hyperactivity of renin−angiotensin system
Paradoxical hypertension	Sharp increase in BP during or at the end of dialysis session	Adrenergic hyperactivity Increased Ca ion levels Dialytic removal of anthyhypertensive agents Cushing reflex Vasopressin hypersecretion (?)
Dialysis-refractory hypertension	BP > 160/90 on at least three occasions in 1 month and/or the need for antihypertensive therapy	Misjudgment of "dry body weight" Hyperactivity of renin−angiotensin system Autonomic dysfunction Secondary hyperparathyroidism

BP, blood pressure.

Table 22.3 Clinical data after 6−12 months of maintenance hemodialysis

	Young patients (mean age 44.9 ± 12) Mean ± SD	Aged patients (mean age 68.2 ± 3) (Mean ± SD)
Height (m)	1.65 ± 1.10	1.64 ± 0.07
Weight (kg)	65.9 ± 13.5	63.6 ± 6.5
Surface area (mq)	1.73 ± 0.19	1.7 ± 0.09
Systolic pressure (mmHg)	149 ± 19.2	158.4 ± 23.6
Diastolic pressure (mmHg)	94.0 ± 9.9	86.5 ± 9.1
Mean arterial pressure (mmHg)	113.7 ± 12.3	109.2 ± 11.9
Heart rate	75 ± 6	*68 ± 5

* $P < 0.05$.

Ten patients from each of the two groups of hemodialysis patients contemporaneously performed hormonal, hemodynamic, and echocardiographic investigations. The main results of the study are reported in Table 22.4. Our data in aged uremic patients with hypertension are substantially in agreement with those reported by Messerli et al. [17] in elderly patients with essential hypertension. In fact, as shown in Table 22.4, the reported mean values of the clinical and hemodynamic data of our hemodialysis patients documented that cardiac output, plasma volume, and PRA were significantly lower in elderly patients as opposed to younger ones, whereas total peripheral resistance, plasma NA and left ventricular end-diastolic volume were higher in the former than the latter group. In addition, BP tended to be less stable in elderly hemodialysis patients than in younger hypertensive patients and in normal subjects.

The pattern of hypertension in elderly CAPD patients is quite similar to that of hemodialysis patients [53]. According to some retrospective studies, most of the patients who began CAPD with normal blood pressure and without antihypertensive medication tended to remain at this status. Approximately, 40−50% of hypertensive uremic patients at the start became stable normotensive after 12 months of CAPD [53,54]. This technique, consisting of three cycles of isotonic and one cycle of

Table 22.4 Hemodynamic variables and left ventricular function (before dialysis)

	Young patients Mean ± SD	Aged patients Mean ± SD
MBP (mmHg)	114.3 ± 12.3	109.7 ± 11.9
Cardiac index (1/min per m²)	4.5 ± 1.3	*4.07 ± 0.9
Stroke index (ml/m²)	58 ± 16	50.6 ± 18
TPR index (units)	31 ± 6.2	28 ± 5.1
LV end-diastolic volume (ml/m²)	110 ± 32	131.7 ± 29
Ejection fraction (%)	56.9 ± 12	61.2 ± 11
Vcf (circ/s)	1.31 ± 0.3	1.34 ± 0.2
Plasma noradrenaline (ng/liter)	225 ± 16	255 ± 26
PRA (ng/AI ml per hour)	3.1 ± 0.5	*2 ± 0.42

MBP, mean blood pressure; TPR, total peripheral resistance; LV, left ventricular, Vcf, velocity circumferential shortening; PRA, plasma renin activity.
* $P < 0.05$.

hypertonic dialysate per 24 hours, usually results in a negative water balance of 1.5–2 liters and a sodium loss of 198–264 mmol. This allows the patients to have a liberal intake, while sodium and water overload are rarely a problem. However, the loss of ultrafiltration capacity may occur with time on CAPD [54]. Hence, the proportion of patients on antihypertensive medication remained at approximately 30–50%. At times, a few CAPD patients had uncontrollable hypertension with standard antihypertensive treatment after 1 year.

Hypertension is very frequently encountered after renal transplantation and approximately 50% of such patients have a high blood pressure. Posttransplant hypertension has multifactorial mechanisms which involve the diseased native kidney, various graft diseases, and therapeutic procedures [55]. We have already stated that renal transplantation is very rarely performed in ESRF patients aged over 65 years and so this matter will not be dealt with here.

Intradialytic hypotension
Dialysis patients are prone to stressful, recurrent, and persistent symptoms which have a significant impact on their general well being. Some symptoms such as tiredness, headache, and itching are nonspecific and fail to respond to any therapy [56]. Other symptoms, including intradialytic hypotension, are potentially reversible.

Dialysis-induced symptomatic hypotension is the most frequent side-effect observed during hemodialysis sessions. Such episodes have been on the increase, in spite of the impressive improvement of RRT know-how. This is possibly as a result of several independent factors, most important of which are the rapid fluid withdrawal during the shortened treatment time, the increasing age of the patients, and multimorbidity of the dialysis population [57,58]. The overriding importance of age in the high frequency of dialysis-induced hypotension is clearly demonstrated in the French Diaphane Registry [57] and this is also documented in our study, as reported in Table 22.1. Moreover, the hemodynamic consequences of dialysis-induced hypotension can be particularly dangerous in elderly uremic patients. In fact, in such patients, together with the "classical" symptoms of hypotension which include inexplicable anxiety, nausea, vomiting, and pallor, other manifestations of cardiovascular instability may occur. Sudden and profound hypotension with a loss of consciousness, angina pectoris, and transient cerebral ischemic attacks may appear [58,59]. The aetiology of dialysis-induced hypotension is, according to clinical and experimental data, very complex and multifactorial. It is generally accepted that during hemodialysis the compensatory vasoconstrictive response to rapid volume depletion is blunted. The various mechanisms responsible for this abnormal response are listed in Table 22.5. According to our suggestion [58], the pathophysiology of dialysis-induced hypotension may be subdivided into two major categories:

1 factors related to the dialytic mode that are identical in both young and older patients;
2 factors related to patient characteristics.

Table 22.5 Pathogenetic factors in dialysis-induced hypotension

---

Factors related to the dialytic mode

Intravascular volume contraction: amount and speed of fluid removed by ultrafiltration

Plasma refilling rate: related to plasma oncotic pressure and the hydration of the interstitial space

Sodium balance

Acute interference with vascular smooth-muscle tone: biocompatibility of dialytic materials, acute phase reaction, temperature changes, acetate

Acute dysfunction in the sympathetic neural reflex

Factors related to patients' characteristics

Poor nutritional status

Myocardial abnormalities

Chronic dysautonomia

The alterations in the arterial wall and in cardiovascular reflex, due both to aging and to uremia, as described in the previous pages, play an important role in this subgroup of mechanisms.

In a recent study on 55 RRT patients (34 under 60 years and 21 over 64) we found that the higher incidence of dialysis-induced hypotension in geriatric patients (see Table 22.1) may be statistically attributable to a poor nutritional status, to the presence of left ventricular abnormalities, and to an ANS dysfunction [60]. In fact, older patients had a lower blood urea nitrogen generation rate and protein caloric rate (PCR) than younger patients during similar dialysis conditions (Table 22.6). Moreover, there was a significantly inverse correlation between PCR and the frequency of symptomatic hypotension (Fig. 22.5).

Several studies have pointed out that wasting and malnutrition are common in dialysis patients, especially in elderly ones. A poor dietary-protein intake may influence the refilling rate of plasma volume during fluid removal, as happens during hemodialysis [61]. A hypocaloric diet results in a decrease in the sympathetic nervous system activity with a plasma NA diminution [62]. Aging itself, as previously described, produces a decreased response to ANS stimulation. Finally, left ventricular dysfunctions are very frequently encountered in elderly uremic patients; we know both from experimental studies and clinical observations [63,64] that these heart dysfunctions may be associated to dialysis-induced hypotension.

The development of orthostatic hypotension sometimes complicates the treatment of ESRF by CAPD. The cause is usually excessive sodium removal via the dialysate relative to the dietary sodium intake, leading to the gradual development of sodium depletion [65].

Table 22.6 Mean values (and SD) of various biochemical parameters and Valsalva ratio in two different age groups of hemodialysis patients

	Young patients	Aged patients
Hematocrit (%)	30.2 ± 1.1	29.2 ± 2.1
Sodium (mmol/liver)	141.5 ± 2.1	142 ± 2.3
Potassium (mmol/liter)	5.2 ± 0.7	5.2 ± 0.6
Calcium (mg/dl)	9.8 ± 0.5	$9.3 \pm 0.3*$
Blood urea nitrogen (mg/dl)	89.8 ± 13.9	78.7 ± 13.8
Total serum protein (g/dl)	6.7 ± 0.6	6.4 ± 0.7
Urea generation rate (mg/min)	6.1 ± 1.2	$5.4 \pm 0.6*$
Protein catabolic rate (g/kg per 24 hours)	1.2 ± 0.3	1.0 ± 0.3
Valsalva ratio	1.4 ± 0.3	$1.13 \pm 0.1*$

$* P < 0.05.$

Therapeutic considerations

The goal of antihypertensive therapy in elderly dialysis patients is to obtain normal BP without compromising coronary circulation and brain perfusion [26], and without favoring intradialytic hypotension.

Owing to the overriding importance of sodium−water retention in the genesis of hypertension, a strict volume control with a correct "dry body weight" is indispensable in treating hypertensive dialysis patients [66]. Dry body weight has traditionally been defined as the weight at which the uremic patient is edema-free and without orthostatic tachycardia and hypotension. This clinical concept, however, does not consider the patient's cardiovascular status and the possibility that a mild fluid overload can fail to provoke detectable edema. In our opinion [44], the postdialysis/cardiothoracic ratio, urea space determination, and/or an ultrasonographic measurement of the inferior vena cava diameter may be important tools for optimal dry body weight estimation. In dialysis-resistant hypertension, antihypertensive drugs ought to be used. Taking into account the characteristics of circulation in elderly uremic patients as previously described, we think that a small or moderate dosage of β-blockers, centrally acting drugs, calcium channel blockers, and angiotensin-converting enzyme inhibitors represent the safest and most active drugs. Beta-blockers may be useful for elderly patients by exerting a cardio protective effect and reducing angina but they are unadvisable in patients with heart block, severe peripheral vascular disease, and chronic obstructive pulmonary disease [67]. Centrally acting drugs show a better hemodynamic behaviour than β-blockers but they may cause depression and aggravate thirst. Calcium channel blockers are very effective in decreasing BP without reflex tachycardia and orthostatic hypotension [68]. Finally, angiotensin-converting enzyme inhibitors may also be very active in low-renin hypertension as they are well tolerated and have fewer side-effects [69]. Calcium entry blockers and angiotensin-converting enzyme inhibitors, apart from their high cost, may be the choice drugs for elderly uremic patients.

The treatment of intradialytic hypotension includes laying the patients down with upraised legs and the reduction of the ultrafiltration degree. If hypotension persists and becomes more serious, an appropriate volume of saline, hypertonic sodium chloride, or plasma expanders must be administered. Red cell transfusion may be useful in geriatric patients with cardiac impairment.

The prevention of dialysis-induced hypotension is the major goal of maintenance dialysis. Investigations for its pathophysiology may be very important in reducing this very distressing intradialytic symptom. As the major factor in dialysis-induced hypotension is plasma volume depletion, the degree of tissue hydration, basically an accurate assessment of the patient's dry weight, represents the first and most important parameter in obtaining normal intradialytic and stable interdialytic BP. Dry body weight is not a fixed parameter but needs to be adapted to changes in the patient's nutritional status. Moreover, a strict control of chronic fluid overload appears to reduce cardiac workload and ventricular dysfunction [70].

Severe anemia and a poor nutritional status have to be eliminated when possible. Moreover, the administration of antihypertensive drugs immediately before the dialysis session ought to be avoided [44]. As regards the dialysis prescription, ultrashort and aggressive ultrafiltration should be performed only on a few elderly uremic patients. Hemofiltration or hemodiafiltration may be a valid alternative to standard acetate hemodialysis in elderly patients who are particularly prone to symptomatic hypotension and have ANS dysfunction [38]. However, one of the requirements for the use of the above techniques is a very high blood flow rate to the hemodialyzer, which is sometimes very difficult to achieve in elderly patients. In elderly patients with impaired left ventricular function, bicarbonate dialysis or acetate-free biofiltration is preferable to standard acetate hemodialysis. These blood purification techniques, in fact, obtain a more efficient peripheral vasocontrictive effect during ultrafiltration: there is a more stable BP, a significant improvement in myocardial contractility, and a reduction in the hemodynamic consequences of arterial hypoxemia [71]. Finally, if none of these techniques sufficiently improves cardiovascular instability, CAPD has to be taken into consideration. The only theoretical cardiovascular drawback to CAPD seems to be the lack of parasympathetic function improvement; it is also known that a deficit in vagal function may be correlated to sudden cardiac death in elderly patients [72].

Table 22.7 Some guidelines for reducing intradialysis symptomatic hypotension

The careful determination and maintenance of correct dry body weight

The correction of the underlying pathophysiologic mechanisms (anemia, poor nutritional status, and so on)

The withdrawal of antihypertensive drugs immediately before dialysis

An adequate dialysate sodium (140−145 mmol/liter)

The avoidance of ultrashort and aggressive ultrafiltration

Morning dialysis or fasting dialysis when postprandial hypotension occurs

Hemofiltration or hemodiafiltration when autonomic dysfunction arises

Bicarbonate dialysis when hepatic dysfunction and/or cardiomiopathy are present

CAPD

To conclude, Table 22.7 sums up some of the precautions that ought to be observed during hemodialysis in elderly uremic patients.

References

1 McGeown MG. Chronic renal failure in Northern Ireland 1968−70. A prospective survey. Lancet 1972;i:307−310.

2 Widt DG. Series editor's comments. Geriatric Hypertens 1987;42:56.

3 Report from the European Dialysis and Transplant Association Registry. Demography of Dialysis and Transplantation in Europe in 1985 and 1986: Trends over the previous decade. Nephrol Dial Transplant 1988;3:714−727.

4 Jacobs C, Diallo A, Balas EA, et al. Maintenance haemodialysis treatment in patients aged over 60 years. Demographic profile, clinical aspects and outcome. Proc EDTA−ERA 1984;21:477−489.

5 Mion C, Oules R, Canaud B, et al. Maintenance dialysis in the elderly. A review of 15 years' experience in Languedoc-Roussilon. Proc EDTA−ERA 1984;21:490−509.

6 Graziani G. Personal communication.

7 Mailloux LU, Bellucci AG, Mossey RT, et al. Predictors of survival in patients undergoing dialysis. Am J Med 1988;84:855−862.

8 Piccoli G, Quarello F, Bonello F, et al. Peritoneal dialysis in elderly patients. In La Greca G, Chiaromonte S, Fabris A, et al. eds. Peritoneal Dialysis. Milano: Wichtig Editore, 1985:275−283.

9 Westlie L, Umen A, Nestrud S, et al. Mortality, morbidity and life satisfaction in the very old dialysis patient. Trans Am Soc Artif Intern Organs 1984;30:21−30.

10 Associazione Nazionale Emo-Dializzati. Censimento dei servizi di dialisi e trapianto italiani al 31 Dicembre 1987,
Milano 1988.

11 Maiorca R, Vonesh E, Cancarini GC, et al. A six-year comparison of patient and technique survival in CAPD and HD. Kidney Int 1988;34:518−524.

12 Shah B, First MR, Munda R, et al. Current experience with renal transplantation in older patients. Am J Kidney Dis 1988;12:516−523.

13 Taube D, Cameron JS, Challoh S. Renal transplantation in older patients. In Nuñez JFM, Cameron JS, eds. Renal Function and Disease in the Elderly. London: Butterworths, 1987:529−537.

14 Schaefer K, Asmus G, Quellhorst F, et al. Optimum dialysis treatment for patients over 65 years with primary renal disease. Survival data and clinical results from 242 patients treated either by haemodialysis or haemofiltration. Proc EDTA−ERA 1986;21:510−523.

15 Rosenthal J. Aging and the cardiovascular system. Gerontology 1987;33(Suppl. 1):3−8.

16 Weisfeldt ML. Aging of the cardiovascular system. N Engl J Med 1980;13:1172−1174.

17 Messerli FH, Sundgaard-Riise K, Ventura HO, et al. Essential hypertension in the elderly: haemodynamics, intravascular volume, plasma renin activity, and circulating catecholamine levels. Lancet 1983;ii:983−986.

18 Gribbin B, Pickering TG, Sleight P, et al. Effects of age and high blood pressure on baroreflex sensitivity in man. Circ Res 1971;29:424−431.

19 Veith RC, Featherstone JA, Linares OA, et al. Age differences in plasma norepinephrine kinetics in humans. Gerontology 1986;41:319−324.

20 Lindner A, Charra B, Sherrard DJ, et al. Accelerated atherosclerosis in prolonged maintenance hemodialysis. N Engl J Med 1974;290:697−701.

21 Editorial. Uraemia, lipoproteins, and atherosclerosis. Lancet 1981;ii:1151−1152.

22 Pickering TG, Gribbin B, Oliver DO. Baroreflex sensitivity in

patients on long-term hemodialysis. Clin Sci 1972;43: 645–652.

23 Campese VM, Romoff MS, Levitan D, et al. Mechanisms of autonomic nervous system dysfunction in uremia. Kidney Int 1981;20:246–253.

24 Naik RB, Mathias CJ, Wilson JL, et al. Cardiovascular and autonomic reflexes in haemodialysis patients. Clin Sci 1981; 60:165–170.

25 London GM, Fabiani F, Marchais SJ, et al. Uremic cardiomyopathy: an inadequate left ventricular hypertrophy. Kidney Int 1987;31:973–980.

26 Chobanian AV. The influence of hypertension and other hemodynamic factors in atherogenesis. Prog Cardiovasc Dis 1983;26:177–196.

27 Kapoor W, Snustad D, Peterson J, et al. Syncope in the elderly. Am J Med 1986;80:419–428.

28 Simpson DM, Wicks R. Spectral analysis of heart rate indicates reduced baroreceptor-related heart rate variability in elderly persons. J Gerontol 1988;43:21–24.

29 Lipsitz LA, Fullerton KJ. Postprandial blood pressure reduction in healthy elderly. J Am Geriatr Soc 1986;34: 267–270.

30 Robbins AS, Rubenstein LZ. Postural hypotension in the elderly. J Am Geriatr Soc 1984;32:769–774.

31 Pfeiffer HA, Weimberg CR, Cook D, et al. Different changes of autonomic nervous system function with age in man. Am J Med 1983;75:249–258.

32 Esler H, Jackman G, Bobik A, et al. Determination of norepinephrine apparent release rate and clearance in humans. Life Sci 1979;25:1461–1470.

33 Collins KJ, Exton-Smith AN, James MH, et al. Functional changes in autonomic nervous responses with aging. Age Ageing 1980;9:17–24.

34 Arora KK, Atkinson MK, Trafford JAP, et al. Changes in glucose tolerance, insulin, serum lipids and lipoprotein in patients with renal failure on intermittent hemodialysis. Postgrad Med J 1973;49:293–296.

35 Massry SG, Goldstein DA. Role of parathyroid hormone in uremic toxicity. Kidney Int 1978;13:539–542.

36 Lewis LM, Flechtner TW, Kerkay J. Determination of plasticizer levels in serum of hemodialysis patients. Trans Am Soc Artif Intern Organs 1977;23:566–571.

37 Kachny WD, Hogg AP, Alfrey AC. Gastrointestinal absorption of aluminum from aluminum containing antiacids. N Engl J Med 1977;296:1389–1390.

38 Zucchelli P, Sturani A, Zuccalà A, et al. Dysfunction of the autonomic nervous system in patients with end-stage renal failure. Contr Nephrol 1985;45:69–81.

39 Zucchelli P, Sturani A, Degli Esposti E, et al. Hemodialysis in contrast to CAPD, improves parasympathetic function in ESRD patients. Trans Am Soc Artif Intern Organs 1983;29: 617–622.

40 Editorial. Coronary artery disease in hypertensive. Lancet 1988;ii:1461–1462.

41 Vincent F, Amend WJ, Abela J, et al. The role of hypertension in hemodialysis associated atherosclerosis. Am J Med 1980; 68:363–369.

42 Charra B, Colemard E, Cuche M, et al. Control of hypertension and prolonged survival on maintenance hemodialysis. Nephron 1983;33:96–99.

43 Zucchelli P, Zuccalà A, Degli Esposti E, et al. Pathophysiology and management of hypertension in hemodialysis patients. Contr Nephrol 1987;54:209–217.

44 Zucchelli P, Santoro A, Zuccalà A. Genesis and control of hypertension in hemodialysis patients. Semin Nephrol 1988;8:163–168.

45 Zucchelli P, Zuccalà A, Santoro A, et al. Management of hypertension in dialysis. Int J Artif Organs 1980;3:78–84.

46 Weidman P. Pathogenesis of hypertension associated with chronic renal failure. Contr Nephrol 1984;41:47–65.

47 Folkow B. The haemodynamic consequences of adaptive structural changes of the resistance vessel in hypertension. Clin Sci 1971;41:1–13.

48 Vanhoute PM. The endothelium-modulator of vascular smooth-muscle tone. N Engl J Med 1988;319:512–513.

49 Deray G, Perudlet MG, Devynck MA, et al. Plasma digital is like activity in essential hypertension or end-stage renal disease. Hypertension 1986;8:632–638.

50 Koomans HA, Roos JC, Dorhout Mees EJ, Delawi JHK. Sodium balance in renal failure. A comparison of patients with normal subjects under extremes of sodium intake. Hypertension 1985;7:714–721.

51 Degli Esposti E, Boero R. Chiarini C, et al. Blood pressure behaviour in hemodialysis patients treated for 10 years. Int J Artif Organs 1983;6:121–126.

52 Vertes V, Cangiano JL, Berman LB, et al. Hypertension in end-stage renal disease. N Engl J Med 1969;280:978–981.

53 Stablein DM, Hamburger RJ, Lindblad AS, et al. The effect of CAPD on hypertension control: A report of the National CAPD registry. Perit Dial Bull 1988;8:141–144.

54 Cassidy MJD, Heaton A, Rodger RSC, et al. Endocrinological and haematological aspects of CAPD. In Gokal R, ed. *Continuous Ambulatory Peritoneal Dialysis*. Edinburgh: Churchill Livingstone, 1986:265–290.

55 Wouthier M, Verlerstraeten P, Pirson J, et al. Prevalence and causes of hypertension late after renal transplantation. Proc EDTA–ERA 1982;19:566–571.

56 Parfey PS, Vavasour HM, Henry S, et al. Clinical features and severity of non-specific symptoms in dialysis patients. Nephron 1988;50:121–128.

57 Degoulet P, Reach I, Di Giulio S, et al. Epidemiology of dialysis induced hypotension. Proc EDTA–ERA 1980;17: 133–138.

58 Zucchelli P. Hemodialysis-induced symptomatic hypotension. A Review of pathophysiological mechanism. Int J Artif Organs 1987;10:139–144.

59 Petitclerc T, Drüeke T, Man NK, et al. Stabilité cardiovasculaire en hemodialyse. In Grosnier J, Funck-Brentano

JL, Bach JF, *et al.*, eds. *Actualites Nephrologiques de l'Hopital Necker.* Paris: Flammarion Med Sciences, 1986: 345–363.

60 Gattiani A, Baldelli MV, Santoro A, *et al.* Tolleranza cardiovascolare al trattamento emodialitico cronico negli uremici anziani. Progresso Med 1987;43:325–328.

61 Koomans HA, Geers AB, Dorhout Mees EJ. Plasma volume recovery after ultrafiltration in patients with chronic renal failure. Kidney Int 1984;26:848–856.

62 Esler M, Skews H, Leonard D, *et al.* Age-dependence of noradrenaline kinetics in normal subjects. Clin Sci 1980;60: 217–219.

63 Leunissen KML, Cleriex EC, Janssen J, *et al.* Influence of left ventricular function on changes in plasma volume during acetate and bicarbonate dialysis. Nephrol Dial Transplant 1987;2:99–103.

64 Mall.G, Rambousek KR, Neumeister A, *et al.* Myocardial interstitial fibrosis in experimental uremia. Implications for cardiac compliance. Kidney Int 1988;33:804–811.

65 Zucchelli P, Chiarini C, Degli Esposti E, *et al.* Influence of continuous ambulatory peritoneal dialysis on the autonomic nervous system. Kidney Int 1983;23:46–50.

66 Gotch FA. Dialysis of the future. Kidney Int 1988;33(Suppl.24):S100–S104.

67 Danforth J, Ports TA. Using beta blockers after MI in the elderly. Geriatrics 1985;40:75–85.

68 Krebs R. Adverse reactions with calcium antagonists. Hypertension 1983;5(Suppl.II):125–129.

69 Williams GH. Converting-enzyme inhibitors in the treatment of hypertension. N Engl J Med 1988;319:1517–1525.

70 Wizeman V, Kramer N, Thormann J, *et al.* Exercise-induced ventricular dysfunction: reversible by hemodialysis. Trans Am Soc Artif Intern Organs 1984;30:567–570.

71 Henrich WL, Hunt JM, Nixon JV. Increased ionized calcium and left ventricular contractility during hemodialysis. N Engl J Med 1984;310:19–23.

72 Billman GE, Schwarts DJ, Stone LH. Baroreceptor reflex of heart rate: A predictor of sudden cardiac death. Circulation 1982;66:874–881.

Index